Stuttering Intervention

A Collaborative Journey to Fluency Freedom

Second Edition

David Allen Shapiro

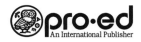

PRO-ED, Inc.
An International Publishe
8700 Shoal Creek Boulevar
Austin, Texas 78757-6897
800/897-3202   Fax 800/397-7
www.proedinc.com

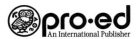

© 2011, 1999 by PRO-ED, Inc.
8700 Shoal Creek Boulevard
Austin, Texas 78757-6897
800/897-3202   Fax 800/397-7633
www.proedinc.com

Library of Congress Cataloging-in-Publication Data

Shapiro, David A. (David Allen), 1954-
    Stuttering intervention : a collaborative journey to fluency freedom /
David Allen Shapiro. -- 2nd ed.
        p. ; cm.
    Includes bibliographical references and indexes.
    ISBN 978-1-4164-0487-3
    1. Stuttering—Treatment.   I. Title.
[DNLM: 1. Stuttering—therapy.   WM 475 S529s 2011]
RC424.S553 2011
616.85′5406—dc22
                                                    2010015927

Art Director: Jason Crosier
Designer: Jan Mullis
This book is designed in ITC Giovanni and News Gothic.

Printed in the United States of America

1 2 3 4 5 6 7 8 9 10   20 19 18 17 16 15 14 13 12 11

To Kay, Sarah, and Aaron Shapiro, who are the light of my life and the finest friends anyone could ever have;

To all comrades—people who stutter, families, clinicians, and others— who are willing to work with and learn from each other; and

To my grandparents, Hattie and Joseph Lyman, in whose memory I find inspiration to dream, to journey, and to try to make a difference. ▥

Contents

Unit I ▦ Stuttering in Relief: A Foundation for Intervention

Chapter One
The Nexus of Stuttering: An Introduction   *2*

Chapter Two

The Onset, Development, and Nature of Stuttering   *31*

Chapter Three

Etiology of Stuttering: Past and Present   *72*

Unit II ▥ Central Intervention Assumptions

Chapter Five
Personal Constructs and Family Systems: Intrafamily Considerations   148

Chapter Six

Interdisciplinary Teaming and Multicultural Awareness:
Extrafamily Considerations *181*

Chapter Seven

Stuttering Modification and Fluency Shaping:
Psychotherapeutic Considerations *205*

Unit III ⠿ Assessment and Treatment Strategies with People Who Stutter: A Life Span Perspective

Chapter Eight

Preschool Children: Assessment and Treatment *236*

Chapter Ten

Adolescents, Adults, and Senior Adults Who Stutter: Assessment and Treatment *371*

Unit IV ⬚ The Clinician: A Paragon of Change

Chapter Eleven
The Clinician and the Client–Clinician Relationship   *444*

Chapter Twelve
Professional Preparation and Lifelong Learning:
The Making of a Clinician   *465*

Foreword

There is hope for people who stutter. That is the message at the heart of this comprehensive, scholarly, and moving textbook aimed at helping both students and practicing clinicians develop the skills they need to become valuable partners in the therapy process for people who stutter. In the past, studies have shown that many speech–language pathologists are not confident in their skills for working with people who stutter. The reasons for their discomfort are numerous, though many of the issues can be described in terms of two key problems: a lack of training about the procedures and processes involved in successful stuttering intervention and, more fundamentally, an underlying lack of understanding of the nature of the disorder and the daily challenges faced by people who stutter.

This book, written by an individual who is both an experienced clinician and a person who has lived with stuttering, deftly addresses both of these concerns and proves that speech–language pathologists do not need to fear this disorder. The text presents necessary background about fluent and disfluent speech, clear explanations of the factors that affect the development and maintenance of the disorder, concrete strategies for evaluating and treating stuttering in different age groups, a strong theoretical background that helps clinicians conceptualize the disorder, a comprehensive and integrated perspective on the effect stuttering can have on people's lives, meaningful links to other disciplines that can support and enhance our interactions with our clients, direct suggestions about how clinicians can develop their skills, and thoughtful guidance about how to cultivate a genuine sense of empathy for people who stutter and their families. Just as importantly, the book does all of this using Dr. Shapiro's gentle and accessible prose, which captures the reader's interest and commitment from the very first page.

The result is a deeply touching and intensely personal companion that will help speech–language pathologists move toward a promising future of understanding of and empathy for people who stutter. The lessons clinicians learn through this book will help them develop the key clinical and personal skills they need to help their clients make meaningful changes in their speech—and in their lives as a whole.

Early in the first chapter, Dr. Shapiro writes that "communication is a uniquely human experience." This book conveys a sense of how stuttering can affect every aspect of that human experience, balanced with a detailed demonstration of how people can overcome those challenges through personal growth and the support of a caring, expert practitioner. Several times throughout the book, Dr. Shapiro reflects on the notion that the therapeutic process can be viewed as a "journey." This metaphor not only embodies the changes experienced by the speaker throughout the course of treatment but also captures the clinician's growth and the intimate relationship that can be shared between the clinician and the client in treatment. The book provides numerous suggestions for how both parties can further their progress along this journey and move toward the freedom highlighted in the book's title.

The book takes a long-term view of change—for both the client and the clinician—starting with the hesitant first steps of a beginner, moving to the gradual growth and expansion of skills experienced during the treatment process, and, finally, over time, achieving ultimate mastery over the disorder. Above all, the text conveys two profoundly hopeful messages: that people who stutter of all ages can make positive changes in their lives, and that speech–language pathologists can expand their understanding of the disorder in order to help their clients reach their goals.

The value of Dr. Shapiro's accomplishments in this book cannot be overstated, and I believe that this book reaches heights that few others have achieved. Put simply, there is a tremendous amount of information that speech–language pathologists need to learn about stuttering and about people who stutter before they are ready to become effective partners in their client's journey. As faculty and stuttering specialists, we often despair of ever being able to communicate all that we want clinicians to know. This book comes as close as any book about stuttering that I've ever read to conveying the "big picture" while still keeping an eye on the all-important details of basic human interaction and daily life. It provides students and experienced clinicians alike with historical perspectives, theoretical underpinnings, balanced and respectful interpretations of the literature, real-world experiences with tested treatment strategies, personal opinions and perspectives of the author and his clients, and numerous examples of practical applications—in other words, all of the underlying knowledge and clinical sensitivity they will need to become truly effective therapists and valued partners in the therapy process.

As a professor who has used the first edition of this excellent book in my classes and referred to it countless times in my own research and writing, I can say that this second edition represents a profound enhancement to an already outstanding text. Dr. Shapiro has expanded nearly every aspect of the book. The result is a monumental achievement that not only builds on the themes that were addressed so beautifully in the first edition but also incorporates many new topics that are critical for a deep understanding of the stuttering disorder, including new and emerging treatment strategies, evidence-based practice and the evaluation of treatment outcomes, the value of self-help and mutual aid, clinical training and specialization, global perspectives on the nature and treatment of the stuttering disorder, and much more. Each subject is handled with the same grace and sincerity as the next, and throughout the book, the clear prose is a pleasure to read.

Beyond increasing knowledge, empathy, and understanding, this book leaves its reader with a strong feeling of satisfaction and accomplishment. I believe that the growing sense of comfort and confidence that clinicians gain through this book will give them the foundation they need to achieve true clinical excellence, enabling them to help people who stutter overcome the challenges of their disorder and pursue their life goals. Thus, the ultimate outcome of Dr. Shapiro's achievement in writing this book is a better life for people who stutter.

J. Scott Yaruss, PhD, CCC-SLP, ASHA Fellow
Board-Recognized Specialist in Fluency Disorders
Associate Professor and Director of Master's Degree
    Programs in Speech–Language Pathology
University of Pittsburgh
Pittsburgh, Pennsylvania

Preface to the First and Second Editions

Preface to the Second Edition

In essence, this second edition is a love story. It is about uniting one's head with one's heart and giving freely the gifts that effective clinicians have. What brings us together, and what brings us together with people who stutter and their families, might be coincidence if not serendipity. Each of us is pursuing a career in communication sciences and disorders and a specialized interest in stuttering intervention for various reasons. Nevertheless, the message to which we commit and that which we impart is absolutely essential: Indeed it is the birthright of every person to be able to use speech and language freely and to enjoy communication freedom. Yet, at a certain point, the message of communication sciences and disorders transforms into a medium for an even larger message: When gathered with a common interest and shared focus, we create an opportunity to realize the best of human potential. In fact, there is probably nothing that we cannot accomplish when we are willing to shift perspective so as to consider alternative points of view and to learn and grow together. This is our calling; this is our passion. It is through this passion that we express and demonstrate our confidence in the human condition and in each other. Perhaps to my last breath, I will know that life is about love, and love is about giving, and laughing, and learning in every moment; this is living.

Since the first edition of this book was published, I have lived and learned so much. I could not have imagined that the first edition would be received so positively and with such a wide audience, both nationally and internationally. Early on, one of the reviewers indicated that the book would serve not only as guide for fluency assessment and treatment, but also as a guide for our clinical profession of speech–language pathology as a whole. Another reviewer commented that one of the most positive elements was that the book was filled with real and instructive stories of clients' challenges and successes in communication and in life. A third noted that the message (i.e., one of humanness) radiates through both the book's content and its manner of expression. This second edition has remained true to these themes, while significantly expanding its scope to account for what we and our discipline have learned over the ensuing decade. Let me explain.

In the preface to the first edition, I underscored the moments of magic that occur within the process of fluency intervention. Also, I highlighted the questions that clinicians tend to ask. Like the first edition, this edition is divided into four units. Unit I provides a conceptual foundation for clinical intervention, with chapters addressing the uniqueness of the book and concepts that are essential for understanding stuttering and people who stutter (Chapter 1); the onset, development, and nature of stuttering and related literature (Chapter 2); the etiology of stuttering from past and present perspectives (Chapter 3); and other disorders of fluency (Chapter 4). Unit II focuses on the central and guiding assumptions that ground the design of effective intervention, including intrafamily considerations (i.e., personal constructs and family systems; Chapter 5), extrafamily considerations (i.e., interdisciplinary teaming and multicultural perspectives; Chapter 6), and psychotherapeutic considerations (i.e., stuttering modification and fluency shaping, with exemplar treatments; Chapter 7). Unit III, the largest and most substantive section of the book, addresses assessment and treatment across the life span with people who stutter. These chapters discuss preschool children (Chapter 8); school-age children (Chapter 9); and adolescents, adults, and senior adults who stutter (Chapter 10). Finally, Unit IV addresses the clinician from multiple perspectives by focusing on the clinician and the client–clinician relationship (Chapter 11) and the roles of professional preparation and lifelong learning (Chapter 12), all of which are essential to becoming and being a clinician.

This edition also covers the significant advancements that have been made over the last decade. These advancements include but are not limited to the following: evidence-based practice, the Lidcombe Program, data from longitudinal investigations of the onset and development of stuttering, risk factors to distinguish between transient and chronic stuttering, neurophysiological research, genetics and twinning research, theoretical explanations for stuttering from Western and non-Western perspectives, other fluency disorders, multicultural considerations in research and treatment for stuttering, electronic devices with altered auditory feedback, neuropharmacology, severity rating and impact assessment, assessment and treatment of children who stutter and have co-existing disorders, collaboration with parents and teachers, confronting and overcoming bullying and relapse, demographic shifts of aging and implications for fluency intervention, revision in training standards, models of clinical and supervisory development, specialization and globalization, self-help and mutual aid, national and international foundations and associations, and international and electronic websites and congresses. This edition thus reflects the most current thought across multiple disciplines as applied to assessment and treatment of people who stutter across the life span.

As with the first edition, ease of reading was one of the principles guiding the book's design and writing. The book is as gender neutral as possible and avoids cumbersome pronoun constructions such as *she or he* and *her or his*. People who stutter are referred to as *he* and student clinicians and professional speech–language pathologists are referred to as *she*. The rationale is that the majority of people who stutter are male; the majority of speech–language pathologists are female.

As I end this preface—which appears at the beginning of the book but was written last—I am experiencing mixed emotions. This book has taken on a life of its own and has become my friend. I have looked forward to our regular interaction, and though I am happy to see the fruits of my labor, I am a bit sorry that this interaction is about to end. My friend and I have spent a lot of time together. We have shifted perspective; we have been companions through significant personal, national, and global events. We have challenged each other; we have comforted each other. We have looked into each other's eyes and, at the most challenging moments, confessed, "I believe in you." We have given to each other selflessly and we have both learned and grown. We are older and, I think we would agree, a tad wiser for the wear.

As I prepare to share these words and this journey with you, I find myself reflecting on the sentiments of my daughter, Sarah Shapiro. In her high school commencement speech, she said:

> As we cross the stage today, we must remember that each and every one of us matters. As we enter a world of uncertainty, we must be guided and strengthened by life's certainties. To me, life's certainties are love, language, and faith. There is no problem too great

that love cannot resolve. There is no weapon more effective than the spoken and written word. And there is no greater promise for tomorrow than faith.

With these thoughts, I thank you—student clinicians, speech–language pathologists, and people who stutter and their families, all comrades—for the opportunity to focus on a labor that is an expression of love, on a product that is a process in progress, and on a mission that is second to none: to enable everyone to enjoy and to relish communication and fluency freedom.

I celebrate you as you embark or continue on your path to understand stuttering and to design and implement assessment and treatment with and for people who stutter. As you reflect on people who stutter and their families, speech–language pathologists, and other colleagues across allied educational, human service, and medical disciplines, remember that "each and every one of us matters." I encourage you to dialogue with others who also are committed to stuttering intervention. Talk about what you are learning: the excitements, the challenges, the fears. We are in this mission together. You are welcome to contact me at Western Carolina University (shapiro@email.wcu.edu) to share your experiences and those of your clients and their families. I applaud you; I am confident that you are doing your best to do well and that, in the process, you are doing "good." Good luck to you.

Preface to the First Edition

The word *therapist* rarely is used today in speech–language pathology and audiology. I like that word. It comes from the Greek root *therapeuein*, meaning "comrade in a common struggle." This book is designed for all comrades, including student clinicians and professional speech–language pathologists, who are committed to understanding stuttering and people who stutter. Stuttering continues to be one of the most perplexing communication disorders. People who stutter and their families are the beneficiaries of our best clinical and scientific efforts to unveil the mysteries of stuttering, as well as our source of motivation to approach the challenge of informed and effective intervention with insight and vigor.

Over the past 2 decades alone, more than 1,400 articles and 30 books have been written about stuttering (Culatta & Goldberg, 1995). Some present a compendium of knowledge to date about stuttering. Others emphasize precise measurements of stuttering and related behaviors. Still others transform these data into intervention strategies based on a particular clinical philosophy. The purpose of this book is to present a specific point of view—i.e., a unique approach to intervention with people who stutter, based on what is known about learning and communication, speech and language fluency, stuttering, and people who stutter. You might say, "Aha! This book presents a recipe." It does not. It shares with you some of my ideas and what I do. I am convinced that as clinicians, we have an obligation to share with each other what we do, the rationale for what we do, and accountability for what we do, in order to ensure the highest quality of service for our clients and maximum growth for our profession. The procedures presented are what I find successful. You, the reader, are free to sift through, select, change, or even drop any of the procedures according to the strengths and needs of your individual clients or your own theoretical orientation, as long as what you do, why, and your accountability are clear. This book tells a story. Every good story has a moral. This story has two. First, design and implementation of intervention with people who stutter are not arbitrary events. Assessment and treatment are based on decision rules that are guiding principles to effective and reliable intervention. Second, the future for people who stutter is, and must be, sincerely viewed as bright and optimistic. This interpretation is based on promising clinical data and an understanding of the impact that the clinician's attitude has on the success of the treatment experience.

You might have noticed that this is not a traditional textbook. It has had no less than a 20-year gestation. Over this period of time, my professional motivation has been maintained by working continuously as a speech–language pathologist providing assessment and treatment services to people of all ages who stutter and their families. Also, in teaching undergraduate and graduate courses in communication disorders (including stuttering), supervising clinical practica required for professional preparation of speech–language pathologists, and providing workshops for literally thousands of professional clinicians in the field, I continue to address a series of predictable questions, including (a) What is stuttering? (b) What is known and not known about stuttering and people who stutter? (c) How do I distinguish stuttering from normal speech disfluencies? (d) How do I assess people who stutter? (e) How do I treat people who stutter? and (f) How do I work with the families and significant others of people who stutter? Such families, teachers, and allied service providers, among others, continue to ask (g) What can I do to facilitate the process of intervention and development of long-term communication independence by the person who stutters? This book is intended to address these and other questions. Specifically, the book addresses, outlines, and accounts for an individualized, collaborative approach to assessment and treatment (within the framework of communication systems) across the life span *with* (i.e., not *for*) people who stutter. This is done from an interdisciplinary perspective and with sensitivity toward multicultural and otherwise diverse realities.

It is said that lightning does not strike the same place twice. It should be said, however, that magic in fluency intervention strikes at least three times. Magic, used here, is the overpowering quality within the process of effective interpersonal communication (i.e., clinical intervention) that distinguishes and enchants the event as a quintessential human experience. The first time magic strikes is when a clinician first experiences the gestalt, the "aha!," the predictable shift in a clinician's focus from oneself (i.e., What do I do if the parent begins to cry? What should I do if my behavior management techniques don't work for the young child? What do I do if the adult client asks me something I don't know?) to the client (i.e., When the child denies that he stutters, is this child unaware or emotionally unprepared to address the issue? When the client fails to complete her assignment, does this mean that she truly forgot, as reported, or is this client unmotivated? What is the clinical significance of what the client is not saying?). This shift in focus from oneself to the client typically is built upon a foundation of academic and clinical knowledge and successful clinical experience and renders the process of intervention thoroughly enjoyable and rewarding. Magic strikes a second time when, within a supportive and open clinical relationship, the client experiences, perhaps for the first time, either controlled or spontaneous fluency. As will be seen, fluency shaping—i.e., more behaviorally oriented techniques (e.g., choral reading with slower, gentler, and more natural sounding speech)—will render all people who stutter temporarily fluent. This experience can offer a client a glimmer of fluency freedom that can be powerfully motivating. From this experience, I have seen clients laugh and cry with the mixed emotions of joy, fear, and wonderment of their fluency future.

Magic strikes a third time when the families of people who stutter feel that they are sincerely cared for and understood, actively involved in the process of intervention, and contributing meaningfully to the communication improvement of their family member who stutters. Expressions of thanks are frequent, and family bonds within a communication system are strengthened. When magic has struck three times, it strikes a fourth.

At this point, clinicians, clients who stutter, and their families are communicating and learning with and from each other. At an earlier time, a colleague and I described the ability to shift perspective as "the hallmark of communication" (Shapiro & Moses, 1989). This type of communication is professionally gratifying, if not exhilarating. I have found these experiences to be communicatively intimate, rendering the dialogue among the participants within the clinical interaction both timeless and placeless. It has not been uncommon for me to lose track of time and place because of my focus on and communication with a person who stutters and the family. I continue to be intrigued by and concerned about the number of clinicians who have completed programs of graduate study, yet fail to experience this magic. Although the printed word has limitations in conveying the multidimensionality of the clinical experience, I hope this book helps impart the magic of fluency intervention to you.

To this point, it might seem that my motivation for writing this book is strictly professional. That is a major part, but not the whole story. This book also has a personal motivation. I was anything but communicatively independent for nearly a quarter of a century. I stuttered miserably for many years and experienced frequent disappointments in scheduled treatment. I have enjoyed fluency freedom for nearly 20 years and perhaps am making up for lost time. In a way, I feel it is unfortunate that I must credit myself for most of my own progress. My commitment to write such a book is in part the settlement of a debt—to myself. I inform my many clients that I will expect them to return the favor, in a way of their own design, to the field or to an individual who might not have been as fortunate and who is still in pursuit of the fluency that seems so elusive. I have always been one to put my actions where my mouth is, and to lead by example so that others may do as I do, rather than do only as I say. Indeed I know firsthand what it is like to be unable to speak, to only dream of enjoying the freedom of speech enjoyed by so many others. More than a freedom, I have come to believe that fluent speech is one's natural right. I have become convinced from the many clients and their families I have worked with, as well as the feedback I received from former students, that my ideas need to be written. I remain positive by nature and believe that every experience, particularly the most challenging, becomes meaningful and instructive. So, this book is my way of integrating my academic and clinical training; my experiences (both professional and, as appropriate, personal); my own positive, collaborative, whole-person, systematic, and systems-based approach to individualized and interdisciplinary intervention with persons who stutter; and yes, my way of saying thanks. I believe that ultimately our legacy will be our caring for and dialogue with others who also are seeking to improve the human condition and to make even better the communicative world in which we all live.

As you begin reading *Stuttering Intervention: A Collaborative Journey to Fluency Freedom*, and thereby your own journey to understanding stuttering and people who stutter, it is helpful to know what to expect along the way. As I indicated earlier, this book is intended for all student clinicians and professional speech–language pathologists who are interested in and committed to designing and implementing effective intervention with people who stutter. This book may be used in upper-level undergraduate or graduate-level courses addressing disorders of speech fluency, including stuttering. It may be used in one semester or across a two-semester sequence. Furthermore, the book may serve as a clinical guide for practitioners who are looking for a clinical method that is practical, directly applied, reliable, and accountable, while based upon theoretical concepts and research across human service disciplines. The concepts and content in the book are presented developmentally in such a way that earlier chapters serve as the instructional foundation for later chapters.

The book contains four units. Unit I contains Chapters 1 through 4 and provides the reader with a conceptual foundation for clinical intervention. Chapter 1 introduces the reader to the uniqueness of this book and to concepts that are critical for understanding stuttering and people who stutter. Chapter 2 addresses the onset, development, and nature of stuttering and reviews related literature. Chapter 3 covers the etiology of stuttering from past and present perspectives and conveys how present thinking relates to ideas we once believed to be true. Chapter 4, the last in Unit I, helps clinicians distinguish and differentially diagnose stuttering from other disorders of fluency, some of which are not mentioned in any other book to date in speech–language pathology. Unit II contains Chapters 5 through 7 and addresses central and guiding assumptions that are critical to the design of effective intervention. Chapter 5 addresses intrafamily considerations (i.e., personal constructs and family systems); Chapter 6, extrafamily considerations (i.e., interdisciplinary teaming and multicultural perspectives); and Chapter 7, psychotherapeutic considerations (i.e., stuttering modification and fluency shaping), including exemplar forms of treatment. Unit III, the largest and most substantive of the book, contains Chapters 8 through 10, which address assessment and treatment across the life span with people who stutter. Chapter 8 focuses on intervention with preschool children; Chapter 9 with school-age children; and Chapter 10 with adolescents, adults, and senior adults. Finally, Unit IV contains Chapters 11 and 12, which address the clinician from multiple perspectives. Chapter 11 focuses on the clinician and the client–clinician relationship. Chapter 12 discusses the roles of professional preparation and lifelong learning as critical processes for developing and maintaining effective speech–language pathologists.

One additional point of information is necessary. Ease of reading was one of the principles guiding the design and writing of this book. For this and other reasons, the book is as gender neutral as possible. When it was not possible—and to avoid use of cumbersome pronoun constructions such as *she or he* and *her or his*—people who stutter are referred to as *he* and student clinicians and professional speech–language pathologists are referred to as *she*. This rationale is based on the documentation that the majority of people who stutter are male; the majority of speech–language pathologists are female.

As you begin your own journey, I encourage you to dialogue with your colleagues in speech–language pathology who, like yourself, are working to understand stuttering and people who stutter. Talk about what you are learning—the excitements, the challenges, the fears. In our shared commitment to providing the best intervention services possible, I would love to hear your reactions, as well as those of your clients and their families, to the material presented here. Feel free to contact me. I can be reached at Western Carolina University, Department of Communication Sciences and Disorders, Speech and Hearing Center—McKee G-30, Cullowhee, NC 28723. Good luck.

Acknowledgments

This book represents the ongoing support of many good people. First, I am grateful to the administration at Western Carolina University, which, since my arrival in 1984, has provided institutional resources and opportunities enabling me to grow professionally and to commit to serving our community, both locally and globally. Completion of this book is only the most recent manifestation of that ongoing support. Particularly, I want to thank Drs. John Bardo, Chancellor; Kyle Carter, former Provost; Linda Seestedt-Stanford, Dean, College of Health and Human Sciences, Interim Provost and Senior Vice Chancellor; and Billy Ogletree, Head, Department of Communication Sciences and Disorders. I am thankful to have such nurturing colleagues and proud to be a part of WCU's community of scholarship. I am thankful also for the support and ongoing interest in this work among the faculty and students in Communication Sciences and Disorders and other disciplines. Thanks to my colleagues at Občanské sdružení LOGO (Brno, Czech Republic) for welcoming me into their professional community and for providing the drawing that appears as Figure 9.3. Thanks to Joseph Agius, David Daly, Charles Healey, Judith Kuster, and Scott Yaruss for valuable editorial suggestions on an earlier version of this manuscript. Thanks to Beth Rowan, Melissa Tullos, and others at PRO-ED for believing in and encouraging this project from the beginning, and to Sue Carter for contributing unparalleled editing skills.

Second, a project such as this becomes a family affair at some point. I cannot even imagine undertaking such a challenge, no less completing it, without the love and support of my best friend for life, Kay, who more than anyone else has stood by me and understood and encouraged my need to write this book, all the while putting up with me. Thanks to the two finest children ever, Sarah and Aaron, who have been my best teachers since they were born and are now responsible young adults, and of whom I am absolutely proud. Looking into the eyes of Kay, Sarah, and Aaron, and even thinking of their voices, I experience both grace and inspiration. Thanks to my parents, Alice and Sidney Shapiro, and my parents-in-law, Esther and Calvin Slattery, for their positive influences throughout this project. Thanks to friends, including Mil and Barbie Clark, Bill and Karen Clarke, Frank and Sandi Cooper, Cliff and Ellen Faull, Chuck deKrafft, Isabella Reichel, Phil Schneider, Anne-Marie Simon, and David Westling, for ongoing support and expressions of kindness.

Last, I owe a debt of gratitude to the many people who stutter and their families who have contributed to our knowledge of fluency disorders and who put their confidence in our hands to help guide their collaborative journey to fluency freedom. May we always be deserving of their confidence; may we always nurture their dreams; and may we always help each other work toward improved communication and thereby global understanding and world peace.

Unit I

Stuttering in Relief

A Foundation for Intervention

Chapter One

The Nexus of Stuttering

An Introduction

It is difficult for those who have not possessed or been possessed by the disorder to appreciate its impact on the stutterer's self-concepts, his roles, his way of living. (Van Riper, 1982, p. 1)

The Face of Stuttering

Picture a young boy preparing to make his first phone call to a girl he has become fond of at school. You, the reader, can recall your own similar experiences. He waits until his family is out of earshot. To a young boy, this experience is so significant that he wishes not to offer explanation to his surely disbelieving parents and siblings. Boys are supposed to think that girls have cooties. Not this boy. He dials her phone number, but disconnects the call before the ring begins because he is not quite ready yet. Regaining his composure, all the while rehearsing, "Hello, this is . . .," he redials. "This time I really am going to do it," he thinks to himself. "I am ready." Before he can change his mind, the phone begins to ring. It seems to the boy an eternity between the end of the first ring and the beginning of the second. Finally, a voice answers, "Hello." This voice is very important to the boy. It could be the girl's father, mother, brother, or sister. Or it could be a wrong number. To the boy, the bearer of the voice represents someone important to the girl. The voice again says, "Hello." The boy begins to say the first sound in Hello. He says, "H. H. H." Try as he might, all that come out are little inaudible puffs of air. "Hello! Hello! Hello!" the voice repeats with increasing impatience. While the boy continues his valiant attempts, he hears, "Oh, these damn pranks!" The phone goes dead. This is stuttering.

The same boy, some years later, prepares at great length for his turn to recite a poem in eighth-grade English class. He knows the poem well. He memorizes it and recites it alone and with his family. He always does his best and is a serious student. He particularly wants to do well on this day because Nancy is in his class. He likes Nancy a lot. He thinks she knows it, although he has never told her. When she recited her poem the day before, the boy smiled at her and told her that she did great. The boy feels relatively confident, although he knows that he never can seem to predict his speech fluency. He takes his place at the front of the room. The teacher says, "Begin." "There once was . . . a . . . a . . ." Oh, dread! Horror! "Why does this have to happen now?" the boy thinks. "Why always to me?" After several attempts, the boy hears some students chuckling; others move uncomfortably in their seats. The teacher interrupts, "You do know your poem, don't you?" "Yes sir," the boy responds. "Now let's all be patient," the teacher continues. "We know that our presenter today tries as hard as the rest of us. We need to show him that we are listening and that we are interested." The boy wishes that he could be somewhere else, anywhere else. Time seems to stand still. The boy feels that he is taking too long. Everybody is waiting. He sees Nancy looking away. "She can't even look at me," he thinks. This is stuttering.

The boy is now a young man in high school who rarely speaks because of embarrassment frequently associated with his stuttering. After much forethought and measured anticipation, he collects his courage and asks a young woman to accompany him to the basketball game on Friday evening. His speech is so disfluent. He tries to relax, but his face contorts. He speaks haltingly. He knows that his speech sounds more like a growl. He sees her beautiful face first tense, then turn into an amused, uncomfortable grin. She tells him she is busy. "Thanks all the same." Both look down, anywhere but at each other, with only fleeting eye contact. This is stuttering.

Later still, the man and his wife are expecting their second child, who they know will be a boy. They agree that the name Aaron is their favorite. The name has an additional significance for the man because of its biblical association, particularly to the Book of Exodus. Moses stuttered and brought his brother Aaron with him as his spokesperson. But the man knows that the initial vowel (A) will occasionally be difficult for him to say. Even before the boy is born, the man pictures himself introducing his son and blocking on his name. He rehearses over and over, "Aaron. Aaron Joseph. This is my son, Aaron." Joseph is to be the son's middle name in honor of the man's grandfather. "Maybe I should name him Joseph Aaron," he thinks, "since Joseph would be easier for me to say, and Joseph provides a transition to say Aaron, unlike saying Aaron Joseph. Or maybe I should just replace the name Aaron with another containing an initial consonant. Who would ever know?" But how could he raise his son, knowing fully that his given name was to be Aaron, but his father decided to call him Kevin, or Seth, or Robert? That would be the ultimate avoidance, if not a permanent penalty, for a boy and his father. This is me. This is stuttering.

This is the face of stuttering. Stories such as these are relived daily by people who stutter. Communication is a uniquely human experience. Stuttering, a significant disorder of communication, reminds people who stutter of their particularly human limitations. Stuttering has a significant impact on one's life:

> Once it has taken hold, after a period of insidious growth, almost every aspect of the person's existence is colored by his communicative disability. Ease in verbal communication is a vital prerequisite for more than marginal existence in any modern culture such as ours. Stuttering is not merely a speech impediment; it is an impediment in social living. (Van Riper, 1982, pp. 1–2)

Stuttering, as we will see, potentially influences all aspects of one's communication and one's life, as well as the lives of others who communicate with people who stutter.

About This Book

This book is based on the conviction that stuttering is both a multidimensional and manageable composite of behaviors, thoughts, and feelings. Successful intervention must take into account not only the individual who stutters but virtually all persons within that individual's communication system. This collaborative enterprise requires that the person who stutters be actively engaged in all aspects of the intervention process, and be treated as whole and able. The communication environment, as well as the communication itself, becomes the object of study. Overt (i.e., directly observable behaviors) and covert (i.e., internalized thoughts and feelings) manifestations of communication are considered, if not addressed, equally. The primary focus of intervention, and the source of ongoing motivation, is success—what the person who stutters can, rather than cannot, do. The approach is tailored to each individual's unique communication strengths and needs; is consistent with what we know about communication, learning, change, and the role of the communicator in the change process; is responsive to lessons learned from people who stutter, families, clinicians, and allied professionals; is committed to an interdisciplinary perspective; and results in positive change by speakers of all ages within communication systems. This approach is in immediate and direct contrast to traditional forms of intervention in which people who stutter are only passively engaged, are the sole focus of treatment, and are treated as disabled or disordered. Such a narrow and negative focus results in treatment that is lacking in its relatedness to one's real communication strengths and needs (i.e., lacking in ecological validity) and therefore does not generalize to contexts outside of the clinical environment. The approach embraced by this book includes the following principles:

- The person who stutters is a whole person who communicates within a communication system, not a disabled person in isolation.
- The intervention process is multidimensional and collaborative, necessarily involving the client, clinician, members of the communication system, and allied professionals, rather than unidimensional and solely an interaction between the clinician and client.
- The clinician facilitates participation by other members of the interdisciplinary team rather than focusing exclusively on the client–clinician relationship.
- The client is an active and critical member of the interdisciplinary team, necessarily involved in all aspects of intervention planning, implementation, evaluation, and follow-up, rather than a passive participant who follows the direction of the clinician.
- Treatment focuses on the fluent aspects of communication, not just the disfluency. While numbers do not tell the whole story, 15% or 20% disfluency typically renders a speaker significantly disfluent—which means that 80% to 85% of the individual's speech is fluent. The client first focuses on how to do more of what he already is doing right. Only then are the disfluencies targeted and eliminated. This process (fluency facilitation) is in contrast to a primary focus on disfluency (and the resulting perspective of rehabilitation).
- Transfer (i.e., generalization) begins from the first contact with the client as opposed to near the end of scheduled treatment.
- Relapse is inevitable, so clients are prepared to handle it productively and with fluency facilitating control. Traditionally, relapse has not been addressed, and the client experiences surprise and communicative defenselessness when it occurs.
- Communicative change is realistic, desirable, and possible at any age within communication systems.
- Stuttering (behaviors, thoughts, and feelings) reflects in part the consequence of active and alternative choices.
- Measured fluency is only one of many indicators of success and evidence-based practice. Other indicators include one's demonstrated sense of communication freedom and acceptance of oneself as a person and as a communicator.
- Early intervention with young children is a form of prevention.

⟲ Regular assignments designed with, not for, clients are a critical form of treatment that occurs between scheduled sessions.

⟲ Multicultural considerations in assessment and treatment are invited, nurtured, and addressed.

⟲ Intervention with senior adults who stutter provides a positive, inviting, and enlightening opportunity.

⟲ Stuttering is a universal challenge, one that enables people across the world to unite and focus on a common area of concern. This view was recently expressed by a consortium of 17 coauthors representing 15 countries across six continents:

> As a profession, we are one. We are united by our universal commonalities, our challenges, and our beliefs. Efforts such as this bring people together from diverse lands, enabling us to explore our common goal of improving the lives of people who stutter. We set an example to other groups around the world for how seemingly insoluble problems can be addressed by constructive and positive means, indeed by communication. That is our business—no, that is our calling—using our freedom of speech to construct a greater understanding, a more harmonious existence, and a more peaceful world. That is our wish. (Shapiro et al., 2004, p. 136)

The objectives of this book, therefore, are to address, outline, and account for individualized assessment and treatment across the life span with (not for) people who stutter within communication systems. The book takes an interdisciplinary perspective and demonstrates particular awareness of and sensitivity toward multicultural, international, and otherwise diverse realities. There are at least two additional overriding objectives. One is to inspire you, the reader, to want to know even more about stuttering and to feel a professional calling to work with people who stutter. Another is to highlight effective clinical methods that you might already be using so as to encourage their further use. Blood (1995b) noted, "Sometimes validation of the techniques people are using already is as important as the creation of new techniques" (p. 177). You will see that this last objective is parallel to a procedure that I will be recommending for intervention: highlighting what a client already is doing right that is conducive to fluency or fluency facilitating control so as to help him know how to do more of what he is already doing right.

Definitions

Fluency

There seems to be little disagreement that when people stutter, they are not talking fluently. Listeners tend to be reliable and accurate in distinguishing individuals as belonging to the category of people who stutter or people who do not stutter (Bloodstein & Bernstein Ratner, 2008). Defining stuttering and identifying with precision individual instances of stuttering, however, prove to be more difficult and less reliable (Brundage, Bothe, Lengeling, & Evans, 2006; Tetnowski & Schagen, 2001).

Starkweather (1984) suggested that because we categorize speakers on the basis of their relative speech fluency, we have erroneously assumed that fluency is the absence of stuttering. He indicated several problems with such a temptingly simple definition. First, stuttering behaviors vary in how fluent they are. People who stutter demonstrate different degrees of fluency at different times and when compared to each other. Furthermore, the therapy goal referred to as "fluent stuttering" seeks to achieve a less effortful, less abnormal, less disruptive, and briefer form of disfluency. Therefore, defining fluency as the absence of stuttering is counterintuitive. Instead, fluency should be defined in terms of effort and temporal duration. Second, people who stutter do not stutter all of the time. In fact, most of their speech is free of stuttering. However, this nonstuttered speech varies in its degree of fluency. People who stutter tend to speak more slowly than people of the same age and sex who do not stutter. People who stutter have the same normal nonfluencies as people who do not stutter. The nonstuttered speech of people who stutter also is less fluent when they expend effort and time on fluency tricks such as circumlocution (i.e., word changing) to avoid stuttering. Finally, people who do not stutter demonstrate times of increased and decreased fluency for reasons of health, fatigue, perceived stress, level of conviction, and so forth. Their nonfluency is characterized by varying degrees of filled pauses, hesitations, false starts, and repetitions of sounds, words, and phrases. Furthermore, fluency is a continuous rather than a dichotomous variable; speech (with or without stuttering) can be more or less fluent, demonstrating differences in the relative effort or ease with which speech is produced.

Starkweather (1984) indicated that in our own speech, we recognize fluency by the ease and rapidity with which words are produced and disfluency by production that is slowed down by unexpected effort. In the speech of others, however, we cannot directly feel how easy or difficult speech production is. We must infer ease of speech fluency from observable events, including the rate (i.e., units per time) at which speech is produced and the continuity (i.e., smoothness) of its output. Both speech rate and continuity are influenced by the information load of the utterance. Information load refers to the "level of uncertainty associated with a transition from one location in an utterance to the next" (Starkweather, 1984, p. 34). Because of the influence of information load on speech fluency and the influence of syntactic structure and word frequency on information load, one must consider a distinction between speech fluency (i.e., motor speech production) and language fluency (i.e., word finding and sentence formulation) (Starkweather, 1984, 1987, 2002a). *Semantic fluency* refers to the ease of retrieving from a large pool of lexical items (i.e., vocabulary words) for reference to many different concepts. *Syntactic fluency* refers to the ease with which speakers construct complex sentences containing linguistically complex structures. *Pragmatic fluency* refers to both knowing and demonstrating what one wants to say within and in response to a variety of situational constraints. *Phonologic fluency* refers to the ease of producing long and complex strings of sounds within meaningful and complex language units.

The location of stuttering and normal disfluency is influenced by language. For example, stuttering is more likely to occur at clause boundaries, on longer and less frequently used words, and within the context of greater information load and syntactic complexity (Bloodstein & Bernstein Ratner, 2008; Logan, 2003; Logan & Conture, 1995; Yairi & Ambrose, 2005; Yaruss, 1999b). These and other influences of language on stuttering, such as the influence of language planning, formulation, and production on the stuttering of children and adults, will be reviewed shortly. The point is that speech fluency and language fluency are different, and that most people who stutter demonstrate language fluency. Such people can stutter severely (i.e., demonstrate deficient speech fluency) and still have a large repertoire of productive vocabulary (semantic fluency), the ability to construct complex sentences (syntactic fluency), knowledge of what sentences are appropriate given the uniqueness of specific conversational and situational constraints (pragmatic fluency), and knowledge of how sounds are produced and combined in meaningful sentences (phonological fluency). So stuttering is not a disorder of language fluency.

Starkweather (1987, 2002a) decried the traditional practice of evaluating stuttering only by counting the frequency of disfluent words and by observing qualitative characteristics, such as associated struggle. He recommended that the assessment of stuttering should contain an analysis of speech fluency including rate, rhythm, and the ease with which the person speaks, as well as the continuity of the speech. Taking into account Starkweather's contributions, Ham (1990) offered the following definition:

> Fluency is deviant when planning and/or execution effort is excessive, when disconti- nuities occur at a frequency and/or to a degree inappropriate for speaker age, or when speech rhythm is atypical or occurs in such a way as to impede or disrupt the speech production. (p. 8)

Implicit challenges here are distinguishing between a fluency deviation and stut- tering (Guitar, 2006; Manning, 2010; Yairi & Ambrose, 2005) and understanding the nature of stuttering, each individual client's personal story, and measurement of change as progress (ASHA, 2006; Manning, 2004; Schneider, 2004; St. Louis, 2001a). A closer look at disfluency follows.

Disfluency Versus Dysfluency

Disfluency and *dysfluency* are terms that have been used to refer to breaks in the for- ward flow of speech. Some have referred to *disfluency* as the nonfluent speech of people who do not stutter, and the nonstuttered yet nonfluent speech of people who do stut- ter. *Dysfluency* has been used to refer to the stuttered speech of people who stutter, and the stuttered speech of people who do not usually stutter (Ham, 1990). Making these distinctions, however, has resulted in a theoretical encampment of limited practical util- ity. Starkweather (1987) argued that speech fluency consists of more than just continu- ity (i.e., smoothness), including effort and rate as well. Disfluency and dysfluency are inadequately descriptive because they do not specify the dimension in which fluency is disrupted. Furthermore, such terms suggest that speech fluency is a dichotomous vari- able (speech either is or is not fluent), rather than continuous (speech varies in its degree and nature of fluency). Cooper (1993c) aptly stated,

> Time and effort are being wasted speculating on whether a discrete behavior is a stut- tering behavior on the basis of data obtained in assessments of behaviors devoid of any consideration of the affective and cognitive milieu in which the behavior occurs. I am hopeful we have seen the last of studies concerned with differentiating a "disfluency" from a "dysfluency" on the basis of a series of sophisticated psychoacoustical measure- ments of vocalizations made without respect to the subjects' histories and their affective and cognitive states at the moment of assessment. (pp. 377–378)

Increasingly, the distinction between disfluency and dysfluency is being dismissed. Nico- losi, Harryman, and Kresheck (2004), for example, defined disfluency as an "alternative spelling for dysfluency" (p. 102).

Thus, *disfluency* is not distinguished from *dysfluency* in this book. The term *disfluency* will be used to refer to all moments of fluency breakdown (Bloodstein & Bernstein Rat- ner, 2008). All events relating to stuttering and people who stutter will be identified, to the extent possible, with terms that generate molecular descriptions.

Stuttering

As noted earlier, there is no universally accepted definition of stuttering. Culatta and Goldberg (1995) concluded that if 10 speech–language pathologists were put in a room, 11 definitions of stuttering would emerge. The divergence of definitions reflects at least a lack of agreement in the attributes considered significant by the definers, as well as differing hypotheses about the etiology of stuttering upon which the definitions are based (F. H. Silverman, 2004). Each definition reflects the kernels of truth considered to be most salient to the author. Wingate (1988) indicated that the reason stuttering is so poorly understood is precisely that so much has been written about it, noting that "the intrinsic mystery of the disorder has been embellished by the many efforts to explain it" (p. 3). Wingate's observation seems to be even more relevant today.

Bloodstein (1990) summarized that traditionally there have been three alternative types of definitions. The first is the observer's perceptual definition—that is, stuttering is whatever observers or conversational partners hear or see it to be. The second is a standard, or dictionary, definition that defines stuttering by other words (e.g., *repetition*, *prolongation*, *struggle*, etc.), each of which is defined by other words. The third is the perceptual definition of people who stutter—that is, stuttering is whatever people who stutter feel their own stuttering to be. Each definition is significant in its impact on the conversational experience. However, Bloodstein acknowledged that speech–language pathologists, in their frequent attempts to count stuttering blocks, have ignored the significance of what the person who stutters perceives to be his own stuttering. Furthermore, clinicians and researchers have assumed that stuttering must be reliably countable. Bloodstein indicated that "it may be that stuttering is inherently indeterminate, uncertain, and relative. If so, it should not surprise us that we have not been able to find a definition that allows us to identify unequivocally when or whether a person stutters" (p. 393). More recently, Bloodstein and Bernstein Ratner (2008) aptly concluded, "It is, of course, within the realm of possibility that not only incidents of stuttered speech, but even individuals who stutter, may prove impossible to characterize in every case with absolute unambiguity" (p. 10).

It seems obvious that the acoustic event (i.e., the listener perception) allows for greater precision in measurement than the personal or subjective experience of the person who stutters. Perkins (1990b) asked, "But does that warrant continued use of listener judgments as valid, or even useful, when the acoustical signal has been demonstrated incontrovertibly to be all but devoid of information about what the stutterer considers to be stuttering?" (p. 404).

Our purpose in reviewing these attempts to define stuttering is more than a semantic exercise. The significance of definitions and the process of their construction become clear when one considers the extent to which such definitions establish the foundation for theories, therapies, and research. Perkins (1990a) indicated that "a definition of stuttering should not only be an explicit reflection of assumptions about the disorder, it should define one's understanding of its basic nature" (p. 370). He expressed concern that invalid definitions generate invalid therapy, theory, and research:

> Definitions, theories, therapies, and research all have underlying assumptions, albeit sometimes obscure. When assumptions are shared, then definitions, research, theories, and therapies are unified in a common conception. Each is logically related to the others. Although each is necessarily predicated on some assumption, these assumptions are not always the same. When they are not, as is currently the case for stuttering, then definitional, investigatory, theoretical, and therapeutic domains become unrelated in ways that impair, if not nullify, progress in all domains. Being conceptually disconnected from each other, advances in one domain are not likely to generalize readily to the others. (p. 370)

Perkins (1990a) identified a resulting disjunction between biologically based research and clinical practice:

> The therapies currently in vogue are all related to stuttering as learned, or at least modifiable, behavior. Conversely, research into the nature of stuttering almost entirely reflects the conviction that it is a biologically based disorder with probable genetic origin. This research has not only become disconnected from theory for the most part, but it also now has little relation to therapy. (p. 371)

Given the varying assumptions about the nature and cause of stuttering, it would seem futile to attempt a definition here. Yet our brief review of definitions reveals more than conflicting assumptions; it shows the evolution of our professional thinking about stuttering. Further, we can see that existing definitions fall roughly into one of three different categories—descriptive, explanatory, and combined descriptive/explanatory. The word *roughly* is used deliberately. Few definitions are purely descriptive or explanatory. Most contain elements of both. These categories, in fact, might better be viewed as anchor points at the two ends of a continuum, with most definitions falling somewhere in between. Some definitions are more heavily descriptive, some more heavily explanatory. A few examples are given for illustration.

Descriptive Definitions of Stuttering

Descriptive definitions respond to the question, "What does a person do when he stutters?" These definitions tend to list a variety of audible and occasionally visible behaviors. However, most definitions mention repetitions of sounds and syllables and prolongations of speech sounds (F. H. Silverman, 2004). The following definition is descriptive:

> For introductory purposes stuttering can be defined as a higher frequency of sound, syllable, and one-syllable word disfluency (more irregular in rhythm and averaging two to four repetitions per instance) and prolonged sounds or postures of the speech mechanism. There may be a disruption of air flow or phonation between repetitions, or a schwa-sounding vowel may be substituted for the correct one in the repetition of a syllable. There may be other signs of increased tension in the lips, jaw, larynx, or chest as well as accessory movements of bodily parts not closely associated with speaking. A covert feature of stuttering includes expectation of difficulty and frustration, which lead to avoidance and inhibitory behaviors—reactions that can be described by older children and adults and that may be mentioned by a preschool child. In the latter we can only assume that covert reactions accompany the development of overt behaviors and are more likely to be present the longer the problem exists. In keeping with the social nature of speaking, as stuttering persists, the person's self-concept is influenced by the speaking problem, and unadaptive attitudes develop. (Gregory, 1986, p. 5)

Explanatory Definitions of Stuttering

Other definitions tend to be more explanatory, or etiological, in nature, addressing the question, "Why does a person stutter?" They attempt to provide etiological justification for the composite of behaviors, feelings, and thoughts. Such definitions tend to limit the objectivity of speech–language pathologists' observational skills (Culatta & Goldberg, 1995) and run the risk of prejudicing the study of stuttering through presumption of a known cause (Wingate, 1988):

> The fact of the matter remains that the cause of stuttering—its essential nature—is unknown. Efforts made toward understanding the nature of stuttering are only obstructed by investigations mounted from a motivation to support conjectures. Unfortunately, a considerable amount of stuttering research bears this onus. (Wingate, 1988, p. 5)

Culatta and Goldberg (1995) expressed concern that definitions with initial biasing statements, such as "stuttering is a learned disorder which . . ." or "stuttering is an emotional disorder which . . ." or "stuttering is a neurologically based disorder which . . . ," might lead clinicians to force clients into categories inappropriately. Furthermore, Culatta and Goldberg advised that clinicians cannot, and perhaps should not, escape from their beliefs, but should avoid prejudgment. The following are examples of explanatory definitions:

> ⬚ "Stuttering is a symptom in a psychopathological condition classified as a pregenital conversion neurosis." (Glauber, 1958, p. 78)

☒ "Stuttering, then, is a child's conscientious effort to speak acceptably despite a deep conviction that he cannot do so . . . . We may call stuttering a severe form of speech consciousness." (Bloodstein, 1958, p. 38)

☒ "Stuttering is the consequence of the young child speaking with his mother and father. In his words he sought their appraisal of him. In his utterances he asked to be known and to be understood. In their reply they told of his unacceptability in his current verbalized form." (Travis, 1971, p. 1009)

Combined Descriptive/Explanatory Definitions of Stuttering

The third category of definitions contains both descriptive and explanatory elements. For example, Van Riper (1982) indicated that "stuttering occurs when the forward flow of speech is interrupted by a motorically disrupted sound, syllable, or word or by the speaker's reactions thereto" (p. 15). This definition highlights the audible or otherwise directly visible aspects of stuttering, emphasizes the reactions of the person who stutters, and implies that the cause of stuttering is a disruption in the motor sequence required to produce speech.

Another definition with both descriptive and explanatory elements was proposed by Wingate (1964):

1. (a) Disruption in the fluency of verbal expression, which is (b) characterized by involuntary, audible or silent, repetitions or prolongations in the utterance of short speech elements, namely: sounds, syllables, and words of one syllable. The disruptions (c) usually occur frequently or are marked in character and (d) are not readily controllable.

2. Sometimes the disruptions are (e) accompanied by accessory activities involving the speech apparatus, related or unrelated body structures, or stereotyped speech utterances. These activities give the appearance of being speech-related struggle.

3. Also, there are not infrequently (f) indications or report of the presence of an emotional state, ranging from a general condition of "excitement" or "tension" to more specific emotions of a negative nature such as fear, embarrassment, irritation, or the like. (g) The immediate source of stuttering is some incoordination expressed in the peripheral speech mechanism; the ultimate cause is presently unknown and may be complex or compound. (p. 488)

This definition characterizes stuttering as a disruption of speech fluency taking the form of audible or silent repetitions or prolongations that are frequent or marked in character and not readily controllable. Sometimes the disruption is accompanied by unusual movements of the speech mechanism or other body structure. People who stutter report negative emotional reactions to their disfluent speech. This definition is particularly significant in its specificity, in introducing the concept of the "involuntariness" (i.e., being out of control) of the speaker, and in acknowledging that the cause is unknown. The involuntary aspect of disfluency again was addressed as a critical diagnostic indicator by the World Health Organization (1977) and Perkins (1990a, 1990b), among others. More recently, the speaker's experience of involuntariness was interpreted to include potentially negative affective, behavioral, and cognitive reactions from the speaker and from those within the environment, as well as limitations in the speaker's participation in daily activities and overall quality of life (WHO, 2001; Yaruss, 2001; Yaruss & Quesal, 2001, 2004b, 2006, 2008).

A third definition of stuttering containing descriptive and explanatory elements was presented by Nicolosi et al. (2004):

1. Disturbance in the normal fluency and time patterning of speech. Primary characteristics include one or more of the following: (a) audible or silent blocking; (b) sound and syllable repetitions; (c) sound prolongations; (d) interjections; (e) broken words;

(f) circumlocutions; or (g) words produced with an excess of tension. Associated behaviors or secondary characteristics include the habitual use of speech musculature or of other body parts which a stutterer uses along with the primary characteristics; thought to be initiated to release, conceal, or modify the dysfluency. The disturbance may be at the level of neuromuscular, respiratory, phonatory, or articulatory mechanisms. Dysfluencies are so numerous that they exceed the normal number or degree for the individual's age, sex, or speaking situation.

2. Involuntary repetition and prolongation of speech sounds and syllables, and fluency interruptions that the individual struggles to end. (p. 295)

This definition presents highly specific behavioral components and introduces the idea of etiology as a timing disturbance. Furthermore, reference is made to events occurring at, and involving functions within, the neuromuscular, respiratory, phonatory, or articulatory mechanisms.

Stuttering Defined

So, what is stuttering? A frugal response would be "all of the above." Indeed, any current definition of stuttering borrows heavily from present and past comrades in the assessment and intervention of speech fluency and stuttering. The three definitions to which I align most closely are those presented by Guitar (2006), Cooper (1993c), and Yaruss and Quesal (2004b).

Guitar (2006) defined stuttering as follows:

Stuttering is characterized by an abnormally high frequency and/or duration of stoppages in the forward flow of speech. These stoppages usually take the form of (1) repetitions of sounds, syllables, or one-syllable words, (2) prolongations of sounds, or (3) "blocks" of airflow and/or voicing in speech. . . . Similarly, a speaker who is stuttering usually reacts to his repetitions, prolongations, or blocks by trying to force words out, or by using extra sounds, words, or movements in his efforts to become "unstuck" or to avoid getting stuck. . . . The child who begins to stutter goes through many of the same feelings of surprise, frustration, embarrassment, and fear. These feelings, in combination with the difficulty he has in speaking, may cause the stutterer to limit himself in school and social situations and at work. (p. 13)

Guitar, using terminology from Van Riper (1982), distinguished between core behaviors and secondary behaviors. Core behaviors are the basic, involuntary, observable behaviors of stuttering, including part-word and whole-word repetitions, sound prolongations, stoppage of air, and so forth. Secondary behaviors are the learned reactions to the core behaviors. Secondary behaviors include escape behaviors (i.e., attempts to exit the stutter and finish the word, such as eye blinks, head nods, interjection of sounds, etc.) and avoidance behaviors (i.e., attempts to prevent stuttering, such as pauses, word changes, hand movements, etc.). Also addressed are the feelings and attitudes of people who stutter. Guitar noted that negative feelings (e.g., shame, embarrassment) may precipitate stuttering, and stuttering may precipitate negative feelings. Therefore, the feelings related to stuttering may be as much a part of the disorder as the observable behaviors. This definition is highly descriptive and inclusive without offering prejudgment about etiology.

Cooper (1993c) captured the essence of stuttering when he stated, "Stuttering is a diagnostic label referring to a clinical syndrome characterized most frequently by abnormal and persistent dysfluencies in speech accompanied by characteristic affective, behavioral, and cognitive patterns" (p. 382). Cooper indicated that the three distinct types of stuttering (i.e., developmental, remediable, and chronic perseverative) result from multiple coexisting and interacting physiological, psychological, and environmental factors. Cooper stated that these stuttering types are multifaceted and consist of characteristic *a*ffective, *b*ehavioral, and *c*ognitive components (the ABCs of stuttering). The significance of any one of these components to an individual who stutters varies over time. Assessment and treatment of people who stutter, therefore, must address the affective, behavioral, and cognitive components.

Yaruss and Quesal (2004b) described stuttering in terms of "(a) the observable characteristics of the speech difficulty (impairment), (b) the functional communication difficulties experienced in the speaker's everyday life (disability), and (c) the impact of the stuttering disorder on the speaker's overall quality of life (handicap)" (p. 37). This description reflects the influence of the World Health Organization's (1977, 1980) older framework and recognizes that stuttering is affected by both internal and external factors and can involve more than observable behaviors. Yaruss and Quesal (2004b; see also Yaruss, Pelczarski, & Quesal, 2010) also highlighted the World Health Organization's (2001) movement away from listing the consequences of diseases and disorders to describing components of health (i.e., the International Classification of Functioning, Disability, and Health; ICF) in terms of body structure and function, activities and participation, and personal and environmental contextual factors. Impairment of body structure may be revealed in neuroanatomical differences; impairment of body function may be revealed in the involuntary behaviors that characterize stuttering. Activity limitation may impact functional communication (e.g., being unable to initiate conversations); participation restriction may impact the individual's quality of life (e.g., reluctance or refusal to participate in educational, social, or other daily activities). Personal factors, such as the speaker's affective, behavioral, and cognitive reactions, are particularly significant because they contribute to, if not determine, the speaker's experience of activity limitation or participation restriction. Yaruss et al. (2010) indicated that a speaker who reacts negatively to his stuttering would be more likely to avoid speaking situations and engage in other behaviors that restrict his daily activities. Environmental factors include the speaker's support systems (e.g., therapists and family members), reactions of others (e.g., acceptance and nurturing vs. bullying and teasing), and influences of different speaking situations (e.g., positive environmental reactions vs. negative environmental reactions). Moving away from an emphasis on health problems, more current terminology focuses on health experiences, both positive and negative. The term *disability* is therefore used more broadly now; the term *handicap* is no longer used. This shift in emphasis and terminology makes it possible to describe both (a) fluency and stuttering and (b) positive and negative aspects of the speaker's experiences of fluent and disfluent speech. Yaruss and Quesal (2004b) indicated that the current emphasis on health experiences invites attention to and understanding of the communication experience on the bases of both internal (i.e., affective and cognitive) and external (behavioral) elements. Discussing the importance of understanding the personal experience of communication and stuttering, they noted, "Although many of these feelings are regarded as negative (e.g., embarrassment, fear, anxiety, shame), there are also some positive feelings that can be identified as a person learns to cope with stuttering (e.g., hope, acceptance, optimism)" (p. 47).

For our purposes, *stuttering* refers to individualized and involuntary interruptions in the forward flow of speech and learned reactions thereto interacting with and generating associated thoughts and feelings about one's speech, oneself as a communicator, and the communicative world in which one lives. Etiology, yet unknown, is conceptualized as relating to the interaction of physiological, psychological/psychosocial, psycholinguistic, and environmental factors. Stuttering occurs within the context of communication systems, thus affecting and being affected by all persons who communicate with the person who stutters. Stuttering is a diagnostic label referring to a complex, multidimensional composite of behaviors, thoughts, and feelings of people who stutter. Whether for clinical or research purposes, stuttering should not be studied and cannot be understood without consideration of the person who stutters, the social contexts within which the person communicates, and the interaction of communicative demands and individualized capacities for speech fluency. The implications of this brief definition and its elements will unfold in the following pages. The nature of stuttering will be addressed in Chapter 2; etiology and theoretical explanations in Chapter 3; and thoughts and feelings of people who stutter and the significance of communication systems in Chapter 5. For now, suffice it to say that understanding the assumptions underlying the thoughts, feelings, and behaviors of people who stutter and of the members of their communication systems is critical. Stuttering does not occur in a communicative vacuum. It must be understood and addressed, therefore, within an individualized, social, and communicatively meaningful context.

Other Terms

A number of other terms are often used to describe aspects of fluency, disfluency, and stuttering. These include, among others, *frequency, duration, severity, disfluency type*, and *associated* or *secondary behaviors* (Conture, 1990, 2001). *Frequency of stuttering* refers to the number of instances of stuttering per unit of speech (e.g., 100 words of reading or conversational speech). *Duration of stuttering* refers to the temporal length, usually in seconds for clinical purposes, of an instance of stuttering, often averaged over a randomly selected sample of several instances of stuttering within a speaking context (e.g., reading or conversational speech, word or sentence repetition, etc.). *Severity of stuttering* refers to the degree of stuttering demonstrated by a person who stutters. When terms such as *mild, moderate*, or *severe* are used to indicate the severity of a stuttering instance or the stuttering observed as a whole, such terms should be defined to the extent possible. *Type of speech disfluency* refers to any within-word or between-word hesitations, interruptions, pauses, prolongations, repetitions, and stoppages that are observed in a person's speech. Associated or secondary behaviors are those speech behaviors that occur with relative consistency during and in learned response to instances of stuttering. These include filler expressions such as "Let me see" and circumlocutions (word changes), as well as non-speech behaviors, such as pitch changes, eye blinks, head shakes and turns, and hand movements.

More Than Just Terminology

Stutterer Versus Stuttering

Our frequent references to people who stutter as "stutterers" in clinical and research contexts is of considerable concern to me. You might say, "What's wrong with that word?" Some might assume that my concern is merely of semantic origin. It is not. The word *stutterer* equates the person with the disorder. When a person who stutters is asked to describe himself by sharing his personal story (Kent, 1989–1990) or point of view (Williams, 1957), his most frequent responses are, "I stutter" or "I am a stutterer." Indeed, people who stutter come to view themselves as a disorder, focusing more on the *dis*order than the dis*order*, on the *dis*ability than the dis*ability*. I maintain that clinicians too often focus more on the *dis*fluency than the dis*fluency*. Even more worrisome to me is when professionals share a negative and fractured view of people who stutter. Referring to a person as a stutterer implies that the disorder captures the essence of the person. The person who stutters is a boy or girl, man or woman, son or daughter, father or mother, boyfriend or girlfriend, spouse, friend, person who goes to school or work, a valued member within a family system and larger community—not just a person who stutters. This is not to minimize the impact that stuttering has on the perceptions and experiences of one who stutters. However, we need to understand how a person who stutters views himself as a person and as a communicator in order to facilitate his understanding, acceptance, and growth in these areas (Corcoran & Stewart, 1998; Crichton-Smith, 2002; Gabel, Blood, Tellis, & Althouse, 2004; Hayhow, Cray, & Enderby, 2002; Manning, 2004; Yaruss & Quesal, 2006, 2008).

When we professionals refer to our clients as stutterers, we tend to acknowledge only one aspect of the person and enable or facilitate maintenance of a narrow view of and by the person who stutters. How often do we say about a client to professional colleagues, "He is a stutterer," or "I've got to get downstairs now to the clinic. My stutterer is coming in"? Our choice of words reflects our assumptions and attitudes about ourselves, our work, and the people we serve. It might be a valuable and instructive exercise to take note of how you and others refer to each other in the language you use. Later, we will address the significance of hearing and understanding how a person who stutters refers to himself in expressing his point of view (Manning, 2004, 2010; Rabinowitz, 2005; Schneider, 2004; St. Louis, 2001a; Williams, 1957; Yaruss & Quesal, 2006, 2008). We will also address the dangers of using a "deficit ledger" (Kent, 1989–1990) in our approach to assessment and intervention with people who stutter. Kent warns that "increasing fragmentation of our clinical perspective—specialization is one word for it— can make the disorder come into focus even as the person goes out of focus" (p. 5). More respectful and empathic use of language views the whole person with dignity (Rush & The League of Human Dignity, n.d.) and is consistent with legislation mandating accommodations and guaranteeing rights for people with exceptionalities (e.g., Americans with Disabilities Amendments Act of 2008; Individuals with Disabilities Education Act of 1990 [IDEA]; Individuals with Disabilities Education Improvement Act of 2004; No Child Left Behind Act of 2001; Rehabilitation Act of 1973).

A simple equation might help remind us of the relationship between our assumptions and the language we use. A person who stutters is an individual with a unique past, present, and future. Stuttering is a composite of behaviors, feelings, and attitudes. You might say that stuttering = disorder; stutterer (or, more appropriately, person who stutters) = person. Therefore, stutterer ≠ disorder. Thus, in this book we deliberately put the whole and able person first by referring to "people who stutter" rather than "stutterers." Doing all we can to preserve and celebrate the dignity of the person we are serving and striving to understand is a professional imperative; it is doing what is right. Paradoxically, Dietrich, Jensen, and Williams (2001) and St. Louis (1999) found that person-first labels (person who stutters) and direct labels (stutterer) did not differ in their degree of negative association among clients, parents, students in communication sciences and disorders, and the general public. Negativity or stigma associated with stuttering appears to be more robust than the terms we use. Nevertheless, I remain convinced of the importance of asserting the person before the disorder in our language and thought and of the urgency to impact public perception of stuttering and people who stutter.

Categorical Versus Noncategorical Behaviors

When defining fluency, we distinguished between dichotomous (categorical, discrete) and continuous (noncategorical, nondiscrete) variables. We tend to think of speech as fluent or stuttered, incorrectly assuming that these represent categorical behaviors. In fact, both represent noncategorical, or continuous, variables, which are more appropriately represented along a continuum. It may be tempting to think of the following as categorical variables: fluency/disfluency, stuttered speech/nonstuttered speech, normalcy/abnormalcy, order/disorder, ability/disability, truth/falsehood, hot/cold, day/night, and so forth. In reality, however, each pair of terms reflects continuous variables; each contains numerous points along a continuum. We will experience a parallel challenge when we attempt to categorize and represent the behaviors, thoughts, and feelings of people who stutter. At best, we will define each as molecularly and scientifically possible. However, professional judgment cannot and should not be ignored in the clinical context. Conture (1990) reminded us that "(a) there are no known objective, listener-independent criteria for identifying instances of stuttering or classifying children as stutterers versus normally fluent speakers and (b) there is no consensus among experienced clinicians and researchers regarding behavioral definitions of stuttering in childhood or classification of children as stutterers" (p. 3).

In fact, efforts are ongoing to identify early childhood stuttering (Ambrose & Yairi, 1999; Yairi & Ambrose, 2005; Yairi & Seery, 2011) by distinguishing "stuttering-like disfluencies" (SLDs) from other disfluencies (ODs). *Stuttering-like disfluencies* include part-word repetitions (i.e., sound and syllable repetitions; e.g., *a-and, f-five, ba-baby, mo-mo-mommy*), single-syllable word repetitions (*but-but, and-and, she-she-she*), and disrhythmic phonation (sound prolongations and blocks—audible or inaudible sound prolongations; *wwwwwhere, looooook*). *Other disfluencies* include interjections (extraneous sounds of one or more units; *um, um-um, uh, er, hmmm*), multiple-syllable word and phrase repetitions (repetitions of segments longer than one syllable or one word; *because-because, Once up—once upon, I was—I was going*), and revision or abandoned utterances (instances in which an utterance is modified in a way that does not change the general content or is not completed. An example of a revision: *I was—I am going, I want the ball—red ball, she gave him—he gave her*. An example of an abandoned utterance: *Yesterday I went—hey what's that over there, I want another . . .*). The distinction between stuttering-like disfluencies and other disfluencies is important; stuttering-like disfluencies occur more frequently in the speech of people who stutter than in the speech of people who do not stutter. Other disfluencies are typical at comparable levels in the speech of both groups (Yairi & Ambrose, 2005).

Children who stutter (23 to 59 months) demonstrated mean stuttering-like disfluencies of 11.30 ($SD = 6.64$) per 100 syllables spoken. Normally fluent children (27 to 58 months) demonstrated mean stuttering-like disfluencies of 4.48 ($SD = 2.41$) per 100 syllables spoken (Yairi & Ambrose, 2005). Yairi and Seery (2011) reported that children who stutter demonstrate stuttering-like disfluencies as much as 10 times more frequently than children who do not stutter. Also, whereas total stuttering-like disfluency constitutes approximately two thirds (66%) of the overall disfluency (stuttering-like disfluency and other disfluency combined) for children who stutter, stuttering-like disfluency constitutes approximately one quarter (24%) of the overall disfluency for children who do not stutter. Among children who stutter, stuttering-like disfluencies are significantly more frequent, are longer in duration, and involve more physical tension than those among children who do not stutter. A study of stuttering-like disfluency in Dutch-speaking children yielded similar findings (Boey, Wuyts, Ven de Heyning, De Bolt, & Heylen, 2007). The accuracy and validity of using stuttering-like disfluencies for differential diagnostic purposes increase significantly when larger speech samples (i.e., at least 600 syllables) are collected and when later, rather than earlier, portions of the speech sample are analyzed (Sawyer & Yairi, 2006). These findings hold significant promise for early intervention efforts.

Despite the diagnostic potential of measuring stuttering-like disfluencies, however, we must always bear in mind that clinical interpretations are to a certain extent tentative. This does not mean that we should be reluctant to exercise informed professional judgment. On the contrary, our judgment must be fully informed, demonstrating both flexibility and accountability. We must be receptive to incoming information, including alternative and challenging perspectives. We also must demonstrate accountability, documenting the observable aspects of the clinical process that inform our clinical rationale.

Fluency Facilitating Controls Versus Tricks

People who stutter learn that stuttering is variable and intermittent. Van Riper (1982) noted,

> The very intermittency of the disorder compounds the problem. One of our clients said it well: "I can't get used to it. I can't get used to it. I wish I were blind or deaf or crippled. Then I'd always be that way and though it would be hard I could finally accept it. But the way it is, I talk all right for a bit and then get clobbered. I hope I can talk; I fear I can't; sometimes I can; sometimes I can't. I'm always torn." (p. 2)

Stuttering varies by time, situation, and language factors. It is important to note, before we turn to fluency facilitating controls and tricks, that several special conditions immediately eliminate, or at least significantly reduce, stuttering. These include, among others,

- choral reading—reading the same text at the same time with a speaker who is fluent
- lipped speech—speaking without voicing
- whispered speech—speaking with greatly reduced volume
- prolonged speech with or without delayed auditory feedback—speaking with an increase in segment duration
- rhythmic speech—speaking with a regularly recurring cadence in response to a rhythmic stimulus, such as the beat of a metronome or finger tapping
- shadowing—repeating what someone else is saying immediately but not in chorus
- singing—replacing the suprasegmentals, or pitch, juncture, intonation, and so forth, of speech with those of song
- slowed speech—reducing the rate by increasing pause time
- other speech conditions—speaking in the presence of a loud bilateral masking noise (i.e., 90 dB), speaking with altered pitch (i.e., increased or decreased fundamental frequency), speaking alone, or speaking with a nonhuman listener (G. Andrews et al., 1983; Bloodstein & Bernstein Ratner, 2008; Guitar, 2006; Ham, 1999; Tanner, 2003; Williams, 1978)

We will address how such special conditions can be used in the clinical setting for differentially diagnosing stuttering from other disorders of fluency and for facilitating success that generates motivation among people who stutter. Because we know stuttering to be variable (changing based on special conditions), individualized (nonidentical—no two people demonstrate the same stuttering), and intermittent (not consistent), yet predictable (people who stutter report knowing when they are going to stutter), we need to distinguish between fluency facilitating controls and tricks.

Fluency facilitating controls, discussed in detail in Chapters 8, 9, and 10, are clinical procedures used to alter the fluency of one's speech. These procedures are communicatively reliable and useful, based on what we know about communication and the role of the communicator, and intended to foster independent communication skills.

Some examples are cancellations, pull-outs, and preparatory sets (Bloodstein & Bernstein Ratner, 2008; Guitar, 2006; Van Riper, 1973), analysis and facilitation of fluency, and speech with soft articulatory contacts and slight prolongation.

Fluency tricks, by contrast, are behavioral adjustments that temporarily improve fluency, are communicatively unreliable, and potentially form communicative dependence. Such tricks are based on expediency and are not consistent with what we know about communication and the role of the communicator. As noted, they improve fluency only temporarily and often become part of the learned reactions referred to as associated or secondary behaviors (Bloodstein & Bernstein Ratner, 2008; Guitar, 2006). Some examples are changing the nature of one's speaking (e.g., demonstrating a more proper or formal presentation), one's accent (e.g., sounding British or French), one's pitch (e.g., raising or, more typically, lowering the fundamental frequency of one's voice), and so forth. These changes are not only temporary but also have secondary risks, including damage to the vocal cords (e.g., nodules, contact ulcers, etc.). Other tricks include interjecting to feign the temporary loss of thought (e.g., "Let me see," "How do you say it," etc.) or movements of the body (e.g., hand, head, foot, whole body, etc.) associated with the anticipation of disfluency. Such tricks have the potential of reducing communicative effectiveness of the message being conveyed. A few anecdotes will illustrate how communication tricks can detract from the effectiveness of the communication message.

Many years ago, I moved to Connecticut to begin my career as a speech–language pathologist. In search of fluency facilitating controls, I still occasionally resorted to tricks for expediency. When talking with a gentleman from England who was to become my landlord, my fluency seemed out of control and I attempted circumlocution (avoiding certain words by selecting others) and phrase insertion to feign lapse of thought (e.g., "Now what was I saying?") and word retrieval difficulty (e.g., "Let me see. What is that word?"). Circumlocution is a challenging task for a speaker. Not only are less feared words substituted for more feared words, but there is an eye-for-an-eye condition (a noun must be substituted for a noun, a verb for a verb, etc.). Van Riper (1982) indicated that such word selection facilitates the development of very large vocabularies as a result of habitual substitution and that the speech of people who circumlocute is "so tortuous and strangely imprecise that a listener must work hard to comprehend its meaning" (p. 132). I cannot recall my exact words today, but I do remember responding in an awkward manner when the landlord asked me, "What do you do professionally?" Having some expertise in working with people who stutter, I tried not to blow my cover and stuttered expertly all over the well-meaning soul. I tried to convey that I was new in my career; hence the gentleman should be merciful in his determination of the monthly rent. After responding to this man's questions, while trying my best to manage my fluency and his impression, I remember what seemed like an interminable silence. The man furrowed his brow, pulled with one hand on his gray beard and wiped his balding head with the other, looked at me sadly, and said, "Young man, what you just said was remarkably cryptic." He was right. Such tricks, without intervention, often have a snowball effect and become part of an individualized behavioral repertoire.

Some years later, a college student came to me to assess his stuttering. His speech was remarkably fluent with a pronounced southern accent, and he demonstrated outstanding interpersonal and social skills. He later revealed that his fluency was dependent upon the accent, one that he had affected to perfection. He referred to this manner of speaking as "hillbilly speech." His vowels were lengthened into diphthongs, consonants were produced with gentle articulatory contacts, pitch had tremendous variation, and juncture was so minimized as to approximate the melody of song. His speech was only fluent as long as he maintained this pattern. He said that this fluency trick was limiting to him in certain conversational contexts and that he felt like an impostor. He desired, and eventually achieved, more reliable and versatile fluency facilitating controls.

In an advanced stage of stuttering, the associated sequence of secondary behaviors may seem to the untrained observer to be simply bizarre, if not haphazard. However, longitudinal or retrospective analysis of such behaviors indicates their development to be highly systematic and somewhat strategic. The following scenario illustrates this pattern. Some years ago, when working as a speech–language pathologist in the public schools, I met with Alan, a 17-year-old in his junior year of high school. When asked a direct question about his classroom activity, Alan tightly closed then opened his eyes, turned his head abruptly to the left, violently threw his head back again, closing his eyes tightly, and rapidly opened and closed his mouth without any audible sounds, all the while demonstrating significant eye, jaw, facial, and neck tension. Bringing his head forward and opening his eyes, still rapidly opening and closing his mouth, Alan then alternated raising his left and right arms, slightly raising himself from his chair while maintaining a seated position, turning himself in the opposite direction of the hand raised. Arm movements became increasingly abrupt with his hand each time, barely missing the back of his head. Verbalizations were rapid when fluent and punctuated by rapid interjection of schwa (i.e., *uh*) preceding monosyllabic sentence-initial words (e.g., *uh-uh-uh-uh-uh-I*) and repetition of subsequent consonant–vowel combinations (e.g., *wuh-wuh-wuh-wuh-wuh want*). Intermittent verbalization on inhalation was less disfluent, yet strained and monotone.

On the surface, Alan indeed demonstrated a bizarre behavioral repertoire. Upon closer scrutiny, however, Alan's behaviors made sense. At an earlier time in his life, closing his eyes was likely to prevent a disfluent episode. When the novelty of that relatively discrete behavior (closing his eyes) and its effect ended, he revised the behavior (tensing then opening his eyes) to achieve the desired outcome. Because the effect of this revised behavior again was temporary, he then chained (i.e., added on) another slightly more noticeable, yet still relatively discrete, behavior (turning his head to the left) to prevent the anticipated experience and consequence of disfluency. This cycle of behavior revision and acquisition continues (e.g., tilting the head back, moving and tensing his mouth, lifting his arms, turning his body) until, in this case, Alan seemed to most conversational partners to be virtually dancing, if not thrashing, in his chair.

This story does have a happy ending. Before Alan graduated from high school the following year, he successfully completed the two highest objectives on his personalized hierarchy. Specifically, he demonstrated reliable yet controlled fluency facilitating techniques in two new contexts without exhibiting the overt associated behaviors. These contexts were working for a political representative in his home state and establishing a dating relationship with a young woman. The intervention process effected improvements in academic success, personal hygiene, personal motivation, professional aspiration, social adeptness, and interpersonal family and school relationships, as well as heightened communication independence. How such changes can be achieved will be addressed in Chapters 9 and 10.

While the behaviors of people who stutter might seem superficially alike and generally bizarre, they are uniquely sequenced, synchronized, and executed, almost like the wind-up of a professional pitcher. Van Riper (1982) clarified the development of such behaviors as follows:

> Most adult stutterers pass through a whole series of different reaction patterns before they develop the final set which is as unique as their fingerprints. At 4 years of age, the stutterer may have only syllabic repetitions; at five, postural fixations. By his 11th birthday he could be retching and gasping; by his 16th, his speech may also be punctuated by long pauses. When he is 30, all of these behaviors may be in his stuttering repertoire, and

there may also be some head-jerks. But some of these behaviors may also be suddenly discarded or replaced by others less abnormal. We knew one man, at the age of 70, who stopped the struggling and avoiding of many years, and began to stutter easily and with the syllabic repetition of his childhood. He told us he was too tired and too old to stutter so hard any longer. (p. 112)

Van Riper (1982) analyzed further the hierarchical development of such behaviors and described why one behavior is used first and another second or third:

We have been able to watch this aspect of the disorder develop in only a few cases, but it is our impression that there are two factors determining the sequence of the various be-haviors. First, the final hierarchy often reflects the order in which the coping behaviors were acquired. Those the stutterer adopted first are those that occur first in the sequence; those developed last are the final ones to be tried out as he struggles to utter the word. Second, the behaviors may occur in the order of their social visibility or listener wince-value. Thus the stutterer may use the least conspicuous coping behavior first. If this fails, he uses one that is just a bit more visible or abnormal, and so on until finally he gives up trying to hide his difficulty. It is then that he shows his most bizarre struggle. (p. 113)

Negative Stereotypes, Bias, and Misinformation: Implications for the Clinician

In spite of the volumes written about stuttering and people who stutter, negative ste-reotypes, bias, and misinformation continue to be held by classroom teachers, princi-pals, nurses, pediatricians, professors, the general public, and, most woefully, certified speech–language pathologists (Cooper & Rustin, 1985; Crowe & Walton, 1981; Dorsey & Guenther, 2000; Lass et al., 1992, 1994; Ragsdale & Ashby, 1982; Ruscello, Lass, & Brown, 1988; E.-M. Silverman, 1982; F. H. Silverman & Bongey, 1997; St. Louis & Lass, 1981; Turnbaugh, Guitar, & Hoffman, 1979; C. L. Woods & Williams, 1971, 1976; Yairi & Carrico, 1992; Yairi & Williams, 1970; Yeakle & Cooper, 1986). Typically, people who stutter are stereotyped as submissive, nonassertive persons who are tense, insecure, and fearful. Attribution of such negative personality traits tends to increase with greater degrees of observed stuttering behavior. Conversely, Gabel (2006) found that people who stutter mildly (less noticeably) are perceived more positively than those who stutter more severely (more noticeably). Also, people who stutter who attend therapy are per-ceived more positively than those who do not. Guitar (2006) indicated that since listen-ers play a major role in shaping the attitudes of people who stutter about themselves as people and communicators, changing the negative attitudes of people who stutter can be a major focus in treatment. This conclusion is indisputable. Equally urgent, it seems, is to identify the rampant misinformation and bias among potential conversational part-ners, particularly speech–language pathologists, and to effect change among these per-sons (Cooper & Cooper, 1985, 1996; Dorsey & Guenther, 2000; Manning, 2004, 2010; Reichel & St. Louis, 2004, 2007; St. Louis, Reichel, Yaruss, & Lubker, 2009).

Interaction Between Clinicians' Attitude and Treatment Outcome
G. Andrews et al. (1983) reported that "the speech–language pathology profession en-tertains negative views about stutterers as persons and holds pessimistic views about the benefits of therapy" (p. 234). They further stated,

This research refers to the U.S. speech–language pathology profession, but it is our im-pression that speech–language pathologists in England, Canada, and Australia have similar views. For 20 years there has been good evidence that stutterers, as people, are no different from anybody else. For 10 years there has been good evidence that a planned and disciplined approach to therapy is effective. Yet these negative stereotypes persist, unsupported by empirical evidence. The authors of this review are neither stutterers nor speech–language pathologists and are at a loss to understand how such negative stereotypes can continue to be believed. We can only surmise that some academics who teach speech–language pathologists have not assimilated the new knowledge and have continued to teach the diagnosogenic/mental health approach to stuttering that was current 30 years ago. (p. 234)

I share the concern expressed by others regarding the negative stereotypes about people who stutter and misinformation about stuttering. Indeed, the level of misinformation about stuttering became all too clear to me when a graduate student of mine conducted a systematic survey of freshmen, sophomores, juniors, and seniors (not studying speech–language pathology) at a regional comprehensive university (K. Nichols, 1987). She discovered that 30% of the respondents believed that stuttering can be contracted from intimate sexual contact. I am most concerned when I learn of speech–language pathologists' negative biases and stereotypes toward stuttering and people who stutter, along with overall pessimism about the potential benefits of treatment (Cooper & Cooper, 1985; Manning, 2004, 2010; St. Louis & Durrenberger, 1993; Yaruss, 1999a; Yaruss & Quesal, 2002; Yaruss, Quesal, & Murphy, 2002; Yaruss, Quesal, Reeves, et al., 2002). Over many years in the workshops I present, I have frequently heard sincere frustration and discouragement from speech–language pathologists regarding the outcomes of their best treatment efforts with people who stutter. Speech–language pathologists report feeling otherwise well trained, yet uncomfortable addressing the needs faced by people who stutter and lacking in the necessary clinical and interpersonal (counseling) skills. In the face of persistent negative bias and stereotypes, I am concerned about what we are accomplishing in university training programs, particularly if we are only affecting clinicians' knowledge (cognitive domain) and behaviors (behavioral domain) to the exclusion of feelings and attitudes (affective domain) (Yaruss, 1999a; Yaruss & Quesal, 2002). Concerted efforts are being made to mitigate negative stereotyping of stuttering and people who stutter in graduate-level fluency disorders classes by curricular adjustment and instructional focus (Reichel & St. Louis, 2007) and by training in emotional intelligence (Reichel, 2005, 2007; Reichel & St. Louis, 2004); preliminary results are positive and invite continued inquiry.

Stuttering, it seems, presents unique challenges and confusion. As will be seen, the clinician must feel confident and competent to address clients' communication past, present, and future from multiple perspectives (cognitive, affective, social, academic, professional, etc.). I am concerned when I see published recommendations, albeit well meaning, that the client be given "a realistic if not pessimistic perception of how successful therapy is going to be" (Starkweather, 1993, p. 163). While a realistic perspective is essential for all participants to embark on effective and individualized treatment, a measure of sincere optimism must be foremost. I do not dispute that our profession must be mindful of how we present ourselves to the public and, in so doing, must avoid explicit and implicit guarantees of treatment results (ASHA, 2010). Nevertheless, a critical ingredient for successful treatment is lacking when the clinician does not sincerely feel good about what she is doing and the potential benefits of treatment.

In discussing three critical variables (in addition to client motivation in the therapy process) for successful treatment with people who stutter, Daly (1988) listed the attitudes and expectations of the clinician as primary. He underscored that "the clinician's attitudes toward stuttering and people who stutter have as much to do with the successful treatment of this disorder as the methods selected for therapy" (p. 34). The clinician must believe in the client, just as the client must believe in the clinician. Daly found support in the literature on terminally ill cancer patients, which indicated that a positive attitude toward treatment was a better predictor of treatment outcome than the severity of the illness. Daly urged clinicians to be positive, patient, and persistent with clients who stutter, and to err in the direction of optimism rather than pessimism. After years of working with clients who stutter, he concluded, "Clinical experience repeatedly demonstrates that intelligent persons will expend effort and energy in treatment only when they expect substantial results" (pp. 34–35). The clinician must not take lightly the responsibility to understand and manage the client's attitude as well as observable symptoms of disfluency. Surely the clinician's attitude affects that of the client.

It would behoove all clinicians to review carefully the Bill of Rights and Responsibilities for People Who Stutter (International Fluency Association and International Stuttering Association, 2001). Its mission is clear:

> The Bill is written to foster attitudes and actions whereby individuals who stutter are provided the opportunity to fulfill their aspirations and to lead successful, productive lives. It recognizes the dual responsibility of listeners and society to create the environment in which people who stutter can develop their aspirations and talents, and of people who stutter to advocate better understanding and to become active partners in their own futures.

The impact of the clinician's attitude on the client's success was eloquently and powerfully conveyed by former speech–language pathologist Joysa Gale Post, who became a client after incurring a cerebral vascular accident at age 29 (Post & Leith, 1983). Ms. Post's article should be required reading for all student clinicians and practicing speech–language pathologists. After regaining her communication skills, she told of the frequent disappointment that she experienced with her speech–language pathologists, offering a number of valuable suggestions. These included conveying sincerity, empathy, caring, enthusiasm, and patience; possessing and demonstrating requisite knowledge in clinical competence and confidence; dressing professionally; maintaining a sense of humor; designing informed, meaningful, and purposeful treatment; and respecting the dignity of the client as a valuable and whole person; among many others. Ms. Post concluded, "Many clinicians just do not realize how much clients like me depend on them for moral support as well as professional treatment. We want you to care about us as well as care for us" (p. 26).

Our attitude toward and knowledge about stuttering and people who stutter are at least as critical as the services we provide. We can facilitate the process of communication intervention and the development of communication competence by our attitudes, aspirations, and actions, or we can impede such an endeavor. Negative bias about stuttering and people who stutter and pessimism regarding the value of treatment are counterproductive. Let us not become another obstacle for people who stutter. Rather, in our knowledge, beliefs, and actions, let us lead the way, realistic and sincerely optimistic, to facilitate fluent futures.

Misinformation Begets Misinformation

Another instance in which misinformation seems persistent is in the frequent advice that professionals in education and allied medical services give to concerned parents of children beginning to stutter. The advice usually takes the form of, "Don't worry about it. He will outgrow it." First, telling a parent not to worry is futile, if not insensitive and inappropriate. When you read the fine print, indeed, worry is within every parent's job description! Second, although the child may well "outgrow it" (i.e., recover spontaneously without treatment; Yairi & Ambrose, 2005; Yairi & Seery, 2011), some children develop stuttering—perhaps unnecessarily. Ignoring the issue has proven to be a misguided clinical decision with far-reaching consequences. Managing the communication of a young child within the child's communication system through relatively indirect intervention procedures (i.e., knowledgeably facilitating fluency while not drawing attention to the disfluency, as will be discussed in Chapter 8) is not the same as ignoring the issue. Many well-meaning people who intend to ignore the disfluency have exacerbated the problem by heightening the child's awareness of fluency breakdown and related feelings. Note, however, that preschool children are more aware and aware earlier (as young as 3 years old) of stuttering than previously thought (Ezrati-Vinacour, Platzky, & Yairi, 2001; Langevin, Packman, & Onslow, 2009; Vanryckeghem, Brutten, & Hernandez, 2005; Yairi, 2004; Yairi & Ambrose, 2005). Also, clinical trials are revealing positive results for a direct form of intervention delivered by parents that deliberately increases the young child's awareness of stuttering and related self-monitoring skills (Bernstein Ratner & Guitar, 2006; Harrison, Onslow, & Rousseau, 2007; Onslow, Packman, & Harrison, 2003; S. Woods, Shearsby, Onslow, & Burnham, 2002), albeit within a positive, inviting, and nurturing context. My own impressions are consistent with these findings after completing training in the Lidcombe Program and after dialoguing with and directly observing numerous clinicians affiliated with the Australian Stuttering Research Center in Sydney, Australia.

Another source of misinformation, not often addressed, are the consumers, the community of people who stutter. Yaruss, Quesal, and Murphy (2002), from a survey of 200 members of the National Stuttering Association (the largest self-help group for people who stutter in the United States), identified both positive and negative opinions about resources and services that are available to them. Significantly, 20% responded that they would "wait and see" if their child might outgrow stuttering before seeking an evaluation by a speech–language pathologist. Others responded that they would contact a psychologist or primary care physician before consulting a speech–language pathologist. These results highlight the pervasiveness of misinformation and the need for public information that is accurate and current about evaluation and early intervention.

The "wait and see" phenomenon clearly is not new. Guy, a man of 63 years with whom I worked clinically for 2 years, said during a televised broadcast,

> My parents shielded me, like any parent would do. And I had seen doctor after doctor and they had always said, "Leave him alone. He'll get over it. Just don't worry with it." Well, I got to be 60 years old and I never had gotten over it. So, I began to think, "When in the world am I supposed to get over this thing?"

During the course of treatment, Guy achieved controlled, reliable fluency and met his objectives of being able to order dinner for his wife, introduce himself on the golf course, and lay read in church. His level of fluency was maintained during the follow-up period of 2 years. The type of intervention Guy received in his later years, after a half-century of unsuccessful treatment, will be discussed in Chapter 10.

Pervasiveness of Negative Stereotypes, Bias, and Misinformation

Why such negativity persists about stuttering and people who stutter is not easily explained and is certainly not justified. Likewise, negative interpretations are not confined to the professional literature or service delivery. One need only to look at the arts and literature within and across cultures to determine that negative stereotypes, bias, and misinformation about stuttering are pervasive. F. H. Silverman (2004) noted, "One way to gain a little insight into how persons who have a fluency disorder are viewed in a particular culture is to observe how they are portrayed in the arts and literature of that culture" (p. 32). For example, representations of stuttering and people who stutter depicted in children's literature, novels, movies, dramas, opera, and newspaper headlines have been analyzed (D. Anderson, 1995; Benecken, 1995; Bushey & Martin, 1988; Tanner, 2001, 2003).

Bushey and Martin (1988) reviewed 20 works of children's fiction in which a character stutters. They found that stuttering typically was represented as severe with visible struggle (i.e., frequent behavioral symptoms described as speechless, choking, and painful), increasing with emotional upset and nervousness (e.g., talking with strangers, in class, and with authority figures), and learned primarily in an unhealthy home and parental environment (e.g., parental separation or divorce, distant or uninterested parents, death of a parent). Of most concern, however, was that in not a single book was the child being seen or recommended to be seen by a speech–language pathologist. Only one depicted a child receiving professional services (that of a psychiatrist). In others, the stuttering disappeared when the character achieved physiological maturity, gained inner strength, or began to think about or help other people. In other words, stuttering was not depicted as treatable, and characters who stutter were depicted as physiologically immature, weak, or self-involved. About stuttering in children's literature, Bushey and Martin (1988) concluded,

> The appearance of these nonspecific, unsystematic, and highly improbable "cures" for stuttering reflected in children's fiction suggests that many people may not view stuttering as a routinely "treatable" problem, and further, that many people may harbor the view that when the unhealthy psychological milieu surrounding stuttering is made healthy, the stuttering will disappear. (pp. 249–250)

Similarly, Benecken (1995) reviewed 19 movies, 23 novels, and 13 children's books and found that people who stutter are portrayed as unattractive males, neurotic or even psychopathologic, and in subordinate roles, characterized by the following:

> a rather soft, unattractive, rather frail, pinched, subordinating, perhaps thinking about murdering somebody, sexually deprived, possibly perverted man with pimples or nibbled fingernails, if of a tall build, then with a baby face. Mostly he is not married or still as a mother's darling in unsolved symbiosis. . . . Not as I actually expected, the clown or the idiot. His bondage is the central issue, he subordinates himself, and normally he isn't acknowledged, but gets beaten. Almost never do you find a stuttering man in a happy leading position, as father and husband, to say nothing of a hero. (p. 548)

Presenting a somewhat different perspective, D. Anderson (1995) reviewed historical perceptions of stuttering as reflected in the arts, specifically films, operas, and novels:

> It cannot be denied that stuttering has been associated with comedy over the centuries. Interpretation is often up to the reader or to the audience, but most of the characters discussed are comic characters, not buffoons. It is striking that these authors, and their societies, do not depict stutterers as members of some societal "underclass": they are a lawyer, a trusted advisor to an aristocrat, a humble but well-loved sailor, and a respected and erudite musician. . . . Perhaps these fictional portrayals argue that the often encountered stereotype of the stutterer may be held more by stutterers themselves than by society. (pp. 569–570)

Tanner (2001, 2003) concluded that books, films, and television typically portray a simplistic view of stuttering, yet that view can powerfully influence society's perception of people who stutter:

> This simplistic view portrays the person who stutters as a humorous, anxious, and befuddled character whose speech disorder can be easily eliminated. When literature and media do address the cause of the disorder, it usually has a psychological theme, related to anxiety, repressed anger, or sexual dysfunctions. Although people who stutter may experience anger at people's insensitive remarks and rude behaviors, stuttering is not

caused by repressed anger. Neither is stuttering linked to any type of sexual dysfunction. It is not the manifestation of an oral or any other type of fixation. Without exception, in literature and media, frustration is shown to increase the amount and severity of stuttering. (Tanner, 2003, pp. 54–55)

In any case, stereotyping confers lower status and power to the person being stereotyped: "People who stutter are typically less valued by society than fluent speakers" (Tanner, 2003, p. 55). Fiske (1993) cautioned that power and asymmetries in control encourage stereotyping and that stereotyping maintains power. A central theme in this book is empowerment, where all participants collaborate, learn, and grow with a shared purpose and mutual respect. Recent empirical efforts are looking to build an understanding of the epigenesis of stereotypes and stereotyping (MacKinnon, Hall, & MacIntyre, 2007). Perhaps once understood, stereotyping will be discarded in favor of more promising human qualities.

The Impact of Stuttering

Stuttering and intervention with people who stutter potentially can have a global impact. Spoken communication is a complex, dynamic experience between at least two conversational partners. Both published and anecdotal records indicate that stuttering, a significant and universal disorder of communication, continues to intrigue and fascinate, if not elude, student clinicians, professional speech–language pathologists, and clinical researchers. In light of other human problems, including poverty, hunger, disease, and war, one might question why so much time and energy should be devoted to the alleviation of an individual's communication disorder. The answer is not as simple as might be suggested in a brief response. It has to do with heightening one's communication competence within a communicative milieu and strengthening the effectiveness of communication within and between all potential conversational partners. Another part of the response has to do with social consciousness, feeling in part responsible for the ills that afflict others—being committed to searching for solutions, realizing in a communicative sense that we might be our brothers' and our sisters' keeper. Perhaps such an influence on individuals and those with whom we communicate could reduce the human problems of intolerance and injustice, thus positively impacting the problems noted above.

A multinational consortium of authors (Shapiro et al., 2004) identified the assumptions, methods, and ultimate lessons learned and purposes served by clinicians who treat people who stutter in diverse nations across six continents. The impact of stuttering, and particularly intervention with people who stutter, was expressed clearly by over 300 clinicians. The following sentiments are representative:

- If you are at peace with yourself, you'll be in peace with the world around. (France)
- Communication ability is a freedom of a human being; If you can bring peace in your own mind, you can bring peace into the world; I see stuttering therapy as one of the many possibilities to decrease human suffering. (Germany)
- To accept the stuttering, to know oneself, helps the person to deal with life. (Iceland)
- The reason why I treat people who stutter is to help them to live easily in this society. (Japan)
- Love is the most important. (The Netherlands)
- Above all—at once getting to know one's self, one's body, one's behavior, one's goals, one's emotions, one's family, and one's role in this family. (Poland)
- To achieve harmonization of the personality of the client who stutters; to enable people who stutter to adapt and function in society. (Russia/Ukraine)

⚇ To change misconceptions, promote tolerance, and provide a verbal gift to which everyone is entitled. (South Africa)

Understanding stuttering is difficult. I do not believe that "those who have not possessed or been possessed by the disorder" (Van Riper, 1982, p. 1) cannot work effectively with people who stutter. As will be seen, personal experience can sensitize, but it also can bias. Above all, we need to understand the uniqueness of each person who stutters as a person and as a communicator, a member of a communicative network. The potential complexity and unique magnitude of stuttering might lie in its impact on individual speakers and all people with whom they communicate. Stuttering potentially affects all communicative and psychoemotional aspects of a person (Corcoran & Stewart, 1998; Crichton-Smith, 2002; Gabel et al., 2004; Hayhow et al., 2002; Jezer, 1997; Rabinowitz, 2001, 2005; St. Louis, 2001a).

Stuttering and Articulation

Stuttering can affect the articulation of one's speech. A person who stutters might demonstrate inappropriate articulatory targets—that is, forming a posture with the articulators that is not appropriate for the target sound within the target word. For example, if a person who stutters is trying to say the *b* in "The boy is . . .," the appropriate target would be the voiced bilabial plosive (*b*). If this person were observed to be blocked with an open mouth and the back of the tongue raised, this back, velar position (*g, k*) would be considered inappropriate. People who stutter often do not realize they are blocking on the wrong sound. If they are going to block, they should block on the right sound! Most people who do not stutter repeat syllables by retaining the correct vowel within the repetition (*bo, boat*). People who stutter tend to repeat an inappropriate vowel (*buh, buh, boat*).

Another intriguing phenomenon is the impact of articulation on stuttering. Clients repeatedly report finding certain sounds harder to say and more likely to result in stuttering. Over the years, numerous people who stutter have sought treatment in anticipation of stuttering when saying their wedding vows ("I do"); others have sought help to be able to say their name. I am working with a college sophomore who said that she is tempted to change both her name and her major because of predictable stuttering when saying the initial sounds of both. At present, the impact, or co-occurrence suggesting predictability, of articulation or phonological errors on stuttering, particularly among young children, is controversial (Bernstein Ratner, 1995; Bloodstein & Bernstein Ratner, 2008; Paden, 2005; Yairi, 2004; Yairi & Ambrose, 2005; Yaruss & Conture, 1996) and is receiving empirical attention, as will be discussed in the next chapter.

Stuttering and Language

There is a reciprocal relationship between stuttering and language; stuttering affects language and language affects stuttering. As noted, word substitution, or circumlocutions, often result from the ability of people who stutter to predict the words on which they will and will not stutter (as well as the people with whom and situations within which they will and will not stutter). Van Riper (1982) discussed how people who stutter develop word fears and indicated that because of their need for synonyms, "some stutterers have developed supervocabularies" (p. 154). This is an influence of stuttering on language.

Language also influences stuttering (Bloodstein & Bernstein Ratner, 2008; Starkweather, 1987; R. V. Watkins, 2005; Williams, 1978; Yairi, 2004; Yairi & Ambrose, 2005; Yaruss, 1999b). Stuttering occurs more often at the beginnings of sentences; on words positioned early in a sentence than on words positioned later; on nouns, verbs, adjectives, and adverbs (lexical words) than on function words for adults; on conjunctions and pronouns than on nouns and interjections for children; on longer than shorter words;

on words beginning with consonants than with those beginning with vowels (a pattern hypothesized to be related more to the nature of the English language than to stuttering); on the first syllable of the word than on later syllables; on less frequently used words (but only when the sentences are syntactically more simple); on stressed than on unstressed syllables; at points of high information load (i.e., propositional value); on words toward the beginning of long sentences than on the same words when they are at the beginning of short sentences; on emotionally loaded material than on emotionally neutral material; at locations where language formulation is occurring, and so forth. We will take a closer look at the impact of language on stuttering in the next chapter.

Stuttering and Voice

Stuttering also affects voice. Consider the strain observed in the voice of a person who stutters trying to say the *a* in *apple* or the *h* in *hello*. The voice cracks and bursts of air are audible, sounding like frying bacon. This is vocal fry. Or consider the increase in pitch that accompanies vocal strain, rendering a prolongation with rising pitch. Just like a guitar string that tightens or shortens, the vocal cords tense or shorten, causing the pitch increase. This is vocal tension. Or consider the increased volume (i.e., loudness) often observed when a person who stutters struggles through a block, without use of fluency facilitating controls. These moments of increasing loudness render the voice, in musical terms, crescendo if not fortissimo. This is vocal intensity. Clearly other vocal (pitch, intensity, quality, melody, resonance) and suprasegmental (juncture, sequence, duration, rate, rhythm, prosody) aspects of speech are affected as well.

Stuttering and Functioning in Society

Stuttering affects one's participation within socially and culturally determined roles, as demonstrated by the following individuals: the boy who must cope after the caller disconnects the phone because the boy cannot say hello; the woman who must cope after she is passed over for promotion because she cannot speak fluently to her subordinates; the man who must cope with the fact that he chose factory work to avoid speaking; the girl who must cope after ordering vanilla ice cream because she knows she will be unable to say "strawberry" in front of her boyfriend; the child who must cope after responding "I don't know" to a question from the teacher because he cannot say the answer fluently even though he knows it well; the young man who must cope when a young woman turns him down for a date after he struggled valiantly with the invitation; and the aspiring model who must cope after withdrawing from the competition because she cannot interact fluently with the judges. Stuttering rallies coping skills and potentially affects the psychological and emotional makeup, educational achievement, and professional aspiration of people who stutter. Guy ordered dinner for his wife in a restaurant for the first time in their 40-year marriage after 2 years of fluency treatment. He reported feeling in control for the first time. "For the first time in my life, I feel like I can wear the pants in this family." While this statement would raise more than an eyebrow from a context of gender equity (Shapiro, 1994b) and heightened awareness and appreciation of nonsexist language, it also conveys the impact of stuttering on a person's functioning within society.

   Numerous empirical investigations of personal accounts from people who stutter have painted a picture of suffering (i.e., helplessness, shame, fear, avoidance, and stigma) and limitations in life (employment, education, and self-esteem) (see Corcoran & Stewart, 1998; Crichton-Smith, 2002; Hayhow, Cray, & Enderby, 2002; J. F. Klein & Hood, 2004; Klompas & Ross, 2004). A challenge in treatment is to enable others to shift from being a victim to a victor, one who has overcome obstacles and learned about oneself and grown in the process. Joy can follow sadness just as sunshine follows a storm. A key is being open to each client's story, being present and understanding change. As will be seen, fluency freedom is only one of several critical indicators of treatment outcome. Discussing indicators of change and success, Manning (2004) stated: "For the clients we are helping, it may be that the best measure of successful change and eventual outcome is indicated by whether or not we understand the client's story and whether or not we meet the client's goals rather than our own" (p. 64).

Alan Rabinowitz, an internationally known scientist, conservationist, naturalist, and explorer, shared the following: "Catching jaguars and tigers, negotiating with presidents and dictators—that's the easy stuff. The challenge for me has been living with the little stuttering, insecure boy inside, the boy who'd come home from school every day and yearn for the darkness and safety of his closet" (2005). Despite years of suffering caused by stuttering and painful, albeit well-meaning, influences of family and clinicians, Rabinowitz promised himself to be the voice of his beloved animals, those who listened attentively to him without judgment or impatience and with whom he felt he could communicate successfully. Without Rabinowitz's voice, the animals would have been annihilated by human hands. Reflecting on his own personal journey, Rabinowitz wrote,

> I will always believe that stuttering is a special little gift granted to certain people in this world, a little key that opens a part of the human psyche that would not have been opened otherwise. But the truth is that every stutterer has to come to this realization in their own time, in their own way, if they do at all. (2005)

For clinicians, Rabinowitz added the following: "If you are willing to journey the long, arduous, often frustrating path of helping those who stutter, then you will help change the world for many young people. And your reward is that, in doing so, you will share in their gift" (2005). This gift, this transcendence, this journey from being the victim to being the victor—this is success. This personal journey to success is the focus of this book.

Stuttering and Interpersonal Relationships

Stuttering also affects the emotions and dreams of all members of the communication system within which a person who stutters communicates. Mothers and fathers ask, if not plead (by their questions and silence), to be reassured that they did not cause their child's stuttering and that there is hope for their child's fluency future. Guy's wife, a most dignified and polite woman, tearfully expresses concern that she is being misjudged as bold because she speaks for Guy, while in fact she is terribly shy. The wife of a new client candidly expresses her desire to help the process of her husband's fluency enhancement, but is fearful that once he becomes communicatively independent, "he won't find me attractive any longer." Interestingly, her feelings of perceived attractiveness were related to the extent and contexts in which she felt needed. Stuttering affects interpersonal relationships and reminds us that intervention is not just with a person who stutters, but with all people within the communication network. This might involve spouses, boyfriends, girlfriends, young and adult children and siblings, relatives, parents, teachers, coworkers, and allied educational (counselors, music directors, coaches, etc.) and medical (physicians, nurses, counselors, therapists, etc.) personnel. Several months ago, I began working with a college junior who until that time had only spoken with her mother about her stuttering. In her 19 years, I was only the second person with whom she risked talking about stuttering; she had never pursued treatment before. She has enjoyed a very successful beginning of treatment. At the fourth week in treatment, she asked if her mother, who lives several hundred miles away, could meet with us. At that meeting, she said to her mother, "It will be difficult, but I know I can do this" (i.e., achieve fluency freedom). This is success. Her mother tearfully expressed her excitement and gratitude, sharing her belief that God had led her daughter to readiness for treatment and success. Pursuing treatment indeed is an expression of the client's faith; working with people who stutter is a responsibility of considerable magnitude. This is interpersonal relationships at their best.

Chapter Summary

This chapter introduced the nexus (i.e., the essence or core) of stuttering and the perspective that stuttering represents a multidimensional and manageable composite of behaviors, thoughts, and feelings. The person who stutters should be viewed as a whole, unique person and communicator, functioning within a communication system. Intervention should actively involve not only the client but also other members of the communication system and the interdisciplinary team. Assessment and treatment emphasize communication strengths rather than weaknesses and focus on facilitation rather than rehabilitation. Clinicians must understand their clients' assumptions about communication and themselves as communicators because these represent filters through which the clients interpret and anticipate interactions within their communication world.

While there seems to be general agreement that people are not talking fluently when they stutter, actual definitions of fluency and stuttering are based inherently on the individual's assumptions about the nature and etiology of stuttering. Fluency is viewed along a continuum reflecting the ease with which speech is produced, rather than as a dichotomy reflecting the presence or absence of stuttering. In addition, fluency involves both speech fluency and language fluency, with the latter including semantic, syntactic, pragmatic, and phonologic fluency. Most people who stutter exhibit language fluency but have deficits in the area of speech fluency. A brief historical review of definitions of stuttering revealed that most definitions describe stuttering, explain why stuttering occurs, or fall somewhere in between, containing both descriptive and explanatory elements. For the purposes of this book, stuttering is defined as individualized and involuntary interruptions in the forward flow of speech and learned reactions thereto interacting with and generating associated thoughts and feelings about one's speech, oneself as a communicator, and the communicative world in which one lives. Etiology, yet unknown, is conceptualized to relate to the interaction of physiological, psychological, psychosocial, psycholinguistic, and environmental factors.

Concern was expressed over the use of the word *stutterer* rather than the phrase "person who stutters." *Stutterer* reduces the individual person to a simple description of the disorder, rather than recognizing each as a whole person functioning within many roles in today's society who also happens to stutter. As professionals, we need to be aware of the assumptions and associations connected to the terms we use to refer to others. These terms may be indicative of negative stereotypes and bias, which can have a detrimental effect on intervention. In particular, a pessimistic view of the outcome of therapy may be communicated to the client. Instead, clinicians must hold and communicate a sincerely optimistic view and be ready to provide moral support and encouragement as a part of skillful and sensitive intervention.

Because stuttering potentially affects every aspect of a person's life, intervention with (not for) the person who stutters should encompass all areas of speech–language and communication. For example, stuttering may affect articulation when the person shapes the articulators into a posture that is inappropriate for the sound on which he is experiencing a block. Tendencies toward circumlocution may result in the development of "supervocabularies." Stuttering also may affect voice as the person tenses the vocal cords while trying to utter a sound. In addition, stuttering may affect the individual's functioning in society and interpersonal relationships. People who stutter make choices based on their perceived relative ability to handle certain social situations, thereby affecting professional aspirations and educational achievements. Because interpersonal relationships are affected, intervention impacts not just the person who stutters, but others within his communicative network as well.

Stuttering has a profound impact on one's life. W. Johnson (1930) articulated the impact of stuttering on his life:

> I am a stutterer. I am not like other people. I must think differently, act differently, live differently—because I stutter. Like other stutterers, like other exiles, I have known all my life a great sorrow and a great hope together, and they have made me the kind of person that I am. An awkward tongue has molded my life. (p. 1)

Communication is central to our humanity. Van Riper's (1972) words continue to inspire and challenge speech–language pathologists today:

> When we deal with speech, we deal with the essence of man. Only human beings have mastered speech. It is what sets us apart from all other species. Because we can speak, we can think symbolically; and it is this which has enabled man to conquer the world and space and every other creature. Dimly we believe or at least hope that someday it may enable us to master ourselves. (p. 5)

Chapter One Study Questions

1. Many definitions exist for stuttering. How would you answer the question, "What is stuttering?" when asked by a client, parent, or another professional? How might stuttering affect not only a person who stutters, but also his communicative partners?

2. Negative attitudes toward stuttering and people who stutter continue to exist among the general population, allied health and education professionals, and, woefully, student clinicians and professional speech–language pathologists. Why do you think such negative attitudes persist, and what can be done about this situation? What can you do as a speech–language pathologist? How do negative attitudes (and their amelioration) relate to ASHA's Code of Ethics (ASHA, 2010) and Scope of Practice in Speech–Language Pathology (ASHA, 2007d)? What are the implications of providing focused training in emotional intelligence in graduate-level fluency disorders courses (Reichel, 2005, 2007; Reichel & St. Louis, 2004, 2007)?

3. Clinical intervention is a multidimensional experience involving a variety of key participants. In what ways might the thoughts, feelings, and attitudes of each participant impact each other and the process and outcome of treatment?

4. People who stutter develop a variety of techniques to cope with stuttering. What are some of these techniques? How do they impact the behavioral, cognitive, and affective domains? How are such techniques addressed in intervention? Why is it important for clinicians and clients to understand the difference between fluency facilitating controls and communication tricks?

5. Bloodstein and Bernstein Ratner (2008) stated, "It is, of course, within the realm of possibility that not only incidents of stuttered speech, but even individuals who stutter, may prove impossible to characterize in every case with absolute unambiguity" (p. 10). What are the implications of this statement for clinical research and intervention? How might this statement impact definitions and theories of stuttering and the interventions that result from them? How does Bloodstein and Bernstein Ratner's

statement regarding the unavoidable ambiguity of stuttering compare with that of Onslow ("The realm of the clinician is unambiguous moments of stuttering"; 2004, p. 9) and the concept of "stuttering-like disfluencies" (Ambrose & Yairi, 1999; Yairi & Ambrose, 2005; Yairi & Seery, 2011)?

6. Yaruss and Quesal (2004b, 2006, 2008) and Yaruss et al. (2010) highlighted the World Health Organization's (2001) transition from listing the consequences of diseases and disorders to describing components of health in terms of body structure and function, activities and participation, and personal and environmental contextual factors. How might such a transition impact our understanding of stuttering, stuttering intervention, people who stutter, and the communication environment? How might such a transition impact our assumptions and practices in stuttering research and intervention?

7. Dietrich et al. (2001) and St. Louis (1999) found from empirical analysis that person-first labels ("person who stutters"), compared to direct labels ("stutterer"), do not lessen negative beliefs, attitudes, or reactions. Since the degree of negativity is no different (i.e., degree of negativity is independent of the labels we use), should we refer to people as "stutterers," rather than "people who stutter"? What are the implications of using the word *stutterer* as opposed to the phrase *person who stutters*? How might the language we use impact our professional effectiveness as speech–language pathologists?

8. Preschool children are more aware and aware earlier (i.e., as young as 3 years old) of stuttering than previously thought (Ezrati-Vinacour et al., 2001; Langevin et al., 2009; Vanryckeghem et al., 2005; Yairi, 2004; Yairi & Ambrose, 2005); clinical trials are revealing positive results for a direct form of intervention delivered by parents that deliberately increases the young child's awareness of stuttering and related self-monitoring skills (Bernstein Ratner & Guitar, 2006; Harrison et al., 2007; Onslow et al., 2003; S. Woods et al., 2002). What are the implications of these findings? How do these findings inform treatment of preschool children who are beginning to stutter through indirect intervention? How do they inform treatment through more direct means?

9. Tanner (2001, 2003) concluded that books, films, and television typically portray a simplistic view of stuttering (i.e., people who are humorous, anxious, befuddled, angry, and dysfunctional). In what ways (both positive and negative) do the media influence society's perception of people who stutter? How might our cornerstones of culture (theatrical performances, literature, and mass media) contribute to the perpetuation of negative stereotypes and misinformation? How might such resources be used for constructing a more accurate picture for public consumption? What are the implications of Fiske's (1993) interpretation of stereotyping as an expression of power that controls people and limits their freedoms, outcomes, and lives? What are the implications for our role as speech–language pathologists?

10. Rabinowitz (2005) reflected on his life as a communicator and the painful journey that resulted in personal triumph. Given what you know about the potentially pervasive impact of stuttering, how can something as painful as stuttering be viewed as "a special little gift granted to certain people in this world," and how can it be the key to opening a part of the human psyche that would not have been opened otherwise? What is transcendence? What is success? Whether or not you are a person who stutters, how might you have experienced a personal journey that led you from being the victim to being the victor? How might such experiences enable you to relate to the experience of stuttering and to serve in your role as a speech–language pathologist?

Chapter Two

The Onset, Development, and Nature of Stuttering

Our unending questions and our ceaseless doubts in no way discredit our profession or our discipline. They may well be among our greatest assets. . . . Nevertheless, honesty demands that we own up to our bewilderment—bewilderment about the nature of human communication and its disorders, bewilderment about the treatment of those disorders, bewilderment about how services should be delivered and about who should deliver those services and how much they should be prepared. Like all bewildered people, we ask many questions and ask them over and over again. . . . So long as we continue to ask questions we are honest, alert, alive, and in good health, no matter how bewildered. A traditional toast proclaims, "To life!" However redundant, I would add, "To bewilderment!" I can think of no more suitable salute to this discipline, to this profession, and to this association. (Flower, 1985, pp. 24–25)

Knowledge and Assumptions Ground Understanding

An understanding of stuttering—of how it begins and develops, its nature, how it has been viewed historically, and current theoretical explanations regarding its etiology—is a critical foundation for a clinician to develop confidence and competence in designing and implementing effective intervention with people who stutter. In Chapter 1, we emphasized the importance of cohesion within and across assumptions underlying stuttering-related domains, including definitions, theories, therapies, and research. A lack of such cohesion impedes the treatment process and the extent to which advances in one domain generalize to others. A clinician's understanding of stuttering is necessary to develop and refine such assumptions.

These assumptions form a clinician's personal construct, a dynamic and generative perspective or point of view on communication, stuttering, and people who stutter. All

31

clinicians have a personal construct about their profession and the roles and responsibilities of the participants within it. In fact, all people have, albeit often implicitly, personal constructs regarding all aspects of life. More to the point, not all clinicians are explicitly aware of their own assumptions, thus risking the relatedness between what they know, or assume to be true, and what they do, or how they design and implement assessment and treatment. For example, many clinicians assume that stuttering must be understood on the basis of overt (i.e., observable behaviors) and covert (i.e., internalized thoughts, feelings, and beliefs) phenomena, that the person who stutters should, and is able to, participate actively in the change process, and that stuttering occurs within communication in social settings. Add to these assumptions a person who stutters and who demonstrates negative, if not destructive, feelings and attitudes toward himself as a communicator. It makes little clinical sense in such a case to embark on a program of strict fluency shaping, in which speech behaviors are addressed to the exclusion of feelings and attitudes, the person who stutters is only passively engaged in the treatment process, and all activities focus on the treatment setting. This is lacking in ecological validity with respect to the person being served and inhibiting transfer to meaningful communicative contexts.

I am concerned that the treatment just described is frequently implemented. The design of such treatment is unrelated to the unique strengths and needs of the person who stutters and the assumptions held by the clinician and the client. One's knowledge and assumptions form the basis for interpreting events and planning and implementing assessment and treatment. Williams (1957) indicated the centrality of clients' and clinicians' assumptions when he stated, "It is recognized that one cannot discuss a 'way of thinking' about a particular problem such as stuttering without implying, either implicitly or explicitly, certain assumptions about the nature of that problem" (p. 390). Amplifying the clinical importance of these assumptions, W. Johnson (1939) stated, "So long as an individual retains and operates on assumptions regarding stuttering and speech, which are characteristic of stutterers, he will not become the sort of individual we refer to as a normal speaker" (p. 172).

Understanding stuttering also requires knowledge of how stuttering has been conceptualized and treated in the past. F. H. Silverman (2004) warned that clinicians who remain unaware of how stuttering has been treated in the past (and, I would add, how stuttering begins and develops, its nature, and theories about its etiology) are more likely to use intervention strategies that have been shown repeatedly to be of little long-term value. These strategies, he cautioned, may produce rapid reduction in stuttering severity, "but the vast majority of clients on whom they are used are likely to relapse within 5 years following termination of therapy" (p. 120). The purpose of this and subsequent chapters in Unit I is to provide a foundation for such an understanding. The onset, development, and nature of stuttering are covered in this chapter; the etiology of stuttering, from past and present perspectives, is discussed in Chapter 3; and other fluency disorders are outlined in Chapter 4.

The Onset and Development of Stuttering— Developmental Classifications

There is little debate that stuttering behaviors change and develop over time. However, why a large number of children who begin to stutter cease to do so without treatment is still not understood. Estimates of such cases vary considerably (23% to 80%— G. Andrews et al., 1983; 36% to 79%—Bloodstein & Bernstein Ratner, 2008; 20% to 80%—Guitar, 2006; 17.8% to 94%—Van Riper, 1982). The differences in the reported rates of spontaneous recovery can be explained by several factors. Many studies are based on retrospective self-reports of people who stutter. These people may have been told by their parents that they stuttered, but in actuality may have been no more disfluent than children who do not stutter (Guitar, 2006). Van Riper (1982) indicated that retrospective reports regarding the child's age and related conditions at the time of stuttering onset contain error because of parents' lapses in memory, need to respond to frequent questions about what caused the disorder, and erroneous assumption that correlation infers causality (i.e., assuming that one event causes another because the events occur at or near the same time). Furthermore, sample sizes and methodologies have varied across studies (Guitar, 2006), and there have been ambiguities in the defining characteristics of stuttering and spontaneous recovery (Bloodstein & Bernstein Ratner, 2008).

More recent studies of spontaneous recovery (Kloth, Kraaimaat, Janssen, & Brutten, 1999; Mansson, 2000; Yairi & Ambrose, 1999, 2005) have identified children who stutter at or near their onset of stuttering and used a consistent longitudinal methodology that followed them over time without treatment, resulting in greater consistency of reported spontaneous recovery (i.e., 70%–74%). Kloth et al. reported a rate of 70% spontaneous recovery after following 23 children for 6 years; Yairi and Ambrose (1999) reported a 74% rate of spontaneous recovery after following 84 children over at least 4 years. Mansson (2000) studied the entire population of children on the Danish island of Bornholm who were born in 1990 and 1991; 1,021 of the 1,042 were screened for speech and language problems by age 3 years. Following 53 children who stutter for 2 years, this study revealed a 71% rate of spontaneous recovery. These children were followed for an additional 7 years, and the rate of spontaneous recovery increased to 80% (some of the children received treatment after screening at age 5 years, which was 2 years post-onset of stuttering). The remainder of this section addresses the onset and development of stuttering in those children who continue to stutter.

Stuttering is a dynamic composite of behaviors, thoughts, and feelings. Van Riper (1982) indicated that new behaviors replace or join the original ones. The new behaviors can be understood only within the context of how they developed. Ham (1990) stated that changes in stuttering behavior are affected by altered motor skills, self-awareness, reactions to the disfluency, and reactions to the responses of others. Many attempts have been made to describe the evolution of stuttering on the basis of developmental stages. While such attempts provide valuable descriptions of behavior, they inevitably fail because there are clients whose speech behavior and development of stuttering cannot be classified neatly into predetermined categories. Developmental classification systems oversimplify behavior, representing continuous variables as if they were unidimensional and dichotomous in nature. As noted in Chapter, 1, this simplification is unrealistic and fails to represent adequately the multidimensionality inherent in human communicative behavior. Van Riper indicated his discomfort with existing classification schemes, including his own, and described attempts to design such systems as "sheer folly" (1982, p. 92). Trying to account for all people who stutter and the uniqueness of communication behaviors, developers of classification schemes could generate an infinite number of minimally differentiated categories. Van Riper (1982) cautioned, however, as follows:

> This does not mean that the beginning stutterer should be treated in the same way we would treat him after he has learned to struggle or avoid. It means that our treatment should fit his needs as shown by his current behaviors, including their history; it should not be a prescribed treatment appropriate only to the child's classification in a developmental category. (p. 92)

Given these caveats about the limits of classification, such systems nevertheless do provide valuable descriptions for building understanding among professional clinicians:

It is essential to know how stuttering frequently develops in order to have a point of comparison for detecting the uniqueness in each client's experience. The categories must not be interpreted as confining or rigid; they provide a general picture that serves as a point of departure. Haynes and Pindzola (2008) underscored this point and warned against "hardening of the categories." Clinicians must maintain flexibility, addressing each person on the basis of individual strengths and needs.

Before we turn to more recent work on the emergence of stuttering, several examples of earlier classification systems are summarized below in order to build an understanding of how stuttering emerges and to provide historical perspective. The classification systems presented here—from Bluemel, Froeschels, Van Riper, and Bloodstein, respectively—are from cross-sectional investigations. As noted earlier, our knowledge has heightened considerably in light of more recent, longitudinal, investigations of how stuttering behavior begins and develops over time (Yairi & Ambrose, 2005; Yairi & Seery, 2011). As you review these developmental classification systems, you will notice similarities but also different areas of emphasis. These systems are provided as snapshots, or pictures to which your client's behavior might be compared, but not as a template into which the behaviors of individual clients should be forced. We will then review the more current longitudinal studies of the onset and development of stuttering and what we know about differential diagnostic indicators of children who are at greater risk of continuing to stutter and those who are not.

Bluemel

Bluemel (1932, 1935, 1957), a medical doctor, introduced the terms *primary* and *secondary* stuttering, still heard today, to distinguish two stages of the disorder. *Primary stuttering* refers to the incipient stage, consisting of easy, effortless repetitions of the first word or syllable of a sentence, behaviors that are intermittent yet recurring. *Secondary stuttering* begins after a period of no observed disfluency for several years or after the child is made aware of or embarrassed by the stuttering. Secondary behaviors are more forceful and consistent. They reflect learned fears and contain specific motor behaviors; they are characterized by physical effort, use of starters and synonyms, attempts to conceal stuttering, and observed fear of letters, words, people, and related speech contexts. Bluemel viewed stuttering as a habit learned as a consequence of conditioning. Intervention to discover the answer to "the riddle of stuttering" (1957) was, he believed, to be found in psychotherapy.

Froeschels

Froeschels (1956, 1964) indicated that the onset and development of stuttering can be observed as a consistent progression from initially effortless syllable and word repetitions that become more rapid, irregular, tense, and inhibited. Speech rate increases at first and then decreases as the disfluency worsens, generating avoidance reactions and deliberateness from the child. Froeschels distinguished between *tonic* and *clonic* types of stuttering. *Tonic stuttering* is characterized by hard pressure and tension (i.e., sustained contraction of the speech muscles), often resulting in breathing interruption, grimaces, and clenching; *clonic stuttering* is more repetitive and oscillatory, resulting in syllable and sound repetitions.

Van Riper

Van Riper (1982) expanded on Bluemel's (1932, 1935) work, adding a transitional stage between primary and secondary stuttering and an entire fourth category. After reviewing client folders, Van Riper (1982) reported that 41 of the 44 longitudinal cases (93%)

followed from onset of stuttering to maturity and 187 of the 256 shorter term cases (73%) fell roughly into one of these four tracks of development. For each track, he described the patterns of onset and development.

Track 1 Onset. Track 1 was the most frequent pattern of development—48% of the longitudinal histories (21 of 44) and 55% of the shorter observations (141 of 256). Children in this track begin speech development with normal-sounding speech fluency, rate, and articulation. Stuttering begins gradually between 2.5 and 4.0 years of age with long periods of remission. These children demonstrate the greatest inconsistency in development, showing a behavior characteristic of the most advanced form one day, and then returning to gentle syllabic repetitions or normal disfluency the next. Behaviors characteristic of this track include frequent gentle syllabic repetitions (without schwa, averaging 3 to 5 per word) on initial and function words. Repetitions occur in clusters, followed by considerable normal fluency. No tension or tremors are noted. The child demonstrates no awareness of or frustration over the disfluency and no speech-related fears. Therefore, the child talks without any perceived interference.

Track 1 Development. Syllable repetitions increase in rate and frequency, and their rhythmic pattern becomes less regular. Prolongations start to appear at the end of the repetitions and begin to demonstrate increased disruption (i.e., tension, tremor, and struggle). Vowels within the repeated syllables begin to be prolonged. Pitch increases indicative of laryngeal tension during prolongation often are observed. Prolongations move forward, from the final repeated syllable of a series to the initial syllable. Frustration and concern become evident, and there is a general overflow of tension, indicated by facial contortion, retrials, and decreased speech output. As this pattern develops, word fears and avoidance occur. These fears lead to sound fears, then situation fears. Repetitions and prolongations increase in frequency and complexity, becoming silent fixations with associated struggle behavior. Breathing during speech is interrupted, and speech rate slows considerably. Eye contact is interrupted and avoidance tactics are observed as a consequence of fear. The child shows embarrassment over speaking and therefore develops reluctance. Ultimately, patterns of stuttering behavior, both overt and covert, become stabilized and stereotyped. Stuttering enters into the child's self-concept, affecting personality factors and catalyzing defenses.

Track 2 Onset. Track 2 was the second most frequent pattern of development—25% of the longitudinal histories (11 of 44) and 12% of the shorter observations (31 of 256). The onset of stuttering is gradual but occurs later, coinciding typically with delayed and disorganized onset of connected speech (phrases or sentences are not observed until between 3 and 6 years of age). Development of stuttering is steady, without remission. Unlike the child in Track 1, the child in this track was never very fluent, demonstrating irregular and rapid rate of speech and relatively poor articulation. Syllabic repetitions, the majority of which are monosyllabic words, are hurried and irregular. Later, there are more silent gaps and hesitations, revisions, and interjections. Disfluencies tend to occur on first words and longer words, and generally distribute throughout the sentence and on content words. The pattern of speech is more variable, typically demonstrating broken speech with hesitation and gaps even when there is no disfluency. Prolongation and fixation are rare, but children demonstrating this pattern of development may silently preform or preposture an initial sound, particularly a vowel, occurring in the first word in a sentence. Children demonstrating this pattern seem to be free of frustration, tension, and tremor. Awareness, fear, struggle, and avoidance develop more slowly than in Track 1.

Track 2 Development. Disfluent behaviors remain relatively the same, but their rate and frequency increase. Long strings of syllabic and whole-word repetitions of increasing rate develop. The child's awareness of disfluencies increases slowly and there is little development of situation fears, avoidance behaviors, sound or word fears, or loss of eye contact. When fears are present, situation fears are more likely than word or sound fears. Overall speech output tends to increase, albeit in a disorganized way, with primarily repetitive, arrhythmic forms of disfluency. In a later stage, compulsive and perseverative (i.e., runaway) repetitions increase in rate, tension, and pitch, resulting in overall unintelligibility. The speaker seems unable to terminate the repetitions until the exhalation is finished. The eyes appear fixed or glazed, and the speaker reports a clear awareness that something dreadful and involuntary is happening to him. Others have described the speech behavior in this stage as *cluttering* (see Chapter 4 for a review of this disorder).

Track 3 Onset. Only 11% (5 of 44) of Van Riper's (1982) longitudinal cases and 5% (13 of 256) of his shorter observations demonstrated Track 3 patterns. At any age after the establishment of connected, fluent speech, a child in this track demonstrates a sudden, acute onset of disfluency, often following a traumatic experience. Development of stuttering tends to be steady, with few remissions. Articulation is normal. At first, stuttering is confined to the beginning of an utterance after a pause and takes the form of tense, prolonged fixation of an articulatory posture. Struggle ensues, usually at the level of the larynx. Breathing during speech is interrupted, and vocal fry (bubbling, cracking type of low-pitched phonation) is common, combined with struggling and forcing. Tense musculature tremors, awareness, and frustration develop almost immediately. General speaking fear and specific situation and word fears develop rapidly, as do speech-related frustrations. Speaking rate tends to slow. Nonstuttered speech sounds fluent.

Track 3 Development. The frequency and complexity of forms of disfluency increase and are accompanied by observed frustration and retrials. Lip protrusions and tongue fixations appear, as do prolongations of initial sounds. Repetitions follow prolongations; each repetition begins with a slight prolongation of the first sound. As tension and tremors increase, facial contortions, jaw jerking, and gasping are observed. Frustration and interruptor devices become prominent. Speech rate slows and speech reluctance increases. The child develops avoidance patterns and intense fears of words and sounds. Severity increases, resulting in bizarre forms of disfluency. Eye contact is interrupted. Nonstuttered speech becomes irregular and hesitant; nonvocalized tense blocks become frequent.

Track 4 Onset. Only 9% (4 of 44) of Van Riper's (1982) longitudinal cases and less than 1% (2 of 256) of the briefer observations demonstrated Track 4 patterns. Stuttering usually begins later than in the other three tracks. As in Track 3, stuttering begins suddenly after several years of fluency. Initial disfluencies often are repetitions of whole words and phrases, rather than syllables that later become observed. Lengthy repetition of words already spoken combines with gaps and pauses. Remissions are rare and the behaviors acquired early change little over time. Articulation and rate are essentially normal. These children seem aware of their stuttering and listener reactions. Stuttering occurs most frequently on first words and content words but rarely on function words. The child demonstrates little evidence of fear or frustration and remains talkative.

Track 4 Development. The frequency of stuttering increases, but the pattern remains stable. Unlike those in other tracks who pass through phases and develop a repertoire of different avoidance and release reactions, those in this track tend to be monosymptomatic. Avoidance and release reactions, therefore, are not common. Stuttering seems to be undisguised, with few consistent loci. While the child demonstrates keen awareness of stuttering behavior, there is little evidence of fear. Eye contact remains uninterrupted. These children are talkative and open about their stuttering but do not demonstrate being negatively affected by it.

Bloodstein

Bloodstein (1960a, 1960b) reviewed the case records of 418 people who stutter between 2 and 16 years of age, from which he proposed four phases in the development of stuttering that appear to be typical but not universal (Bloodstein & Bernstein Ratner, 2008). These phases, according to Bloodstein, are reference points along a continuum, indicating that the development of stuttering is a continuous and gradual process. Many people who stutter correspond to one of the phases; others might be in transition between two phases.

Phase 1. During the preschool period (between 2 and 6 years of age), disfluency is highly episodic, observed for weeks or months between intervals of normal speech, and noticed mostly under conditions of communicative pressure or emotional arousal. The dominant form of disfluency is whole-word repetition at the beginning of sentences, clauses, and phrases and on content and function words. Evidence of concern or frustration by the child is infrequent and fleeting.

Phase 2. Children in Phase 2 tend to be elementary school age, but such patterns have been observed in children as young as 4 years and in people who have reached adulthood. Disfluencies become chronic, with few intervals of normal speech, thus affecting the child's self-concept. Disfluency occurs mainly on content words, with less tendency to stutter on initial and whole words. There is little evidence of concern (i.e., no evidence of avoidance tactics or word, sound, or situation fears). Stuttering worsens during excitement or rapid or demanding speech.

Phase 3. Phase 3 is typically observed in late childhood and early adolescence (approximately 8 years to adulthood). Stuttering becomes more specific to situations, words, or sounds. Circumlocutions and substitutions emerge as an escape from impending frustration. Avoidance of speech situations is not observed. Little or no evidence of fear or embarrassment is apparent. The distinguishing feature of this phase is that the person speaks freely, despite advanced development of stuttering. Reactions tend to be more irritation than shame or anxiety.

Phase 4. Although typically seen in later adolescence and adulthood, this phase may be recognized in later childhood (i.e., 10 years). In this last phase, stuttering is characterized by fearful anticipation of stuttering; feared sounds, words, and situations; frequent word substitutions and circumlocutions; and avoidance of speech situations and other indications of fear and embarrassment. This phase is characterized by emotional reactions and interference with life activities. Sensitivities and disguises are a significant cause of impairment in social relationships and avoidance of social interaction.

Summary—Onset and Development of Stuttering— Developmental Classifications

The foregoing developmental classification systems, or snapshots, indicate that stuttering usually begins gradually during the preschool years and only infrequently in adults. When stuttering persists, the behaviors, thoughts, and feelings that characterize stuttering change and develop with the passage of time and interaction within a social context. Typically, stuttering begins with repetitions of sounds and syllables or prolongations. Most people who stutter develop struggle or avoidance reactions as a consequence of frustration, embarrassment, and fear.

There are risks in sharing snapshots, however. Namely, in presenting this information, some will adhere strictly to the track or phase concept, attempting to fit clients into categories that do not fit them (like trying to put square pegs into round holes), failing to realize the uniqueness of each person who stutters and the stuttering experience itself. We must not abandon current developmental representations of stuttering, yet we must not become prisoners of them. Wall and Myers (1995) indicated that implicit in a stage approach to developmental stuttering is the tenet that stuttering, particularly in children, gets worse when left untreated. They verified this premise in "a good many" (p. 84) clinical cases. They cautioned, however, that holding too rigidly to a stage approach excludes other possibilities. They urged readers to remember that stuttering can remain unchanged or show great periodicity and fluctuation, that symptoms can remit spontaneously, that stuttering may be severe at onset, even in early childhood, and that stuttering may be mild in adults.

Others have offered similar cautions. Bloodstein and Bernstein Ratner (2008) indicated that the presence of secondary symptoms does not mean that the child is habitually fearful of speaking and that childhood disfluency, anticipatory preparation, and emotional reaction are inevitable, yet not sufficient, to define stuttering behavior. As noted in Chapter 1, we must not misinterpret continuous variables, such as stuttering, as dichotomous. Wingate (1976) also indicated that progression concepts only present stuttering as becoming worse and do not provide for conditions of no change, fluctuation, or improvement. Furthermore, he objected to the assumed yet unsubstantiated positive correlation between age and severity (see also Schwartz, Zebrowski, & Conture, 1990; Yairi & Ambrose, 1999, 2005; Yairi & Seery, 2011) and suggested the abandonment of developmental labels or stages in favor of precise description of simple or complicated patterns. Wingate argued, "In fact, we have absolutely no grounds for predicting either course or destination for any case of stuttering" (1976, p. 67). Van Riper (1982) also emphasized the benefits of "molecular" description, which is defined both qualitatively and quantitatively, over "molar" identifications, which he called "gross categories" and "wastebasket phrases" (pp. 14–17). Van Riper reminded clinicians and researchers to exercise caution in interpreting developmental patterns of stuttering that are based on cross-sectional data. He also identified longitudinal investigation of the onset and development of stuttering as a critical need facing our field.

The Onset and Development of Stuttering— Longitudinal Investigations

One of the most comprehensive series of longitudinal investigations addressing the early development of stuttering is being conducted by Yairi and colleagues (Yairi, 2004; Yairi & Ambrose, 1999, 2005) at the University of Illinois Stuttering Research Program, with participants at other locations in the United States, Israel, Sweden, and the United Kingdom. These studies are focusing on changes that occur in stuttering over time and differentiating characteristics of persistent and naturally recovered subtypes of stuttering. Children younger than 6 years of age who stuttered less than 1 year were assessed regularly between 3- and 6-month intervals for durations of 4 to 8 years. A total of 190 children who stutter, 50 nonstuttering control children, and 450 parents participated in the investigations. Audio- and video-recorded speech samples and parent interviews provided the core data. Notably, the development of stuttering is not presented in terms of stages; there is evidence of a strong genetic component as well as extensive behavioral variability in the onset of stuttering.

Onset of Stuttering

As noted, developmental classifications emphasize relative uniformity in the onset of stuttering. In contrast, the University of Illinois Stuttering Research Program studies reveal substantial variability in the age, type and severity, and conditions at onset. The mean age at onset was 33 months (68% of the onsets occurred before age 3 years, 85% occurred by 3.5 years, and 95% occurred before 4 years), approximately 9 months earlier than the composite mean age of onset from previous investigations. In other words, "children under age 3 have the greatest risk for beginning to stutter. . . . There appears to be a critical period that rarely allows stuttering to occur prior to age 2, even though the child is talking, and relatively infrequently after age 4" (Yairi & Ambrose, 2005, pp. 78–79).

In contrast to the traditional view that stuttering onset is mild and gradual (i.e., gradual appearance, effortless repetitions of syllables and words, lack of physical tension, lack of awareness and affective reactions related to stuttering), these longitudinal studies revealed that 30% of the children experienced sudden onset within a single day, and 40% experienced sudden onset over no more than 3 days. Intermediate onsets (between 1 and 2 weeks) occurred with 33% of the children; gradual onset (more than 2 weeks) represented the smallest group at 25%. Male and female children were distributed similarly across the three types of onset patterns (i.e., severe, intermediate, and gradual); however, the differences in percentage between the two genders in each onset pattern remained close to the 2:1 male to female ratio. Most parents rated their child's initial stuttering as moderate (45%) or severe (20%); only 35% rated their child's stuttering onset as mild (Yairi, 2004).

Traditional views hold that stuttering typically begins in otherwise relatively uneventful environmental circumstances. In contrast, again, these studies revealed that in 50% of the cases, stuttering began in uneventful circumstances; but at least the same proportion revealed conditions of stress at onset (14% experienced illness or physical fatigue just before onset, 40% experienced emotionally upsetting events, and 50% experienced language stresses, such as fast-developing vocabulary and word-finding difficulty).

Older conceptualizations assert that stuttering begins with mild and easy repetitions of sounds and syllables that are nearly indistinguishable from normal disfluency. The University of Illinois Stuttering Research Program studies show that although repetition of initial syllables and short words is universal, frequently observed symptoms near onset in many children are complex, diverse, and "advanced," including prolongations and articulatory fixations, multiple repetitions with tension (i.e., repetitions were more tense and contained at least twice the number of repeated units compared to children who do not stutter), tense sound prolongations, complete silent blocks, respiratory irregularities, and complex secondary characteristics. On the basis of these and other data, Yairi and Ambrose (2005) concluded, "Consequently, views of the early stage of stuttering as involving complex, diverse phenomena have been replacing long-held views of its onset and development as a simple, uniform, linear phenomenon. We do not believe, however, that early stuttering is fundamentally different from advanced stuttering" (p. 12).

Approximately half of the parents reported that their children experienced physical components at onset, including abnormal, visible tension or movement of the face, eyes, lips, tongue, jaw, and neck, and tense movement of the head or limbs. There were no differences in the types or frequency of such secondary characteristics observed between boys and girls at onset. Given that half the children demonstrated early physical components and half did not, Yairi and Ambrose (2005) cautioned that such signs might not be indicative of more advanced stuttering. Severity ratings by the investigators revealed symptoms that were most often moderate (45%) and less often mild (27%) or severe (28%). Note the similarity between the investigators' severity ratings and those of the parents. More than 20% of the parents indicated that the children were aware of their disfluency; some recalled specific comments from the children, such as "I can't talk." Research procedures utilizing puppets (one fluent and one disfluent) revealed that approximately 10% of preschool children within 1 year of onset were aware of their speech disfluency (Ambrose & Yairi, 1994; Ezrati-Vinacour et al., 2001; Yairi & Ambrose, 2005; Yairi & Seery, 2011).

Development of Stuttering

In contrast to the traditional view of uniform, linear, stepwise progression of stuttering that increases in severity and abnormality, the University of Illinois studies "definitively and objectively illustrated that early stuttering generally does not follow a rule, but may begin as sudden or gradual, mild or severe, with or without disrhythmic phonation and accessory physical characteristics, and with or without emotional reactions to it" (Yairi & Ambrose, 2005, p. 150). Variability is also the hallmark of the development of stuttering beyond its onset.

Longitudinal investigations have highlighted the importance of understanding the phenomenon of spontaneous or natural recovery on several grounds. Being able to distinguish between children whose stuttering will recover versus those whose stuttering will persist facilitates the assessment of relative risk (e.g., high, moderate, low, or no risk of chronic stuttering) and guides clinical intervention (i.e., decision rules for the design of differential and individualized clinical intervention strategies). The course and relative persistence of stuttering may be guided more by genetic factors than by characteristics of speech, physiology, home environment, or other variables (Ambrose, Yairi, & Cox, 1993; Bloodstein & Bernstein Ratner, 2008; Yairi & Ambrose, 2005). The developmental patterns revealed by the University of Illinois studies are based on 89 children younger than 6 years of age whose stuttering was first identified within 1 year of onset and followed at 6-month intervals for 2 years and yearly thereafter for 4 to 12 years. Of these 89 children, the stuttering of 70 ultimately recovered naturally (84% of girls, 77% of boys), while the stuttering of 19 persisted (16% of girls, 23% of boys).

The longitudinal data indicated that most of the children who recovered did so within the first 3 years of onset. Rate of recovery dropped sharply after 3 years of onset, but some did recover between 3 and 5 years post-onset; none recovered naturally after 5 years of onset. The percentages of children who recovered naturally at different times post-onset are as follows: 1 year, 12%; 2 years, 31%; 3 years, 63%; 4 years, 74%; 5 years, 79%. Therefore, a child who has just begun to stutter has a 65% to 80% chance of natural recovery between 3 and 5 years post-onset (i.e., 20%–35% chance of persistence). After 2 years of stuttering, the chance of natural recovery is 47%; after 3 years of stuttering, the chance of natural recovery is 16%; after 4 years of stuttering, the chance of natural recovery is 5%. Females tended to recover more frequently than males (male to female ratios are 3.75:1 for persistent stuttering and 2.33:1 for natural recovery) and more quickly than males (females who recovered did so by 3 years post-onset; most males who recovered also did so by 3 years post-onset, but some continued to recover up to 5 years post-onset) (Yairi & Ambrose, 2005, pp. 170–172).

Longitudinal disfluency profiles of children whose stuttering recovered and children whose stuttering persisted can be formed on the basis of stuttering-like disfluencies (SLDs—part-word repetitions, single-syllable word repetitions, and disrhythmic phonation) and other disfluencies (ODs—interjections such as *um* and *uh*, revisions or abandons, and multiple-syllable word and phrase repetitions). Frequency of SLDs was not significantly different between the two groups of children within the 6-month post-onset period. After 6 months post-onset, however, children whose stuttering persisted demonstrated significantly more SLDs than did children whose stuttering naturally recovered. Interestingly, ODs, which remained static over time, failed to distinguish the two groups of children during any time interval. These results suggest that SLDs should receive particular attention in assessment, in follow-up, and in the consideration of prognostic indicators; ODs may not be as useful as indicators of stuttering severity and prognosis. Yairi and Ambrose (2005) highlighted one exception. During the third year of stuttering, ODs (particularly interjections) were significantly more frequent among children whose stuttering persisted than for children whose stuttering naturally recovered.

More precisely, the SLDs either declined gradually or remained static and then declined gradually for children whose stuttering persisted. In contrast, SLDs declined sharply after 7 to 12 months of stuttering for children whose stuttering naturally recovered. Yairi and Ambrose (2005) highlighted the clinical implications:

> A considerable drop in any of the SLD types may be a good indicator of recovery, but children who persist may also experience fluctuations in the severity of their stuttering. In terms of disfluency counts, then, the best predictor is a decrease in all SLD types, which approach normal limits within 6 to 18 months following onset. In other words, if substantial recovery is not seen within this time period, chances for natural recovery decrease. Early stuttering is highly variable, and predictions of recovered versus persistent pathways, based on disfluency profiles alone, are still difficult to make accurately early in the course of the disorder. The more significant finding, however, is that such recovery shows strong signs within the first 12 months of stuttering. Based on current data, we need to examine more than disfluency levels to obtain optimal early prediction. (p. 178)

These longitudinal investigations challenge traditional views that stuttering increases in duration and complexity over time. Duration of disfluency typically has been considered a significant risk factor (Cooper & Cooper, 2003; Riley, 1981, 2009). From a subset of children in the University of Illinois studies (20 children, 10 who ultimately recovered and 10 who persisted), Throneburg and Yairi (2001) and Yairi and Ambrose (2005) reported that the mean length of repetitions and silent intervals between repeated units for children who ultimately recovered tended to be longer than for those whose stuttering persisted, but these differences were not statistically significant. They also reported that the duration of disfluencies remained relatively constant for children whose stuttering persisted over a 3-year period. Yairi and Ambrose (2005) indicated that these findings do not support traditional assumptions that longer blocks and prolongations predict persistence of stuttering and that repetitions become more rapid, irregular, and longer when stuttering continues. They conceded, however, that "one cannot ignore the fact that some children who persist eventually develop more severe problems" (p. 181).

Traditional views hold that secondary symptoms are a reflection of advanced stuttering. However, Yairi and Ambrose (2005) revealed that physical concomitants often are observed near onset among both children who recover and those who persist. However, the number of head and facial movements tends to decrease over time, as the frequency of disfluency decreases. Yairi and Ambrose (2005) noted,

> Although a large number of physical concomitants close to the onset of stuttering does not appear to be a warning sign of persistent stuttering, a decreasing trend over time may be a positive sign of recovery, and absence of minimal change of physical concomitants within a year could be a warning sign. (p. 182)

Summary—Onset and Development of Stuttering—Longitudinal Investigations

The data from the University of Illinois Stuttering Research Program are complex yet, when taken as a whole, provide a compelling if not provocative perspective regarding the onset and development of stuttering. The majority of children who stutter peak in stuttering severity typically within the first few weeks or months of onset, after which overt symptoms subside. Within the first 4 years of onset, the decline results in natural recovery in approximately 75% of the children. Children whose stuttering naturally recovered early and who maintained fluency for at least 6 to 10 months tended not to relapse. Most children whose stuttering recovered, however, tended to stutter for longer periods, with recovery occurring slowly and gradually beginning during the first year and continuing for up to 3 years post-onset; some continued into the fourth and fifth year. Yairi and Ambrose (2005) characterized the stuttering of children who recovered as a pattern of asymmetry, with a brief beginning and ascending phase, followed by a relatively prolonged declining phase. Natural recovery occurred more frequently and earlier among girls than among boys.

Children whose stuttering persists represented the minority. They demonstrated a fairly stable level of SLDs during the first year (in contrast to the typical drop in SLDs during the first year among children whose stuttering recovered). Yairi and Ambrose (2005) highlighted the importance of learning when the child's stuttering first began and not assuming that it began just before the referral (i.e., there might have been a delay between the onset of stuttering and the referral). They also cautioned not to assume that relative severity shortly after onset predicts the course of stuttering; rather, later severity is a better indicator of persistent stuttering.

To this point, the results of the University of Illinois longitudinal investigations of early stuttering have challenged traditional perspectives on the onset and development of stuttering. The importance of these studies resides in a clearer articulation of risk factors—those that might distinguish a child whose stuttering will recover without treatment (i.e., natural recovery, transient stuttering) from a child whose stuttering will not (i.e., persistent or chronic stuttering).

Risk Factors to Distinguish Transient and Chronic Stuttering

Yairi and Ambrose (2005) identified primary, secondary, and other risk factors in regard to transient versus chronic stuttering (see also Chapter 8).

Primary Risk Factors

⬚ *Family history.* Children tend to follow the pattern of their family's history of persistence or recovery. When a child has close family relatives whose stuttering persists, the child's stuttering is more likely to persist. Also, when a child has close family relatives whose stuttering has recovered, the child's stuttering is more likely to recover.

⬚ *Gender.* Boys are at greater risk for stuttering incidence and persistence than girls. Girls recover after a shorter history of stuttering than boys. Yairi and Ambrose (2005) suggested that a 1-year history of stuttering without improvement indicates a greater risk for a girl's stuttering to be persistent than for a boy's stuttering.

⬚ *Age of onset.* Persistence tends to be associated with later age of onset. Children whose stuttering persists begin to stutter 3.5 months later than those whose stuttering recovers.

⬚ *Stuttering-like disfluencies.* Children whose stuttering naturally recovers tend to demonstrate reduction in SLDs within the first year of onset. Those whose stuttering persists tend to demonstrate a more stable degree of SLDs. A downward trend in the number of SLDs within the first year of onset, therefore, is interpreted as a positive prognostic indicator for ultimate recovery.

⌨ *Duration of stuttering*. Natural recovery tends to occur within 3 years of onset. Stuttering that persists beyond the first year is viewed as indicating a higher risk for persistence, particularly for girls.

⌨ *Disfluency length*. Severity of stuttering at the earliest stage of stuttering is not a predictor of persistence or recovery. However, continuing disfluency, particularly with more than three units of repetition, suggests higher risk. Yairi and Ambrose (2005) recommended assessing both the extent and frequency of disfluency, particularly during the first year of stuttering. They posit that the duration of disfluent events does not differentiate children whose stuttering will persist from those whose stuttering will recover (disputing previous claims that longer blocks and prolongations indicate persistence). They also noted that children whose stuttering recovered demonstrated an increase in the duration of silent intervals between repeated units, indicating normalization, or repetitions that are slower in tempo.

⌨ *Sound prolongations and blocks*. Except during the first few months of the disorder, sound prolongations and blocks tend to predict persistence of stuttering. Reduction in the percentage of sound prolongations tends to predict recovery; increase in the percentage of sound prolongations tends to predict persistence.

Secondary Risk Factors

⌨ *Stuttering severity*. Stuttering severity near the time of onset is not a predictor of persistence or recovery (i.e., children whose stuttering recovered demonstrated stuttering as severe as or more severe than children whose stuttering persisted). However, severity in relation to extent of stuttering history may be predictive (i.e., severe stuttering that continues for more than the first few months indicates a greater risk of persistence).

⌨ *Head and neck movements*. As with initial stuttering severity, the number and degree of head and neck movements near onset were not predictive of persistence or recovery. Within the first 12 months, however, children whose stuttering recovered demonstrated reduction in head and neck movements; those whose stuttering persisted did not show this reduction. Yairi and Ambrose (2005) concluded that children who do not demonstrate substantial reduction in the number and severity of secondary characteristics within the first year of onset are at higher risk for persistent stuttering.

⌨ *Phonological skills*. Children whose stuttering persists tend to demonstrate lower phonological skills early in their history of stuttering (stuttering may emerge in children who have poor phonological skills). Within the second year of stuttering, however, the deficit in phonological skills tends to disappear, as does the predictive power of phonological skills. Yairi and Ambrose (2005) cautioned that phonological skill alone is insufficient to predict stuttering outcome; it may be more predictive in combination with other factors.

⌨ *Expressive language skills*. Close to stuttering onset, language skills alone did not predict persistence or natural recovery. Young children who stutter tend to demonstrate language skills that are at or above average expectations. Yairi and Ambrose (2005) suggested that in some children, stuttering may emerge in conjunction with developmentally advanced language abilities. Similarly, the course of children's language development is not a clear prognostic indicator, despite the observation that atypical language development was observed in some children whose stuttering persisted.

Other Risk Factors

⌨ *Concomitant disorders*. Concomitant disorders (e.g., physical, emotional, learning, speech–language, behavioral, cognitive, psychological, attentional, medical) tend to contribute to the persistence of stuttering.

⌨ *Awareness and affective reactions*. Yairi and Ambrose (2005) noted that there is no evidence that the child's awareness of stuttering or emotional reaction to it shortly after onset is a predictor of persistence. However, they stated that emotional reactions of the child or parents could have secondary effects and interfere with recovery. For that reason, they suggested that such reactions be addressed and serve as a factor in recommending intervention.

Most children who begin to stutter recover naturally. Given the issues of resource allocation and clinical efficacy, clinicians should reserve direct treatment for those who stand to benefit the most—children who are at greatest risk. Those at lower risk are not to be ignored; they should receive parent counseling and other forms of indirect intervention. All young children who are beginning to stutter should receive a thorough communication evaluation and subsequent reevaluations, accompanied by parent education about childhood stuttering; children whose stuttering does not abate after 14 to 18 months should receive a priority for direct fluency intervention, addressed in Chapter 8. The clinician must also bear in mind that risk assessment is not infallible. Yairi and Ambrose (2005) advised, "The clinician must always inform parents that, as yet, nobody can accurately predict the development of stuttering in a given child" (p. 359).

The Nature of Stuttering

While interacting with people who stutter and their families, clinicians are asked many questions. This section presents a snapshot of stuttering and effective treatment to help the clinician respond in an informed way to some of the most frequently asked questions. Others have presented more complete portraits of stuttering and its treatment (G. Andrews et al., 1983; Bernstein Ratner & Healey, 1999; Bernstein Ratner & Tetnowski, 2006; Bloodstein & Bernstein Ratner, 2008; Conture & Curlee, 2007; Guitar, 2006; Kalinowski & Saltuklaroglu, 2006; Yairi & Ambrose, 2005; Yairi & Seery, 2011; Van Riper, 1982); the brief sketch provided here is based on these works. Keep in mind that each individual client who stutters may or may not exhibit any of these characteristics.

Types of Disfluency

There are several classification schemes for identifying types of disfluency; some of the most widely used typologies are briefly described here. Williams, Darley, and Spriestersbach (1978) presented a classification system containing eight types of overt forms of disfluency. Today considered the classic forms of disfluency, they include interjections of sounds, syllables, words, or phrases (e.g., *uh, er, hmmm, well, you know*); part-word repetitions (*buh-boy, guh-guh-girl*); word repetitions (*I-I-I, was-was-was*); phrase repetitions (*I was—I was going*); revisions (*I was—I am going*); incomplete phrases (*She was—and after she got there he came*); broken words (also called disrhythmic phonation) (*g-oing, b-oy*); and prolonged sounds (also called tension pause) (*sssssssee sssssssaw*).

As noted previously, one of the most prominent metrics used for assessing and diagnosing stuttering is the number of stuttering-like disfluencies (SLDs) per a given number of words or syllables spoken (Ambrose & Yairi, 1999; Yairi & Ambrose, 1999, 2005; Yairi & Seery, 2011). Yairi and Ambrose (2005, pp. 96–97) classified SLDs (1–3, below) and other disfluencies (4–6, below) as follows:

1. part-word (i.e., sound or syllable) repetitions (e.g., *a-and, f-five, ba-baby, mo-mo-mommy*);

2. single-syllable word repetitions (*but-but, and-and*);

3. disrhythmic phonation (i.e., audible or inaudible sound prolongations or blocks, identified within words, including unusual stress, intonation, or breaks);

4. interjections (extraneous sounds of one or more unit, e.g., *um, um-um*; note that interjected words and phrases, such as *like, well,* and *you know,* are not considered disfluencies and, therefore, are counted only as words and not as interjections);

5. multiple-syllable word and phrase repetitions (repetitions of segments longer than one syllable or one word, such as *because-because, once up—once upon, I was—I was going*); and

6. revision or abandoned utterances (i.e., utterances that are modified yet retain the original content, such as *I was—I am going, She gave him—he gave her, I want the ball—red ball,* or utterances that are not completed, such as *Yesterday I went—hey, what's that over there?*).

Categories and systems for classifying disfluencies have proliferated, as have resulting challenges in terms of their usefulness for measuring, diagnosing, understanding, and treating stuttering (Einarsdottir & Ingham, 2005). Despite interrater reliability issues (Bloodstein & Bernstein Ratner, 2008), such systems can be useful for categorizing and describing, and thereby understanding, fluent, disfluent, and stuttered speech. At least as critical to a comprehensive understanding of stuttering is realizing that the overt elements—those that are observed or heard directly—do not tell the whole story, particularly among people for whom stuttering has become advanced or chronic. Stuttering also is manifested in more covert elements—the associated experiences (i.e., feelings, attitudes, fears, avoidances, anxieties, shame, embarrassment, and phobias) that directly impact both one's anticipation of and interpretation of events that inform perceptions of oneself as a person and as a communicator (Craig, Blumgart, & Tran, 2009; Guitar, 2006; Hayhow, Cray, & Enderby, 2002; International Fluency Association and International Stuttering Association, 2001; Irwin, 2007; Manning, 2004, 2006, 2010; Plexico, Manning, & DiLollo, 2005; Stewart & Richardson, 2004).

Symptoms, Prevalence, and Incidence

What do we know about the speech of young children and particularly the symptoms of stuttering at its onset?

Preschool children typically demonstrate speech disfluencies, including word and phrase repetitions, interjections, and revisions. In other words, disfluency is the norm for young children. Being able to distinguish between typical childhood disfluencies and those of incipient stuttering is an essential skill for speech–language pathologists. We know that children who stutter tend to demonstrate more within-word disfluencies (e.g., sound or syllable repetitions, sound prolongations, broken words, etc.) than children who do not. In fact, disfluencies that fragment the word (within-word disfluencies) are more likely to be perceived as stuttering than those that do not (i.e., between-word disfluencies such as whole-word repetitions, revisions, and incomplete phrases) (Bjerkan, 1980; Guyette & Baumgartner, 1988). This is what Van Riper (1982) meant when he said, "It is the broken word that characterizes the majority of the stutterer's difficulty. Stuttering interruptions to the forward flow of speech are primarily intra-morphemic; normal disfluencies are primarily supra-morphemic" (p. 13). Again, although commonalities are observed among people who stutter, the onset, development, and features of stuttering are unique to each individual.

When does stuttering develop and what is the likelihood of recovery?

The majority of children who stutter begin stuttering between ages 2 and 5 years. A person can begin to stutter at any age, however. Stuttering begins in adulthood only in rare cases. When it does, its onset typically is sudden and represents a distinct subtype of the disorder (e.g., subsequent to emotional trauma, intracranial trauma, etc.) (Attanasio, 1987a; Haynes & Pindzola, 2008; Mahr & Leith, 1992; Theys, van Wieringen, & De Nil, 2008; Wingate, 1983). Subtyping of stuttering is receiving focused attention for the sake of improving our knowledge base, theoretical constructs, research strategies, and assessment and treatment decisions, and for predicting the relative course of stuttering (i.e., transient or persistent stuttering) and determining effective treatment approaches (Seery, Watkins, Mangelsdorf, & Shigeto, 2007; Yairi, 2007; Yairi & Ambrose, 2005).

Regarding the onset of stuttering, G. Andrews (1984) stated, "On the basis of data presently available, half the risk of ever stuttering is passed by Age 4, three quarters by Age 6, and virtually all by Age 12" (p. 8). More recently, however, Yairi and Ambrose (2005) found that the mean age for stuttering onset was 33 months, about 9 months earlier than the composite of data published in 11 previous reports (Yairi, 1997). Finding a similar pattern for boys as for girls, Yairi and Ambrose (2005) reported,

> Over half (59%) of the stuttering onsets occurred during the third year of life (24–35 months). By 42 months of age, over 85% of onsets had occurred, increasing to 95% by age 4 years. Thus, only 5% of the children in this study began to stutter after age 4. . . . It is apparent that a majority of onsets occur from 2 to 3½ years of age at the present time. (pp. 54–55)

Yairi and Ambrose (2005) concluded from longitudinal findings that children under 3 years of age have the greatest risk for beginning to stutter (i.e., 60% of the children who stutter began prior to age 3 years and more than 85% by age 3.5 years.). They noted also a critical period for stuttering in that children rarely begin to stutter prior to age 2 years or after age 4 years. The risk of persistent stuttering is greater among boys (1.5%) than among girls (0.5%). And, whereas G. Andrews (1984) reported that 75% of the risk for beginning to stutter is passed by age 6 years, Yairi and Ambrose (2005) asserted that a significantly greater degree of risk is passed at earlier ages.

How prevalent is stuttering and what is its lifetime incidence?

The *prevalence* of stuttering (total number of cases at or during a specified time, determined from cross-sectional studies and retrospective surveys) in prepubertal schoolchildren is approximately 1% and generally drops in postpubertal schoolchildren. No reliable prevalence figures are available for adults who stutter. However, if prevalence continues to decline after puberty, the figure for adults would be less than 1% (i.e., 0.8%) (G. Andrews et al., 1983; Bloodstein & Bernstein Ratner, 2008; Curlee, 2007; Guitar, 2006; Guyette & Baumgartner, 1988; Moscicki, 1984; Yairi & Ambrose, 2005). The *incidence* of stuttering (total number of people who have stuttered at some point in their lives, or lifetime incidence; Bloodstein & Bernstein Ratner, 2008) lasting longer than 6 months is approximately 5%. The difference between incidence (5%) and prevalence (1%) indicates that most people who stutter recover from it (Bloodstein & Bernstein Ratner, 2008; Guitar, 2006). Yairi and Ambrose (2005) noted that the 5% incidence figure can be broken down further. Given that approximately 80% of children who ever stutter recover, "the incidence of recovered stuttering is about 4%, and the incidence of persistent stuttering is 1%. The last figure equals the prevalence, usually measured by looking at persistent adults" (p. 298). Certain special conditions resulting from perinatal brain damage, including mental retardation, epilepsy, cerebral palsy, and other syndromes, reveal a higher than expected prevalence of stuttering. Deafness is the only condition associated with a lower than expected prevalence of stuttering (G. Andrews et al., 1983; Bloodstein & Bernstein Ratner, 2008; Guitar, 2006; Van Riper, 1982). However, several studies have addressed disfluencies in manual communication, including repetitions, hesitations, interjections, and extraneous movements found in signing and finger spelling (Montgomery & Fitch, 1988; F. H. Silverman & Silverman, 1971; Snyder, 2006; Whitebread, 2004; see also Chapter 4 of this volume).

Does stuttering incidence vary by gender, class, nationality, or ethnicity?

The ratio of males who stutter to females who stutter is approximately 3:1. This ratio tends to increase with age (Bloodstein & Bernstein Ratner, 2008; Guitar, 2006; Guyette

& Baumgartner, 1988). Craig and Tran (2005a, 2005b) reported approximate ratios (i.e., male to female) of 3:1 for 2- to 10-year-old children who stutter, 4:1 for 11- to 20-year-old individuals who stutter, 2:1 for 21- to 49-year-old adults who stutter, and 1.4:1 for adults over 50 years of age who stutter. It is unclear why the ratios narrow for the oldest groups of people who stutter. Estimates of age of onset, based on retrospective and cross-sectional data, vary. G. Andrews et al. (1983) reported age of onset to be the same for both sexes, whereas Yairi (1993) and Yairi and Ambrose (2005) reported onset for girls to be 6 months earlier than that for boys. However, it appears that girls recover more frequently and quickly than boys. Some have suggested that this tendency might reflect a genetically controlled and milder form of stuttering in girls (Drayna, 2005, 2006; Kidd, 1984; Yairi, 1993, 2006; Yairi & Ambrose, 2005). Constitutional explanations abound, suggesting that the sex ratio in stuttering may reflect the broader congenital vulnerability of males compared to females (e.g., more infant mortality, birth injury, susceptibility to childhood diseases); environmental explanations suggest differences in parental and societal attitudes toward and reactions to boys and girls (Bloodstein & Bernstein Ratner, 2008).

Stuttering is found in almost all peoples and cultures (Bloodstein & Bernstein Ratner, 2008; Haynes & Pindzola, 2008; Van Riper, 1982). Some say the prevalence among different cultural and national groups is nearly the same (Wingate, 1983), while others suggest greater prevalence among middle- and upper-middle-class families. While the prevalence of stuttering in Western and other technologically advanced cultures (including Japan, China, and India) is reported to be approximately 1%, that of other countries reportedly is greater than 1% (the population of Korea; the Kawakiutl, Nootka, and Salish Indians of Canada; the Idoma and Ibo tribes of West Africa [i.e., the Igbo people in Nigeria and Cameroon]; and schoolchildren in Dakar, Senegal, and Accra, Ghana) or less than 1% (the Mundugumar, Arapesh, Tchambuli, Manus, Dobuan, New Hanover, Tabor, and Kamamentira tribes of New Guinea; the Aborigines of Australia; Polar Eskimos; the Bannock and Shoshone tribes of the United States; and Polynesians) (F. H. Silverman, 2004). Reflecting on the universality and variability of stuttering, Bloodstein and Bernstein Ratner (2008) suggested that a richer question is whether there are cultural differences in the incidence of the disorder:

> Those who have collected these data believe that it is possible that stuttering is a significant comment on the culture that produces it. To say that there are many stutterers in a given society is possibly to say that it is a rather competitive society that tends to impose high standards of achievement on the individual and to regard status and prestige as unusually desirable goals, that it is sternly intolerant of deviancy, and that, as a by-product of its distinctive set of cultural values, it in all likelihood places a high premium on conformity in speech. Alternatively, these prevalence differences may reflect differences in the culture's identification of typical and impaired speakers, or of genetic variability that can differentiate some communities (particularly those that are less likely to be mobile and thus are more genetically homogenous) from others. (p. 109)

Does stuttering result from one's environment?

Environmental factors are of great interest because of their potential role in causing stuttering and inhibiting its remission. Conversely, environmental factors might have an important role in preventing stuttering from occurring, even in people who have such a predisposition. As noted previously, certain conditions ensuing from perinatal brain damage are associated with a higher than expected prevalence of stuttering. Indicating that perinatal brain damage appears to be the only environmental event causally related to idiopathic or developmental stuttering, G. Andrews et al. (1983) stated,

> There are no other established facts about the more obvious features in a stutterer's environment that might point to the cause or maintenance of stuttering, be they family

structures, race, socio-cultural factors, or parental characteristics. Stutterers appear to come from the same environment as do nonstutterers, with one exception; they come from families with an excess of stuttering relatives. (pp. 228–229)

Research has also focused on the occurrence of environmental stresses near the onset of stuttering. Yairi and Ambrose (2005) found that 14% of the children in their study experienced physical stresses (e.g., illness or surgery requiring hospitalization, respiratory problems, asthma, acute illness) and over 40% experienced emotional stresses (e.g., divorce of parents, moving, death of a pet, birthdays, sibling rivalry, family vacations, or difficult day-care situations). Additionally, approximately 36% of the children experienced behavioral or developmental stress or change, such as toilet training, giving up favorite "blankies" or bottles, family rivalry, and more. In other words, general stresses were reported for almost half of the children close to the time of stuttering onset. No significant difference was identified between the genders, refuting the notion that more males than females stutter because of the extra stress put on males. Yairi and Ambrose (2005) reported, "Our data indicate that physical or emotional stresses might play an active role in stuttering onset. If a child possesses predisposing (i.e., genetic) factors to stutter, aggravating physical or emotional stresses might very well trigger the onset" (p. 63).

What is the role of genetics in stuttering?

People often ask if stuttering is inherited or caused by genetic factors. People do not inherit behaviors. Rather, we inherit genes, and genes interact with environmental factors (i.e., life circumstances, socioeconomic status, cultural or religious beliefs, birth order, temperament, illness, etc.), the combination of which influences behavior. Yairi and Ambrose (2005) presented a clear example of how genes must interact with environmental influences for genetic expression to occur. They noted that two neighbors may buy the same variety of strawberry plants, each with genes for producing large, red, juicy berries. One neighbor plants them in a sunny location with rich soil and ample moisture. The other neighbor plants them in a dry, shady corner, in poor soil. The first condition allows the genes (i.e., the behavioral potential) to be expressed, resulting in a bountiful crop. The second condition prevents the genes from being expressed, resulting in a poor crop.

There are a few basic terms and tenets of genetics research. The behavior or characteristic that may be expressed, given the combination of genetics and the necessary and sufficient environmental conditions, is the *phenotype* (e.g., rich strawberries, stuttering). The underlying genes, which may or may not be expressed (i.e., the sum total of one's genetic inheritance), are referred to as the *genotype*. Many genes reside on each chromosome; one copy of each chromosome is inherited from the mother (23) and one copy from the father (23). The genotype transmits susceptibility to an array of phenotypes (e.g., speech–language disorders, stuttering). However, the interaction of genes with environmental conditions is complex, rendering prediction of genetic expression (e.g., whether a child will stutter or not, based on the necessary and sufficient combination of genetic and environmental factors) imprecise, at best. Yairi and Ambrose (2005) underscored how challenging it is to identify the contribution of a single gene or of multiple genes because of their interaction with each other and the environment. They stated,

If the overall liability to stuttering is the summation of all the genetic and environmental agents that can affect this phenotype, then it is possible for an individual to have a number of factors and not stutter, but have parents, siblings, or children who do stutter. It may be that individuals in families with stuttering do not all have the same set of factors; there may be one or more primary genes that are involved in virtually all stuttering, but the remaining contributors probably vary at least to some extent. . . . One or more genes may contribute to the underlying susceptibility to stuttering, and may have wider effects, affecting susceptibility to other disorders as well. These genes may also interact with other genes to cause a variety of phenotypic effects. Conditions that sometimes co-exist with stuttering, such as phonological disorders, attention deficit, or even asthma, could possibly stem from this interaction. (pp. 287–288)

The challenge to genetics research, therefore, is to isolate the genes that transmit susceptibility to stuttering and to determine the necessary and sufficient combination or combinations of genes and environmental conditions that cause the onset and development of stuttering, as well as the subtypes of genetic and environmental conditions that render distinctly different onset and development patterns. To address this challenge, genetic researchers analyze family trees, twin pairs, and adoptions. In family studies, the genetic characteristics of family members expressing a trait (i.e., the phenotype, or stuttering) are compared with those who do not. In this way, the chromosomal location of the gene or genes that influence stuttering can be identified. Fairly consistently, family studies have revealed that stuttering *probands* (i.e., people who stutter around whom relatives are assembled and studied) are found to have a greater incidence of stuttering relatives than that of the general population. The risk to first-degree male relatives of an individual who stutters is about 5 to 10 times that in the general population, and it does not matter whether the proband, or individual who stutters, is male or female (Ambrose et al., 1993; Janssen, Kloth, Kraaimaat, & Brutten, 1996; Viswanath, Lee, & Chakraborty, 2004). Reviewing the literature from 1924 to 1983, Yairi, Ambrose, and Cox (1996) reported that percentages of people who stutter who have a family history of stuttering ranged from 20% to 74%, while the nonstuttering comparison groups with a family history of stuttering ranged from 1.3% to 42%. Similarly, Yairi and Ambrose (2005) reported that of the 123 families of people who stutter, 69% (85/123) reported a positive history for stuttering in the family; 31% (38/123) did not report a positive family history for stuttering. The pattern is clear—people who stutter are more likely than people who do not stutter to have relatives who stutter (Bloodstein & Bernstein Ratner, 2008; Guitar, 2006). Yairi and Ambrose (2005) provided additional information based on their persistent and recovered subtypes—88% (21/24) of the families of children with persistent stuttering had a positive family history for stuttering, and 63% (49/78) of the families of children with recovered stuttering had a positive family history for stuttering. Yairi and Ambrose (2005) summarized, "In other words, families of children who stuttered persistently were more likely to have at least one stuttering relative than families of children who recovered" (pp. 291–292).

In twin studies, researchers attempt to distinguish the relative influence of genetics and environment. Identical (*monozygotic*) twins have identical genes. Fraternal (*dizygotic*) twins are genetically like any other siblings, sharing up to half of their genes. Any greater similarity in the traits of identical twins as opposed to fraternal twins generally is at-tributed to the role of inheritance (Guitar, 2006). Twin studies of stuttering indicate that there is more concordance of stuttering in identical twins than in fraternal twins. This means that stuttering occurs more often in both members of identical twin pairs than in both members of fraternal twin pairs, supporting the notion that a predisposition for stuttering is inherited. For example, Howie (1981) reported 63% concordance for monozygotic pairs and 19% concordance for dyzygotic pairs. Interviewing 91 twin pairs (38 monozygotic, 53 dizygotic) identified through the Australian Twin Registry, Felsenfeld et al. (2000) found 45% concordance for monozygoic twins and 15% concordance for dizygotic twins. Cases of discordance among identical twins, or when only one member of an identical twin pair stutters, however, suggest environmental as well as genetic influences. These and other data indicate that a predisposition to stutter might be influenced by genetic factors (Ambrose, Yairi, & Cox, 1993; G. Andrews et al., 1983; Cox,

1988, 1993; Felsenfeld, 1996, 1997, 2002; Felsenfeld et al., 2000; Van Riper, 1982). Kidd (1984) argued that "an inherited neurologic susceptibility underlies most cases of stuttering" (p. 149), yet concurred that stuttering is determined by both nature (inherited factors) and nurture (environmental influences). Felsenfeld et al. (2000) estimated that 70% of the phenotypic expression (likelihood that one or the other twin will stutter) is attributable to genetic factors; 30% is attributable to environmental factors. Similarly, G. Andrews, Morris-Yates, Howie, and Martin (1991) reported that 71% of the liability to stutter is determined by additive genetic influences; 29% is attributable to an individual's unique environmental influences. Ooki (2005) estimated that as much as 80% (in males) and 85% (in females) of the liability of phenotypic expression is attributable to additive genetic factors; 15% (in females) and 20% (in males) is attributable to unique environmental factors.

Yet another way to investigate the relative contribution of genetic and environmental influences on stuttering is to study the families of children who stutter who were adopted shortly after birth. A higher proportion of stuttering among biological relatives of adopted children who stutter would suggest genetic influences; a higher proportion of stuttering among the adoptive relatives would suggest environmental influences. Such studies are rare, partly because birth records of adoptions are hard to access. Bloodstein and Bernstein Ratner (2008) presented information on a small sample (N = 13) of people who stutter who were interviewed about their adoptive families (information about the biological families was not available; Bloodstein, 1961). Of the 13 people who stutter, 4 had a history of stuttering in the adoptive family, which is greater than chance occurrence. The small sample size precludes generalization of these findings, however. Drayna (1997) and Felsenfeld (1997) found that stuttering is more related to whether an individual's biological parents stutter than to whether the adoptive parents stutter. Clearly, both genetic and environmental factors impact the etiology, familial incidence, onset, and development of stuttering; genetic factors appear to contribute more than environmental factors.

Another dimension to understanding the genetics of stuttering is biological genetics. Such investigations are referred to as "linkage studies," where DNA (deoxyribonucleic acid, the chemical inside cell nuclei that carries the genes) is extracted from body tissue samples for the purpose of locating and analyzing the gene or genes that may implicate stuttering. Then, forms of known marker genes are identified on the chromosome or chromosomes of interest. When a marker gene form is co-inherited with stuttering (i.e., when the marker gene form is linked to stuttering by co-inheritance), the implication is that the gene contributing to stuttering is on or near the same chromosome as the marker gene (Yairi, 2006). Various studies are providing promising evidence of implicated chromosomes, or at least chromosomes of interest. Studying members of the Hutterite population in North Dakota, who do not marry outside of their own community and who therefore have a relatively homogenous gene pool, N. J. Cox and Yairi (2000) linked chromosomes 1, 3, 5, 9, 13, and 15 with stuttering. Shugart et al. (2004) studied 68 families throughout North America and Europe and implicated 18 markers on chromosome 18. Riaz et al. (2005) studied 46 families in Pakistan, where marriage between cousins is common and considered highly desirable, and implicated chromosomes 1, 5, 7, and especially 12. Drayna (2005), at the National Institutes of Health, has been studying a single 100-member family in the northwest province of Cameroon, of which 45 individuals stutter. One of the family members, a colleague and personal friend of mine, explained that the family is so large because of polygamous customs, and that all of the family members live in close proximity. Drayna (2005) reported that while this family is remarkable, it is not unique. In the same province of Cameroon, four additional families (ranging from 25 to 80 members each), nearly half of whose members stutter, are being studied. Preliminary results link chromosome 1 with stuttering (Levis, Ricci, Lukong, & Drayna, 2004). Yet another study, this one of families of European descent in the United States, Sweden, and Israel, has linked chromosome 9 with the broad category of "ever stuttered" (i.e., persistent and recovered stuttering) and chromosome 15 with persistent stuttering. The strongest marker for males only occurred on chromosome 7 and for females only on chromosome 21. This study suggested two possible genetic pathways to stuttering. The first was evidence of linkage on chromosome 12, dependent upon linkage on chromosome 7 (the region on chromosome 12 is close to that reported for the Pakistani families). The second was evidence of linkage on chromosome 2, dependent upon linkage on chromosome 9 or negative linkage on chromosome 7 (the region of chromosome 2 also has been linked with autism, suggesting direction for research into stuttering subtypes) (Suresh et al., 2006; Yairi, 2006, Yairi & Ambrose, 2005). These and other studies suggest that an inherited chromosome or combinations of inherited chromosomes, mixed with individualized and generative combinations of environmental influences, impact the susceptibility to, onset of, and course of stuttering.

What factors other than speech are part of stuttering in its developed form?

In advanced stages, stuttering typically has both overt and covert features. Much of the observed escape and avoidance behaviors of advanced stuttering are overt attempts to cope with the emission of speech disfluency. In addition to speech disfluencies, stuttering may be characterized by speech and voice abnormalities (e.g., narrow pitch range, vocal tension, lack of vocal expression, muscular lags and asynchronies) that can be detected in nonstuttered speech. In one study, even the fluent (i.e., nonstuttered) speech of people who stutter was judged to be more disfluent than that of people who do not stutter (Lickley, Hartsuiker, Corley, Russell, & Nelson, 2005). These traits may be a function of stuttering or may reflect impairment in phonation, respiration, neuromotor coordination, or cortical integration (Bloodstein & Bernstein Ratner, 2008; Guitar, 2006; Haynes & Pindzola, 2008; Van Riper, 1982).

Bloodstein and Bernstein Rather (2008) reviewed the symptomatology of chronic stuttering, which is summarized here. It is important to note, however, that what is presented is a composite group portrait, not necessarily fully reflective of any particular individual who stutters. Each individual who stutters will be both like and unlike the group portrait in unique ways. The moment of stuttering has been analyzed from acoustic and physiological descriptions, associated symptoms, and attitudes and adaptations. Acoustic and physiological descriptions addressed respiration, phonation, and articulation. Disordered breathing while stuttering (i.e., breathing was not disordered when not speaking) included antagonisms between abdominal and thoracic breathing, irregular respiratory cycles, prolonged expirations or inspirations, cessation of breathing, interruption of expiration by inspiration, and phonation upon inhalation. Phonatory abnormalities included irregular vocal fold vibration, excessive and irregular activity of laryngeal muscles, delay in laryngeal activity prior to disfluencies, inappropriate vocal fold adduction or abduction with respect to the spoken target, and observed vocal tension (i.e., vocal fry, hoarseness, breathiness). Irregularities in articulation were addressed through electromyographic, aerodynamic, spectrographic, and other studies. Electromyographic studies revealed excessive or uncoordinated muscle activity during stuttered words and silences, potentially implicating muscles that are responsible for movement of the tongue, lips, upper and lower jaw, and larynx. Aerodynamic studies revealed peaks, elevations, and irregular states of intraoral air pressure during stuttering, reflecting attempts to speak while airways were restricted, and precipitous drops in intraoral air pressure during silent intervals. Spectrographic studies revealed a decrease in the duration and amplitude of vowels within stuttered speech during transitions between sounds, sometimes perceived as a neutral vowel (schwa) replacing the intended vowel, and reduced lip rounding within coarticulatory movements. Other studies revealed reduced time between repeated segments within stuttered speech, rapid articulatory movement at the moment of release from a stuttering block, jaw movement that was not coordinated with onset of vocalization (i.e., sometimes preceding, sometimes behind vocalization), and repositioning of articulators prior to release from the stuttering posture.

Associated symptoms were identified as overt, physiological, and introspective concomitants. Overt concomitants include tension and movement expressed on the face (e.g., rapid or irregular blinking or other eye movement, wrinkling of the forehead, sudden exhalation, distortions of the mouth and jaws, quivering of nostrils, irregular movement of the tongue), head, hands, arms, legs, feet, and torso; interjected speech fragments (sounds, syllables, words, and phrases); vocal abnormalities (irregularities in speech rate, vocal quality, inflection, pitch); and physical reactions (flushing, perspiration). Physiological concomitants include irregular eye movements, increases or decreases in heart rate, tremor, and increased alpha-wave cortical activity. Introspective concomitants include feelings of frustration, vocal involuntariness and being out of control, muscular tension (within the speech apparatus, affecting the muscles of articulation, phonation, and respiration; or elsewhere in the body), and affective involvement (ranging from uneasiness to panic, frustration, embarrassment, and anxiety).

Bloodstein and Bernstein Ratner (2008) noted that attitudes, assumptions, and methods for coping that develop as a consequence of stuttering must be understood as a key part of stuttering symptomatology. Many people who stutter report feeling innately unable to speak and that stuttering is shameful, unpleasant, and threatening. As a consequence, specific words, sounds, and situations become feared. People who stutter come to perceive listeners as critical, impatient, embarrassed, and pitying. The self-concept of a person who stutters comes to be equivalent with "stutterer." Many people design strategies to cope with stuttering. Some avoid feared words, using synonyms or circumlocutions. Others avoid feared situations and may restrict verbal output and social relationships. Some people who stutter adopt an unnatural persona (e.g., clowning, bravado) so as to conceal their fear of speaking. Stuttering potentially influences and restricts all aspects of one's life, including personal, social, academic, and vocational areas (Craig et al., 2009; Hayhow et al., 2002; Plexico et al., 2005; Stewart & Richardson, 2004). Indeed, people who stutter go to great lengths to cope with stuttering. A client of mine tearfully recalled telling her boyfriend repeatedly, "Never mind," rather than let him observe her stuttering. She confessed, "He's going to think I don't care, when I really do." The pain from anticipated humiliation of stuttering was far greater than that from misrepresentation and miscommunication. Rabinowitz (2005) recalled putting a lead pencil through his hand in order to avoid reading aloud in class; he was rushed to the hospital just prior to his turn to read. The pain from anticipated humiliation of stuttering, he recalled, was far greater than that received from any bodily injury.

Differences Between People Who Stutter and Those Who Do Not

What is known about the intelligence of people who stutter?

Children who stutter tend to score a .5 standard deviation lower on verbal and nonverbal tests of intelligence and lag 6 months behind their peers in school performance (G. Andrews et al., 1983; Guitar, 2006; Guyette & Baumgartner, 1988). How to interpret these findings remains controversial. Some have argued that the measured deficit might be a result of stuttering rather than a cause of it. This interpretation seems plausible given the emphasis on verbal skills in both traditional intellectual and educational assessment and the emotional consequences of stuttering on a person who stutters. However, the studies revealing that people who stutter perform more poorly on verbal and motor subtests are interpreted by some as suggesting that stuttering might be related to inadequacy in linguistic and motor domains (Guitar, 2006). Additionally, stuttering tends to increase under conditions of increased and competing cognitive and linguistic engagement, requiring a person who stutters to focus on one aspect of the required task despite the conflicting task demands. Given this line of argument, it might be predicted that a greater deficit in cerebral functioning (deficient resources underlying both linguistic and motor performance) would predict stuttering. Indeed, it is the case that intelligence is negatively correlated with stuttering (i.e., as level of intelligence goes down, the prevalence of stuttering goes up). People with intellectual disabilities, including mental retardation, typically demonstrate more than the 1% prevalence of stuttering found among the general population (i.e., 14 of the 16 prevalence figures reported by Bloodstein & Bernstein Ratner, 2008, were above 1%, ranging from 1.4% to 20.3% prevalence of stuttering among people with intellectual disabilities). Van Borsel et al. (2006) reported prevalence of stuttering in special needs classrooms in Belgium to be four times that found in the general school population. In other words, lower intelligence does seem to correlate with and predict a greater prevalence of stuttering. However, it is both unfortunate and inaccurate when people assume that stuttering correlates with and predicts a lower level of intelligence; this is flatly wrong.

Yairi and Ambrose (2005) reported a study in which children who stutter were administered the *Arthur Adaptation of the Leiter International Performance Scale* (Arthur, 1952) to determine if each child's nonverbal skills were within normal limits and comparable to the child's verbal skills. The scores of children who stutter were above normal limits. However, distinguishing between children whose stuttering was transient and those whose stuttering was persistent proved to be instructive. The recovered group had a mean score above normal limits; the persistent group achieved the lowest mean score, albeit still within normal limits. Thus a lower score on this scale may predict persistence of stuttering, implying that children whose stuttering is transient have more cognitive resources or neural resilience than do children whose stuttering is persistent (Guitar, 2006). In any case, the clinical relevance of differences in measured intelligence among children who stutter is equivocal at best. As noted, there is no difference in the intelligence of people who stutter when compared to those who do not except that the former group demonstrates a slight measured gap in early intellectual and educational assessment. This gap is likely a consequence of stuttering rather than a cause of it. Yairi and Ambrose (2005) cautioned, "The different or poorer performance for people who stutter may simply represent skills at the lower end of the normal range, as a result of how their brains function due to stuttering (or to other disorders that may tend to co-occur with stuttering)" (p. 269). Bloodstein and Bernstein Ratner (2008) cautioned further that "an average difference of several IQ points is more important theoretically than practically" (p. 230).

Do people who stutter have a different personality?

As early as the 4th century B.C., theories postulated that stuttering results from disordered personality, emotional conflicts, and psychoneurosis. Aristotle wrote in his book *Problemata* that stuttering results from nervousness and a form of fear that creates coldness (cited in Seery et al., 2007; Wingate, 1997). As noted in Chapter 3, theories of stuttering as an expression of psychopathology persisted and became particularly popular in the early 20th century (Brill, 1923; Glauber, 1958). Early-20th-century theories postulated that stuttering reflects psychosexual fixation originating from unconscious and unsatisfied conflicts and needs. These unresolved issues were traced to neurotic and dysfunctional personalities of parents. Bloodstein and Bernstein Ratner (2008) noted that such theories have declined; Yairi and Ambrose (2005), by contrast, see a renewed interest in theories that associate stuttering with personality. Previous studies have analyzed many characteristics of people who stutter, including social adjustment, oral and anal eroticism, passive dependency, obsessive-compulsive traits, hostility and aggression, guilt, somatization (i.e., conversion reactions), self-concept, aspiration and achievement drive, body image, role perception, handwriting, color preference, language style, anxiety, conditionability, defense preference, rigidity, suggestibility, locus of control, and self-monitoring ability, among others (Bloodstein & Bernstein Ratner, 2008). The prevailing interpretation is that people who stutter, as a group, do not demonstrate emotional maladjustment or specific personality characteristics and do not show differences on measures of neurotic behavior. However, people who stutter do show more problems in social adjustment (e.g., low self-esteem and willingness to risk failure, avoidance of social contact requiring speaking with others, insecurity); such adjustment problems, however, are more likely a result of stuttering rather than a cause of it (Bloodstein & Bernstein Ratner, 2008; Guyette & Baumgartner, 1988; Yairi & Ambrose, 2005). Even though theories of deep-seated neurosis and psychiatric intervention have been abandoned by current professionals who are knowledgeable about the disorder, the legacy of such theories and interventions continues to impact how stuttering is viewed today. The World Health Organization's *International Classification of Diseases* (ICD-10; WHO, 2010) lists stuttering and stammering (the equivalent term used throughout the United Kingdom) in a chapter titled "Mental and Behavioral Disorders." Under the heading "Behavioral and Emotional Disorders with Onset Usually Occurring in Childhood and Adolescents," stuttering (F98.5, p. 227) is described just before cluttering (F98.6) and other disorders (F98.8, e.g., attention-deficit disorder without hyperactivity, excessive masturbation, nail biting, nose picking, and thumb sucking). The imprint of history is indelible and resists, if not defies, revision. Indeed we have our work cut out for us.

Several researchers have studied the relative temperament of people who stutter. Preliminary findings suggest that preschool children who stutter tend to have more negative attitudes about speaking, temperaments that are more sensitive and inhibited, and hypervigilant (i.e., less distractible) and less adaptable profiles (J. D. Anderson, Pellowski, Conture, & Kelly, 2003; Ezrati-Vinacour et al., 2001; Yairi & Ambrose, 2005). Similarly, Schwenk, Conture, and Walden (2007) found that preschool children who stutter are less adaptable to change than preschool children who do not stutter; but they also found that preschool children who stutter are more distractible, rather than less. Some hypothesize that children who are born with sensitive temperaments are more vulnerable to stuttering, become more sensitive as a consequence of stuttering, and are more easily aroused by stimuli but also more inhibited when confronted by unfamiliar people or situations (Conture, 2001; Guitar, 2006; Oyler, 1996; Seery et al., 2007; Yairi & Ambrose, 2005). Others posit that children who stutter are more likely to be raised in families that are more pressured, less harmonious, and more socially withdrawn than those of children who do not stutter. Also, it is possible that characteristics of temperament interact with language ability and other aspects of communication, emotions, heredity, and environmental experiences to predispose, precipitate, or perpetuate stuttering (Seery et al., 2007; Yairi, 1997; Yairi & Ambrose, 2005). Expansions of our understanding of how such potential causal elements interact may lead to a better understanding of stuttering in terms of prevention, assessment, diagnosis, interpretation, and alleviation—and, at least as important, a better understanding of people who stutter.

Do children who stutter show a different pattern of speech development?

Interest in the relationship between stuttering and speech sound production has been increasing due to at least three observations: frequent co-occurrence of articulation/

phonological disorder and early stuttering, influence of specific speech sounds on the location of stuttering, and possible impact of central speech planning of sounds on the occurrence of stuttering (Paden, 2005). As noted previously, stuttering onset usually occurs during the third year (i.e., between ages 2 years and 4 years), coinciding with rapid and complex physical, motor, cognitive, and linguistic (including phonological) development. Prevalence figures for co-occurrence of stuttering and speech sound disorders vary: 15% to 50% (Bloodstein & Bernstein Ratner, 2008), 32% (Arndt & Healey, 2001), 30% to 40% (Cantwell & Baker, 1985; Wolk, Edwards, & Conture, 1993; Yaruss, LaSalle, & Conture, 1998), and 45% (Blood, Ridenour, Qualls, & Hammer, 2003). The variance in these figures can be attributed to differences within and across investigations (e.g., sample size, age and gender distribution of the participants, procedures and test materials, definition of stuttering and articulation or phonological disorder). Importantly, however, estimates for co-occurrence of stuttering and phonological disorders among young children vary (usually between 30% and 35%), whereas expected incidence of phonological disorders in the general population is between 2% and 6%. Clearly a larger percentage of children who stutter have speech sound production errors, and phonological impairment is the most common coexisting speech problem among children who stutter (Paden, 2005).

Paden (2005) also highlighted previous research related to phonology and stuttering: Studies of adults who stutter revealed that consonants are implicated more often than vowels. However, phonetic attributes (i.e., consonants or vowels) are only one factor that influences the location of stuttering. Other factors are word position (earlier in sentence), grammar (content rather than function words), and syntax (syntactic elements and complex structures). Among children, phonological difficulty did not influence occurrence of stuttering; severity of stuttering did not change the types of articulation errors observed. However, those who stutter more severely did have more sound production errors than those who stutter less severely. The most common phonological error pattern for children who stutter and for those who do not stutter is cluster reduction. Children who stutter tend to progress more slowly in phonological acquisition than those who do not stutter; also, children whose stuttering persisted progressed more slowly than children whose stuttering recovered. Children whose stuttering persisted were also significantly poorer in phonological acquisition than children who did not stutter. There were no differences in the order of mastery of phonological targets among children whose stuttering persisted, those whose stuttering recovered, and children who did not stutter. Therefore, phonological acquisition alone is not sufficient for distinguishing between children who stutter and those who do not stutter or for predicting the course of stuttering (natural recovery or persistence).

Paden (2005, pp. 229–230) offered a series of interpretations about the co-occurrence of phonological involvement and stuttering among children who stutter. Shortly after onset, children who stutter lag behind in phonological development (order of mastery of phonemic targets and word-formation strategies). The phonological development of children whose stuttering persists lags behind that of children whose stuttering naturally recovers; this delay tends to disappear within 2 years after stuttering onset. Despite the delay observed, phonological development alone is insufficient to predict the course of stuttering. The phonological development of children who stutter and those who do not is similar (i.e., the difference is one of delay, not deviance or disorder).

Do children who stutter show a different pattern of language development?

Researchers have long maintained that children who stutter are slower at developing language and have more language learning impairments than children who do not stutter

(Bloodstein & Bernstein Ratner, 2008; R. V. Watkins, 2005). Current investigations continue to maintain such perspectives (Arndt & Healey, 2001; Wingate, 2001). Most early investigations were conducted using a variety of standardized tests to compare the language abilities of children who stutter with those who do not (G. Andrews et al., 1983; Bernstein Ratner, 1997; Guyette & Baumgartner, 1988; Wingate, 1983). More recently, surveys of speech–language pathologists have indicated high levels of co-occurrence of speech–language disorders among children who stutter. Arndt and Healey (2001) reported that 44% of the children on speech–language caseloads had concomitant language or phonological problems requiring clinical attention. Similarly, Blood, Ridenour, Qualls, and Hammer (2003) reported that approximately one third of the children receiving clinical service for stuttering also demonstrated receptive or expressive language problems, including ones relating to syntax, semantics, and pragmatics.

As noted, there is increasing empirical interest in the relationship between stuttering and speech sound production. Similarly, the literature reveals increasing empirical interest in the relationship between stuttering and linguistic variables. Interest in the nature of this relationship is being fueled by the predictable impact of grammatical complexity and language planning or production processes on the location of stuttering. For example, young children are more likely to stutter in sentences that are more grammatically complex than in sentences that are less grammatically complex (Logan & Conture, 1995; Yaruss, 1999b). Evidence from investigations with adults who stutter indicates that grammatical form class impacts the location of stuttering as well; stuttering was observed more frequently on content words (nouns and verbs) than on function words (prepositions and pronouns). More recently, however, the grammatical form class (content–function variable) is being viewed as less relevant to stuttering. Current thinking suggests that stuttering is more likely on either a content word or a phrase-initial function word that precedes a content word than in other phrase locations (R. V. Watkins, 2005).

In contrast to previous investigations, nearly all of which utilized standardized tests, the University of Illinois Stuttering Research Program used spontaneous language samples to assess the relationship between stuttering and linguistic variables in young children who stutter (R. V. Watkins, 2005). These children were identified as close to stuttering onset as possible and monitored longitudinally for several years to distinguish between those whose stuttering naturally recovered and those whose stuttering persisted. To enable comparison with previous investigations, the researcher also administered sections of the *Preschool Language Scale* (PLS; Zimmerman, Steiner, & Pond, 1979), which addresses language/auditory comprehension and expressive language abilities. The language comprehension and expression of children who stutter (both recovering and persistent), close to onset of stuttering and during the two subsequent visits (1 year and 2 years post-onset), was found to be well above average. However, the PLS scores for both groups of children dropped in the third visit (i.e., 2 years post-onset), approaching the test average; the scores for the persistent group were slightly lower than those of the recovered group. Importantly, however, both groups of children who stutter demonstrated advanced language abilities; the clinical utility of the potential gap between the persistent and recovered group cannot be determined because of the global nature of the PLS. Subsequently, the Illinois researchers analyzed the children's spontaneous 1,000-word samples and compared them to normative expectations for mean length of utterance (an index of grammatical ability), number of different words (an index of vocabulary skills), and developmental sentence score (an index of grammatical ability). As a group, again, the children who stutter performed at or above normative expectations for expressive language skills. Further, there was no difference in expressive language abilities at the time of stuttering onset between children whose stuttering persisted and those whose stuttering recovered. The young children who stutter, contrary to previous reports, were found to be capable language users.

Other investigations have yielded the finding that the receptive and expressive language abilities of young children who stutter are at or above normative expectations, in both English-speaking (J. D. Anderson & Conture, 2000; Miles & Bernstein Ratner, 2001; Nippold, 1990; S. W. Silverman & Bernstein Ratner, 2002; R. V. Watkins, Yairi, & Ambrose, 1999) and German-speaking (Hage, 2001; Rommel, Hage, Kalehne, & Johannsen, 2000) communities. Subsequent analyses of a subset of children in the Illinois studies revealed that language proficiency was maintained over time and the course of stuttering history. Also, the children whose stuttering recovered tended to decelerate in expressive language production over time. R. V. Watkins (2005) clarified that the children did not demonstrate language difficulty. Rather, they began to use sentences of average length and a diversity of vocabulary that would be expected for other children of the same chronological age. Children whose stuttering persisted maintained higher than expected expressive language over time. Similar findings were indicated among German-speaking children (Hage, 2001).

It is challenging to propose summary statements about the relationship between linguistic factors and stuttering. Indeed, it is easier to describe evidence of this relationship than to explain it. We cannot say that language development among children who stutter is vulnerable. The frequently cited figures of co-occurrence might be an artifact of the standardized instruments used, methodological issues, differences in the experimental participants (e.g., age, socioeconomic status, life experiences, general exposure), and the relative time post-onset of stuttering. R. V. Watkins (2005) clarified that studies of language ability close to stuttering onset and those of language ability after stuttering has developed are asking different questions; the different results may be attributable to different pathways of language acquisition or adaptations in expressive language to reduce stuttering events, both of which could predict a less favorable expressive language performance for children who stutter. It does seem, however, that early advanced language abilities may be a risk factor for stuttering or, according to R. V. Watkins (2005), may be a by-product of some other risk factor (e.g., perhaps advanced language development in one domain, such as syntax or semantics, creates difficulty with fluency when ability in other domains, such as motor abilities, is less advanced).

In summary, the Illinois studies reveal that linguistic strength often coexists with speech production challenges within young children, that both children whose stuttering persisted and those whose stuttering recovered demonstrated expressive language abilities at or above normative expectations, that expressive language abilities tend to reduce toward average as a child's stuttering recovers, and that language ability alone is not sufficient to predict the future course of stuttering. R. V. Watkins (2005) emphasized that many young children seem to have language abilities that exceed their abilities for fluent speech production and that the hypothesis that sophistication in one developmental area (e.g., language) is gained at the expense of facility in another development area (e.g., motor control) must be systematically evaluated. Furthermore, she argued against limiting or artificially manipulating language that is provided to preschool children and emphasized the importance of including language development in investigations of children who stutter and considering the role that advanced expressive language abilities may play in the onset and early development of stuttering. Ongoing research is exploring the possibility of a trade-off of linguistic resources (i.e., advanced language at the expense of speech motor skill) that might contribute to the risk of persistent stuttering (Anderson et al., 2005; Seery et al., 2007; R. V. Watkins, 2005; R. V. Watkins et al., 1999; Yairi, 2007; Yairi & Ambrose, 2005). Insights from ongoing and future investigations into child language and stuttering may illuminate different pathways for early childhood stuttering and may provide useful directions for understanding stuttering and its subtypes.

Is the brain or central nervous system of people who stutter different from that of people who do not stutter?

Early records implicating the brain in patients with head injury date back to Egyptian texts of the 17th century B.C. Theories of the brain as the center of conscious experience and cognitive processing are attributed to Hippocrates in the 5th century B.C. (Guenther, 2008). In the 1860s, French neurologist Pierre Broca made the landmark discovery that damage to the left inferior frontal gyrus of the cerebral cortex, now known as Broca's area, results in severe deficits in language expression (loss of speech output, with relatively spared ability to perceive speech), or Broca's aphasia. In another landmark discovery a decade later, German neurologist Carl Wernicke found that damage to the posterior superior temporal gyrus of the left cerebral hemisphere, now known as Wernicke's area, results in an inability to comprehend spoken language (with relatively intact, albeit nonsensical, speech output), or Wernicke's aphasia.

More recently, the brain has been implicated in stuttering. In the 1920s, the cerebral dominance theory of Sam Orton and Lee Travis, which will be reviewed in Chapter 3, indicated that stuttering results from the brain's failure to achieve lateral dominance of the speech centers and handedness. Early studies using electroencephalography (EEG) indicated that people who stutter tend to have more activity on the right side of the brain during speech, particularly during stuttered speech, than people who do not stutter. Also, people who stutter tend to have more right-hemisphere dominance for speech and language, while the general population tends to have more left-hemisphere dominance for speech and language. In addition to shedding light on the origins of stuttering, EEG studies have suggested that hemispheric lateralization in people who stutter is malleable and impacted by treatment. Various studies have shown that right-handed adults who stutter can demonstrate a shift from a relatively high degree of right-hemisphere brain activity during speech to relatively high degree of left-hemisphere activity during speech as a consequence of treatment (Boberg, Yeudall, Schopflocher, & Bo-Lassen, 1983; Guitar, 2006; Ingham, Cykowski, Ingham, & Fox, 2008; W. H. Moore, 1984). Guitar (2006) indicated that this apparent shift in brain activity could also be attributable to a reduction in negative, right-hemisphere emotions after treatment, which could lessen the relative amount of right-hemisphere activity.

A more recent technology, the measurement of cerebral blood flow (CBF), indicates a greater degree of brain activity, or neuronal firing, with increases in the blood supply to the brain in a given time period. An increasingly sophisticated line of radioactive tracers has been injected into the bloodstream of people who stutter, with subsequent interpretation of the amount of radioactivity emitted. Early CBF studies showed that a greater degree of right-hemisphere activity shifted to the left hemisphere after injection of haloperidol (Wood, Stump, McKeehan, Sheldon, & Proctor, 1980) and less left-hemisphere dominance (i.e., reduction in cerebral blood flow in left superior and middle temporal gyri) among people who stutter for motor initiation and speech motor control (Pool, Devous, Freeman, Watson, & Finitzo, 1991). The Pool et al. study utilized single photon emission computed tomography (SPECT), a relatively new form of technology at the time that had significant resolution limitations.

Improvements in technology have led to better understanding of the brain function of people who stutter. Imaging improved with the advent of positive emission tomography (PET; i.e., injecting tracers into the arterial bloodstream and then recording their flow throughout the brain) and with functional magnetic resonance imaging (fMRI), magnetoencephalography (MEG) recording, and transcranial magnetic stimulation (TMS). As summarized by Ingham et al. (2008), findings revealed functional differences among people who stutter during stuttered speech, including overactivation in the right frontal operculum, right anterior insula, and supplementary motor area, and deactivation in the bilateral auditory association areas and left putamen. Structural differences in the cerebral anatomy of people who stutter include "(1) a loss, reversal, or reduction of asymmetry between cerebral areas long known to exhibit structural asymmetry in normal populations, (2) aberrant features of white matter tract connectivity and tract size, and (3) abnormal patterns of perisylvian cortical folding including aberrant sulcal patterns and increased gyrification" (p. 63).

Yet another potential difference being studied in the brains of people who stutter is neurochemical. Dopamine is an important neurotransmitter that plays a critical role in motor functioning, including fluent speech. Even a slight imbalance in neurotransmission, as demonstrated by the influence of different neuropharmacological agents (i.e., prescription medications; see Remington & Fagan, 2007, for a review of drug-induced stuttering), can disrupt the fluency of both people who stutter and those who do not stutter. There is evidence to suggest a hyperdopaminergic state (i.e., a greater level or uptake of dopamine activity) in the brains of people who stutter. Haloperidol, a medication used to suppress the symptoms of Tourette syndrome (see Chapter 4), has been found to improve the fluency of people who stutter by serving as a dopamine antagonist (i.e., slowing or normalizing the neurotransmission or uptake of dopamine). However, its possible side effects (e.g., drowsiness, sexual dysfunction, excess limb movement, risk of a permanent neurologically based movement disorder—tardive dyskinesia) contraindicate its use as an intervention for stuttering. Guitar (2006) reported that haloperidol reduced the tension in his own stuttering, "allowing the blocks to seemingly melt in my mouth" (p. 427), but that the side effects, including always being on the verge of falling asleep and wiggling his legs uncontrollably, were hard to bear. Medications with the same purpose and function as haloperidol, with similar side effects, are risperidone and pimozide. More recent studies with improved controls are looking at other medications that reduce the uptake of dopamine (e.g., olanzapine, pagoclone; Maguire, 2007; Maguire, Franklin, et al., 2010; Maguire, Riley, Franklin, & Gumusaneli, 2010; Maguire et al., 2004), thus reducing stuttering behavior, with fewer side effects (Ingham, 2010, challenged the methodology and results of the Maguire, Franklin, et al., 2010, randomized clinical trial for pagoclone). Other medications (e.g., theophylline; Movsessian, 2005) have increased the level of dopamine release in the brains of people who stutter, thus increasing stuttering behavior. While controlled studies of neuropharmacological intervention for stuttering are ongoing (e.g., Bothe, Davidow, Bramlett, & Ingham, 2006; Stager et al., 2005; see Saxon & Ludlow, 2007, for a critical review of neuropharmacological intervention for stuttering), neurological structures being implicated by alterations in dopamine neurotransmission include Broca's area, Wernicke's area, insula, amygdala, and basal ganglia, among others.

The preponderance of neuroanatomical research has been conducted on adult males who stutter (e.g., Braun et al., 1997; Brown, Ingham, Ingham, Laird, & Fox, 2005; Cykowski et al., 2007; De Nil & Kroll, 2001; Foundas, Bollich, Corey, Hurley, & Heilman, 2001; Fox et al., 1996; Giraud et al., 2008; Ingham, 2001; Jancke, Hanggi, & Steinmetz, 2004; Neumann et al., 2003; G. M. Schulz, Varga, Jeffres, Ludlow, & Braun, 2005; Sommer, Koch, Paulus, Weiller, & Buchel, 2002; K. E. Watkins, Smith, Davis, & Howell, 2008). Subsequent neuroanatomical research should include children who stutter (Chang, Erickson, Ambrose, Hasegawa-Johnson, & Ludlow, 2008), as well as adult females who stutter and people who have recovered from stuttering (Ingham, Ingham, Finn, & Fox, 2003).

Variability and Predictability of Stuttering

What commonalities are there among people who stutter?

Several patterns are generally characteristic of people who stutter, including anticipation, consistency, and adaptation; certain language traits; and fluency inducing conditions and fluency inhibiting conditions.

First, people who stutter predict with accuracy the words on which they will stutter (*anticipation*) and, upon repeated readings of the same passage, tend to stutter on the same words each time (*consistency*), yet demonstrate a decrease in the overall frequency of stuttering across the passage (*adaptation*) (Bloodstein & Bernstein Ratner, 2008; Guitar, 2006). Bloodstein and Bernstein Ratner referred to the conditions under which stuttering diminishes (e.g., adaptation, response-contingent stimulation, white noise and other forms of altered auditory feedback) as "controversial phenomena" (p. 283). Of these conditions, we will address only adaptation. Bloodstein and Bernstein Ratner noted that the rate of adaptation decreases as the time interval between successive readings increases, that passage length does not seem to impact adaptation, that there is little transfer of adaptation to readings of different material, and that adaptation is found among both children and adults who stutter, yet to individually varying degrees (i.e., some show a high degree of adaptation, some show a small degree of adaptation, and some show increased stuttering with repeated readings). The evidence seems to support the association between less severe stuttering and a greater tendency to adapt (Bloodstein & Bernstein Ratner, 2008).

Second, certain language-related factors are predictable. Most adults who stutter do so more frequently on consonants; on sounds in the word-initial position; in contextual speech (vs. isolated words); on content words (i.e., nouns, verbs, adjectives, and adverbs, as opposed to function words, such as articles, prepositions, pronouns, and conjunctions); on longer words; on words of greater uncertainty; on words at the beginnings of sentences; and on stressed syllables. School-age children who stutter tend to follow the same predictable language-related patterns as adults. Preschool children have been found to follow a distinctly different pattern. They tend to stutter on pronouns and conjunctions, rather than on nouns, verbs, adjectives, and adverbs. Their forms of disfluency tend to involve repetitions of parts of words and monosyllabic words at the beginning of the sentence, rather than repetitions, prolongation, or blocking of sounds at the beginning of words (Bloodstein & Bernstein Ratner, 2008; Guitar, 2006). Yairi and Ambrose (2005), however, reported on the basis of longitudinal investigations that forms of disfluency vary among young children shortly after stuttering onset. Young children may demonstrate the predictable repetitions of initial syllables and short words, but they may also present with sound prolongations and articulatory fixations with visible tension and awareness, which are typically interpreted as characteristics of advanced or chronic stuttering.

Third, several fluency inducing conditions have been identified. Stuttering is immediately eliminated in choral, lipped, prolonged, or rhythmic speech, as well as during shadowing, singing, and instructions to slow down. Stuttering is more gradually eliminated by response-contingent stimulation. Immediate reduction of stuttering is observed when the person who stutters speaks alone (when no other person is present) or with rhythmic movement, delayed auditory feedback, masking, change in pitch, or whispering. More gradual reduction of stuttering results from haloperidol, EMG feedback from speech muscles, and adaptation (reduction in baseline stuttering upon repeated reading of the same material). Other conditions that markedly reduce or eliminate stuttering include speaking when relaxed, to an animal or an infant, in a dialect, or while simultaneously writing, swearing, or receiving reinforcement for fluent speech (Bloodstein & Bernstein Ratner, 2008; Guitar, 2006). In general, stuttering is temporarily reduced when one is speaking in a nonhabitual or novel manner, including altered speaking rate, pitch, voice quality, accent, intonation, and vowel duration; and when one is using conversational interjections, nonverbal movements, and deliberate impersonations (F. H. Silverman, 2004).

Fluency inhibiting conditions, in which a temporary increase of stuttering is observed, include (with some reported variation) speaking on the telephone, saying one's name, telling jokes, repeating a message that was not understood, waiting to respond, speaking to authority figures, speaking to a relatively large audience, and attempting to conceal stuttering, among others (F. H. Silverman, 2004; Van Riper, 1982; Young, 1985). These patterns of variability and predictability are critical in the differential diagnosis of stuttering from other disorders of fluency, which will be reviewed in Chapter 4.

Patterns that characterize stuttering have been used by speech–language pathologists to verify whether a person really has a fluency disorder or is malingering (Bloodstein, 1988; Shirkey, 1987). For example, Shirkey was asked to verify the stuttering of a 33-year-old man accused of a series of sexual assaults on young girls and one woman. In a previous trial, he was acquitted based on observations that he was a person who stutters and that none of the victims reported that the attacker stuttered. In order to determine the veracity of the suspect's stuttering during interrogation, Shirkey analyzed his communication-related attitudes and speech fluency patterns during conversation and reading, observing adaptation and consistency effects. While most of the suspect's patterns were typical of stuttering, exceptional, if not contrary, observations included appropriate vowels during syllabic repetitions, inability to speak fluently using a rhythmic speaking pattern and external stimulus, and increased frequency of stuttering during prolonged speech and simple linguistic tasks. Shirkey concluded that the suspect's stuttering was legitimate, yet with significant, but not atypical, variability. Partly on the basis of that variability (that the suspect could have spoken fluently at the scene of the crime), the suspect was convicted and sentenced to 101 years in prison.

Bloodstein (1988) was asked to verify the stuttering of a suspect in his 30s accused of armed robbery whose defense was that, as a person who stutters, he could not have said fluently, "This is a stickup. Get down on the floor and don't make a move or I'll blow your head off." Bloodstein analyzed the suspect's feelings and attitudes in addition to anticipation, adaptation, consistency, and adjacency effects; loci of stuttering; and effect of masking noise and contingent stimuli. Bloodstein concluded that the suspect's stuttering was legitimate, thus contributing to testimony leading to an anticipated acquittal. Both Shirkey (1987) and Bloodstein (1988) raised important questions regarding our profession's ability to diagnose malingering in stuttering and encouraged research efforts to improve current methods. Fake stuttering (pseudostuttering), notably, is a deliberate component of treatment programs (Van Riper, 1973); it has also been used by political prisoners during interrogations (more processing time enables prisoners to prevent contradictions and minimize information given) (Lew, 1995).

Treatment of Stuttering

What does the clinical literature tell us about designing effective treatment?

Few topics have garnered more attention in the allied health-care professions since publication of the first edition of this book than evidence-based practice (Bernstein Ratner,

2005a, 2006; Bothe, Ingham, & Ingham, 2010; Dollaghan, 2004; Ferguson, 2008; Fey & Justice, 2007; C. J. Johnson, 2006; Kamhi, 2006; Kent, 2006; Manning, 2006; Meline, 2006; Pietranton, 2006; Plante, 2004; Robey, 2004; St. Louis, 2006; Yaruss, 1998, 2001; Yaruss & Pelczarski, 2007; Yaruss & Quesal, 2004a). *Evidence-based practice* refers, in short, to "combining research and reason to make treatment decisions" (Kamhi, 2006, p. 255). One might ask why such an explicit focus should be necessary within a helping profession that is guided by a cogent Code of Ethics (ASHA, 2010), Scope of Practice (ASHA, 2007d), and Preferred Practice Patterns for the Profession of Speech–Language Pathology (ASHA, 2004c). The answer has to do with the reality that, despite a commitment to hold paramount the welfare of people we serve professionally, some clinicians use treatments that are outdated, unsupported by well-designed clinical research, or untested on sufficient numbers of individuals (ASHA, 2004a, 2005b; Bloodstein & Bernstein Ratner, 2008). Yet, we must remember that it is possible—and essential—to be both data based and clinically creative, theory driven and person centered, externally valid and internally consistent, grounded and aspiring, concrete and personally relevant. Manning (2001) underscored the degree to which ours is a profession not of science *or* art, but rather science *and* art:

> Waiting to make clinical or even scientific decisions until we can base all of our choices on satisfactory empirical evidence would result in, at the most, clinical gridlock and, at the least, a lack of spontaneity and creativity during the process of treatment. . . . There is a tendency for social scientists to rely on investigative models used in the "hard" sciences, a strategy that often works well. It can also result in investigative strategies that study a phenomenon one variable at a time and a gross oversimplification of human behavior. Effective clinicians must do more than that as they attend to many variables and help a person change with the context of their world. Furthermore, clinical decisions are made in real-time, often without all of the information we would like to have. . . . Plainly, there is no excuse for failing to base clinical decisions on good data or documenting the efficacy of our investigation. On the other hand, much of what experienced, wise, and effective clinicians do has a great deal to do with artistry. What takes place during treatment is considerably more complex than what can be accepted in the laboratory. . . . The treatment of fluency disorders should be challenging and fun. It should also be exciting, for to the degree that we as clinicians enter the process, model the behavior we want to change, take risks with our clients, and even experience setbacks with them, we grow as well. (p. xx)

More recently, Manning (2006) cautioned that we should not unduly restrict treatment goals in compliance with a narrow view of evidence-based practice:

> I believe that effective treatment is about far more than decreasing the number of times that someone stutters. Successful therapy is also closely tied to the quality of stuttering, the quality of fluency, and the speaker's ability to communicate and problem solve. Successful therapy also has to do with being able to live a life that is unrestricted, even if it occasionally involves stuttering. As it turns out, many people who stutter can become better communicators than nonstuttering adults. (p. 128)

Similarly, Manning (2006) noted that the standardization associated with treatment efficacy can inhibit best practice:

> It is good for us to be able to demonstrate that what we do when we try to help people really does work (see Guidelines for Practice in Stuttering Treatment, ASHA, 1995). But in order to do efficacy research, things must be controlled and variables must be standardized. I would argue, however, that the very act of such control and standardization makes therapy, especially stuttering therapy, less effective. The less spontaneous, dynamic, and evolving the relationship is, the less effective the therapy is likely to be.

If we package the therapy into a protocol or manual that follows a prescribed sequence for each person, the flow of therapy is likely to be grotesquely distorted. Standardizing a treatment may make it easier to "teach" and easier to evaluate statistically to justify support from agencies who are paying for therapy. But it does not make it better. (Manning, 2006, pp. 137–138)

Fey and Justice (2007) discussed the importance of making informed clinical decisions on the basis of at least three sources of evidence: external evidence from published research; internal evidence from careful evaluation of client and family characteristics, their willingness to participate, and their preferences; and internal evidence from examination of clinician preferences, professional competencies and values, and workplace values, policies, and culture. These sources suggest six steps for making intervention decisions that are well grounded in evidence-based practice:

1. Develop a four-part clinical question that focuses on the client and family, the intervention being considered, comparisons with other treatments, and desired outcomes (i.e., PICO, P = patient/patient group or problem, I = intervention being considered, C = comparison treatment, O = desired outcome).

2. Find the internal evidence that pertains to the question (e.g., attending to client/family values, desires, circumstances; clinician knowledge about the disorder and the client; and clinician experience and theoretical knowledge).

3. Find the external or published research evidence.

4. Critically evaluate the external evidence on the basis of relevance to the clinical question being asked and levels of evidence (from most to least credible, these are randomized controlled trials with consistent study outcomes, a single randomized control trial with a narrow confidence interval, non-randomized quasi-experimental trials or single-subject experiments that document consistent study outcomes, studies of multiple individuals who receive the same treatment, single case studies, and expert opinion).

5. Integrate the internal and external evidence.

6. Make the clinical decision by applying the evidence, and evaluate the outcome of the decision.

Fey and Justice (2007) advised clinicians not to view evidence-based practice as limiting or restrictive. Rather, they acknowledged that the evidence to support our clinical decisions is often unavailable, requiring us to make decisions based upon a comprehensive understanding of relevant theory and basic research and careful attention to internal evidence. New clinical ideas often follow such careful examination. Evidence-based practice does require clinicians to examine their approaches and to distinguish between those for which we do have, and those for which we do not have, evidence grounded in clinical studies. In general, clinicians need to be constructively skeptical about the practices we use and to be vigilant in seeking evidence in the literature and monitoring the outcomes of their interventions.

Bernstein Ratner (2006) similarly argued that clinical skills must grow with the application of currently available data, not just from personal, educational, and clinical experience. Also, clinicians must consistently seek new information to improve therapeutic effectiveness:

To this end, clinicians must be data seekers, data integrators, and critical evaluators of the application of new knowledge to clinical cases. Thus, even if something appears to work, new information may assist the therapeutic process to work better. We cannot afford, and our clients cannot afford, for therapy to be less efficient or effective than it might be given the state of research available to us. (pp. 257–258)

Kent (2006) reminded clinicians that a commitment to the clinical endeavor requires a commitment to current best evidence, clinical expertise, and client values:

> Clinical experience, like client values, needs to be considered seriously. . . . In my view, theory is highly important, and it is unfortunate that research evidence is sometimes construed as theory neutral or theory irrelevant. Research is rarely theoretically neutral, given that theory is important to connect facts and to formulate testable hypotheses. Theory is a compass that directs research efforts in promising directions, and it is critical for the synthesis of the components of all research, including clinical research. Moreover, theory is critical to clinical practice, right down to the level of the individual client. . . . The practitioner who is armed with research evidence, clinical experience, and an awareness of consumer values probably operates with a theory that integrates the various sources of information into a best understanding of the disorder and its management. . . . To be sure, some individual clinicians will be better than others in virtually all specialties, but this admission does not release us from the obligation to identify assessments and interventions that meet rigorous standards of benefit to our consumers. One of the desired outcomes of EBP is that continuing professional education will be increasingly founded on research evidence, which will enhance the accountability of clinical services. . . . In preparing clinicians, academic programs must do what they have always done—provide the knowledge base and develop the interpersonal skills that enable the clinician to work effectively with an ever-changing group of clients in an ever-changing world of clinical service economics. (p. 269)

Fey (2006) noted that evidence-based practice involves more than research-based evidence: "I would argue that clinicians who fail to consider client and clinician factors and attend only to research-based evidence are not doing EBP" (p. 318). Fey also stressed the importance of "evaluating internal evidence and merging it with evidence from research" (p. 318).

Bloodstein and Bernstein Ratner (2008, pp. 338–343) presented 12 specific criteria for successful treatment:

1. The method must be shown to be effective with an ample and representative group of people who stutter (i.e., focus is on measured change, based upon predetermined criteria; e.g., 70%, 80%, or 90% reduction in stuttered behavior compared to pretreatment, or posttreatment stuttering levels below 5%).

2. Results must be demonstrated by objective measures of speech and nonspeech behavior, such as frequency of stuttering or rate of speech (i.e., before, during, and after treatment, rated by judges other than the clinician/experimenter).

3. Reports of success must be based on repeated evaluations and adequate samples of speech (i.e., measurement in the clinic immediately following treatment is not sufficient; repeated pretreatment measures are recommended for comparison).

4. Improvement must be shown to carry over to speaking situations outside the clinic (i.e., audio or video recordings made before and after treatment may not represent transfer and maintenance over time and place).

5. Stability of results must be demonstrated by long-term follow-up (i.e., 18 months to 2 years in novel settings and with unfamiliar people; measurement in the clinic with familiar clinicians often is invalid).

6. Control groups or conditions must be used to show that reductions in stuttering are due to treatment (i.e., natural fluctuation and spontaneous recovery are not reflections of treatment; control conditions, such as a waitlist or alternative interventions, are necessary to identify a positive treatment effect).

7. The speech must sound natural and spontaneous to listeners (i.e., large reduction in stuttering severity is insufficient unless accompanied by speech naturalness).

8. Clients must be free from the necessity to monitor their speech (i.e., reduction in severity is insufficient unless paired with reduced attention to maintain it).

9. Treatment must reduce not only stuttering behaviors, but related thoughts and feelings as well (i.e., measurement must address behaviors, thoughts, and feelings).

10. Success of a program must not be inflated by ignoring dropouts (i.e., outcome data based only on participants who complete the program artificially inflate the program's success; clients who discontinue treatment for unavoidable reasons should be distinguished from those who did not achieve the target objectives).

11. The method must be effective when used by any qualified clinician (i.e., a large and diverse pool of clinicians must administer the treatment).

12. The method must be successful over time (i.e., effectiveness must withstand the test of time as the program matures and its novelty subsides).

Using a preliminary version of these criteria, Bloodstein (1981) proposed that only prolonged speech and precision fluency shaping produce significant long-term benefits. Attitude therapy, rhythmic speech, and airflow therapy were found to be of some benefit, but to a lesser degree. Hours of therapy correlated positively with treatment outcome (G. Andrews et al., 1983; G. Andrews, Guitar, & Howie, 1980). More recently, however, Yairi and Ambrose (2005) concluded, "There are no current, comprehensive, widely accepted theories of stuttering that provide clinicians with basic understanding of why they do what they do in therapy in light of the nature of the disorder" (p. 403). They also stated that clinical efficacy research in stuttering does not yet permit scientifically based endorsement of specific clinical methods. Similarly, discussing the limitations of current theories as sources of treatment, Onslow (2004) advised (somewhat provocatively), "Do not do any therapy that is based on a theory of stuttering (at least not just now)" (p. 10). Onslow (2004) directed clinicians to base treatment on scientific research and to use only evidence-based treatment practices. Given the evolving nature of our scientific basis and the challenge facing every clinician to identify those behaviors that are both internally relevant to the communicator and externally measurable, Yairi and Ambrose (2005) wrote, "We advocate the view that treatment of stuttering should be theory-driven, reflecting the clinician's beliefs about the nature of the disorder, with clear understanding of why specific procedures are applied and a clear rationale for sensible alternatives" (p. 401). This conclusion seems to represent the current state of thinking for the clinician working with people who stutter.

In summary, evidence-based practice is about using the best available information and resources to enable people to realize their own potential. It is about doing all we can to identify those outcomes that are most meaningful to each individual and to identify the most effective elements of treatment. Yet, as we become increasingly comfortable with evidence as the basis of practice, we must make sure that the person we are serving is not moved to the background as evidence is moved to the foreground. Let us always keep the person we are serving in the foreground, without distraction or compromise. Evidence emphasizes the known and the knowable; this is important. Evidence, however, fails to reckon with the unknown, that which approaches, or more likely exceeds if not transcends, the limits of science and what is known about the human condition. The fact remains that some successes are not predictable on the basis of the evidence. Other successes are not reflected by the evidence being collected. Consider the following account.

Five years ago, Natalie, my family's friend and my wife's colleague, was in a serious car accident (Cool, 2005; Elders, 2006; Reinhardt, 2005). Comatose, with numerous broken bones, traumatic brain injury, and a damaged brain stem, Natalie faced a grim prognosis. Her family was told by the physicians that her chances of coming out of the coma were about 1 in 1 million. Should she ever wake up, they were told, she would be severely disabled and unable to function independently. Medical science had reached its limit. Natalie's family is prayerful; their source of support, the way they view the world, their personal construct, is one of faith. Natalie had been on life support for 8 days. On Good Friday, the family was told that they would need to face the decision to remove life support after Easter. I remember; I was among the friends assembled at the hospital. Defying the evidence, Natalie awoke on Easter Sunday. Following physical, occupational, and speech therapy, Natalie left the hospital to return home, not after 18 months, as predicted, but 2 months after her accident. Having relearned to walk, talk, eat, and more, Natalie returned to work 8 months after the accident. The physician was quoted as saying, "I believe that a higher power was looking out for her, because I never would have predicted that she'd walk or talk again." Another physician described her as "an Easter miracle." That Easter miracle has shared her story with my graduate seminar on professional issues on several occasions. She chronicled her recovery, sources of support, and her inner strength. She recalled when she was in the earliest stage of rehabilitation, in bed and unable to communicate. Her medical folder was left on her lap, where she could read but not react to the words "lost cause." There are times when, despite the most scientific, controlled, and rigorous published evidence, one cannot know.

Consider also Jake and Jennifer. Both are college students who stutter, with whom I am currently working. Jake had five previous unsuccessful treatments, failed out of a major university due to events related to his stuttering, and has coexisting psychiatric challenges. Jennifer never had treatment previously and defined herself on the basis of her stuttering. Treatment includes documentation of changes in the affective, behavioral, and cognitive domains, as outlined in Chapters 7 and 10. Nevertheless, I question if those data, or any data, can fully reflect the spirit or implications of the change process. Do they reflect the human phenomenon of courage, what it takes to stand up after failed treatment and to try yet again, or to risk vulnerability and embarrassment when seeking a trusted clinician? Do the data collected, while reflecting remarkable commitment and successful use of fluency facilitating controls, reflect the spirit behind Jake's words? He said, "Now that I am experiencing fluency success, I am more outgoing, ask questions in class, raise my hand to volunteer an answer, and talk with teachers. It improves your life; you're happier as a person. It enables me to do things I previously was not willing to do." Do the data reflect Jennifer's remarkable change as a communicator, that she is simply and elegantly using language for so many different purposes, where she previously would have remained silent? These are no small victories. As will be seen, both clients are beating the odds (i.e., negative prognostic indicators, reviewed in Chapter 10). The data, even the best data, may not capture the "*joie de vivre*" (Prutting, 1985, p. 6) that is at the essence of communication success.

Let's consider evidence a little further. Do the data necessarily reflect the process, or might the process occasionally transcend the data, so that the composite parts being measured, once reassembled, are qualitatively different from the integrated whole? Might the data emphasize what is done—the procedure—rather than how the procedure is delivered or is defined by the uniqueness of each clinician and each client? One of my colleagues in physical therapy shared with me her fear of the loss of human connectedness that our student clinicians might be learning as they blur the distinction between the person being served and the data being collected, or when they sit in front of computers and "communicate" virtually as if the computers were people. My colleague recalled a dying young woman in the Intensive Care Unit, where the woman was heavily monitored. Everyone was watching the monitors; no one was holding the woman's hand, making eye contact, or connecting with her in any way. My colleague also recalled a physical therapy student talking about having spent the previous 2 weeks working on a research paper at his computer. He offered no mention of patient contact, which he had also experienced over the previous 2 weeks, or growing as a clinician. Computers and research, for this student, were viewed as the heart of his preparation for becoming a physical therapist. Are there implications for professional preparation for speech–language pathology and, specifically, for stuttering intervention? A touch of a hand, a pat on the back, a wink of an eye, an irreplaceable smile; this is real communication. Do the data we collect and the evidence we assemble reflect communication at its essence? Do data and evidence appreciate communicators for what and who they genuinely are?

As we move through the 21st century—increasingly defined by technological developments and information advancement—one thing remains true: There simply is no replacement for direct person-to-person interaction. May we always retain life, wisdom, and knowledge as we go about our business with people who stutter and their families. The words of T. S. Eliot (1934, p. 179), from "Choruses from 'The Rock,'" ring prophetic, timeless, and essential to our roles as people, as communicators, and as servants of others:

> Where is the Life we have lost in living?
> Where is the wisdom we have lost in knowledge?
> Where is the knowledge we have lost in information?

Summary—The Nature of Stuttering

Traditionally, overt stuttering has been thought to include at least eight forms of disfluency: interjections, part-word repetitions, whole-word repetitions, phrase repetitions, revisions, incomplete phrases, broken words, and prolonged sounds. More recently, six types of disfluency have been used for assessment and diagnosis: stuttering-like disfluencies (part-word repetitions, single-syllable word repetitions, and disrhythmic phonations) and other disfluencies (interjections, multisyllable word and phrase repetitions, and revisions or abandoned utterances).

The majority of children who stutter begin stuttering between 2 and 4 years of age, often demonstrating more within-word disfluencies (e.g., sound or syllable repetitions, sound prolongations, broken words) than children who do not. Prevalence of stuttering is about 1%; incidence is about 5%. The ratio of males who stutter to females who stutter is approximately 3:1 (2:1 close to stuttering onset) and increases with age, although some cultural variation is reported. Girls appear to recover from stuttering more frequently and quickly than boys. Until recently, the environment of people who stutter was thought to be the same as that of those who do not, except that those who stutter have more relatives who stutter. However, recent longitudinal research suggests that physical or emotional stresses may play a role in stuttering onset, when combined with genetic predisposing factors. The contribution of genetics to the onset of stuttering is being studied by analyzing family trees, twin pairs, and adoptions. Genetic influences contribute as much as 70% to 85% of the likelihood that one will begin to stutter; the remainder of the variance (15%–30%) is attributable to environmental influences. Features of stuttering, both overt and covert, were reviewed. Compared to people who do not stutter, those who stutter demonstrate a small measured deficit on verbal and nonverbal tests of intelligence, a controversial finding that may be interpreted as a result of stuttering, rather than a cause of it. People who stutter do not demonstrate emotional maladjustment. One current line of research, however, is addressing relative temperament. Preliminary findings are tentative if not equivocal. It is possible that temperament interacts with language ability and other aspects of communication, emotion, heredity, and environment to predispose, precipitate, or perpetuate stuttering. Children who stutter tend to progress more slowly in phonological acquisition than those who do not stutter; children whose stuttering persists progress more slowly than children whose stuttering recovers. No difference was found in expressive language abilities at the time of stuttering onset between children whose stuttering persisted and those whose stuttering recovered. Young children who stutter were found to be capable language users; in fact, often children who stutter were found to have receptive and expressive language skills at or above normative expectations. Neither phonological nor expressive language skills, however, are sufficient to predict the course of stuttering.

Both neurophysiological (i.e., overactivation in the right frontal operculum, right anterior insula, and supplementary motor area, and deactivation in the bilateral auditory association areas and left putamen) and neuroanatomical (i.e., patterns of cerebral asymmetry, connectivity and tract size, and cortical folding and gyrification) differences are being investigated among adults who stutter. Neurochemical differences are being investigated as well; preliminary findings are revealing a greater level or uptake of dopamine activity in the brains of adults who stutter. People who stutter demonstrate the effects of anticipation, consistency, and adaptation; specific influences of language on stuttering; and fluency inducing and fluency inhibiting conditions. The commonalities among people who stutter have been used for differential diagnosis. Finally, specific criteria and evidence-based procedures were discussed in relation to the designing of effective treatment.

Chapter Summary

Because assumptions about stuttering and people who stutter can affect the intervention process, clinicians must be aware explicitly of their assumptions and must understand how stuttering begins and develops, its nature, how it has been viewed historically, current theoretical explanations of its etiology, and other fluency disorders. This chapter provided an overview of the onset and development of stuttering (using both developmental classifications and longitudinal studies), risk factors to distinguish transient and chronic stuttering, the nature of stuttering, and what the clinical literature tells us about designing effective treatment.

While developmental classifications can be helpful in understanding how stuttering develops, clinicians must remember that each client is unique and should not and cannot be fit into rigid categories. Instead, these categories should be used as snapshots to which individual clients' experiences can be compared. The classification schemes of Bluemel, Froeschels, Van Riper, and Bloodstein were reviewed. Bluemel described stuttering as consisting of two stages, primary and secondary stuttering. Primary stuttering is characterized by easy, effortless, intermittent repetitions of the first word or syllable in a sentence; secondary stuttering is characterized by more obvious physical effort, use of starters and synonyms, attempts to conceal stuttering, and observed fears. Froeschels described a similar progression, but differentiated between easy syllable and sound repetitions (clonic types of stuttering) and more rapid, tense behaviors involving muscle tension, interrupted breathing, and facial tension (tonic types of stuttering).

Van Riper expanded Bluemel's classification system, adding two more categories. The most frequently occurring pattern of development is Track 1, characterized by gradual, inconsistent development of stuttering between the ages of 2.5 and 4.0 years, with long periods of remission. Typical behaviors include frequent gentle syllable repetitions on initial or function words. In Track 2, rate and frequency of repetitions increase and are accompanied by prolongations and pitch increases. Tension and frustration become evident, and word and situation fears develop. In Track 3, stuttering typically appears abruptly after a traumatic experience and develops steadily with few remissions. Tense, prolonged fixations, struggle, and breathing interruptions are common. In Track 4, stuttering appears suddenly after long periods of fluency. Repetition of whole words on first and content words is typical, with little observed fear or frustration.

Bloodstein proposed four phases of stuttering reflecting developmental points along a continuum. Phase 1 occurs typically between 2 and 6 years of age under conditions of stress or emotional arousal and is characterized by whole-word repetitions at the beginning of sentences, clauses, and phrases, as well as on content and function words. Phase 2 typically emerges during the elementary school years, where disfluency notably occurs on content words, becomes chronic, and affects how the child views himself as a communicator. Phase 3 is observed in late childhood or early adolescence, with disfluency typically linked to certain situations, words, or sounds. Circumlocutions and substitutions are observed; however, the person continues to speak freely. Finally, Phase 4 is seen in late adolescence or early adulthood and involves sound, word, and situation fears. Behaviors may include word substitution and situation avoidance, and fears and embarrassment become evident.

These conceptualizations of the onset and development of stuttering have been challenged by more recent longitudinal investigations conducted at the University of Illinois, which have revealed greater variability in the age, type and severity, and conditions at onset. Mean age at onset was 33 months (68% of the onsets occurred before age 3 years, 85% by 3.5 years, and 95% before 4 years). Stuttering onset was not found to be mild and gradual, in uneventful circumstances; rather, 30% of the children experienced sudden onsets within a single day and 40% within 3 days. Gradual onsets (i.e., more than 2 weeks) represented the smallest group (25%). At least half of the children experienced eventful circumstances (e.g., physical fatigue, emotional upset, language stress) shortly before onset. Symptoms near onset included articulatory fixations, multiple repetitions with tension, tense sound prolongations, silent blocks, respiratory irregularities, and visible facial, head, neck, or limb tension. This is in contrast to the earlier view, which postulated mild, easy repetitions nearly indistinguishable from normal fluency. Furthermore, children demonstrated awareness of their disrupted speech far sooner than had been assumed.

The Illinois studies also revealed that the majority of children who stutter peaked in severity within the first few weeks or months of onset, after which overt symptoms subsided (in contrast to the earlier view that stuttering tends to worsen over time). Natural recovery (i.e., recovery without treatment) occurred in 75% of the children within 4 years of onset. Those children who naturally recovered and maintained fluency for at least 6 to 10 months tended not to relapse. Natural recovery occurred more frequently and earlier among girls than among boys. Nevertheless, children whose stuttering persists represented the minority.

The Illinois studies also yielded valuable information in the form of primary, secondary, and other risk factors to distinguish transient and chronic stuttering. Primary factors include family history (i.e., children tend to follow the pattern of their family's history for persistence or recovery), gender (boys are at greater risk for stuttering incidence and persistence than girls), age at onset (persistence tends to be associated with later age of onset), stuttering-like disfluencies (children whose stuttering naturally recovers tend to demonstrate reduction in stuttering-like disfluencies), duration of stuttering (natural recovery tends to occur within 3 years of onset), disfluency length (continuing disfluency, particularly with more than three units of repetition, indicates higher risk for persistence), and sound prolongations and blocks (continuing sound prolongations and blocks tend to predict persistence). Secondary factors included stuttering severity (severe stuttering that continues for more than the first few months indicates greater risk of persistence), head and neck movements (children who do not demonstrate substantial reduction in the number and severity of secondary characteristics within the first year of onset are at greater risk for persistence), phonological skills (lower phonological skills early in the history of stuttering tend to predict persistence of stuttering, but this likelihood wanes during the second year of stuttering), and expressive language skills (close to stuttering onset, language is not predictive of persistence or recovery, but stuttering may emerge for children with developmentally advanced language abilities). Other factors include concomitant disorders (other disorders tend to contribute to persistence) and awareness and affective reactions (the child's awareness of stuttering or emotional reaction to it tend not to predict persistence or recovery).

Finally, after presenting several perspectives on the onset and development of stuttering and related risk factors, this chapter summarized the nature of stuttering, including types of disfluency; symptoms, prevalence, and incidence; differences between people who stutter and those who do not; and variability and predictability of stuttering, in addition to implications related to designing effective treatment. Frequently occurring questions were posed and addressed, leaving clinicians with a standing challenge.

Chapter Two Study Questions

1. Throughout this chapter, many questions were raised about the onset, development, and nature of stuttering. For example: What risk factors distinguish transient stuttering from chronic stuttering? How does stuttering vary by gender, class, nationality, and ethnicity? What factors other than speech are part of stuttering in its developed form? How would you address these and the other questions raised?

2. An explicit understanding of one's assumptions is essential for effective assessment and treatment with people who stutter. What are your assumptions about the onset, development, and nature of stuttering, and how might these impact your intervention with people who stutter? How have your assumptions about stuttering and people who stutter changed as a result of reading this chapter?

3. Several developmental classification systems were discussed in this chapter. In what ways might they be clinically useful, and why? What do you feel are the dangers in using developmental categories when assessing and treating a person who stutters? How do your experiences with young children beginning to stutter relate to the classification systems discussed (compare and contrast)?

4. In what ways do the results of the longitudinal investigations challenge our traditional beliefs about the onset and development of stuttering that resulted from the developmental classifications? How do your experiences with young children beginning to stutter relate to the longitudinal data presented (compare and contrast)? How do the longitudinal investigations enable us to make predictions about the course of stuttering (i.e., persistent or transient)?

5. Why do you think more males than females stutter? What are possible explanations for the more frequent and faster recovery among girls than boys who stutter?

6. In what ways do environmental and genetic factors contribute to the likelihood that a person will stutter? In what ways do these factors contribute to the overt and covert manifestations of stuttering? Why would a person deliberately misrepresent himself and miscommunicate rather than stutter? Why would a person literally stab a lead pencil through his hand rather than stutter? In what ways can a conversational partner understand the experience of a person who stutters? In what ways is it impossible for a conversational partner to understand the experience of a person who stutters?

7. What do we know about the speech and language development of people who stutter? What do we know about the brain and central nervous system of people who stutter (i.e., neurophysiologically, neuroanatomically, neurochemically)? How might this and our other knowledge about the onset, development, and nature of stuttering enable us to predict who will stutter and the course of that stuttering? What knowledge are we lacking about stuttering and people who stutter?

8. While our knowledge of stuttering and people who stutter has grown tremendously in recent years, many inroads are yet to be made. What do we know and what do we need to learn? With all that is known, what might be the reasons for perpetuation of negative attitudes among the general public, allied education and health professionals, and student clinicians and professional speech–language pathologists? How might the confusion about the disorder contribute to the stereotypes, and what can be done about it?

9. Bloodstein and Bernstein Ratner (2008) presented 12 criteria for effective treatment. Which of these criteria do you believe are most and least important and why? In what ways might these criteria impact your treatment? How are these criteria informed by evidenced-based practice? What was meant by this statement, made earlier: "The fact remains that some successes are not predictable on the basis of evidence. Other successes are not reflected by the evidence being collected"? How might the admonition of T. S. Eliot from 1934 be relevant today, both to you and to our profession?

10. W. Johnson (1939) was quoted as saying, "So long as an individual retains and operates on assumptions regarding stuttering and speech, which are characteristics of stutterers, he will not become the sort of individual we refer to as a normal speaker." What are possible implications of this statement for the client, the clinician, and the client–clinician interaction?

Chapter Three

Etiology of Stuttering
Past and Present

You can't connect the dots looking forward. You can only connect them looking backwards, so you have to trust that the dots will somehow connect in your future. . . . Believing that the dots will connect down the road will give you the confidence to follow your heart, even when it leads you off the well-worn path, and that will make all the difference. (Jobs, 2005)

Generally we need to know where we have been to understand how we arrived at where we are and the rationale for where we are going. Intervention with people who stutter is no exception. To this point, we have addressed a number of seminal concepts and reviewed the onset, development, and nature of stuttering. This chapter highlights the evolution of our thinking throughout recorded history about stuttering and people who stutter. This foundation contributes to our understanding of contemporary theories of etiology, which supports and informs related treatment practices.

History of Stuttering: The Past

"If You Stutter, You're Not Alone"

Stuttering and people who stutter are events of historical and contemporary significance. It is of historical interest to know that there have been many prominent and accomplished figures whose stuttering did not hold them back. This information also is of clinical interest and may be used as a positive and motivating influence during assessment and treatment interactions with people who stutter. Famous people who also stutter are receiving increasing attention in publications (Bobrick, 1996; F. H. Silverman, 2004; Van Riper, 1982) and in foundations (e.g., The Stuttering Foundation of

America), associations (National Stuttering Association, Friends: The National Association of Young People Who Stutter), and websites (The Stuttering Homepage). Some of these historical figures are as follows:

Moses (Hebrew prophet)	Dekanawida (Iroquois peacemaker)
Virgil (Roman poet)	Demosthenes (Greek orator)
Aesop (Greek storyteller)	Claudius (Roman emperor)
King Charles I of England	Isaac Newton (British scientist)
Erasmus Darwin (British physician, author, and grandfather of Charles Darwin)	Charles Darwin (British naturalist and author)
Moses Mendelssohn (18th-century German Jewish philosopher)	Charles Lamb (British essayist)
	Arnold Bennett (British writer)
Clara Barton (founder of the American Red Cross)	Cotton Mather (Puritan leader)
	Henry James (American novelist)
Lewis Carroll (British author)	Kim Philby (British spy)
Marilyn Monroe (American actress)	Winston Churchill (British prime minister)
Aneurin Bevan (British labor leader)	Henry Luce (founder of *Time* magazine)
Somerset Maugham (British writer)	Patrick Campbell (British humorist)
Field Marshall Lord Carver (British military leader)	Kenneth Tynan (British drama critic)
George VI (British monarch)	Robert Heinlein (American writer)
Raymond Massey (American actor)	Theodore Roosevelt (U.S. president)
Vladimir Lenin (Russian leader)	George Washington (U.S. president)
Washington Irving (American author)	Napoleon I (French emperor)
Aristotle (Greek orator, philosopher)	Michael Ramsey (Anglican archbishop)

Contemporary figures who stuttered or continue to stutter include the following:

James Earl Jones (American actor)	Anthony Quinn (American actor)
Bob Love (Chicago Bulls basketball player)	Pat Leahy (New York Jets football player)
	Samuel L. Jackson (American actor)
Neville Shute (British novelist)	Kenyon Martin (Denver Nuggets basketball player)
Jonathan Miller (British director)	
Greg Louganis (Olympic diver)	Bill Walton (American basketball star and sportscaster)
Dave Taylor (L.A. Kings hockey player)	
Ken Venturi (American golfer)	Nicholas Brendon (American actor)
John Updike (American novelist)	Ben Johnson (Canadian runner)
Carly Simon (American singer)	Ron Harper (Chicago Bulls basketball player)
Robert Merrill (American singer)	
Bruce Oldfield (British fashion designer)	Margaret Drabble (British novelist)
Joseph Biden (U.S. vice president)	Bruce Willis (American actor)
John Welch (chairman of General Electric)	Tommy John (Yankees pitcher)
Henry Rogers (American public relations pioneer)	Lester Hayes (Oakland/L.A. Raiders football player)
John Stossel (American reporter)	Butch Baird (American golfer)

(*continues*)

Annie Glenn (American public speaker and wife of astronaut John Glenn)	Jimmy Stewart (American actor)
	Chris Zorich (Chicago Bears lineman)
Mel Tillis (American singer)	Sam Neill (New Zealand actor)
Richard Condon (American novelist)	Peggy Lipton (American actress)
Jake Eberts (Canadian film producer)	Tiger Woods (American golfer)
Frank Wolf (U.S. congressman)	Alan Rabinowitz (American explorer, conservationist)
Austin Pendleton (American actor)	
Bo Jackson (American football and baseball star)	Julia Roberts (American actress)

Numerous accounts address the impact of stuttering on the lives of some of these people (e.g., Attanasio, 1987b; Emerick, 1966; J. E. Jones, 2005; J. E. Jones & Niven, 1993; Terry, 1994; Tillis & Wagner, 1984) and others (Carlisle, 1985; Jezer, 1997; Murray, 2008; St. Louis, 2001a). Stuttering and people who stutter have been present at least throughout recorded history. The slogan "If you stutter, you're not alone" appears on buttons and posters distributed by the National Stuttering Association (NSA), the largest self-help and mutual aid organization in the United States. The facts that stuttering is an age-old affliction and that people who stutter are in good company are both clinically relevant. As we have seen, stuttering can negatively impact the self-esteem of people who stutter. The knowledge that people who stutter have been and are successful is both motivating and reassuring to clients of all ages. References to stuttering in ancient texts are of clinical interest in at least two ways. First, it is instructive from a theoretical standpoint to see how stuttering has been conceptualized previously. Some of the older ideas seem to lack contemporary relevance; in others, we can see the root of ideas that prevail to this day. Second, the existence of ancient references to stuttering reinforces the essential point that if you stutter, you're not alone. Many have come before you, and the tales of their experiences can enrich your own.

Stuttering in Egyptian Hieroglyphics

People have attempted to explain stuttering (or *stammering*, the term more commonly used in the United Kingdom) in various ways for over 4,000 years. Egyptian hieroglyphics from around 2000 B.C. included a determinative (symbol or icon) of a figure pointing with one hand to the mouth and the other to the ground (see Figure 3.1; see also Clark & Murray, 1965; Curlee, 1993; Manning, 2010). This symbol is said to represent a reduplicated verb root, *nitnit*, or *njtjt*, interpreted by Egyptologists to mean "to talk hesitantly" or "to stutter" (Clark & Murray, 1965, p. 132; Faulkner, 1981, p. 126). Clark and Murray noted,

> Its basic sense refers to a retarding movement of the walking mechanism, in a figurative sense it refers to the "gait" of talking with the vehicle of the tongue. What was originally a picture of the reluctant retarded stepping of the legs, was figuratively applied to the stepping (walking) movements of the tongue. (p. 132)

The symbols are read from right to left. The verb has the determinative of "walking legs" and is used in the sense of an impediment of movement. With the substitution of the determinative of the person with the hand to mouth, however, the ancient Egyptians successfully conveyed the concept of an impediment to one's speech. The symbols represent the oldest evidence of a speech defect (Clark & Murray, 1965) and may be one of the earliest retrievable references to stuttering (Curlee, 1993; Manning, 2010). This

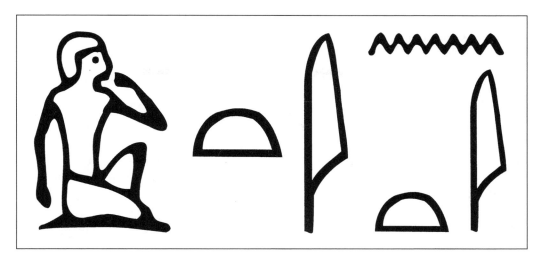

Figure 3.1.   Egyptian hieroglyphics for stuttering. *Note.* Courtesy of the Institute of Egyptian Art and Archaeology, University of Memphis. Reprinted with permission.

would indicate that the disorder of stuttering has affected speakers for as long as human civilization has been recorded.

The symbols are originally from "The Tale of the Shipwrecked Sailor" (De Buck, 1970, p. 100), an Egyptian prose narrative that, on papyrus, was discovered by W. Gole-nischeff and is preserved in Moscow (Clark & Murray, 1965; Lichtheim, 1973). The tale, translated by Lichtheim, tells of a high official returning from a failed expedition who is despondent and fearful about the reception he is about to receive at the royal court. One of his attendants tells him to take courage, and as an example of how a disaster can be turned into a success, tells him of an adventure (being shipwrecked) that happened to him many years before. The attendant advises,

> Now listen to me, my lord! I am not exaggerating. Wash yourself, pour water over your fingers. You must answer when questioned. You must speak to the king with presence of mind. You must answer without stammering! A man's mouth can save him. His speech makes one forgive him. (p. 212)

The attendant tells of being shipwrecked on an island and encountering a large snake. Interestingly, the snake demonstrates a pattern of phrase and sentence repetition, as follows:

> Then he opened his mouth to me, while I was on my belly before him. He said to me: "Who brought you, who brought you, fellow, who brought you? If you delay telling me who brought you to this island, I shall make you find yourself reduced to ashes, becoming like a thing unseen." (pp. 212–213)

After telling the story of the shipwreck, the sailor is comforted by the snake. "Don't be afraid, don't be afraid, fellow; don't be pale-faced, now that you have come to me. It is god who has let you live and brought you to this island" (p. 213). The snake then foretells the sailor's rescue:

> You shall pass month upon month until you have completed four months in this island. Then a ship will come from home with sailors in it whom you know. You shall go home with them, you shall die in your town. (p. 213)

The snake adds words of encouragement: "How happy is he who tells what he has tasted, when the calamity has passed" (p. 213). "If you are brave and control your heart, you shall embrace your children, you shall kiss your wife, you shall see your home" (p. 213). And so it came to be that ultimate joy reigned over temporary sorrow.

Stuttering in the Bible

Other early references can be found in the Bible. Stuttering is mentioned in the book of the prophet Isaiah. He called out against social injustice between 742 and 687 B.C. (May & Metzger, 1962) and proclaimed that private and public lives should reflect confidence in the omnipotence of God: "The heart also of the rash shall understand knowledge. And the tongue of the stammerers shall be ready to speak plainly" (Isaiah 32:4; Jewish Publication Society, 1965, p. 573). The book of Exodus also references stuttering. Exodus recounts the period from 1350 to 1200 B.C. (May & Metzger, 1962) and tells of Israel's emancipation from Egyptian bondage and the establishment of the covenant between God and the people of Israel. Moses is God's agent in delivering Israel from slavery and the mediator of the covenant. Exodus contains evidence suggesting that the historical figure Moses stuttered. When God calls Moses to approach Pharaoh and lead the Jews out of Egypt, Moses protests:

> And Moses said unto the Lord: "Oh Lord, I am not a man of words, neither heretofore, nor since Thou hast spoken unto Thy servant; for I am slow of speech, and of a slow tongue." And the Lord said unto him: "Who hath made man's mouth? Or who maketh a man dumb, or deaf, or seeing, or blind? Is it not I the Lord? Now therefore go, and I will be with thy mouth, and teach thee what thou shalt speak." (Exodus 4:10–12; Jewish Publication Society, 1965, p. 76)

In response to Moses' protests, God instructs Moses to bring Aaron, Moses' brother, as his spokesman.

> Is there not Aaron thy brother the Levite? I know that he can speak well. . . . And thou shalt speak unto him, and put the words in his mouth; and I will be with thy mouth, and with his mouth, and will teach you what ye shall do. And he shall be thy spokesman unto the people; and it shall come to pass, that he shall be to thee a mouth, and thou shalt be to him in God's stead. (Exodus 4:14–16; Jewish Publication Society, 1965, p. 76)

Then, according to the text, Aaron, not Moses, speaks God's words and performs God's signs. Then Moses and Aaron go to Pharaoh, and together they present God's order: "Let my people go" (Exodus 5:1; Jewish Publication Society, 1965, p. 77). As noted earlier, people who stutter generally become immediately fluent when speaking in unison with another person. Moses and Aaron go repeatedly from God to Pharaoh, conveying the respective messages between the plagues. All the while, Moses gradually becomes more the spokesman and Aaron, while present, grows increasingly silent. During the last four plagues, Moses speaks to the people and to Pharaoh, no longer complaining about his speech or seeking Aaron's help. In fact, Moses becomes an eloquent speaker.

How did Moses first begin to stutter? A midrash (a story from the Talmud told by rabbis) explains:

> While Moses was still an infant, the Pharaoh was advised to kill him, for one day, it was predicted, Moses would rise up against him. The Pharaoh at first shrugged, then decided to put Moses to the test. He placed two bowls before Moses, one filled with gold, the other, with hot coals. If Moses chose the gold, he would be slain. Of course Moses reached for the gleaming gold, but an angel intervened and struck his hand. So he grabbed a hot coal and put it in his mouth. And thereafter stuttered. (Goldberg, 1989, p. 71)

Was Moses' pattern of speech disfluency stuttering? In support of this claim, Gruber (1986) analyzed biblical scholars' interpretations of Moses' speech behavior, his dialogue with God, and his eventual confrontation with Pharaoh within the context of systematic desensitization (i.e., increasing levels of challenge gradually to facilitate success and eliminate related anxieties). Gruber noted, "After modifying His initial instructions (Exodus 3:10, 18), by having Aaron speak for Moses (Exodus 4:15–16), Moses eventually is led to do his own talking" (p. 10). Specifically, the designation of responsibilities to Moses and Aaron in their meetings with the Israelite people and Pharaoh is based upon a literal interpretation of God's words:

1. "The Lord said to Moses" (Exodus 4:21; 6:10; 7:1, 14; 8.1)
2. "The Lord said to Aaron" (Exodus 4:27)
3. "The Lord said to Moses and Aaron" (Exodus 6:13; 7:8; 9:8)
4. "The Lord said to Moses, say to Aaron" (Exodus 7:10; 8:5, 16) (p. 11)

Gruber (1986) also highlighted the significant events: Aaron speaks for Moses in the first encounter with the Israelites. Then Moses and Aaron, while speaking together (Exodus 5:1–3), go to Pharaoh, and Aaron utters the words to Pharaoh, having received them from Moses, as directed by God. After this first meeting with Pharaoh, Moses and Aaron return to the Israelites, where Moses speaks for himself and continues to do so in all subsequent meetings with them. With this success, Moses speaks during the second interaction with Pharaoh, although to Aaron (i.e., not to Pharaoh), directing Aaron to cast down the rod before Pharaoh (i.e., that would become a serpent, reflecting God's divine intervention). This verbalization in the presence of Pharaoh is indirect and brief. Then Moses speaks directly with Pharaoh during their third contact and thereafter; Aaron continues to provide support by handling nonverbal tasks (Exodus 7:19; 8:5–6, 16–17; 9:8–10). It is during the seventh encounter with Pharaoh that Moses performs both the verbal and nonverbal tasks (Exodus 10:12, 21–23), demonstrating full independence as a communicator with the Israelite people and with Pharaoh. From this retrospective analysis, early fluency intervention could be viewed as prophetic and divinely inspired. In fact, one could interpret Gruber's presentation as suggesting that God was the first speech–language pathologist. In actuality, we will never be certain that Moses stuttered, despite ongoing biblical analysis (Attanasio, 1997; Marshall, 2003). Regardless, the story of his difficulties with speech is a powerful reminder that stuttering can be seen not just as an affliction but, to quote Rabinowitz (2005), also as a "special little gift" that can be bestowed on very special people.

Siegel (1990) noted that the early rabbis believed that stuttering came directly from God, and he questioned how people can turn to God for strength and understanding if God is the source of the affliction. Siegel concluded that an impediment does not disqualify a person from important work, leadership, or vision:

> We don't have to be perfect to lead rich and ennobling lives. All of us have impediments of one sort or another, but for all of us there is a role to play, there are deserts to cross, people who need our help, in our own time and our own domains, in the circles or semicircles that frame our lives. We may not hear God calling to us directly, but we are surrounded by burning bushes and God is pleading with us, even as Moses pleaded with God, to make holy these places where we walk. (p. VII–12)

Stuttering in Professional Literature

The cause and treatment of stuttering have been foci of speculation for more than 2,500 years. The Greek historian Herodotus (484–424 B.C.) recorded the treatment of stuttering by a Pythian priestess who recommended emigration south to Libya. Hippocrates (450–357 B.C.), the Greek physician known as "the Father of Medicine," commented that chronic diarrhea was common to people who stutter and recommended its cure by varices—dilating or twisting veins, arteries, or lymph vessels. He viewed the cause to be a disturbance in the mingling of the four "humours"—heat, cold, moisture, and dryness. Aristotle (384–322 B.C.), trained as an orator, attributed stuttering entirely to the tongue. Satyrus, the Greek actor, is said to have cured Demosthenes (383–322 B.C.), who stuttered and demonstrated voice and articulation errors, by having him perform voice exercises with pebbles in his mouth while declaiming and walking uphill. Galen (131–201 A.D.) thought that stuttering was caused by debility of the muscles resulting from diminution of heat and used cauterization as a remedy. Avicenna (980–1037 A.D.), a philosopher and physician in Arabia, believed that humidity caused mollification of the tongue and recommended deep inspiration before speaking. Francis Bacon (1560–1626) thought stuttering was caused by refrigeration of the tongue resulting in dryness and immobility, for which he recommended drinking wine "because it heateth."

This is only a sample of the diverse thinking across time. In my review of the history of stuttering, I discovered a number of excellent sources (Bloodstein, 1993; Bluemel, 1957; Clark, 1964; Culatta & Goldberg, 1995; Diehl, 1958; Freund, 1966; Hahn & Hahn, 1956; Lewis, 1899; Murray, 2008; Shames & Rubin, 1986; F. H. Silverman, 2004; Van Riper, 1973, 1982; Wingate, 1976, 1997, among many others). One remarkable article was that of Klingbeil (1939), who described the evolution of etiological concepts and treatments of stuttering from 484 B.C. to 1915 A.D. The following highlights are adapted from these sources. For each contributor, the two dates noted refer to the year of birth and death. When only one date is given, it refers to the approximate time when the theory was published or became known.

Stuttering as an Anatomical Defect

Throughout history, different anatomical structures have been implicated as the cause of stuttering. The tongue has been mentioned frequently. Aegineta (7th century), Menjot (1615–1696), Kustner (1716), and Savary (1812) all ascribed stuttering chiefly to malformation of the tongue. Others holding similar views attempted to reduce the size (Chegoin, 1830) or alter the position (Wutzner, 1850) of the tongue by mechanical methods. Hagemann (1845) recommended placing an *n* sound before each difficult syllable. Hahn (1694–1745) and Morgagni (1682–1771) both argued that the hyoid bone was responsible. Among those blaming the glottis were Yates (1828), a New York doctor and inventor of "the American Method" who recommended raising the tongue tip to the palate while speaking. This method also has been associated with a Mrs. Leigh, whose husband stuttered. She directed an institute using this method. Arnott (1788–1874), a Scottish physician, recommended continuous phonation of *e* between each word to keep the glottis open. Muller (1801–1858), a German physiologist, recommended omission of plosive sounds to keep the glottis open. Hoffman (1818–1892) advocated physical relaxation and elimination of vocal tension. Finally, Graves (1797–1853), an Irish physician, advised directing the attention of the patient away from speech by having him strike an object simultaneously with speaking, in order to keep time. Santorini (1681–1737), an Italian anatomist, believed that an abnormal size of two holes in the middle region of the palate was the cause of stuttering. Others implicated a combination of structures. Thelwall (1764–1834), an English lawyer, differentiated four types of stuttering on the assumed causal basis of the lips, tongue, pharynx, or bronchi, all of which were treated by rhythm. Harnisch (1832) held that the larynx or posterior part of the tongue was responsible and advocated speaking rules governing movement of the tongue and lips.

Stuttering as a Medical Problem Requiring Surgery

Approaches to surgical intervention for stuttering (without the benefit of anesthesia) varied considerably. Aetiuus (1542), a royal physician to Justinian at Byzantium, implicated the tongue and recommended surgical division of the lingual frenum. De Chauliac (1300–1380), a French surgeon, ascribed stuttering to a defect in the tongue, paralysis, or moisture of the nerves or muscles, and recommended embrocations to desiccate the brain and cauteries for the vertebrae. Dieffenbach (1795–1847), a German surgeon, assumed a connection between defective articulation and strabismus (misalignment or asymmetrical movement of the eyes); he advocated making a horizontal section at the root of the tongue and excising a triangular wedge completely across and nearly through it in order to interrupt the innervation, thereby modifying the muscular spasm. Velpeau (1795–1867), a French professor of clinical surgery, held that stuttering originated from an unusual depth of the palate and therefore surgically divided the hyoglossus, geniohyoglossus, and styloglossus muscles. Other French surgeons, including Amussat (1796–1856), Baudens (1804–1857), and Bonnet (1841), surgically divided the geniohyoglossus muscle. Froriep (1804–1861), a German surgeon, utilized an electrical form of intervention and also divided the geniohyoglossus muscle (on one side only). Braid (1795–1860), an English surgeon, excised the tonsils or uvula. Parker (1806–1866), an American professor of surgery, introduced surgical intervention for stuttering to the United States, which was subsequently practiced in New York by Mott (1785–1865) and Post (1806–1866). In general, the German school followed the surgical methods of Dieffenbach, the French followed those of Velpeau, and the English those of Braid. Because of the medical complications associated with surgery (sometimes death) and the minimal improvement reported (less than 5% receiving permanent benefit), the procedures were abandoned.

Stuttering as a Disorder of Articulation

Colombat de l'Isere (1831) viewed stuttering as a result of spasmodic action of the articulators or rigidity of the laryngeal, pharyngeal, and respiratory muscles. For these conditions, he recommended rhythmic vocal gymnastics, focused practice on opposing movements of articulatory muscles, or mechanical devices such as a rhythmic pacesetter, the *muthonome* (metronome). Good (1840) also held that stuttering was the result of defective articulation and that the will should be strengthened to establish better control of the affected muscles. Bishop (1851) proposed that stuttering was the result of attempts to speak without vocal cord vibration, thus indicating disassociation between the articulatory and vocal organs. Others implicating defective articulators included James Hunt (1870) (and his son, also named James Hunt) of England, who recommended disciplined exercise; Bristowe (1879), also of England, who recommended breathing exercises and precise articulation; and Bates (1884), an American, who used various appliances, including a narrow flattened tube of silver applied to the palatal midline to facilitate formation of lingua-palatal sounds. Bates also used a hollow biconvex disk with a projecting silver tube placed between the lips to help with labial and dental–labial sounds, and a belt and spring adjusted over the thyroid cartilage to help with velar sounds. Other treatments intending to add articulatory precision were those of Dupuytren (1817), who utilized speech in a singing tone, marking intervals by movement of the foot; Serre d'Alais (1829), who used forcible pronunciation of every syllable aided by synchronous arm gestures; and Comstock (mid-1800s), a Philadelphia physician who used elocutionary exercises by reading aloud in unison with others.

Stuttering as a Disorder of Respiration

Theories of stuttering as a result of defective articulation often overlapped with those implicating defective breathing. Du Soit (1840) attributed stuttering to spasms of the respiratory system, as did Becquerel (1847), who proposed that the defect was in the respiratory muscles, which permitted air to escape prematurely, and recommended retention and controlled use of breath. Coen (1879) of Vienna viewed stuttering as the result of deficient atmospheric pressure in the lungs or pathological changes in the respiratory system and recommended elocutionary exercises. Findlay (1885) believed that both the respiratory musculature and the structures of articulation and voice were responsible for stuttering, and that gestures could normalize movement of the diaphragm for fluent speech. Similarly, Rouma (1907) advocated the use of arm gestures; the rationale was to facilitate overflow of cerebral activity from the arms to the speech centers. McCormac (1828), an English doctor, recommended deep inspirations and forcible expirations, based on the assumption that stuttering resulted from speaking on emptied lungs. Kingsley (1819–1875), an English orator and writer, recommended on the basis of his own experience of stuttering speaking with an open mouth and full lungs, inhaling at every stop, keeping the tongue down, exercising with weights to help breathing, keeping a piece of cork between the back teeth when speaking, and keeping the upper lip drawn down tightly.

Stuttering as a Disorder of Neuroanatomy or Motor Speech Dysfunction

Theories of articulation and respiration overlapped with those of neuromotor disorder. Erasmus Darwin (1731–1802), an English physician and naturalist (and grandfather of Charles Darwin), held that emotions such as awe and bashfulness interrupted movement of the speech apparatus and recommended softening initial consonants. Itard (1817), a French surgeon, ascribed stuttering to a muscular deficit and used a golden or ivory fork, placed in the cavity of the alveolar arch of the lower jaw, to support the tongue. Rullier (1821) proposed that stuttering resulted from a disproportion between the rate at which the brain produces thoughts and that at which it transfers them to sites of innervation. He argued that the speech organs are unable to function properly because of the high demand placed upon them when profusion of stimuli must be processed so rapidly by the brain. Rullier's thinking introduced an early version of the demands and capacities model, presented later in this chapter. Voisin (1821), a French doctor, held similar etiological views to those of Rullier, but added the treatment recommendation of pressing one's thumb against the chin while speaking. Astrie (1824) also located the cause in some modification of brain action, but recommended precise articulation and use of Itard's fork. Deleau (1797–1862) held that stuttering resulted from organic lesions yielding incomplete cerebral action or deficient innervation, and identified three aspects of stuttering, including faulty tongue action and spasmodic closure of the lips or glottis. His treatment consisted of maximizing visual feedback for precise articulation. Schulthess (1830) identified stuttering as "phonophobia," a spasm of the glottis extending through nerve associations to the speech organs. Bell (1774–1842), a Scottish anatomist, held that stuttering resulted from inadequate capacity of the nerves to coordinate speech, which caused subsequent respiratory disruption, and emphasized the role of the larynx in articulation. Chervin (1867) concluded that the higher brain was responsible for stuttering and recommended education to strengthen the will, imitation, and precise articulation. Guillaume (1868) also implicated the central nervous system and stressed the importance of whispering, lip gymnastics, keeping the tongue in contact with the palate during speech, and taking deep inspirations at every sentence.

Several others attributed stuttering to motor incoordination resulting from central nervous system involvement. Hall-Marshall (1790–1857) spoke of the involuntary action of the reflex spinal center and recommended a continuous, flowing manner of speaking. Rosenthal (1861) blamed the coordinative disorder on an injury received during childhood to the medulla oblongata and recommended rhythmic exercises. Wolff

(1861) held that the nerves or organs themselves were at fault and recommended trying all methods, almost all drugs, and eventually surgical division of the hypoglossal nerve. Finally, Shuldam (1879) proposed the interaction of nervous weakness and muscular spasm and recommended elocutionary exercises of a rhythmic nature and regulation of respiration.

Stuttering as a Psychoneurosis

Mendelssohn (1729–1786), a philosopher, saw stuttering as the result of the collision of too many ideas flowing simultaneously from the brain, and recommended slow reading with systematic disclosure. Others who believed stuttering to be an aspect of psychoneurosis included Lee (1773–1877), an English physician who recommended surgical treatment, and Wyneken (1868), who emphasized building faith in the client regarding the client's ability, speech and breathing exercises, and rhythmic beating of time. Kussmail (1822–1902), a German surgeon, defined stuttering as "lalloneurosis," "disarthria syllabaris," and "intermittent spasmodic neurosis," and recommended strengthening the willpower, breathing and articulatory exercises, and rhythmic speech. Some felt that stuttering was triggered by negative emotions, including dread of speaking or excessive eagerness to speak (Sandow, 1898), fear and anxiety (Steckel, 1908), and embarrassment and lack of confidence (Thome, 1867). Thome, however, also held that stuttering was a function of motor speech and respiratory breakdown. Klencke (1813–1881), a German physician who emphasized the importance of the scientific method as a foundation for intervention, indicated that stuttering represented the person's need for psychological help; he opened an institution for treatment of people who stutter that focused on the unique personality disturbance from which stuttering was thought to originate. As always, treatments varied, including correcting the overt manifestations of stuttering by drill and exercise (Hudson-Makuen, 1910), rest and relaxation (Sandow, 1898), distraction (Bertrand, 1795–1831), and psychoanalysis (Appelt, 1911; Coriat, 1915; Netskatschen, 1909; Steckel, 1908).

Stuttering as a Learned Behavior

The following theorists viewed stuttering as a bad habit or learned behavior. Amman (1667–1724), a Swiss physician, was among the first to state in print that stuttering was a learned behavior and recommended that it be treated by speaking loudly and slowly. Watson (1809), an English instructor, described stuttering as a "vicious habit" and recommended exercise of the speech organs and strengthening the will. Warren (1837) held that stuttering was a habit induced from weakness in and functional irregularity of the nervous system, causing nervous agitation and disruption to the processes of articulation and voice. Merkel (1844), a German anatomist, believed that stuttering was a deeply rooted habit learned from an adynamic state of the speech organs and insufficient will, and should be treated by raising the tone of the whole body, lessening the force of the articulatory organs, and strengthening respiratory function. Kingsley, noted earlier for his treatments emphasizing breath control, held that stuttering was the result of conscious or unconscious imitation. Howard (1879), a speech specialist in New York, proposed that stuttering was a habit in which the glottis contracted, thus contracting the throat because of insufficient pulmonary energy; he recommended relaxation of the chest and throat musculature.

In the latter part of the 19th century, several theorists maintained that stuttering was a learned behavior. Butterfield (1880), a professor of vocal physiology, held that stuttering was a habit-induced spasm of the diaphragm that should be treated by speech and respiratory gymnastics. Alexander Melville Bell (1819–1905), a vocal physiologist and grandfather of the inventor of the telephone, believed that stuttering in any stage of its habit formation could be uprooted by reading aloud in a loud whisper and by counting while breathing to improve pulmonary regularity. Finally, Potter (1882) maintained that the stuttering spasm was a habit induced by defective nerve function that occurred at the stop points on the vocal chain (lips, tongue, larynx, glottis).

Summary—History of Stuttering

Stuttering has continued to fascinate and intrigue throughout history. There is evidence of stuttering from the Egyptian Empire (2000 B.C.) in Egyptian hieroglyphics and from the Bible. Questions about the origin, nature, and treatment of stuttering have been continuous. Explanations for stuttering have included anatomical defects, medical problems requiring surgery, respiratory disorders, neuroanatomical and motor speech dysfunction, psychoneurosis, and learned behavior, among others. The mid-1800s saw unsuccessful attempts to link stuttering and strabismus, as well as frequent implications of the tongue as the cause of stuttering. Mechanical devices and surgery were used to raise or lower the tongue position. The physiological approach was more rational and humane than the surgical or medical approach, and sought to correct defective breathing, vocalization, and articulation. Exercises for breathing, articulation, voice, inflection, elocution, rhythm, continuity, and building multisensory feedback were among the remedies.

It is indeed apparent that our present harvest of theoretical explanations and related treatments were sown in seeds of the past. Goldberg (1989) appropriately referred to historic treatments for stuttering as spanning a period "from pebbles to psychoanalysis" (p. 71). Bluemel's (1957) thoughts are no less current or encouraging today:

> Much remains to be done in the field of disordered speech. . . . The research worker in the speech field need not be discouraged by progress which seems at times to be disappointingly slow. The history of poliomyelitis dates back at least 3500 years, and it was not till 1955 that the Salk vaccine became available. Stammering is as old as language; but now the answer to the riddle of the disorder seems close at hand. (p. 134)

Etiology of Stuttering: The Present

Throughout recorded time to the present day, we continue to ask, "What causes stuttering?" The apparent simplicity of this question is deceptive. The question is asked frequently by people who stutter, their families, and members of the general public. As indicated earlier in this chapter, the professional community, including speech–language pathologists, physicians, surgeons, anatomists, and psychotherapists, has been on this trail for over 40 centuries. Now, we will focus on present or recent thinking. Today, when asked, "What caused your stuttering?" or "What caused (your family member) to stutter?" responses from anecdotal reports suggest that the term *cause* is often assumed to relate to those factors that were immediately present at the time the stuttering was first observed. Let's consider the concept of cause more directly.

Etiology Defined: Three *P*s

Haynes and Pindzola (2008) indicated, "The notion of cause has different meanings depending on its distance from the problem" (p. 18). Indeed, causality implies an ongoing or developmental concept and therefore assumes a time frame that must be specified. Traditionally, etiology has been defined in terms of predisposing, precipitating, and perpetuating factors (i.e., causes; a helpful mnemonic device is to remember the three *P*s).

Predisposing Factors

Predisposing factors are those agents that incline the person to stutter (Nicolosi et al., 2004) and address the question, "What factors cause one person to be at greater risk than another for beginning to stutter?" (F. H. Silverman, 2004, p. 129). An example of predisposing factors, reviewed in the last chapter, is the apparent genetic inclination (predisposition) to stutter; stuttering tends to run in families. However, as will be seen, it might be that environmental or developmental (precipitating) factors or the interactions between predisposing and precipitating factors are the reasons that stuttering surfaces. Another way of looking at the significance of predisposing factors is in their potential link with a third agent (Haynes & Pindzola, 2008). For example, one frequently observed predisposing factor is left-handedness, which has a higher incidence among people who stutter. There is little significance in the left-handedness by itself. However, the implication of basic underlying neurological differences is noteworthy and continues to be the focus of a current line of research. The clinician and diagnostician must be watchful for factors that occur with regularity in association with the stuttering. Such predisposing factors may be instrumental in revealing information regarding the nature of stuttering and people who stutter (Haynes & Pindzola, 2008).

Precipitating Factors

Precipitating factors are those agents thought to have made stuttering surface or those that brought it to its present state (Haynes & Pindzola, 2008; Nicolosi et al., 2004). F. H. Silverman (2004) indicated that these factors address the question, "What actually causes a person to begin to stutter?" (p. 129). Precipitating factors generally are no longer operating, and therefore may or may not be identifiable. Some may debate the value of identifying factors that are not still operating. Haynes and Pindzola pointed out, however, that in each moment, a new set of precipitating factors is created that, acting as characteristics of the past, perpetuates behaviors of the present. They indicated that communication disorders, including stuttering, are not static entities developed at a given point in time; rather, they are dynamic, ever-changing characteristics that are constantly influenced by internal and external factors. Examples of precipitating factors might include rapid growth in speech and language skills during the preschool years, competition among siblings for attention and conversational turns in busy homes, and the social adjustments necessary upon entering preschool and school settings. As will be seen, these factors place increasing demands on children's developing communication skills.

Identification and Interaction of Predisposing and Precipitating Factors

It should be noted that determination of predisposing and precipitating factors in developmental (i.e., idiopathic) stuttering generally is an estimate at best. I am reminded of a young boy with language impairment with whom I worked many years ago. At the time, he said "I can't know" for "I don't know." This led me to consider the distinction between that which is not knowable and that which is not known. Often, although not always, we cannot know the causal link between predisposing and precipitating factors and the occurrence of stuttering. For example, consider the case of a boy who presented a family history of stuttering (a predisposing factor). His stuttering began around the age of 3 years, when his speech and language skills were developing rapidly, his home routine was busy as both parents worked, and he was beginning a part-time preschool program (precipitating factors). The predisposing factors cannot be altered. The clinician worked with the family to reduce the potential influence of the precipitating factors (e.g., facilitating fluent conversation though age-appropriate language content and form in a restructured environment that eliminated interruption and perceived communicative pressure), yet the stuttering persisted.

Ultimately, we cannot know if the child's stuttering would have begun and developed in the absence of the factors noted. How do we explain other children who have similar predisposing and precipitating factors and who develop stuttering with early recovery, or those who do not begin to stutter at all? Perhaps the presence, absence, and outcome of stuttering are independent of the factors identified. Maybe a unique interaction of known or unknown factors is at work. Communication is a complex process, and thus causal factors, including social, learning, motivational, psychological, physiological, and linguistic, among others, may singly or collectively hold the hidden key. Previously, I warned that correlation (events that occur in temporal proximity to one another) does not imply causality (a direct link between two events—one assumed to be a stimulus and the other assumed to be its direct result). I am mindful that attempts to determine predisposing and precipitating factors might appear to be an imprecise science of diagnosis. I am mindful also of the challenging if not provocative findings being revealed by the best of longitudinal research, reviewed in the previous chapter. Yet, I am encouraged by the potential for understanding predisposing and precipitating factors and their interactions to shed some light on the nature of a person's stuttering experience or help to tailor the treatment experience to the uniqueness of each person who stutters.

Therefore, I maintain that pursuing these factors is essential. Sometimes the precipitating factors are easily identifiable, as is their causal connection to the stuttering behavior. An example might be the infrequent cases of abrupt onset of stuttering surrounding a traumatic event. When observed, such cases are typically viewed as a distinct subtype of the disorder (e.g., neurogenic acquired stuttering or psychogenic acquired stuttering; see Chapter 4). Other cases where precipitating factors are clear and causally linked to the communication disorder include instances of cerebral vascular accident (i.e., stroke), vocal abuse, structural anomalies, and certain congenital conditions (Haynes & Pindzola, 2008).

Perpetuating Factors

Perpetuating factors are those variables that are continuing or maintaining the stuttering at the present time (Nicolosi et al., 2004) and address the question, "What causes a person to continue to stutter after the disorder has begun?" (F. H. Silverman, 2004, p. 129). Haynes and Pindzola (2008) indicated that habit strength is a prime perpetuating factor, as the client has made compensations for the stuttering in terms of cognitive and linguistic strategies, motor adjustments, and other modifications. The clinician needs to uncover environmental and physical factors that reinforce, and therefore perpetuate, the disorder. Occasionally, precipitating factors that are still present might serve to perpetuate the stuttering. For example, environmental influences such as criticism of speech, inappropriate linguistic models, unrealistic expectations, and experienced fluency failure may exacerbate the problem and maintain the likelihood of its predictability. Perpetuating factors, unlike predisposing and precipitating factors, are nearly always "knowable."

Although many clients do not recognize the perpetuating factors, they can become aware of them with the assistance of a supportive and knowledgeable clinician. Sometimes the negative feelings and attitudes that result from repeated frustration and embarrassment with stuttering are the most challenging perpetuating factors to alter. Accommodations are made by the person who stutters and others within his communication system (family, friends, classmates, teachers, colleagues, employers, etc.). Thus the dynamics of communication, including how we perceive ourselves and others as communicators, are established that perpetuate or maintain the disorder. The anticipation of fluency failure so often felt by people who stutter in situations perceived to be important (asking someone out for a date, speaking to one's employer, saying one's own name) is understandable given one's history, yet is a barrier to fluency facilitation.

The spouse who continues to order for her husband in restaurants during their 40-year marriage is helping him avoid frustration and embarrassment, yet perpetuating the likelihood that he will continue to be disfluent in that setting. A man of 55 years who reportedly was severely disfluent for his entire life discovered during trial management that he possessed the potential for remarkable fluency. When asked to consider how an improvement in his fluency would affect him as a communicator, he was unable to imagine those possibilities. He said, "I have always stuttered. I cannot imagine what it would be like not to stutter. This is all that I've ever known." This is habit strength. This is what happens when stuttering establishes the perimeters of one's self-concept, of one's personal construct. This is a man who saw himself as a "stutterer." Stuttering was at the heart of his very existence. He reported that in his sleep, he saw himself stuttering in his dreams. Stuttering was the anchor around which all of his life revolved—emotionally, interpersonally, socially, professionally. Indeed, it was hard for him even to consider another paradigm—until he experienced systematic and reliable success in treatment. At the sixth week of treatment, he confessed, "You know, I didn't believe in this stuff at the beginning. But now, I'm hooked."

Perpetuating factors vary with each individual and may be simple or complex, subtle or obvious, malleable or resistant to change. Nevertheless, we can know and must identify these factors in order to facilitate change. The process, as will be seen, is a tender one at times, in that people learn intimate things about themselves and others. Learning constitutes change. Change is sometimes difficult to accept. But a sensitive, caring, and knowledgeable clinician cares for, with, and about the person who stutters, and enters into the process as a comrade in a common struggle.

Theoretical Explanations

What is theory and who needs it? Why do so many courses spend so long on theoretical explanations of stuttering and then shortchange clinical intervention? Why do so many speech–language pathologists and students of stuttering think of theory as the "*T* word," a dirty word, an unrelated and necessary evil on the way to intervention?

For me, theory is like a map. It represents the lay of the land, what is known about a territory, enabling us to navigate through it. With a map, we understand clearly our point of origin, our destination, and our options for embarking on the journey, mindful of our purposes and the challenges along the way. Without such a map, our route may be scenic but circuitous, progressive but indirect, if successful at all. A theory of stuttering represents what we know to date, enabling us to understand the contributions of previous clinical teaching, service, and research; interpret those of the present; and plan for those in the future. A theory of stuttering unites what we think and know with what we do, an obligation too often overlooked by well-meaning clinicians. In other words, each clinician must have her own theory to navigate through stuttering and allied disciplines and to apply what is known from an informed, inquiring, and accountable perspective so that she can recognize the strengths and meet the needs of each person who stutters.

Guitar (2006) explained that a theory unites findings in a systematic way in order to explain past phenomena and to predict future phenomena. A theory about stuttering should explain why one person stutters and another does not, why a person stutters only on some words and in some situations, and why a person who stutters does, thinks, and feels what he does. Guitar defined theory as a formal set of hypotheses that explain a causal relationship in a phenomenon. These hypotheses are tested and, as a consequence, discarded, confirmed, or refined. He indicated, however, that the field of stuttering has not developed sufficiently to have a formal theory of stuttering but, rather, has only theoretical explanations, perspectives, or models, which as yet lack causal links.

Bloodstein and Bernstein Ratner (2008) noted five pressing challenges that are representative but not exhaustive in developing viable theories:

1. Theories must posit the cause of stuttering, yet must take into account the fact that what causes stuttering to emerge may or may not relate to factors that contribute to the development of stuttering (i.e., affective, behavioral, and cognitive) over a lifetime. Also, studying adults may not provide a window for understanding how their stuttering began as children, and understanding what initially causes stuttering may not relate to the most effective treatment, as the experience of stuttering changes over time.

2. Theories must account for the features of stuttering itself and distinguish between stuttering and other forms of speech disfluency.

3. Theories should be able to predict the distributional characteristics of stuttering (i.e., its patterns near onset and as it develops, and conditions under which stuttering worsens or ameliorates).

4. Theories must account for the onset of stuttering, which typically begins between ages 2 and 4 years, during or after a period of fluent and capable speech and language performance, and resulting in the child's awareness of communication difficulty.

5. Theories must account for and differentiate between children who begin to stutter yet recover without treatment (80%) and those whose stuttering persists (20%).

It is no wonder that there are so many theoretical explanations of stuttering, some of which seem complementary and others contradictory. Perhaps this apparent theoretical discord contributes to student clinicians and speech–language pathologists alike occasionally being inclined to dismiss the relevance of theory for understanding stuttering and planning treatment. I must assert again the value of theory as our road map. Theory must be taken seriously—in fact, as an essential part of our commitment to our Code of Ethics (ASHA, 2010) and to client welfare. We must continue to ask ourselves why we do what we do as clinicians, what the origins of those ideas are, and what the available data are to support or refute those ideas. To do anything less is to fall short of our professional obligations. I might assert as well that clinicians must at some point stand back and ask themselves how what they do reflects what they believe and who they are as people and as professionals. Too often, we forget to calibrate our compass, thus discounting the trueness of our map. The evidence-based practice movement only reminds us of our commitment to theory and its direct relatedness to quality service delivery and the integrity of every clinician's personal construct.

Bloodstein and Bernstein Ratner (2008) organized theories of stuttering around the moment of stuttering (i.e., discrete instances of stuttering behavior), etiology (i.e., onset of stuttering), and reformulations of etiology and the moment of stuttering. Using their organizational scheme (see also Bloodstein, 1981; Guitar, 2006), I will discuss six major developmental theories of stuttering (and some representative subtypes): stuttering as the result of a neurotic response, communication failure and anticipatory struggle, learned behavior, physiological deficit, disturbed feedback, and multifactorial causes. The earlier theories (e.g., Freud's repressed need theory) are presented both because they have historical interest and because even though they may have been discarded, some remnant often informs later conceptualizations.

Stuttering as a Neurotic Response

In the early 1900s, Sigmund Freud explained stuttering psychoanalytically, asserting that stuttering satisfies oral or anal erotic needs or represents repressed hostility (repressed need theory). Within this framework, stuttering is seen as an attempt to suppress speech and as a symptom of a deep neurotic conflict. This theory, reviewed by Ambrose (2004), was adapted to suggest that stuttering reflected libido fixation at the oral stage of infant psychosexual development (Coriat, 1928), causing the child to be sensitive and anxious, combined with left-handedness, weak tongue and throat musculature (Blanton, 1931), and anal fixation yielding aggressive characteristics (Fenichel, 1945). Bloodstein and Bernstein Ratner (2008) summarized this theory as follows. Stuttering satisfies an infantile need for oral erotic gratification (i.e., perpetuation of early pleasures from nursing, biting, and oral exploration of objects), satiates anal erotic needs, expresses hostile or aggressive impulses that the person fears to express openly (i.e., hostile forcing out or holding back of words, parallel to hostile expulsion and retention of feces), and reflects an unconscious desire to suppress expression of forbidden wishes and feelings related to oral gratification and the consequent feelings of guilt and anxiety. Beyond the historical value of the repressed need theory, current research (i.e., both adjustment inventories and projective tests) reflects that people who stutter are no more neurotic or maladjusted as a group than people who do not stutter (Bloodstein & Bernstein Ratner, 2008). The repressed need theory is no longer considered valid. Nevertheless, personality, particularly anxiety and temperament, continues to be studied. For example, people who stutter have been found to demonstrate a greater degree of situational anxiety, a finding that can be explained as a consequence of stuttering rather than as a cause of it (Craig, Hancock, Tran, & Craig, 2003).

Stuttering as Communicative Failure and Anticipatory Struggle Behavior

Theories that explain stuttering as communicative failure and anticipatory struggle behavior assume that the person who stutters disrupts the way he speaks because he believes that speech is difficult or that he will fail at speaking. The following theories are reviewed here: diagnosogenic theory, the continuity hypothesis (communication failure theory), and preparatory set (primary stuttering theory).

The Diagnosogenic Theory. W. Johnson's (1958, 1959, 1961) diagnosogenic (or semantic) theory states that stuttering is caused by the parents' or care providers' misdiagnosis of and inappropriate reaction to normal disfluencies in a child's speech, followed by the child's attempts to avoid the disfluencies that are mistakenly assumed to render the child's speech abnormal. Johnson (1942) stated,

> The parents classified their children as stutterers and then proceeded to react to them largely in terms of the implications of the label. These reactions on the part of parents were not confined to inner states of tension and anxiety or chagrin, but usually also involved overt attempts to influence the child's speech behavior and definite communication to the child of the parental evaluations of his speech. (p. 255)

Johnson (1942) further asserted that "highly similar varieties of speech in young children are thus differently evaluated by different parents, and there can be little question that the way in which they are evaluated plays a determining role in the subsequent speech development of the child" (p. 256). He concluded, "Stuttering in its serious forms develops after the diagnosis rather than before and is a consequence of the diagnosis" (p. 257).

Van Riper (1982; see also Bloodstein, 1986) classified Johnson's theory, which was widely accepted in the 1940s and 1950s, as a form of cognitive learning theory. It strongly criticized the environmental events, namely reactions of parents and other listeners, as a direct precipitator of stuttering, and implied that predisposing or constitutional factors were relatively insignificant. Johnson and his associates (1959) observed that children who stutter demonstrated more sound and syllable repetitions, complete blocks, and prolonged sounds than children who do not stutter, with the latter group showing more phrase repetitions, pauses, and interjections than children who stutter. He emphasized the similarities, rather than the differences, across children to stress that stuttering is first in the parent's ear, not in the child's mouth.

In 1988, F. H. Silverman published a paper describing an unpublished study by one of Johnson's graduate students (Tudor, 1939) in which normally fluent children were reported to have been turned into children who stutter. The Tudor study, as we will see, became the topic of much interest, conflicting interpretations, and outrage in the years following Silverman's 1988 article on it. The study ("An Experimental Study of the Effect of Evaluative Labeling on Speech Fluency") was conducted before Johnson proposed the diagnosogenic theory. Those familiar with the study at the University of Iowa referred to it as "the monster study." Silverman asserted that the study holds tremendous historical significance because it is the only direct test of the diagnosogenic theory and provides clinical implications contraindicating the wisdom of increasing children's awareness of their speech hesitations. Others would later question this assessment.

In the study, according to Silverman's (1988) account, Tudor selected six children residing in an orphanage whose chronological ages were 5, 9, 11, 12, 12, and 15 to serve as subjects. All of the children, chosen because of their normal communication development, were told flatly that their speech contained symptoms of a child beginning to stutter and that they should stop this pattern immediately, use willpower, and stop talking unless they could get it right. In addition, the orphanage teachers and matrons were told that the children showed "definite symptoms of stuttering," should be watched closely for speech errors, and should be corrected when such errors occurred. The subjects reportedly experienced negative communicative changes, including decrease in verbal output, rate of speech, and length of utterance; heightened self-consciousness; acceptance that there was something defective in their speech; and nonverbal behavior interfering with the message (e.g., gasping and covering the mouth when speaking, avoiding eye contact, laughing awkwardly, showing embarrassment). Tudor attempted to treat the children and continued to do so for several years, but the communicative changes persisted, and at least one child reportedly continued to stutter (F. H. Silverman, 1988).

The results of Tudor's (1939) study were never disseminated widely because, according to Silverman (1988), the experimenters regretted the experiment and were remorseful about the outcome. Silverman, a former student and research assistant of Johnson, noted that Johnson never published the findings of this study in any of his writings on the diagnosogenic theory, although they directly supported it.

A widely disseminated two-part story on the Tudor study published by the *San Jose Mercury News* in 2001 captured the public's attention with its assertion that Johnson had intentionally suppressed the study in light of the World War II atrocities perpetrated on human subjects by Nazi scientists and physicians (Dyer, 2001a, 2001b). Since 2001, both conventional news media and scholarly publications have addressed two key issues—the scientific validity of the findings and the ethics of the study. While there seems to be general agreement that the study's research design and methods do not reflect current scientific standards, some have asserted that the conclusions of the study support the diagnosogenic theory (e.g., Halvorson, 1999, 2008; Retzinger, 2001; M. J. Retzinger, personal communications, September 28, 2007, June 4, 2008). Others (e.g., Yairi & Ambrose, 2001) have rejected the conclusions of the study, noting, "We have examined the data carefully and found that the study completely failed to demonstrate any support for its conclusions that stuttering could be elicited via labeling" (p. 17). Yairi and Ambrose (2001) reported that neither the judges nor Tudor described the children's posttreatment speech as stuttering and that there was no significant change in disfluency types for any of the four groups (the only exception was the normally fluent group labeled as "stutterers," but the significant increase in interjections could be interpreted as typical of normal speech). In this same group, reanalysis of one of the participants' speech patterns justified a classification of stuttering at the beginning of the study. Several other researchers articulated additional concerns. First, the participants were not representative of U.S. children, having a relatively high incidence of stuttering and lower than average IQs (Bloodstein & Bernstein Ratner, 2008; Van Borsel et al., 2006). Second, control for experimenter bias and consistency of experimental procedures were inadequate (i.e., there were no reliability data), and the follow-up by orphanage staff was inconsistent (Ambrose & Yairi, 2002; Bernstein Ratner, 2001; Yairi & Ambrose, 2001).

The ethical foundation of the Tudor study has been consistently condemned. Yairi and Ambrose (2001) noted, "As for the ethical issue, to conduct research in an orphanage without disclosure of its real purpose, and to attempt to convert normally fluent children into children who stutter, is indefensible" (p. 17). The University of Iowa, as well as the American Speech-Language-Hearing Association, issued a formal apology in 2001 for the experiments, stating that strict policies and procedures today ensure the safety of all human research subjects (Annett, 2001). A 2003 lawsuit brought by Tudor subjects against the state of Iowa was settled out of court in 2007, with the state agreeing to pay a total of $925,000, of the original $13.5 million sought, to the six subjects or their heirs (ASHA, 2007c). Wendell Johnson died in 1965; the orphanage closed in 1975; and Mary Tudor, whose thesis was never published, died in 2006.

Regardless of the scientific validity of the Tudor study and the degree to which it might support the diagnosogenic theory, there is a kernel of truth to Wendell Johnson's conceptualization of stuttering that is still relevant to clinical practice today: Negative labeling can adversely affect behavior, and we as clinicians should be mindful of this fact as we work with clients who stutter (Harrison & Onslow, 2010; Reeves, 2006; Yaruss et al., 2002).

The Continuity Hypothesis. The continuity hypothesis, or communication failure theory, was proposed by Bloodstein (1975, 1984, 1995) and suggests that stuttering develops from normal disfluency that becomes tense and fragmented as the child experiences frustration and failure in attempts to talk. Many types of experiences can lead the child to experience difficulty with speech, including criticism of normal disfluencies, delay in speech or language development, communication disorders, traumatic experience in oral reading, cluttering and reminders to "slow down," and emotionally traumatic events during which the child tries to speak (Bloodstein, 1975, 1984). Guitar (2006) indicated that other aspects of the internal and external environment may add pressure and lead a child to expect failure. These influences may include a perfectionist nature or a high need to perform or meet the perceived standards of others. The level of unconditional acceptance and positive regard within the child's communication environment is critical in influencing the child's attitude and expectations toward himself as a communicator.

Bloodstein (1975) interpreted stuttering as a form of communication failure resulting from anticipatory struggle (i.e., a response to stimuli representative of past speech failure). Bloodstein (1975) indicated that people who stutter "behave as though they have acquired a belief in the difficulty of speech, or of specific speech segments, and appear to struggle against an imagined obstacle in the process of articulation" (p. 4). Tension and fragmentation represent the embodiment of the speaker's doubts about his ability to speak well, heightened by the perception of a critical audience or the memory of past speech failure or pressure. Bloodstein (1975) indicated that most children demonstrate speech tension and fragmentation in their speech, but in children who stutter, this tension is greater. This observation formed the core of the continuity hypothesis.

On the surface, the diagnosogenic theory and the continuity hypothesis sound similar. In both, the child becomes aware of his speech-related tension and fragmentation and desires to avoid it. However, the diagnosogenic theory suggests that the child does so because of the negative reactions of listeners to the disfluency (i.e., the child plays more of a passive role in the evolution of stuttering), while the continuity hypothesis emphasizes the child's own awareness of and increasing concern about his own disfluency (i.e., the child is more active).

Taken to an extreme, Bloodstein's (1975) hypothesis implies that no differential diagnosis can be made on the basis of indicators of developmental stuttering because "most young children stutter" (p. 51). Stuttering becomes a problem only when the child evaluates the breaks in fluency as unpleasant and shows fear, avoidance, and struggle reactions. Bloodstein (1975) concluded,

> Any attempt to make such a "diagnosis" is a futile and meaningless exercise. We can describe his tensions and fragmentations, count them, compare them with norms, find out under what conditions they occur, determine how much of a problem they are for the child or anyone else, and make a judgment about whether he should be getting some help from us because of them. But we cannot tell whether he is or is not a "stutterer." (p. 51)

Bloodstein's (1975) continuity hypothesis and its implications have been challenged by the clinical literature, particularly as clinicians and researchers have become increasingly aware of the importance of differential diagnosis and appropriate early intervention (Bloodstein & Bernstein Ratner, 2008; Gordon & Luper, 1992a, 1992b; Van Riper, 1982; Yairi & Ambrose, 2005; Yaruss & Quesal, 2006, 2008).

Preparatory Set (i.e., Primary Stuttering Theory). Van Riper (1972, 1973, 1982) indicated that stuttering emerges gradually from a child's normal hesitations and repetitions. Such disruptions first occur without effort or apparent awareness by the child, and later become chronic when the child begins to anticipate, avoid, and fear speech and related contexts because of reactions by listeners. Stuttering can originate from learning (environmental), constitutional (organic), or neurotic (emotional) sources. Van Riper (1972) described the onset and development of stuttering using a series of metaphors to represent learning, constitutional, and emotional sources. According to Van Riper (1972), stuttering can come from any of these three sources:

> As the stream leaves Lake Learning, it flows slowly and many a child caught in its current may make it to shore by himself or with a bit of parental or therapeutic help. Some of them are cast up on Precarious Island and become fluent for a time, only to be swept away again by the swift-moving emotional currents from Neurosis Pond. The second stage in the development of stuttering is represented by Surprise Rapids, and the stutterer begins to know that he is in trouble. It isn't hard to rescue him, however, if you know how to do it.
>
> Once he is swept over Frustration Falls, however, he takes a beating from the many rocks that churn the stream. Despite their random struggling, a few make it to shore even at this stage, the third, but they usually need an understanding therapist and co-operative parents to help them. The river flows even faster here, and soon it enters the Gorge of Fear. This is the worst stretch of the whole stream of stuttering, for below it lies the Whirlpool of Self-Reinforcement. Once the child is caught in its constant circling, there is little hope that he will ever make it to shore by himself. Only an able and stout swimmer who knows not only this part, but all of the river of stuttering, can hope to save him. Where does the river end? King Charles the First knows. (p. 277)

Bloodstein and Bernstein Ratner (2008) used Van Riper's (1973) preparatory set in their formulation of the anticipatory struggle hypothesis. Specifically, the preparatory set, or alteration of the block before it occurs, is used to counteract the tendency of the person who stutters to place himself in a tense, fixed, inappropriate articulatory posture in advance of attempting to say a word he fears or believes will be disfluent. (I interpret the alteration as utilizing a deliberate evenness of rate, gentleness of articulation, and naturalness of inflection.) This preposturing influences the relative shape and fluency of the word to follow. The fixed, uncontrolled, muscular, and psychological set effectively guarantees that the word will be spoken disfluently. Conversely, the pre-block alterations described earlier ensure control and enable the person who stutters to say any word without stuttering. Van Riper (1982) offered a tentative explanation that stuttering is related to the difficulty some children experience in mastering the synchronized timing of the motor coordinations required for speech.

Stuttering as Learned Behavior

Within the context of the behavioral sciences, theories that characterize stuttering as learned behavior define the processes by which stuttering is originally learned and maintained and postulate motivational factors, stimulus variables, and reinforcing conditions (Nicolosi et al., 2004). Learning theories can be classified into those that view stuttering as an avoidance response and those that view stuttering as an interaction of at least two behavioral phenomena.

Stuttering as an Avoidance Response. Several theories in this subcategory are reviewed here: conflict theory, operant conditioning theory, and instrumental avoidance act theory. Generally avoidance response theories hold that stuttering is the involuntary outcome of other learned approach–avoidance drives and not itself a learned behavior (Nicolosi et al., 2004).

In Sheehan's (1958, 1975) *conflict theory of stuttering*, stuttering results from a double approach–avoidance conflict between speaking and not speaking and between being silent and not being silent. "The avoidance does not come primarily from the fear of stuttering as such but from the competition between the alternative possibilities of speech and silence, with the stuttering a resultant of this conflict" (Sheehan, 1958, p. 126). When the approach drive is more powerful, fluent speech results; when the avoidance drive is more powerful, disfluency or silence results. When both motivational drives for approach and avoidance of speaking are equally dominant, stuttering results. Theoretically, stuttering reduces the fear underlying the avoidance drive, thus enabling the approach motivational drive to regain dominance.

The *operant conditioning theory* of stuttering states that speech is a behavior subject to operant control by positive and negative reinforcements and punishments. There is no simple cause of stuttering that is maintained on a complex schedule of reinforcement. Shames (1975) stated, "Operant behavior is that behavior whose frequency is a function of its consequences. On certain occasions, certain responses generate consequences in the environment. If these consequences affect the frequency of the behavior that they follow, we are dealing with operant behavior" (p. 267). He indicated that stuttering and disfluency decrease with contingent aversive stimulation through negative reinforcement, and that fluency increases through positive reinforcement. Given the reliability of these observations, Shames noted that conditioning processes are probably active in the onset and development of stuttering. The particular form that these conditioning processes may take in the child's natural environment can only be suggested and have not been experimentally verified.

The *instrumental avoidance act theory* states that stuttering is an acquired response reflecting expectancy, anticipation, adaptation, or anxiety and is motivated by the learned drive of apprehension about the normal disfluencies of speech (Nicolosi et al., 2004). Wischner (1950, 1952) applied the concept of drive reduction (i.e., anxiety) to explain the maintenance of stuttering. Wischner adopted Wendell Johnson's postulates that the child reacts to the parents' misdiagnosis with tension, anxiety, and avoidance. Wischner emphasized, however, that the child is trying to avoid not the normal disfluencies, but rather the consequences that are associated with the original disfluent behaviors (i.e., feelings of anxiety, hurt, and shame). Certain cues precipitate these anxieties, which the person attempts to lessen by avoidance. Because of anxiety reduction, the avoidance behaviors are reinforced and thereby developed and maintained. For example, avoidance behaviors such as interjection of a sound (e.g., *um*) or phrase (e.g., "Let me see") might prevent or stall the moment of disfluency, thus reducing the anxiety reaction that reinforces the avoidance behavior.

Stuttering as an Interaction of Behavioral Phenomena. One theory that interprets stuttering as an interaction of behavioral phenomena is the *two-factor learning theory of stuttering*, also referred to as the *conditioned disintegration theory* (Nicolosi et al., 2004). Two-factor theorists (e.g., Brutten, 1975; Brutten & Shoemaker, 1971) differentiate between classical conditioning (stimulus-contingent learning) and instrumental conditioning (response-contingent learning). Classical conditioning generally describes the conditions within which a person (or other organism) learns to be motivationally or emotionally stimulated by previously neutral stimuli. Classical conditioning increases the number of stimuli that motivate, arouse, or drive a person. Instrumental conditioning generally describes conditions within which a person learns coping responses in order to modify "learned or unlearned drive states" associated with a stimulus context. Brutten and Shoemaker noted, "Classical conditioning leads to the development of relationships between stimuli and motivational states or emotional responses, and instrumental conditioning leads to the development of relationships between stimuli and relatively specific, goal-oriented behaviors" (p. 1055). These authors proposed that the core characteristics of stuttering (such as part-word and word repetitions and prolongations) represent the involuntary breakdown of speech resulting from negative emotional responses that are classically conditioned. (Stress may produce autonomic reactions that disrupt the speech. The negative emotions aroused become classically conditioned with concurrent stimuli.) Secondary characteristics (such as escape and avoidance) are instrumentally conditioned responses (or learned adjustments) of the individual to unpleasant experiences (Nicolosi et al., 2004).

Summarizing the influence of learning on stuttering, Van Riper (1982) indicated, "The different varieties of stuttering reactions, the changes that occur as the disorder develops, the role of situational and verbal cues in its precipitation, all these and many other features of the problem testify to the influence of learning" (p. 284). Van Riper added that it is generally agreed that learning plays at least a part in determining the patterns of advanced stuttering. There is much disagreement, however, regarding the exact role that learning plays.

Stuttering as a Physiological Deficit

Theories that conceptualize stuttering as a physiological deficit, also referred to as *breakdown theories*, characterize the moment of stuttering as an indication of failure or breakdown in the complex coordination required for fluent speech. Most breakdown theories assume that a person who stutters has a constitutional predisposition toward stuttering that is precipitated by psychosocial or environmental stress, and a reduced physiological capacity to coordinate speech. The precise nature of the organic predisposing factors and the role of heredity vary across theorists. Such theorists have postulated perceptual, motor, or central deficits. The following theories are reviewed here: incomplete cerebral dominance, dysphemia, perseveration theory, and brain lesion.

Stuttering as a Function of Incomplete Cerebral Dominance. The theory of stuttering as a function of incomplete cerebral dominance suggests that people who stutter do not show the usual pattern for left-hemisphere dominance. Orton and Travis (Travis, 1978) observed that many people who stutter are left-handed but were deliberately changed to right-handedness by their parents. Orton and Travis hypothesized that ambidexterity or a change in handedness (i.e., incomplete cerebral dominance, or laterality) caused a disruption in the regular flow of nerve impulses to the speech musculature. This disruption caused a conflict between the two hemispheres for the control of speech, taking the form of neuromotor disorganization and mistiming resulting in stuttering.

Dysphemia. *Dysphemia* refers to stuttering conceptualized as a manifestation of an internal condition triggered by illness, emotional or environmental stress, or biochemical imbalance. West (1958) indicated that "stuttering is primarily an epileptic disorder that manifests itself in dyssynergies of the neuromotor mechanism for oral language. Its spasms are precipitated by social anxieties involved in communication by oral language" (1958, p. 197). These anxieties are more likely to be precipitants of stuttering when they take the form of conscious feelings of guilt, particularly related to the topic of the conversation. West, therefore, viewed stuttering as a convulsive disorder involving a relationship between the person who stutters and his conversational partners within a social communicative context.

Perseveration Theory. Perseveration theory states that a person who stutters has an organic predisposition to motor and sensory perseveration of which stuttering is an outward manifestation. Eisenson (1958, 1975) elaborated his interpretation of stuttering as a perseverative phenomenon, indicating that "stuttering is a transient disturbance in communicative, propositional language usage" (1975, p. 426). Speech is implicated because it is the medium for oral language, that which is temporarily disturbed. Eisenson indicated that the majority of people who stutter are constitutionally predisposed to perseverative oral language behavior (i.e., stuttering). While he distinguished between organically predisposed and functional or nonorganic stuttering, his premise was that both are the products of constitutionally predisposed perseveration.

Stuttering as a Consequence of Brain Lesion. Based on high-speed cineradiographic data, Zimmermann (1980a) studied the movements, positions, and timing of lip and jaw structures in the perceptually fluent production of isolated monosyllables by people who stutter, comparing these productions to those of people who do not stutter. The fluent syllables spoken by people who stutter revealed longer duration of movement onset, slower voice onset, longer latency for peak velocity of lip and jaw movements, longer transition times, and greater lip and jaw movement asynchrony. These patterns were evident during perceptually fluent sounds and syllables, and even more evident during stuttered speech. Zimmermann (1980a) postulated that stuttering involves changes in the interaction of laryngeal, supralaryngeal, and respiratory reflexes. This proposal implicates the brain stem as the site of lesion and suggests that stuttering is the consequence of disruption of motor organization, timing, and control (Zimmermann, 1980a, 1980b, 1984; Zimmermann, Smith, & Hanley, 1981).

Stuttering as the Result of Disturbed Feedback
Disturbed feedback (or cybernetic) theory is based on the servomechanism feedback model, in which the ear is the sensor, the vocal organs and motor innervations are the effector, and the brain is the controller. People who stutter are assumed to possess a defective monitoring system for speech. To remain error free, ongoing fluent speech movements require feedback and sensory information. When errors occur, the system corrects itself by searching for the appropriate output until it is achieved. Stuttering is

seen as a consequence of this corrective process, as the absence of a correct standard pattern for production of a syllable or word, or as a perceptual error on the input side of sensory information processing. This theory assumes that the automatic motor sequencing of speech occurs within a closed-loop system in which auditory feedback is critical (Fairbanks, 1954). The feedback systems used to monitor speech potentially have many sources of distortion (e.g., asynchrony or delay of auditory feedback, which can interfere with proprioceptive feedback). Too much feedback distortion and output correction can cause fixation in the system. According to this model, such distortion, interference, and overload can cause stuttering.

Stuttering as a Result of Multifactorial Causes

Multifactorial theories generally posit that stuttering results from a confluence of factors. The following theories are reviewed here: the demands and capacities model, CALMS (cognitive, affective, language, motor, social), the revised component model, the psycholinguistic model, neurophysiological theory, the multifactorial dynamic model, and the dual premotor model of stuttering and cluttering.

Demands and Capacities Model.
In the demands and capacities model, stuttering results if the child's demands exceed his capacities for fluent speech. Fluency is a multidimensional variable composed of continuity, rate, and effort (Starkweather, 1984, 1987). Fluent speech, therefore, is characterized by continuous production, without effort, at an appropriate rate. Both the child's capacities for fluent speech and the demands for fluent speech imposed on the child by listeners and himself are increasing as the child develops. When the demands exceed the child's capacities for fluent speech, stuttering occurs. If the demands are reduced or increased slowly or the child's capacities develop sufficiently, stuttering remits. If the demands continue to outpace the child's capacity for fluent speech, stuttering persists. The continuation of stuttering might be self-perpetuating. In other words, if stuttering continues long enough for the child to develop struggle, tension, and avoidance, his whole approach to speaking is influenced by anticipated fluency failure.

Starkweather, Gottwald, and Halfond (1990) and Gottwald (2010) elaborated the demands and capacities model, indicating that the capacities for fluency fall into four categories: speech motor control (i.e., rate of syllable production and coordination of movement), language formulation (i.e., word-finding, formulation of grammatical sentences, and knowledge of conversational rules), social–emotional maturity, and cognitive skill (i.e., general intelligence and metalinguistic skill). The demands for fluency are those conditions that impose a pressure perceived by the child to speak at a greater rate (i.e., faster) or with greater continuity (i.e., more smoothly). The demands, which increase as the child matures, include time pressure, uncertainty, and avoidance.

Time pressure is imposed when parents or others speak too rapidly in the child's presence, thus conveying the impression that speech time is limited and information is expected to flow rapidly. There is evidence that mothers of children who stutter talk more rapidly and interrupt more often than mothers of children who do not (Meyers & Freeman, 1985a, 1985b), and that a positive correlation exists between the extent to which parents decrease their rate of speech (Gottwald & Starkweather, 1984, 1995) or implement structured conversational turn-taking (Winslow & Guitar, 1994) and the extent to which the child's fluency improves. Negative listener reactions (such as interrupting, finishing the child's sentence, interpreting the child's behavior as negative, telling the child to "hurry up") also impose time pressure. Likewise, using language with the child that includes longer and more complex vocabulary and syntax increases time pressure. Such constructions, which the child attempts to match, are motorically more difficult to plan, time, coordinate, and execute, thus consuming neuromotor resources that would otherwise be devoted to maintaining fluency. Additional sources of time pressure are demand speech (e.g., frequent questions or requests to recite something or recount events), a rushed household or other environment, high levels of excitement or emotionality, and rushed and interrupted patterns of conversational turn-taking. Starkweather et al. (1990) indicated that such demands may convey to the child that neither he nor his conversational contribution is valued. As a consequence, the child feels he is not worthy of much talking time. Self-esteem suffers.

Uncertainty, or any event that might introduce change or disruption, can challenge the child's sense of security, thus placing additional demands on the child's existing capacities for fluent speech. Examples of situations involving high demand are moving into a new house or neighborhood, first separation from parents, birth of a sibling, illness of a parent, change in day-care setting or childcare arrangement, and a household charged with emotionality or tension (Starkweather et al., 1990). The uncertainty of these and other circumstances might leave the child feeling unsure of the consequences of behavior, thus causing him to become hesitant to do or say anything. This uncertainty may worsen the frequency and severity of disfluency.

Avoidance of stuttering or speaking constitutes another demand on the child. Such avoidance might originate from inadvertent negative reactions from listeners, such as tensing when the child stutters and relaxing when the child regains fluency, looking away, filling in for the child, tapping fingers, wrinkling brows, or other behaviors that communicate to the child that his stuttering is undesirable and unpleasant. In addition to perceiving pressure to speak more rapidly and smoothly, some children experience guilt for the discomfort that they feel they have caused their parents or other listeners. Starkweather et al. (1990) concluded,

> We believe that fluent speech is rapid and continuous, and that the capacity to speak fluently increases with maturity. At the same time, the environment, both internal and external, is increasingly demanding of fluency. There is increased pressure to generate more complex ideas within a limited period of time. Parents, reacting to disfluency in the child's speech, may speak more quickly and interrupt more often, and these reactions increase the demands of time pressure even further. In addition, changes in the child's life may lead to increased insecurity and uncertainty of the consequences of speaking.
>
> Finally, the reactions of parents to the child's disfluency may lead increasingly to an attitude of avoidance of disfluency. The gap between these demands and capacities widens or narrows as changes in the demands proceed more or less quickly than changes in the capacities. The capacities stem from speech motor control—programming, timing, and coordination—and from linguistic and social skills, such as language formulation and pragmatic knowledge. Both speech and language fluency impact on the ease with which a child can produce meaningful speech, as reflected in the rate and continuity of the child's utterances. (pp. 28–29)

The appeal to clinicians of the demands and capacities model has endured despite challenges to its inherent constructs. Manning (2000) coordinated a special section devoted to the demands and capacities model in the *Journal of Fluency Disorders*, in which six clinician–researchers (Curlee, Bernstein Ratner, Yaruss, Kelly, Starkweather, and Gottwald) responded to Siegel's (2000) critique of the capacities concept. Siegel argued that because capacities are less observable and therefore less measurable than demands, the construct of performance should replace that of capacities. The respondents asserted that the model remains appealing because of the relative simplicity with which it explains stuttering onset and development, particularly to parents, and because of its parallel to clinicians' orientation (i.e., seeing the entire person and approaching treatment from a multifactorial perspective). The respondents also noted, however, that the nature of scientific investigation requires a controlled approach in which phenomena (i.e., demands, capacities, and others) must be investigated one variable at a time (see also Bothe et al., 2006; Harris, Onslow, Packman, Harrison, & Menzies, 2002; Harrison et al., 2007; Onslow, 2003, 2004; Onslow et al., 2003; Onslow & Yaruss, 2007). Such investigation is, in fact, a present and likely ongoing research focus (e.g., Franken, Kielstra-Van der Schalk, & Boelens, 2005; Huinck et al., 2006; M. Jones, Onslow, Harrison, & Packman, 2005; Yaruss, Coleman, & Hammer, 2006). Starkweather (2002a, 2002b) has also encouraged evidence-based applications and future research on consilience among genetic influences at the physiological, behavioral, and cultural levels.

CALMS: An Integrated Model. In their CALMS model, Healey, Trautman, and Susca (2004; Healey, 2007) asserted that stuttering results from and is maintained by the dynamic interaction between five components: *c*ognitive (thoughts, perceptions, awareness, understanding), *a*ffective (feelings, emotions, attitudes), *l*inguistic (language skills, formulation demands, and discourse complexity), *m*otor (sensorimotor control of speech movements), and *s*ocial (environmental effects of type of listener and speaking situations). This model holds that stuttering is influenced both by motor issues and by how people think and feel about themselves and their stuttering; thoughts, perceptions, feelings, and attitudes impact formulation and delivery of the message and interact with motor, linguistic, and social elements (and vice versa—motor, linguistic, and social elements impact affective and cognitive elements). The five elements combine uniquely for each person who stutters, influencing the frequency, type, and duration of stuttering; the five elements form the roots of stuttering and therefore must be assessed and monitored for change in communication functioning as a part of stuttering intervention. The authors provided guidelines for assessment and quantification of each element of CALMS and a case profile to guide intervention.

Revised Component Model. The revised component model (Riley & Riley, 2000), a revision of the original component model (Riley & Riley, 1979), holds that three main factors contribute to stuttering and are found to be more prevalent among children who stutter. The components include physical attributes (i.e., attending disorder, speech motor control difficulty), temperament factors (high levels of anxiety, self-blame, and self-expectations or perfectionism; low threshold for frustration; and overly sensitive), and listener reactions (disruptive communication environment or negative listener reactions to the stuttering, secondary gains from stuttering, and increased likelihood of teasing and bullying related to the stuttering). Using this model for the assessment and treatment of stuttering among children, Riley and Riley noted the significance of other interactive factors (e.g., linguistic demands, parental or environmental expectations) on the experience of stuttering. The authors noted that the multidimensional nature of stuttering must be central to improving assessment, treatment, and understanding the risk factors that ultimately will lead to an understanding of the causes of stuttering.

Stuttering as a Psycholinguistic (Speech–Language Encoding) Disorder. Psycholinguistic models interpret speech disfluency as reflective of weakness or breakdown in the encoding of syntactic, lexical, phonological, or suprasegmental elements in speech production (Bloodstein & Bernstein Ratner, 2008). One influential psycholinguistic model, referred to as covert repair, assumes that stuttering and all other types of speech disfluency are consequences of self-repairs (Kolk & Postma, 1997; Postma & Kolk, 1993). According to this theory, identification and monitoring of real or perceived errors occur in pre-articulation, or at the level of phonological encoding. Disfluency results from unsuccessful covert repair or correction of speech errors. When covert repair is successful, no speech errors are noticed, but forward movement of an utterance may be impeded, leading to a disfluency. While most speakers make covert repairs at the level of phonological encoding, people who stutter are thought to have a deficit of phonological encoding, which leads to a greater number of phonological errors. These errors, in turn, must be repaired frequently, which leads to stuttering (Ambrose, 2004). An extension of this psycholinguistic model predicts the internal sources of error, the covert repair strategy, and the resulting disfluency type. For example, the disfluency might be a function of (a) a semantic or syntactic formulation error, leading to restarting the phrase and resulting in phrase repetition; (b) a lexical retrieval error, leading to restarting the previous word and resulting in word repetition; or (c) a phonemic encoding error detected before word execution has begun, leading to restarting the syllable from the beginning and resulting in a block or movement arrest (Bloodstein & Bernstein Ratner, 2008). Bloodstein and Bernstein Ratner noted that other psycholinguistic models specify other "core precipitating [tasks] that [trigger] stuttering onset" (p. 52), including syntax encoding (Bernstein Ratner, 1997; Bloodstein, 2006; Bloodstein & Bernstein Ratner, 2008), auditory feedback and syllable planning (Harrington, 1988), linguistic and prosodic feature delays exacerbated by the speaker's perception of time pressure and loss of control (Perkins, Kent, & Curlee, 1991), segmental (lexical, syntactic) and suprasegmental (prosodic-stress, intonation) misalignment (Karinol, 1995), suprasegmental variability encoding (transitions between targets with different stress values; Packman, Onslow, Richard, & von Doorn, 1996), and linguistic planning and motor execution (Howell, 2004), among others.

Stuttering as a Neurophysiological Disorder. Acknowledging that psychological and neurophysiological processes are not independent but, rather, intricately related, De Nil (1999) proposed the interaction of three dynamic levels of influence on all human behavior, including stuttering. Those three influences are central neurological processing; observable behavior or output associated with motor, cognitive, linguistic, social, and emotional factors; and environmental or contextual influences. Output components are multidirectional because feedback is sent and received between sensory mechanisms and central processes. Environmental conditions that impact communication do so through the influence of neurophysiological processing. Because of how each individual person experiences, processes, and filters environmental conditions, central neurophysiological processing varies both across and within people who stutter. Consequently, this dynamic interplay among multiple factors might explain why different people react differently and why people may react differently at different times to life's challenges and opportunities, including stuttering and stuttering intervention. De Nil (1999; see also Smits-Bandstra & De Nil, 2007) applied this model to explain the onset, development, and maintenance of stuttering, supported by research identifying neuromotor and neurophysiological differences between people who stutter and those who do not, and suggested that functional neuroimaging and direct observation of changing task and contextual variables will contribute to our understanding of stuttering and clinical treatment.

Also relevant to the neurophysiological conceptualization of stuttering are studies of hemispheric dominance indicating that people who stutter are more likely to process meaningful linguistic material in the right hemisphere (i.e., demonstrating less left-hemisphere dominance for speech and language than the general population; see Chapter 2). Studies of central auditory processing reveal that people who stutter are poorer at recognition and recall of competing messages and demonstrate reduced pain thresholds for intense auditory stimulation. Studies of motor speech behavior indicate that voice onset times, voice initiation times, and speech initiation times are slower in people who stutter. Muscle activity increases and abductor and adductor laryngeal muscles co-contract during stuttered speech. This co-contraction also occurs during silent periods prior to fluent speech. The fluent speech of people who stutter also demonstrates lower speed and degree of lip and jaw movement as well as greater movement-onset times. These data suggest motor speech, neuromotor, and neurophysiological differences that distinguish people who stutter from those who do not stutter in both fluent and disfluent speech (G. Andrews et al., 1983; Guyette & Baumgartner, 1988).

Stuttering as a Multifactorial Dynamic Disorder. A. Smith (1999) conceptualized stuttering as a directly observable manifestation of a complex interaction between diverse factors within each individual (i.e., genetic, cognitive, linguistic, emotional, environmental) and the speech motor control system. She noted the importance of interpreting stuttering from a nonlinear perspective, citing how onset of stuttering can be swift and severe and how an adult who stutters may shift suddenly from fluent to highly disfluent modes. Borrowing from physical theories of nonlinear dynamics, Smith defined attractor states as self-organizing, consistent, and complex patterns of output that represent an internal system's preference over all possible alternatives. She noted, "Systems with many interacting components can suddenly produce patterns in space and time, and can display nonlinear behavior, that is, a shifting from one pattern of output to another very rapidly" (p. 39). Furthermore, she identified both fluent and nonfluent attractor states between which children move during development. As the child matures and develops typical speech fluency, the attractors for fluent speech are more stable and prominent, resulting in fewer movements toward unstable or disfluent attractors. For people who stutter, a combination of fluent and disfluent attractors remains, maintaining instability in speech (i.e., stability in disfluency) and speech motor breakdown. Smith's proposal that stuttering behavior represents a stable attractor state (i.e., disfluent) is novel in that stuttering typically is thought of as discoordinated. Rather, from a speech motor perspective, Smith suggested that stuttering represents hypercoordination, discoordination, or hypocoordination, each of which is consistent with (i.e., considered a stable representation of) nonlinear, dynamical systems. She argued that stability and instability should not be equated with good and bad, respectively, noting that there are many examples of stable attractor states that are not reflective of healthy functioning (e.g., EEG rhythms in epilepsy, hyperregularity of heart rate associated with heart disease). Similarly, some stable behaviors (e.g., tremor) are not conducive to the forward flow of speech. The dynamics and level of stability of each person's speech motor system interact with multiple factors to determine the level of fluency observed, and this dynamic interaction will vary across and within each person who stutters. Smith stated that although stuttering unfolds in individualized ways, only a limited number of factors interact to impact speech motor performance and fluency. Smith concluded, "Our goal is to understand the dynamic interplay of these factors as the developing brain seeks the stable, adaptive modes of interaction among neural networks that generate fluent speech most of us take for granted" (p. 42).

Dual Premotor Model of Stuttering and Cluttering. Stuttering and cluttering (reviewed in Chapter 4) are disorders of fluency that can occur separately or together. Alm proposed a model to explain the neurological mechanisms of stuttering (2004, 2005, 2007a) and then stuttering and cluttering (2007b). He proposed that speech is a sequential motor behavior in which each segment (e.g., syllable) requires a "go signal" to be initiated. The basal ganglia provides the supplementary motor area with timing information, communicating that the previous segment has been executed and that it is time to release the next segment. According to this model, the brain has two parallel systems for initiation of movement: the medial system (i.e., the basal ganglia and the supplementary motor area), which is more active during spontaneous speech, and the lateral system (the lateral premotor cortex and the cerebellum), which is more active during nonautomatic modes of speech. Alm hypothesized that both stuttering and cluttering result from disturbances in the initiation of speech segments by the medial premotor system. He views stuttering and cluttering as opposite symptoms of the same function, with impaired (i.e., stuttering) versus premature (cluttering) initiation of the speech segments. According to this model, impairments of the medial system may be temporarily bypassed by shifting the responsibility for speech timing to the lateral system during certain speech modes. For example, this model suggests that such shifts to the lateral system take place during the conditions under which stuttering and cluttering are greatly reduced. As noted, conditions favorable to fluency are choral reading, singing, the use of a metronome, and timed-syllable speech. On an admittedly insufficient number of clinical cases, Alm proposed two preliminary disorder subtypes (i.e., stuttering and stuttering-cluttering). He did not, however, apply this model to the assessment or treatment of stuttering or cluttering.

To sum up on the foregoing theoretical orientations toward stuttering, it often seems that the more we study the theoretical map, the more challenging it is to read and to follow. Yet we must remain committed to understanding the territory—the challenges, the alternatives, the comparisons and contrasts, the consistencies and contradictions, and, ultimately, the journey that will enable us to reach our destination and to achieve our objectives. Ambrose (2004) noted that as our theoretical questions have evolved from unidisciplinary to multidisciplinary, unifying what we know has become increasingly challenging. We no longer ask whether stuttering is a function of solely one domain—motor, motor speech, language, genetic, psychological, or learned.

Researchers in fluency are trying to determine how genetics interact with factors of environment, linguistics, time pressure, and excitement or anxiety, among others, to result in a fragile fluency generating system. Ambrose (2004) indicated, as have others, that theory must ultimately explain how many children who stutter severely recover completely without intervention while others stutter for a lifetime despite intervention. Are the physiological components in order, disordered, or dysfunctional? What is the locus of breakdown (e.g., auditory processing, central processing, speech planning)? Where does auditory processing become central language–cognitive processing and where does motor planning begin? Is neural development uneven among people who stutter, with the systems serving speech and language not maturing in the right order or at the right time? Noting that there may be a deficit in the left hemisphere that affects both auditory and motor function, that the right hemisphere may compensate for the left hemisphere, and that one or more of the multilevel sensory and motor systems that plan and execute fluent speech may be fragile, Ambrose proposed the following:

> In persistent stuttering, the left hemisphere system may be wired differently and less efficiently, but may attempt to develop coping strategies, compensating with the right hemisphere. Those who stutter mildly and/or occasionally have successfully developed organized wiring mechanisms to circumvent the problem areas. Those who stutter consistently and/or severely manage to use available pathways but cannot maintain and/or develop consistent new efficient wiring. . . . The neural system of a child who fully and naturally recovers from stuttering may develop unevenly but become indistinguishable from that of a child who is normally fluent. (2004, p. 88)

Non-Western Theories

Up to this point, the theories reviewed have reflected what many consider to be traditional, or Western, thinking. Unless we clinicians remember that our own viewpoint is not necessarily shared by others, we risk tunnel vision at best and treatment that is unrelated to our client's own personal construct and worldview at worst. Among my research fascinations are the assumptions, practices, and lessons from clinicians whose assumptions, constructs, and worldviews are distinctly different from my own (Shapiro et al., 2000, 2004). I am asked frequently by Western colleagues why this information is of interest to me; in many instances, as you will see, I would not adopt the practices of others. I respond to such questions from three perspectives: personally, clinically, and empirically.

Personally: I believe there are many ways of knowing; ours is only one. It is essential that we commit to learning what is known within our discipline, including the diverse schemes for organizing that knowledge. To me, it is at least as essential to commit to learning about the organizational schemes of others. Too many interact only with people who see the world as they do. We stand to benefit our clients by broadening our own perspectives by learning about those of others.

Clinically: I believe that if we are to serve another person, we must understand that person's perspective about the cause, nature, and treatment of stuttering. Presuming (i.e., without verification) that there is congruence in the assumptions between clients and clinicians places at risk the effectiveness of the communication experience, and thereby the clinical process itself.

Empirically: I am fascinated by the relatedness between what clinicians and clients think and what they do. Too often, clinicians and others form impressions, usually negative impressions, about others' assumptions or practices, both in isolation. For example, treating stuttering by offering sacrifices of palm wine, hens, and goats within the context of public chanting and hypnotic states would seem odd at best to many Western clinicians. Similarly, many clinicians would be dubious if told that stuttering is caused by a curse from the gods for misdeeds of a family member or diseased relative. Yet, it would make more sense to a clinician, albeit a departure from one's own thinking, to be told that a client's family offered sacrifices to the gods to gain their approval in order to reverse the curse (i.e., stuttering) imposed due to misdeeds of a relative. The logic of one's behavior often makes more sense when it is interpreted within the context of one's assumptions. I believe clinicians are obligated to seek an understanding of the relatedness between the assumptions and practices of those we are committed to serve. Only then are we in a position to establish a common territory upon which we can build our clinical relationship and strive toward achieving fluency freedom.

Burkina Faso and Cameroon, West Africa—Personal Interviews. In 2005, Moussa Dao (Burkina Faso), Joseph Lukong (Cameroon), and I, while participating in the First African Stuttering Conference in Douala, Cameroon, conducted interviews with 13 indigenous medical practitioners. Of those interviewed, 9 were male and 2 were female; chronological age ranged from approximately 25 to 85 years (official records of birth and chronological age often are not kept). These individuals are revered locally (i.e., they are called "Doctor" or "Native Doctor") because of their unique skills and abilities to remediate a wide range of conditions. In addition to stuttering, conditions treated reportedly included malaria, typhoid fever, mystical disorders, stomach disorders, wounds, epilepsy, male sexual dysfunction, female infertility, headache, diarrhea, dysentery, and rheumatic fever. Typically there are two types of traditional healers—herbalists and diviners. Herbalists are healers who have special training in the medicinal use of plants, herbs, and related natural products; diviners have special abilities endowed by spirits and other transcendent forces. Many traditional healers practice both herbal and divine interventions, depending on the type of condition to be treated. Anecdotal reports and others presented by the World Health Organization indicate that as many as 85% to

90% of the villagers in rural Africa receive intervention by traditional healers. Western medicine is sought only when the individual does not respond to traditional medicine (if it is available). The traditional methods and underlying assumptions typically are kept secret and only handed down from father to son (less frequently from grandmother or mother to granddaughter or daughter), usually within the context of initiation rites. Future herbalists typically accompany their fathers or other male relatives into the bush to learn what plants must be cut and from what location, what part of the plant is to be used, what season the plant must be cut, and what prayer must be said and at what moment in order for the plant to gain its healing influence. Diviners are endowed with supernatural, mystical, and spiritual powers (i.e., healing, recalling otherwise unknown past events, and foretelling the future) from deceased relatives, divine call, and unseen spiritual forces. Usually a family has only one traditional healer, who has three or fewer alternative remedies. Healers often consult among themselves to learn of others' practices. The success of the traditional remedies often spreads by word of mouth.

These preliminary interviews revealed interesting connections between assumptions and practices for stuttering intervention. For example, when stuttering is assumed to result from natural causes (i.e., from the gods), intervention approaches include using herbs and other traditional substances. These include making an ointment or topical treatment from burnt leaves of the kola nut tree or elephant grass, eating insects (*kibem*), drinking a yellow liquid (*kiluh*) from the raffia palm bush root, and drinking water from a waterfall. Such approaches also include taking the child into the bush and, combined with spiritual invocation, singing the melody of, and in rhythm with, one of the indigenous birds. When the cause is assumed to be an evil spirit, which might be due to a misdeed of a relative or a curse from a living person with a grudge, intervention includes offering sacrifices to appease the gods or to counteract the forces of the evil spirit, as well as consulting deceased ancestors through spiritual incantation to request that they remove the stutter from the person afflicted. Additionally, the healers reported that snoring predicts stuttering. Stuttering, they believe, can be acquired through imitation, inheritance, or contagion. When stuttering has been caused by an uncut lingual frenulum, the preferred intervention is to cut the frenulum; when it is caused by disease (e.g., hypertension, meningitides, paralysis), intervention is to bathe daily with a healing plant.

Africa—Published Accounts. Few African accounts of stuttering address indigenous healing practices (Kathard, 1998; Kuster, 2005; Platzky & Girson, 1993). Those accounts that do address healing tend not to relate the intervention directly to the causal assumptions underlying them. Nevertheless, they are valuable for exploring other windows into the discipline of stuttering intervention. For example, causal assumptions for stuttering in Burkina Faso, Cameroon, Ivory Coast, Mali, and South Africa include eating improper foods by the mother during breast-feeding, allowing the infant to look into a mirror, tickling the infant, cutting the child's hair before first words are spoken, seeing a snake during pregnancy, dropping the baby, being bitten by a dog, experiencing other emotional traumas, leaving the baby out in the first spring rain, failing to inform ancestors of imminent childbirth, eating grasshoppers, and offending the "God of Tongues." Interventions include telling the child not to move his feet when talking, hitting the child on the mouth with a dish towel or on the back of the head with the lung of a sheep, holding nutmeg under the tongue, eating fruit that has been pecked by a bird, telling the child not to imitate others who stutter, singing around a wood fire during initiation rites, drinking water from a snail shell but not drinking water from the bottom of a water jar, eating porridge mixed with ground owl's nest, heating a metal tool or knife in a fire and applying it to the lips of a child who stutters, eating a specific green grasshopper (*kimem*) and other green insects (*kibem*), drinking traditional herbs (*kighavir, ghay kiyon, maro-oh, ghan kidzem*) boiled with palm wine and the lungs of a cow (*boofu*), ingesting through the nostrils a yellow liquid from the cola nut tree and the burnt outer layer of the cola nut seed, and drinking seawater and water from a fresh spring.

China and Mexico—Published Accounts. Kuster (2005) reported that traditional interventions in China include hitting the face of a person who stutters when the weather is cloudy, setting fires, and using traditional Chinese herbs. Traditional interventions in Mexico include putting a 20-inch string in the mouth with a pebble attached (i.e., the pebble is to be brought to the mouth only using the lips), singing or trilling with a live cicada (*chicharra*) in the mouth, and moving a spoon up and down in the mouth while a formation of birds flies in the sky.

Summary and Synthesis—Etiology of Stuttering and Theoretical Explanations

What factors render one child more at risk than another for beginning to stutter?

The presence of predisposing constitutional (organic) factors seems to increase a child's risk for stuttering, though to an unknown degree (F. H. Silverman, 2004). Guitar (2006) indicated that it is unlikely that any of these factors directly causes stuttering. The connection between these factors and stuttering may be indirect; their presence may tax a child's communication development, and the resulting frustration and failure may lead to stuttering. However, it is possible that these factors are unrelated to stuttering. Nevertheless, the following constitutional factors seem to present greater risk or predisposition for stuttering:

- Male gender—Boys are more likely than girls to stutter.
- Age between 2 and 5 years—While stuttering can begin at any age, the majority of children who stutter begin to do so between the ages of 2 and 5 years.
- Family history of stuttering—While stuttering can appear in any family, the risk is greater for a child born to a parent who stutters or into a family with a history of stuttering.
- Middle- and upper-middle-class socioeconomic status and certain nationalities—Children from middle- and upper-middle-class families and certain groups from Canada, Korea, and West Africa show greater risk.
- Identical twin—A child who is a twin, particularly an identical twin, is at greater risk than a child who is not a twin. Also, stuttering occurs more often in both members of identical twin pairs than in both members of fraternal twin pairs.
- Brain injury—A child with a brain injury is at greater risk.
- Mental retardation—A child with mental retardation, particularly Down syndrome, is at greater risk.
- Bilingualism—Bilingual children are at greater risk.

Furthermore, children who stutter demonstrate the following group differences when compared to children who do not stutter:

- greater likelihood to have a history of delayed articulation or language development (recall the challenging findings regarding language competence from longitudinal investigations of the onset and development of stuttering; Yairi & Ambrose, 1999, 2005)
- poorer performance on verbal and motor tests of intelligence
- poorer performance on measures of school performance

- ⛭ more problems in social adjustment
- ⛭ less left-hemisphere dominance for speech
- ⛭ slower reaction times
- ⛭ poorer recognition and recall of competing messages
- ⛭ slower speech movements even during fluent speech

Theoretical explanations for the patterns demonstrated by some children to show greater predisposition to stutter include atypical patterns for laterality or handedness (cerebral localization theory), disruption in the motor sequence of the spoken utterance resulting from neuromotor mistiming in the patterns needed for perceiving and producing speech (disorder of timing theory), problems in learning relationships between the desired sounds and the required motor sequences (reduced capacity for internal modeling), and multiple psycholinguistic or neurophysiological factors (multifactorial causes).

Why do people stutter?

Various environmental and developmental factors have been discussed as precipitating causes of stuttering. Again, establishing a causal connection between the factors and the literal beginning of stuttering is a speculative exercise. Guitar (2006) metaphorically compared the developing human brain to a computer:

> Like a computer, the brain can work on several things at once, but like a computer, the more tasks it performs simultaneously, the slower and less efficiently it does each one. . . . The problem of shared resources is more acute in children because their immature nervous systems have less processing capacity to share. . . . Some children are especially at risk for straining their developing resources. Their development of speech and language skills may be delayed, yet they have to compete in a highly verbal environment. Or, their language development may surge ahead of their speech motor control skills, giving them much to say but limited capacity to say it. Such children may become excessively disfluent as other developmental demands outpace their ability to coordinate the complex movements of rapid, articulate speech. (p. 74)

The developmental factors that are thought to present significantly competing demands on the production of fluent speech include the following:

- ⛭ physical development—structural, perceptual, fine and gross motor, sensorimotor, neurological
- ⛭ cognitive development—perceiving, reasoning, imagining, and problem solving
- ⛭ social and emotional development—forming social relationships, coping with stress and arousal, forming self-concept
- ⛭ speech and language development—syntax, semantics, pragmatics, phonology, integration of speech motor skills with linguistic ability

Other demands imposed by the environment include the following:

- ⛭ unrealistic speech-related expectations and standards in the home
- ⛭ internal or external expectations for greater communicative speed or complexity
- ⛭ life events generating uncertainty or insecurity
- ⛭ traumatic or otherwise emotionally arousing experiences

Various theories have been reviewed to explain why people begin to stutter. One such theory rarely claiming support today is that stuttering is a symptom of an unsatisfied repressed emotional need for oral gratification (repressed need theory). Other theories explain the beginning of stuttering as communicative failure and anticipatory struggle. These theories hold that stuttering is precipitated by (a) the parents' misdiagnosis of and inappropriate reaction to normal disfluency (diagnosogenic theory), (b) the child's awareness of and increasing concern about his own disfluency (continuity hypothesis), or (c) the child's reactions to negative listener reactions to his normal disfluencies, which he then comes to fear and try to avoid, in response to which tense prepostures are developed (preparatory set or primary stuttering theory).

Other theories propose that stuttering is a learned avoidance behavior resulting from an attempt to alleviate the double approach–avoidance conflict between speaking and not speaking and between being silent and not silent (conflict theory of stuttering and avoidance reduction), from principles of positive and negative reinforcements and punishments (operant conditioning), or from attempts to prevent the emotionally painful consequences that are associated with the original disfluent behaviors (instrumental avoidance act theory). Other learning theories stress the interaction of at least two behavioral phenomena (two-factor learning theories), including classical conditioning (stimulus-contingent learning) and instrumental conditioning (response-contingent learning).

Still other theories explaining the beginning of stuttering emphasize physiological deficits, also referred to as *breakdown theories*. Some of these also have been used to explain the predisposition to stuttering, including that cerebral dominance for speech production is not present to a sufficient degree (incomplete cerebral dominance); that a disruptive internal condition is triggered by stress or biochemical imbalance (dysphemia); that the person has an internal transient disturbance in language use (perseveration theory); or that stuttering is the consequence of the disruption of motor organization, timing, and control (stuttering as a consequence of brain lesion, or a disorder of timing). Other theories view stuttering as a consequence of a defective monitoring system for speech (cybernetic theory of stuttering) or of related multifactorial causes (demands and capacities model, CALMS, revised component model, covert repair, and psycholinguistic or neurophysiological breakdown, among others). Many other hypotheses for the beginning of stuttering exist and do not fit neatly into any of the categories already noted. F. H. Silverman (2004) identified other factors that can precipitate a breakdown in one's speech fluency, including stress and anxiety, shocks and fright, illness, imitation, emotional or communicative conflicts, demand for fluency exceeding capacity, reduced ability to generate temporal patterns, and dyssynchrony between linguistic and paralinguistic components when the speaker experiences time pressure.

Why do people continue to stutter?

Identifying the perpetuating causes of stuttering tends to be more promising than identifying the predisposing or precipitating factors. Once the predisposing foundation is in place and stuttering has been precipitated, what keeps people stuttering? Several factors have been considered, all of which resist change:

- habituated cognitive, linguistic, and motor adjustments
- maladaptive environmental conditions
- interpersonal dynamics within communication systems
- personal construct of a "stutterer"

A number of theoretical explanations for why people continue to stutter hold that any of the following conditions that predisposed or precipitated stuttering continue to be present: unsatisfied emotional need for oral gratification (repressed need theory); anticipation and fear of stuttering and subsequent struggle to avoid it (communicative failure and anticipatory struggle); learned avoidance behavior to reduce speaking-related conflicts, to respond to environmental reinforcements and punishments, or to prevent painful emotional consequences (stuttering as an avoidance response); learned adjustment to unpleasant experiences (stuttering as an interaction of behavioral phenomena); physiological deficits (breakdowns); disturbed feedback (cybernetic theory); disrupted motor organization, timing, and control (stuttering as a consequence of brain lesion or a disorder of timing); defective monitoring system for speech (cybernetic theory of stuttering); multifactorial causes (excessive internal and external demands on the child's capacity for fluent speech production, psycholinguistic or neurophysiological breakdowns, and covert repair, among others); and environmental factors such as stress, fear, illness, and conflict.

A Personal Postscript on Theory

As I throw my own theoretical hat into the ring, I am reminded of Bloodstein's (1986) admonition: "Anyone who advances a supposedly new idea about stuttering must be put on notice that someone has probably said it before and that someone else will probably disprove it" (p. 130). And, as I weigh the merits of the descriptive and explanatory notions of what predisposes, precipitates, and perpetuates the "riddle" (Bluemel, 1957), the "enigma" (Wingate, 1988), the "tangled tongue" (Carlisle, 1985), the "age-old human anguish" (Bloodstein, 1993), I realize the importance of articulating my own assumptions about stuttering. To that end, I hold that stuttering is a multidimensional neuromotor disruption resulting in asynchronous timing of the simultaneous and successive motor movements necessary for relatively effortless, continuous, and rapid speech. At least as significant, the affective and cognitive dimensions interact with the behavioral, thus impacting the internalized thoughts and feelings of a person who stutters in individualized ways and to varying extents. These statements recognize both the observable and acoustic elements of mistiming and the underlying physiological processes of excessive muscular tension and effort, as well as the significant emotional and cognitive impact that such an experience can have on a person who stutters and his conversational partners. The process of neuromotor control, and thereby maintenance of speech fluency, is influenced by many other multidimensional factors or capacities, including speech and language competence, oral and speech motor coordination (and other fine- and gross-motor control mechanisms), cognitive and learning potential, and social and emotional maturity. My thinking is particularly influenced by Guitar (2006), Yairi and Ambrose (2005), Starkweather et al. (1990), and Van Riper (1982).

Guitar (2006) suggested that constitutional factors predispose a child to stutter and that developmental and environmental factors precipitate the stuttering. He cautioned that in some cases, environmental factors may trigger stuttering in children who have this predisposition. In other cases, the predisposition may be present, but the environment may nurture fluency. These children may never develop stuttering. Therefore, identifying and attributing the role of predisposing and precipitating factors is within "a domain of educated guesses and tentative conclusions" (p. 73). After reviewing the role of heredity, Guitar (2006) indicated that some unknown predisposing genetic factor or factors might act singly or together. Guitar (2006) also noted that as a group, people who stutter differ from those who do not on cognitive, linguistic, and motor tasks. However, many people who stutter do not show these differences, and many who do not stutter perform as deviantly as those who do. Taken together, these differences might or might not be causally related to stuttering. Establishing a causal connection between constitutional factors and stuttering is speculative.

Guitar (2006) proposed relevant developmental (physical, cognitive, social and emotional, and speech and language) and environmental (parents, speech and language environment, and life events) influences that might precipitate stuttering. The impact of developmental factors is supported by the observation that stuttering frequently begins when children are growing rapidly both mentally and physically in the preschool years. Similarly, stresses are often reported in relation to the beginning of stuttering, and remission is frequently reported when these stresses are reduced. Nevertheless, Guitar (2006) acknowledged the apparent ordinariness of the environment: "Conditions at the onset of stuttering are typically not dramatic; the child is usually not under great stress, nor has the child just experienced a traumatic event" (p. 73). Van Riper (1982) made a similar observation:

> In the great majority of the children we have carefully studied soon after onset, we were unable to state with any certainty (or even with some feeling of probability) what precipitated the stuttering. In most instances, there simply were no apparent conflicts, no illnesses, no opportunity to imitate, no shocks or frightening experiences. Stuttering seemed to begin under quite normal conditions of living and communicating. We cannot, of course, be sure of this. Who can look within the inner world of a child? All we can say is that usually we could not account for the onset of stuttering in terms of the conditions surrounding it. In only a fraction of our cases do we feel we identified the circumstances that might have been precipitating. (p. 81)

This apparent contradiction between the intuitive (presumed) and actual influence of environmental factors at the time of onset suggests that constitutional predisposition often plays a part in the first appearance of stuttering and supports the concept of multiple and yet undetermined origins of stuttering. Guitar (2006) described the rapid growth between 1 and 6 years of age as a "two-edged sword" for children predisposed to fluency problems:

> Neurological maturation may provide more "functional cerebral space" that supports fluency, but it also spurs development of other motor behaviors that may compete with fluency for available neuronal resources. An example of such competition is the common observation that children learn to walk first or talk first, but not both at the same time. (p. 75)

Major developmental tasks like talking and walking consume the available resources. For example, children who are learning a new motor skill often are observed to become temporarily disfluent. Guitar (2006) described the conflict between the demands imposed by developmental processes on the available resources as creating "extra noise in their neural circuitry for speech" (p. 82), particularly for children who may be neurophysiologically vulnerable or predisposed to stuttering.

Within this postscript, I have highlighted the following assumptions about stuttering:

- Stuttering is a multidimensional neuromotor disruption in the timing and control of speech-related motor movements.
- Affective and cognitive dimensions interact with the behavioral, thus impacting the internalized thoughts and feelings of a person who stutters in individualized ways and to varying extents.
- Stuttering is caused by the interaction between individually determined, yet unknown, predisposing (constitutional) factors and precipitating (developmental and environmental) factors.
- Stuttering is maintained by perpetuating factors that can and must be identified and systematically eliminated in the treatment process.
- The phenomenology of stuttering can be explained and conceptualized best as a result of the interaction of presumed yet unconfirmed elements, including inherited genetic and neurophysiological components, psycholinguistic processing, covert repairs and consequent learning and avoidances (i.e., affective, behavioral, and cognitive reactions), and mutifactorial elements, including cognitive, affective, linguistic, motor, and social.

Stuttering is triggered by a multisensorily induced cognitive or affective overload (Gottwald, 2010; Manning, 2000; Starkweather et al., 1990). My own notion of the demands that potentially interact with each individual's capacity for fluent speech production is distinct in at least two respects. First, the demands need to be interpreted from a multisensory and multidimensional perspective, including, but not exclusive to, pressures of time, uncertainty, and avoidance (Healey, 2007; Healey et al., 2004; Riley & Riley, 2000). We have become increasingly aware of the risks of presenting any of the following to children: speech models characterized by rapid speech or complex language, negative or impatient listener reaction, demand speech, excessive or busy scheduling, high levels of emotionality, limited turn-taking, dramatic change that challenges the child's sense of security, or other experiences that lead the child to avoid stuttering or the experience of communication in general. One additional item not generally addressed is the impact of multisensory overload—that is, of overburdening the existing avenues of sensory input, particularly the auditory and visual channels (Bloodstein & Bernstein Ratner, 2008; De Nil, 1999; Guitar, 2006; Healey, 2007). As noted earlier, as a group, people who stutter tend to demonstrate less proficiency in recognition, discrimination, and recall of competing auditory messages and slower reaction times when vocal or nonvocal responses are required (G. Andrews et al., 1983). My own observations indicate that some children tend to be more prone to disruption of speech fluency in conditions of auditory and visual bombardment. These have included homes where the television or stereo plays constantly, presenting both auditory and visual noise during all opportunities for conversational interaction. Other common household interferences include noise from the dishwasher, laundry machines, microwave, exhaust fans, oven timers, and phones (both incoming and outgoing calls). In today's world, where technology seems to change by the minute, the same could be said about the potential interference of electronic devices, such as computers, fax machines, pagers, personal digital assistants (PDAs), and cellular phones, among others.

Interferences and interrupters certainly are not limited to the home setting. We know that children who stutter demonstrate poorer performance on measures of intelligence and school performance, whether because of or as a result of stuttering. I have often wondered if the deficit in school performance is exacerbated by auditory or visual overload. I am not aware of literature addressing the differential learning strategies of children and adults who stutter. However, in light of the identified differences among the population of people who stutter, the potential benefits of modified teaching methods are yet to be determined. These methods might include reducing the rate at which verbal instructions are given, allowing for processing time between verbal instructions, and establishing rules for conversational turn-taking to eliminate interruptions.

The environment beyond home and school is rich with potential sources of sensory overload. Consider the following illustration. I visited with a 3-year-old boy and his family at night in a local tourist town known for its constant and timeless activities. We walked past the shops and arcades, all crowded, booming with music, and nearly blinding with bright and colored lights. I observed this young boy's distraction, which took the form of kinetic attention to the auditory and visual stimuli. At the same time, his fluency disintegrated gradually to frequent part-word repetitions, though without any visible tension. These disfluencies were managed successfully by providing models of slow, gentle, normal-sounding speech. When we walked by a "haunted house," a commercial dungeon intended to elicit fear, a masked and costumed man shouted "boo" at us. At this, the boy startled and immediately repeated an initial w four times, equally spaced, without pitch rise but this time with oral and facial tension ("Wuh-wuh-wuh-wuh-why did he do that?"). His speech continued to be speckled with repetitions of similar form for the next 10 minutes, until he was removed from the noise and lights and provided models of normalized speech with more deliberate transitions. Some might argue that it was the fright or the late hour that contributed to the boy's fluency breakdown. Perhaps the fright precipitated the repetitions with oral and facial struggle. Previous to that, however, when bombarded with auditory and visual stimuli, the boy's fluency became increasingly disfluent with repetitions but without any evidence of tension or struggle. This example, while anecdotal, is instructive. I am convinced that we all are prone to sensory overload, particularly children who are constitutionally predisposed to stuttering.

A second distinction in my conceptualization is that demands appear to be cumulative rather than episodic. In other words, the conditions of multisensory overload can be reversed or removed, and the child who is at risk for stuttering may regain fluent speech (Yairi & Ambrose, 2005). However, with repeated exposure to such environments, whether at home, school, day care, camp, or other settings, the child is less able to regain fluency, and the process of reversing the effects of such overload takes an increasingly longer time with results that are more temporary. Perhaps some children within these environments develop buffering mechanisms that shield them from the potentially damaging effects of sensory overstimulation. This concept is not a new one. The literature addressing wartime activity and imprisonment is replete with examples of how sensory bombardment through auditory, visual, and other channels of input has been used to create cognitive and affective overload in order to effect behavioral change (Coan, 1997; Mandela, 1995; Samelson, 2006; Weber, 2007). Perhaps children who are prone to stutter are more likely to experience behavioral, affective, and cognitive disorganization from sensory overload. Those who stutter have been less successful in developing or using strategies to buffer themselves from such overload, thus experiencing the effects of ultimate disintegration of previously organized behaviors, feelings, and thoughts related to communication, specifically speech fluency. Thus, controlling for multisensory stimulation and preventing systemic overload are critical in facilitating fluency in both the prevention and intervention processes (Bloodstein & Bernstein Ratner, 2008; Gottwald, 2010; Guitar, 2006; Healey, 2007; Manning, 2000).

What does all of this mean? It seems likely that there are unique and undetermined predisposing and precipitating factors for each person who stutters. However, we remain unaware of these factors or their combinations and interactions. Also, we remain unaware of how knowledge of such factors might impact prevention and intervention. It seems more than just chance that renders such factors active (necessary and sufficient) for some yet dormant (neither necessary nor sufficient) for others. Yet, current research still cannot determine which combinations of factors are necessary and sufficient. Nevertheless, there seems to be orderliness in both the constitutional and developmental/environmental factor model and the demands and capacities model, among others. Notwithstanding the results of longitudinal investigations reviewed in the previous chapter, we still cannot predict to any satisfactory degree who will stutter and who will not and the developmental course for those who begin to stutter. At this point, some will throw up their hands in utter frustration; others will seize the challenge and the resulting opportunity to make a meaningful contribution to our understanding of stuttering and people who stutter. By virtue of you reading these leaves, I know that we share a commitment as comrades to work and learn with and for people who stutter.

Chapter Summary

Chapter 3 highlighted the evolution of our thinking throughout recorded history about stuttering and people who stutter as a foundation for understanding contemporary theories of etiology, which ground related treatment practices. Famous people from times past and present, all of whom stutter, were identified to illustrate that stuttering is an old affliction and that many successful people stutter. Indeed, stuttering was traced through Egyptian hieroglyphics (2000 B.C.), the Bible (1350–687 B.C.), and professional literature from 484 B.C. to the present day. Theoretical constructions of etiology and treatment have included anatomical defects, medical problems, articulation disorders, respiratory disorders, neuroanatomical or motor speech dysfunctions, psychoneurosis, and learned behavior.

Contemporary interpretations of etiology were defined as the interaction of predisposing factors (agents that incline a person to stutter or put one at greater risk for stuttering), precipitating factors (agents thought to have triggered the stuttering or brought it to the surface), and perpetuating factors (variables that are continuing or maintaining the stuttering at the present time). Six major theoretical explanations for stuttering were reviewed, as follows:

1. Viewed as a neurotic response, stuttering is a consequence of deep repressed needs.

2. As a result of communicative failure and anticipatory struggle, stuttering is explained by (a) the diagnosogenic or semantic theory (stuttering is caused by the parents' or care providers' misdiagnosis of and inappropriate reaction to normal disfluencies in a child's speech, followed by the child's attempts to avoid the disfluencies that are mistakenly assumed to be abnormal); (b) the continuity hypothesis, also referred to as communication failure theory (stuttering develops from normal disfluency that becomes tense and fragmented as the child experiences frustration and failure in attempts to talk); and (c) preparatory set or primary stuttering theory (stuttering emerges gradually from a child's normal hesitations and repetitions and becomes chronic when the child begins to anticipate, avoid, and fear speech and related contexts because of reactions by listeners).

3. As a learned behavior, stuttering is explained as an avoidance response or as an interaction of behavioral phenomena. Avoidance response explanations include (a) the conflict theory of stuttering and avoidance reduction (stuttering is the result of a double approach–avoidance conflict between speaking and not speaking and between being silent and not being silent); (b) operant conditioning (speech is a behavior subject to operant control of positive and negative reinforcements and punishments); and (c) instrumental avoidance act theory (stuttering is an acquired response reflecting expectancy, anticipation, adaptation, or anxiety and is motivated by the learned drive of apprehension about the normal disfluencies of speech). As an interaction of behavioral phenomena, stuttering is explained by the two-factor learning theory (which differentiates between classical conditioning, or stimulus-contingent learning, and instrumental conditioning, or response-contingent learning), which states that the core characteristics of stuttering are the involuntary breakdowns of speech resulting from negative emotional responses that are classically conditioned, while the secondary characteristics are instrumentally conditioned responses of the individual to unpleasant experiences.

4. As a physiological deficit, stuttering is explained by (a) the incomplete cerebral dominance theory (stuttering is a result of not showing the usual pattern for left-hemisphere dominance); (b) the dysphemia theory (stuttering is a manifestation of an internal condition triggered by illness, emotional or environmental stress, or biochemical imbalance); (c) the perseveration theory (stuttering is an organic predisposition to motor and sensory perseveration of which stuttering is an outward manifestation); and (d) as a consequence of a brain lesion (brain damage causes changes in the interaction of laryngeal, supralaryngeal, and respiratory reflexes, thereby disrupting motor organization, timing, and control).

5. As a result of disturbed feedback (the cybernetic theory), stuttering results from distortion, interference, or overload of the internal feedback mechanisms to messages received or produced or too much output correction to the internalized distortion.

6. Finally, as a result of multifactorial causes, stuttering is explained by (a) the demands and capacities model (stuttering results as a consequence of the mismatch between the internally or externally imposed demands placed on the child and his finite capacity for

fluent speech), (b) CALMS (stuttering results from and is maintained by the interaction of cognitive, affective, linguistic, motor, and social elements), (c) the revised component model (stuttering results from the interaction of physical, temperament, and listener factors that interact with linguistic, parental, or environmental demands), (d) the covert repair hypothesis (stuttering results from a deficit in phonological encoding, which leads to a greater number of phonological errors, a greater number of corrections, and, ultimately, stuttering), (e) the neurophysiological disorder hypothesis (stuttering results from the dynamic interaction between central neurological processing and observable behavior associated with motor, cognitive, linguistic, social, and emotional factors and environmental or contextual influences), (f) the multifactorial dynamic disorder hypothesis (stuttering results from nonlinear stable attractor states for disfluency), and (g) the dual premotor model of stuttering and cluttering (stuttering and cluttering result from disturbance in the initiation of speech segments by the medial premotor system, i.e., the basal ganglia and the supplementary motor area).

These theoretical explanations were followed by a series of perplexing questions addressing how genetics interacts with factors of environment, linguistics, time pressure, and excitement or anxiety, among others, to result in a fragile fluency generating system. Also addressed were non-Western theoretical explanations for stuttering from Burkina Faso, Cameroon, and other African countries, and China and Mexico.

Finally, based upon the theoretical, clinical, and research foundation presented, stuttering was characterized as a multidimensional neuromotor disruption in the timing and control of speech-related motor movements, an interaction of individually determined yet unknown predisposing (constitutional) factors with precipitating (developmental and environmental) factors, a communication disorder that is maintained by perpetuating factors that can and must be identified and systematically eliminated in the treatment process, and a phenomenology that can be best explained and conceptualized from the delicate and dynamic balance of multifactorial elements. These statements recognize both the observable and acoustic elements of mistiming and the underlying physiological processes of excessive muscular tension and effort, and do not minimize the significant emotional and cognitive impact that such an experience can have and often does have on a person who stutters and his conversational partners.

Chapter Three Study Questions

1. Many people throughout recorded history have stuttered. What relevance is there in this observation to understanding stuttering and people who stutter, and to the processes of assessment and treatment?

2. Written records attest to an awareness of and beliefs about stuttering over at least the past 4,000 years. Also, the professional literature over the last 2,500 years has addressed the etiology and treatment of stuttering. How have previous notions contributed to our present level of understanding? What are the historical underpinnings of our present understanding about stuttering and people who stutter? How has our thinking developed and changed over time? How do you predict that our thinking will continue to develop into the future? What inroads are yet to be made?

3. Etiology was conceptualized as the three Ps. What are the three Ps, and why is a consideration of all three essential for assessing and understanding stuttering and for designing effective intervention?

4. An understanding of theoretical explanations is essential for developing your own theory, which is a foundation for designing effective intervention. How would you

explain the development of our profession's theoretical understanding of stuttering? Given your understanding of the theories and the importance of the three *P*s, what is your theoretical explanation for why people stutter? How might your theory impact your design of assessment and treatment?

5. Selected non-Western theories and practices were reviewed, as were justifications for why understanding non-Western theories is important. Why do you think understanding such theories is important, and in what ways is such an understanding consistent with our commitment to quality service delivery? In what ways might being open-minded serve you as a clinician? In what ways do perspectives (of the clinician, client, and others) contribute to or inhibit clinical effectiveness? In what ways might the ability to shift perspective serve you as a service provider and as a lifelong learner?

6. It is consistent with our professional obligations to ask ourselves regularly why we do what we do as clinicians, what the origins of those ideas are, and what the available data are to support or refute those ideas. Also, we must ask ourselves how what we do reflects what we believe and who we are as people and as professionals. Why must we ask ourselves these questions and in what ways is doing so consistent with our commitment to the Code of Ethics, evidence-based practice, and quality service delivery?

7. Real or perceived reactions of listeners play a significant role in the development of stuttering. Thinking about your own experiences, how have you reacted to the differences of others (including but not limited to stuttering), and how have others reacted to your differences?

8. We have summarized why some people are at greater risk for stuttering (predisposing factors), why people stutter (precipitating factors), and why people continue to stutter (perpetuating factors). How would you explain each of the factors reviewed? For example, why is greater risk experienced by boys, twins, people from middle- and upper-middle-class families, those from certain countries, and so on?

9. Among the multifactorial theories of the etiology of stuttering, much has been written about the demands and capacities model. What evidence (both anecdotal and empirical) supports and refutes this proposal? What citations can you identify both to support and to challenge this proposal? On what basis would you argue for or against this proposal to explain the onset of stuttering or to explain other behavioral phenomena?

10. Many of the theories reviewed focus on the behavioral element of stuttering. In what ways do the theories account for the frequent and significant affective and cognitive elements that accompany the stuttering experience?

Chapter Four

Other Fluency Disorders

The generic use of the term stuttering *can obscure important differences, despite shared symptoms. Not all headaches are the result of brain tumors; not all neoplasms are carcinogenic; and not all disfluencies are stuttering. (Culatta & Goldberg, 1995, p. 23)*

A common misconception is that all abnormal disfluency is stuttering behavior. This chapter distinguishes stuttering from other fluency disorders. Those that will be addressed are cluttering, neurogenic acquired stuttering, psychogenic acquired stuttering, malingering, Tourette syndrome, adductor spasmodic dysphonia, acquired disfluency following laryngectomy, linguistic disfluency, normal developmental disfluency, and other forms of disfluency that resemble stuttering (disfluency in manual communication and disfluency while playing a wind instrument). Familiarity with different fluency disorders is essential to clinical intervention with stuttering.

Cluttering

The term *cluttering* was first used in 1877 by Adolph Kussmaul, a German lexicographer (St. Louis, Myers, Bakker, & Raphael, 2007; Weiss, 1964). Also referred to as *tachyphemia* or *tachylalia* (a Greek term meaning "fast speech"), cluttering is a fluency disorder that begins during early childhood, frequently occurs with stuttering, and is thought to be caused by neurological, linguistic, cognitive, and genetic factors (Dalton & Hardcastle, 1989; Daly, 1986, 1993, 1996; Daly & Burnett,1999; F. H. Silverman, 2004). Referred to as the "orphan" in the family of speech–language pathology because of relative neglect (Weiss, 1964), cluttering has received more attention in the European literature than in the American literature. Acknowledging its "adoption" by the field of speech–language pathology, however, St. Louis et al. (2007) suggested that clinicians "retire that image" (p. 297) and yield to the metaphor of a partly completed jigsaw puzzle. Notwithstanding many "puzzle pieces" yet to be discovered and despite residual reluctance to accept cluttering as a clinical entity (Ryan, 2001), physicians (Arnold, 1965; Froeschels, 1955; Weiss, 1964) and speech–language pathologists (Daly, 1986, 1993; Diedrich, 1984; Myers & St. Louis, 2007; St. Louis, 1996; St. Louis & Myers, 1997; St. Louis, Myers, Faragasso,

Townsend, & Gallaher, 2004; St. Louis, Raphael, Myers, & Bakker, 2003; Tiger, Irvine, & Reis, 1980) increasingly are intrigued by this multidimensional disorder. As interest in cluttering has grown, people who clutter have shared their own personal perspectives (Dewey, 2005; Myers & Kissagizlis, 2007) and networked with the academic and professional communities; as a result of this work, the International Cluttering Association (see Appendix for contact information) was launched at the first International Conference on Cluttering in Katarino, Bulgaria (Myers & Kissagizlis, 2007; Reichel & Bakker, 2009).

As with stuttering, cluttering is difficult to define. Some have defined cluttering as a verbal manifestation of a central language disorder, others as a speech defect, while still others as a combined speech–language disturbance. Representative definitions indicating the comprehensiveness of cluttering follow:

    Cluttering is a speech disorder characterized by the clutterer's unawareness of his disorder, by a short attention span, by disturbances in perception, articulation and formulation of speech and often by excessive speed of delivery. It is a disorder of the thought processes preparatory to speech and based on a heredity disposition. Cluttering is the verbal manifestation of Central Language Imbalance, which affects all channels of communication (e.g., reading, writing, rhythm and musicality) and behavior in general. (Weiss, 1964, p. 1)

    Cluttering [is] a disorder of both speech and language processing which manifests itself as rapid, dysrhythmic, sporadic, disorganized, and frequently inarticulate speech by a person who is largely unaware of or unconcerned about these difficulties. (Daly & Burnett, 1999, p. 224)

    Cluttering is a fluency disorder characterized by a rate that is perceived to be abnormally rapid, irregular, or both for the speaker (although measured syllable rates may not exceed normal limits). These rate abnormalities further are manifest in one or more of the following symptoms: (a) an excessive number of disfluencies, the majority of which are not typical of people who stutter; (b) the frequent placement of pauses and use of prosodic patterns that do not conform to syntactic and semantic constraints; and (c) inappropriate (usually excessive) degrees of coarticulation among sounds, especially in multisyllabic words. (St. Louis et al., 2007, pp. 299–300)

Cluttering has been defined as a disorder of both speech and language processing, often negatively impacting all channels of communication and related behavior, including grammar, reading, writing, handwriting, rhythm, musicality, coordination, and self-monitoring (Diedrich, 1984; Perkins, 1978; Weiss, 1964). Listeners tend to perceive rate of speech and relative naturalness of people who clutter as least acceptable, articulation as relatively more acceptable, and disfluency and language as most acceptable (Myers & St. Louis, 2006; St. Louis et al., 2004). Weiss (1964) is often cited for his iceberg representation (see Figure 4.1) of cluttering as one prominent symptom among multiple deficiencies (delayed speech, dyslalias, reading and writing disorders, disorders of rhythm and musicality, and disorderliness and restlessness), all sharing the common pathological basis of central language imbalance. The constellation of symptoms defines cluttering as a clinical syndrome that is related to, but often independent of, stuttering.

Daly (1993) presented eight quantitative and seven qualitative features of cluttering. Quantitative symptoms are as follows:

1. acceleration of speech rate between and within multisyllabic words
2. short attention span and poor concentration
3. vowel stops or pauses before vowel-initial words without fear or muscular tension
4. six to eight units of repetition of single syllables, short words, and phrases, without apparent concern
5. articulation errors including /r/ and /l/ phonemes, reduction of consonant clusters, or signs of oral apraxia

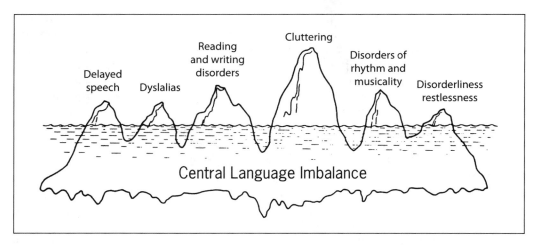

Figure 4.1. Cluttering as one symptom of a central language imbalance. *Note.* From *Cluttering* (p. 7), by D. A. Weiss, 1964, Englewood Cliffs, NJ: Prentice Hall. Copyright 1964 by Allyn & Bacon/ Pearson. Reprinted with permission.

6. vocal monotony (lack of speech melody or intonation)
7. reading errors such as skipping small words, revising text, or poor concentration
8. writing errors such as poor integration of ideas and motor incoordination

Qualitative symptoms are as follows:

1. disorganized speech characterized by abrupt topic shifts, incomplete phrases, and deficient word-retrieval skills
2. verbal transpositions without awareness
3. physical immaturity, clumsiness, incoordination, often appearing inattentive, restless, or hyperactive
4. deficits in musical ability and rhythm, often unable to imitate a simple rhythmic pattern
5. familial pattern of cluttering
6. personality characteristics variously described as impulsive, hasty, restless, hyperactive, careless, impatient, and short-tempered
7. lack of awareness that speech deviates from normal

Daly (1993) concluded that "cerebral dysfunction and/or heredity may play an even more prominent role in cluttering than in stuttering" (p. 185), that "future research will verify that cluttering and LD [learning disabilities] are frequently interrelated" (p. 186; see also Tiger et al., 1980), and that "pure" cluttering is rare. Thus, cluttering and stuttering often occur simultaneously; this pattern has been observed internationally (Miyamoto, Hayasaka, & Shapiro, 2007). On the basis of feedback received from 60 cluttering experts in 21 states within the United States and nine other countries, Daly (2007, 2008) presented a useful checklist, represented in Figure 4.2, to assist clinicians in making a differential diagnosis among people who clutter, people who clutter and stutter, and people who neither clutter nor stutter. The Predictive Cluttering Inventory (PCI) contains 33 items that are indicative of cluttering, each of which is rated between 0 (*never*) and 6 (*always*). Daly (2007) suggested that a score of 120 points (of a possible 198) or above is rare and usually is sufficient to support a diagnosis of cluttering. Scores between 80 and 120 may be indicative of cluttering-stuttering. The two items ranked as most characteristic of cluttering by the experts were 13 (telescopes or condenses words; selected by 93% of the experts) and 1 (lack of effective self-monitoring skills; selected by 90% of the experts). Six other items were selected by at least 80% of the experts as most indicative of cluttering: 2 (lack of awareness of own communication errors or problems; 83%), 18 (lack of pauses between words and phrases; 83%), 11 (articulation errors; 82%), 12 (irregular speech rate, speaks in spurts or bursts; 82%), 3 (compulsive talker; verbose; tangential; word-finding problems; 80%), and 24 (many revisions; interjections; filler words; 80%). On the basis of these expert ratings, Daly (2008) projected that of the disfluent clients evaluated, 2% will be "pure clutterers," 33% will be "pure stutterers," 33% will be "clutterer-stutterers," and 32% will be "stutterers with concomitant problems" (e.g., articulation, language disabilities, motor coordination, attention-deficit/hyperactivity disorder or attention-deficit disorder, hearing loss, speech dyspraxia).

St. Louis et al. (2007) outlined the challenges faced in the assessment and measurement of cluttering, including the lack of precise and behaviorally explicit definitions of cluttering, the variable nature of cluttering (i.e., in form of presentation and over time), and the multidimensional nature of interrelated symptoms of cluttering. St. Louis et al. (2007, p. 315) reported the following symptoms to be important for a differential diagnosis of cluttering:

> excessive typical disfluencies, rapid and irregular speech rate, atypical pauses, neutralization of vowels, over-coarticulated (collapsed) syllables, and atypical co-articulation patterns. Frequently present symptoms include: pragmatic, syntactic/morphological, and lexical (word finding) errors; mazes; consistent developmental misarticulations; distractibility and hyperactivity; and reading and writing difficulties. Occasionally present symptoms include excessive atypical disfluencies and phonological errors.

To organize the assessment information for treatment planning, Daly (2008) presented the Cluttering Treatment Planning Profile, which is a slight modification of the Predictive Cluttering Inventory. The 33 descriptive statements in the Predictive Cluttering Inventory are referred to as "cluttering characteristics" in the Cluttering Treatment Planning Profile, the ratings of which emphasize severity of symptoms (from 6 = *very severe*; 0 = *not a problem*). The scores from the Predictive Cluttering Inventory are transferred directly to the Cluttering Treatment Planning Profile, with directions for structuring relevant data into a framework for identifying strengths and weaknesses by displaying observable behaviors in the four categories. Daly cautioned that, too frequently, there is a tendency to focus exclusively on rate reduction. He recommended that treatment address at least two other carefully selected characteristics in addition to rate.

Daly and Burnett (1999, pp. 242–243) suggested that in addition to reducing rate of speech, areas targeted for improvement might include the following:

1. self-awareness (e.g., use audio and video recordings, provide verbal and multisensory feedback, engage in negative practice)
2. self-monitoring (i.e., use self-corrections; use delayed auditory feedback; engage in self-rating)
3. attention span (measure time on task and number of redirections required, address listening skills and following directions)
4. thought organization and formulation (name attributes, categorize and describe, sequence and tell stories both verbally and in writing)
5. semantics and syntax (unscramble words, sentences, and paragraphs; build vocabulary; engage in naming and cloze activities; frame and combine sentences)
6. pragmatics and social skills (heighten listening skills, use blind board activities, build awareness through direct feedback, role-play social skills, read body expressions and nonverbal messages, tell jokes with proper sequencing and timing)

Predictive Cluttering Inventory (PCI)

Instructions: Please respond to each description section below. Circle the number you believe is most descriptive of this person's cluttering.

Descriptive Statement	Always	Almost Always	Frequently	Sometimes	Infrequently	Almost Never	Never
Pragmatics							
1. Lack of effective self-monitoring skills	6	5	4	3	2	1	0
2. Lack of awareness of own communication errors or problems	6	5	4	3	2	1	0
3. Compulsive talker; verbose; tangential; word-finding problems	6	5	4	3	2	1	0
4. Poor planning skills; misjudges effective use of time	6	5	4	3	2	1	0
5. Poor social communication skills; inappropriate turn-taking; interruptions	6	5	4	3	2	1	0
6. Does not recognize or respond to listener's visual or verbal feedback	6	5	4	3	2	1	0
7. Does not repair or correct communication breakdowns	6	5	4	3	2	1	0
8. Little or no excessive effort observed during disfluencies	6	5	4	3	2	1	0
9. Little or no anxiety regarding speaking; unconcerned	6	5	4	3	2	1	0
10. Speech better under pressure (improves short term with concentration)	6	5	4	3	2	1	0
Speech–Motor							
11. Articulation errors	6	5	4	3	2	1	0
12. Irregular speech rate; speaks in spurts or bursts	6	5	4	3	2	1	0
13. Telescopes or condenses words	6	5	4	3	2	1	0
14. Rapid rate (tachylalia)	6	5	4	3	2	1	0
15. Speech rate progressively increases (festinating)	6	5	4	3	2	1	0
16. Variable prosody; irregular melody or stress pattern	6	5	4	3	2	1	0
17. Initial loud voice trailing off to unintelligible murmur	6	5	4	3	2	1	0
18. Lack of pauses between words and phrases	6	5	4	3	2	1	0

#		6	5	4	3	2	1	0
19.	Repetition of multisyllabic words and phrases	6	5	4	3	2	1	0
20.	Co-existence of excessive disfluencies and stuttering	6	5	4	3	2	1	0
	Language–Cognition							
21.	Language is disorganized; confused wording; word-finding problems	6	5	4	3	2	1	0
22.	Poor language formulation; poor storytelling; sequencing problems	6	5	4	3	2	1	0
23.	Disorganized language increases as topic becomes more complex	6	5	4	3	2	1	0
24.	Many revisions; interjections; filler words	6	5	4	3	2	1	0
25.	Seems to verbalize before adequate thought formulation	6	5	4	3	2	1	0
26.	Inappropriate topic introduction, maintenance, or termination	6	5	4	3	2	1	0
27.	Improper linguistic structure; poor grammar; syntax errors	6	5	4	3	2	1	0
28.	Distractible; poor concentration; attention span problems	6	5	4	3	2	1	0
	Motor Coordination–Writing Problems							
29.	Poor motor control for writing (messy)	6	5	4	3	2	1	0
30.	Writing includes omission or transposition of letters, syllables, or words	6	5	4	3	2	1	0
31.	Oral diadochokinetic coordination below expected normed levels	6	5	4	3	2	1	0
32.	Respiratory dysrhythmia; jerky breathing pattern	6	5	4	3	2	1	0
33.	Clumsy and uncoordinated; motor activities accelerated or impulsive	6	5	4	3	2	1	0

Total Score: _____

Comments: _____

Figure 4.2. Predictive Cluttering Inventory (PCI). *Note.* From "Cluttering: Characteristics Identified as Diagnostically Significant by 60 Fluency Experts," by D. Daly, October 2007, paper presented at the 10th International Stuttering Awareness Day Online Conference—Stuttering Awareness: Global Community, Local Activity. Available at http://www.mnsu.edu/comdis/isad10/papers/daly10/daly10.html. Reprinted with permission.

7. speech production and prosody (reduce rate, use delayed auditory feedback, change inflection and emphasis to alter meaning, contrast statements and questions, highlight verbal punctuation)

8. motor skills (train oral motor skills, recite tongue twisters, improve penmanship)

Similarly, St. Louis et al. (2007, pp. 316–319) recommended a systems approach to intervention for cluttering, suggesting that clinicians select from among nine treatment targets and multiple intervention strategies, depending on the individual client's profile. The targets for improvement include the following:

1. awareness and self-monitoring skills (e.g., audio- and video-record speech to monitor and self-correct, heighten client's sensory awareness of movement during nonspeech and then speech-related motor acts, use computer-generated visual feedback to monitor speech rate, use feedback from listeners, provide feedback among other people who clutter)

2. speech rate, articulation, and intelligibility (slow rate by using delayed auditory feedback, timed syllable speech, and prolonged vowels; use deliberate articulation, pauses, and phrasing; use prosodic variations, accented syllables, shadowed speech, and musical analogies)

3. linguistic and narrative skills (teach and improve elements of story grammar, sequencing of thoughts, turn-taking skills, semantic classification and categorization, word-finding and retrieval, syntactic structuring, and cohesion within and across utterances)

4. fluency skills (use audio- and video-recorded samples for analysis of speech disfluencies and maze behaviors, use strategies noted earlier for rate and language to decrease disfluencies)

5. meta-cluttering skills (identify the unique nature of the client's cluttering; distinguish reactions of self and others to the client's cluttering; distinguish between thought and language organization during moments of clarity and moments of incoherence; use sensory feedback during different rates of speech; compare and contrast the client's cluttered and stuttered speech if the client demonstrates both; and role-play and study the intelligibility, narrative, and pragmatic skills of others)

6. phonatory and respiratory behaviors (mark passages for pauses and breath intake, heighten client's awareness of optimum and exceeded number of words per breath group)

7. family, friend, and employer support (obtain feedback from family and friends during clear and poor communication, recommend participation in group speaking activities)

8. collaboration with other team members (consult with or refer to other specialists as appropriate, e.g., attention-deficit/hyperactivity disorder or learning disability specialists, psychologists, mental health professionals, neurologists)

9. transfer and maintenance

Using St. Louis et al.'s (2007) metaphor, we leave this "unfinished jigsaw puzzle" to address another puzzle, neurogenic acquired stuttering.

Neurogenic Acquired Stuttering

Interest in the sudden or gradual onset of stuttering-like disfluency in adults is long-standing (De Nil, Jokel, & Rochon, 2007; see also Kussmaul, 1877), although related publications were few until the 1970s. Helm-Estabrooks (1999) noted that two papers were published in 1978, one describing 7 patients who acquired "cortical stuttering" after incurring cerebral vascular accident (CVA; i.e., stroke) (Rosenbek, Messert, Collins,

& Wertz, 1978) and another describing 10 patients with "acquired stuttering" after incurring CVA (6 adults) and traumatic brain injury (TBI, 4 adults) (Helm, Butler, & Benson, 1978). Helm-Estabrooks (1999) reported that over the next 20 years, 60 additional cases revealed "neurogenic stuttering" resulting from traumatic brain injury, stroke, extrapyramidal disease, Alzheimer's disease, brain tumor, encephalitis, dialysis dementia, drug toxicity, and anorexia nervosa.

Since that time, interest in the etiology, symptomatology, and treatment of neurogenic acquired stuttering has increased markedly (Caruso, Max, & McClowry, 1999; De Nil, 2007; De Nil et al., 2007; Duffy, 2005; Dworkin, Culatta, Abkarian, & Meleca, 2002; Goberman & Blomgren, 2003; Grant, Biousse, Cook, & Newman, 1999; Guitar, 2006; Mowrer & Younts, 2001; Theys et al., 2008; Van Borsel, Van Lierde, Van Cauwenberge, Guldemont, & Van Orshoven, 1998). Cases of neurogenic acquired stuttering have generally been thought to be rare, but published surveys indicate that the percentage of speech–language pathologists who treat such patients ranges from 27% (Theys et al., 2008) to 36% (Stewart & Rowley, 1996) to 81% (Market, Montague, Buffalo, & Drummond, 1990). Establishing precise incidence and prevalence data is complicated because neurogenic acquired stuttering does not always persist. Also, symptoms of neurogenic acquired stuttering may appear within weeks of onset of the medical problem (often the case with stroke); at times, symptoms do not appear until months later. Sometimes symptoms of neurogenic acquired stuttering are revealed before diagnosis of the medical condition (to be discussed later in this chapter with respect to dementia and tumor). In some cases, developmental stuttering has occurred, worsened, recurred, or even disappeared in the presence of neurological dysfunction (De Nil et al., 2007; Helm-Estabrooks, 1999; Theys et al., 2008). De Nil et al. noted that increased time intervals between diagnosis of the neurological condition and observed fluency disruption interferes with establishing a causal link between the two events; he recommended longitudinal studies of people with neurogenic acquired stuttering.

So what is neurogenic acquired stuttering? Culatta and Goldberg (1995) defined this condition as "the result of an identifiable neuropathology in a speaker with no history of fluency problems prior to occurrence of the pathology" (p. 34). Helm-Estabrooks (1993) offered the following distinction between developmental or idiopathic stuttering and neurogenic acquired stuttering:

> Stuttering refers to disorders in the rhythm of speech in which the individual knows precisely what he or she wishes to say but at the same time is unable to say it because of an involuntary repetition, prolongation, or cessation of a sound. When the behavior first occurs, notably worsens, or recurs in the presence of acquired neurological problems, it is diagnosed as stuttering associated with acquired neurological disorders (SAAND). (p. 207)

More recently, De Nil et al. (2007) stated that "neurogenic stuttering is generally diagnosed when the onset of stutter-like disfluencies occurs following a neurological event, such as head trauma or disease, which disrupts normal brain function" (p. 326). A significant point in these and other definitions of neurogenic acquired stuttering is that the speech disfluency occurs subsequent to nervous system damage and is not accountable in any other way (Duffy, 2005; Rosenbek, 1984). Other terms for disfluencies associated with acquired neurological involvement have included acquired stuttering, cortical stuttering, neurogenic stuttering, late-onset stuttering, and organic stuttering, among others. Frequent reservation is expressed, however, over application of the term *stuttering*, a diagnostic label that identifies idiopathic or developmental disfluency, to the disfluent speech of adults whose adventitious onset following neurological damage is only one symptom of an underlying and identifiable dysfunction. Duffy stated,

> These reservations stem from a desire to avoid: (1) confusing this disorder [neurogenic stuttering] with behavioral, etiologic, and theoretical issues associated with idiopathic childhood stuttering; (2) implying that acquired neurogenic dysfluencies represent strong evidence for a neurogenic basis for developmental stuttering; (3) implying that all dysfluencies associated with acquired CNS damage reflect the same underlying disturbance; (4) implying that all acquired stuttering-like behavior is neurogenic—it can also be psychogenic in origin, even in people with neurologic disease. (p. 354)

The inherent imprecision in our professional lexicon is not a new concern. Rosenbek (1984) identified as a major problem that "too many kinds of disfluency have been called by one name: stuttering" (p. 36). Acknowledging the reservations, I am electing to use the term *neurogenic acquired stuttering*, which is a departure from *neurogenic disfluency*, used in the previous edition of this book, to be more consistent with related references in the professional literature while maintaining explicit reference to the neurogenic etiology and adventitious onset that distinguish this condition from developmental stuttering (Duffy, 2005; Guitar, 2006). Duffy clarified that the term *stuttering* in *neurogenic stuttering* is shorthand for "stuttering-like behaviors" that are similar in only some ways to surface features of idiopathic childhood stuttering. I concur, acknowledging that any such term is a molar or "wastebasket" expression (Van Riper, 1982), relatively limited in meaning by itself and necessitating a more molecular description. The uniqueness of an individual's neurogenic acquired stuttering is determined by the site and degree of lesion. Unlike other speech–language deficits, disfluency by itself is of limited utility in differentially diagnosing the site of lesion (Culatta & Goldberg, 1995; Helm-Estabrooks & Holz, 1998; Rosenbek, 1984). This becomes particularly apparent in light of the evidence that disfluent speech results from damage to most areas of the central nervous system. Rosenbek observed,

> Various kinds of speech and language deficits can be used to help localize where damage has occurred to the nervous system. Neurogenic stuttering, however, may not be one such deficit. It has occurred following damage to the low and high brainstem, to the basal ganglia, cerebellum, left and right cortical hemispheres, and to the white matter (tracts) of the frontal lobes of both the right and left hemispheres. . . . Stuttering has also been reported after frontal, parietal, and temporal lobe lesions within the left hemisphere. About the only sites within the nervous system which have not been associated with stuttering are the occipital lobes of the brain, which are devoted primarily to vision and the cranial nerves once they leave the brainstem. (pp. 42–43)

Others have reported similarly that neurogenic acquired stuttering is associated with damage to most areas of the brain (i.e., right and left hemisphere, including the frontal, parietal, and temporal lobes) and that only the occipital lobes and the cranial nerves once they leave the brain stem are not associated with neurogenic acquired stuttering (Grant et al., 1999; Van Borsel et al., 1998). Disfluency has also originated from diverse neurological events (De Nil et al., 2007; Duffy, 2005; Helm-Estabrooks, 1986, 1999). The following types of events are discussed next: stroke, traumatic brain injury, extrapyramidal disease, dementia and tumor, drug use, and AIDS.

Stroke

Stroke accounts for one of the two most frequent etiologies of neurogenic acquired stuttering (the other is traumatic brain injury; Market et al., 1990; Theys et al., 2008). Stroke results from *thrombosis* (occlusion of a blood vessel by fatty substances and blood platelets), *embolus* (occlusion of a blood vessel by detached tissue from a thrombosis), or *hemorrhage* (rupture of a blood vessel). People who experience a stroke frequently show fluency disruption of abrupt onset on initial phonemes and content words, particularly within conversation. In fewer instances, onset is more gradual and becomes increasingly worse over a span of weeks to months later (Theys et al., 2008). Other contexts affected to a lesser extent include medial phonemes and, even less frequently, final phonemes, function words, automatized sequences, rote paragraphs, singing, and tapped speech. The adaptation effect generally is absent and performance is reduced in carrying a tune, tapping rhythms, block designs from a model, stick designs from memory, sequential hand positions, and three-dimensional drawing (Helm-Estabrooks, 1986, 1993). Disfluency generally is present whether or not stroke co-occurs with other conditions (e.g., aphasia, seizure disorder, secondary motor involvement) (Duffy, 2005; Grant et al., 1999; Helm-Estabrooks, 1986, 1999; Theys et al., 2008). Helm-Estabrooks (1986) indicated that disfluency may be of little relative concern to people with severe aphasia, yet may be a source of frustration inhibiting verbal expression in people with milder aphasia. Therefore, fluency management is influenced by the nature and extent of the language problem.

Traumatic Brain Injury

A common brain trauma is acquired from car accidents. Focal damage is due to compression of the skull, skull fractures, and hemorrhages. Other, more diffuse microscopic damage is possible, resulting in coma or seizure disorders. Closed head injury often results in change or deficit in memory, personality, and cognitive capacity, particularly in abstract thinking. These effects and others from an acquired language disorder might inhibit the treatment process. Helm-Estabrooks (1986, 1993) reported that in such cases, onset of disfluency tends to be gradual. However, Theys et al. (2008) reported results of a clinician survey indicating that of six cases whose stuttering onset and progression were known to have followed traumatic brain injury, five began to stutter suddenly and only one gradually. Typically, disfluency is observed on initial phonemes in conversation and in automatic sequences and rote paragraphs, tapped speech, and singing. Medial and final phonemes and content and function words are affected less. The adaptation effect is observed only rarely, and when observed, is milder (De Nil et al., 2007; Theys et al., 2008). Occasionally, aphasia, seizure disorder, and secondary motor involvement co-occur. As with stroke, performance may be reduced in carrying of a tune, tapping of rhythms, block designs from a model, stick designs from memory, sequential hand positions, and three-dimensional drawing. Despite efforts to distinguish traumatic brain injury on the basis of behavioral patterns, however, injuries resulting from head trauma or other circumstances may have communication-related consequences that cannot be predicted. In two such cases described by Helm-Estabrooks, Yeo, Geschwind, Freedman, and Weinstein (1986), an ambidextrous 21-year-old man who had stuttered since he was 8 years old fell and struck his head, causing right hemiparesis. Following a period of unconsciousness for 10 days, his stuttering disappeared; however, his speech became slower and dysarthric, with slight hypernasality and articulatory imprecision. In another case, a man who stuttered as a child achieved spontaneous fluency by the time he was 8 years old. At 61 years of age, he incurred a stroke with right hemiparesis, resulting in the reappearance of his stuttering. Helm-Estabrooks (1999) indicated that such cases reflect the complexity and multidimensionality of stuttering associated with acquired neurological disorders (SAAND), which render prediction of individual symptoms and response to intervention impossible; indeed, we have much to learn about the brain and its organization related to communication and its disorders, specifically stuttering. Helm-Estabrooks (1999) concluded, "Fluent speaking is, perhaps, the most refined motor act performed by humans, requiring complex coordination of many different muscle groups. It can be sensitive, therefore, to even small changes in neurological status" (p. 265).

Extrapyramidal Disease

Dysarthric-type disfluency in patients with extrapyramidal disease, such as Parkinson's disease, has been referred to as "kinetic stutter" (Sacks, 1995, p. 97). Faulty motor execution gives rise to the characteristic slurred speech and sound prolongations, repetitions, and blocks related to articulatory immobility. Compared to disfluency in other neurogenic conditions, disfluencies resulting from extrapyramidal disease are usually gradual in onset and progressive in nature; they are observed on initial phonemes and content words in conversation, and often on medial phonemes and function words. Occasionally, errors of verbal perseveration and reduced verbal output are observed (Downes, Sharp, Costall, Sagar, & Howe, 1993). The adaptation effect may be present. Secondary motor involvement, aphasia, and buccofacial apraxia generally do not co-occur. Performance is typically reduced in carrying a tune, tapping rhythms, and sequential hand positions (Helm-Estabrooks, 1986, 1993). Others have narrowly described the increased number of disfluencies (i.e., particularly within-word disfluencies) among patients with Parkinson's disease and hypothesized that such increases may be due to changes in dopamine level (i.e., increases or decreases) in the brain (Goberman & Blomgren, 2003).

Dementia and Tumor

Dementia is another progressive disease linked to the onset of disfluency in adults. Several cases of dialysis dementia revealed that after prolonged dialysis for kidney disease, disfluent speech was the first symptom preceding mutism and death (Rosenbek, McNeil, Lemme, Prescott, & Alfrey, 1975). Similarly, a 62-year-old businessman experienced recurrence of childhood stuttering 7 months before other symptoms of Alzheimer's-type dementia, including mild aphasia, cognitive loss, and death within 18 months of the observed disfluency (Quinn & Andrews, 1977). Tumor is related to speech disfluency as well. Helm, Butler, and Canter (1980) reported on a woman of 54 years who had a metastatic brain tumor. Three weeks after symptoms of ataxic gait and right hyperreflexia, she became disfluent on initial phonemes of content and function words, with no evidence of the adaptation effect. Her condition worsened, leading to mutism and eventual death. Helm-Estabrooks (1986, 1999) reported on a man with sudden onset of mildly disfluent speech who was found by the attending physician to have "no positive neurological signs" and who was sent to the hospital's psychiatric unit. The man had a history of good mental health, and the psychiatrists found no basis for his speech disruption. One week later, Helm-Estabrooks (1986, 1999) evaluated the man and detected a slight right facial weakness. Several months later, the man died of a brain tumor. I had an experience similar to that of Helm-Estabrooks several years ago. One of the senior faculty members I had known at our university invited me to guest lecture in his seminar. I noticed that he had become significantly disfluent, forgetful, and awkward in gait and arm movement. Despite prodding from his faculty colleagues to go for a medical examination, he did not go, even after he became distinctly dysgraphic. After his symptoms worsened further, he went for the neurological evaluation, which detected an enlarged inoperable brain tumor. He passed away shortly thereafter; I think of him every time I pass the conference room named in his honor. Helm-Estabrooks (1986) stressed that "onset of stuttering in a well-adjusted adult should be regarded as a possible symptom of neurological disease" (p. 201). Early identification and appropriate referral for neurophysiological evaluation "may be the major contribution made by the speech pathologist in cases of progressive dementia" (p. 202). Helm-Estabrooks (1999) added, "Early diagnosis of SAAND may lead to successful treatment of either a neurological disorder causing stuttering or the communication disorder itself" (p. 265).

Drug Usage

Anecdotal accounts document the co-occurrence of disfluency with the introduction of different pharmacological agents, and elimination of disfluency with removal of the agent. Early reports implicated amitriptyline, a tricyclic antidepressant (Quader, 1977), and theophylline, a bronchodilator used for asthma with a 4-year-old boy (McCarthy, 1981). Another report implicated phenothiazine, a drug used to control both psychosis and stuttering in people with schizophrenia (Nurnberg & Greenwald, 1981). However, the effects were mutually exclusive (i.e., low dosage left patients fluent but psychotic; higher dosage controlled the psychosis but not the stuttering). Subsequent research has resulted in a literature on "drug-induced stuttering" and implicated individual medications, including antidepressants (amitriptyline, dothiepin, desipramine, fluoxetine, and sertraline), neuroleptic agents (propranolol, perphenazine/desipramine combination, chlorpromazine/lithium combination, clozapine, and risperidone), radiopaque contrast medium (metrizamide), and other drugs (theophylline, prochlorperazine, methylphenidate, pemoline, levodopa, gabapentin, clorazepate, and alprazolam, in addition to benzodiazepines, L-dopa, and methylphenidate) (Brady, 1998; Movsessian, 2005; Remington & Fagan, 2007; Rentschler, Driver, & Callaway, 1984; Rosenfield, McCarthy, McKinney, & Viswanath, 1994). An ongoing concern is that most label warnings do not include information about the effects of medications on speech fluency. Indeed, speech–language pathologists are encouraged to inquire about a client's medication, especially if the disfluency is of recent onset (Culatta & Goldberg, 1995; Culatta & Leeper, 1989–1990). Interest in the interaction of prescription medication and stuttering has led another growing literature, that of neuropharmacological intervention for stuttering (see Saxon & Ludlow, 2007, for a critical review of the effect of drugs on stuttering).

AIDS

The human acquired immunodeficiency syndrome (AIDS) virus causes a variety of neurological symptoms reflective of progressive neuropathology. One such symptom is speech disfluency. Fantry (1990) described one of her male patients who, at 27 years old, tested positive for the AIDS virus antibody and developed "stuttering" for the first time. This symptom was concomitant with other, more predictable symptoms, including weight loss, fever, fatigue, diarrhea, difficulty with memory, and "haziness of mind." Fantry reported, "During the clinic visit, the patient was observed stuttering on three separate occasions with no impairment of language function" (p. 38). Another physician (Vinnard, 1990a) labeled the disfluency reported by Fantry as "AIDS-related acquired stuttering" (p. 6). It is unfortunate, however, that Fantry reported neither the speech-related nor psychoemotional characteristics of the patient. Fantry indicated that the disfluency "decreased" after 2 weeks of zidovudine (AZT) treatment and "completely resolved" after an additional 4 weeks of treatment. She also suggested that "certain sites in the brain may have structural or vascular abnormalities that lead to stuttering" (p. 6) and concluded that "it is entirely possible that zidovudine therapy could account for the cessation of stuttering, just as removal of focal central nervous system lesions has relieved acquired stuttering in other patients" (p. 6). The parallel intervention to which

Fantry referred is surgery (Andy & Bhatnagar, 1992; De Nil et al., 2007; Donnan, 1979; Helm-Estabrooks, 1999; Motluk, 1997). Lopez et al. (1994) analyzed and described the "speech motor control disorder" (SMCD) characteristics of six patients infected with the AIDS virus. These characteristics, which are progressive in nature, included irregular articulatory breakdowns in consonants and vowels (in terms of range, rate, and direction of movement), prolongation of phonemes and the intervals between them, dysrhythmia of speech and syllable repetition, greater difficulty initiating than completing single word production, harsh voice, and monopitch and monoloudness (occasionally interrupted by patterns of excessive loudness variation), respiratory and vocal arrest, and slow and effortful cognitive processing associated with motor speed and attentional tasks. The authors concluded that the deficits were the consequence of cerebellar dysfunction, possibly accompanied by basal ganglia deficits. No intervention was used to alter the observed speech-motor characteristics, however.

Cases Defying Clinical Profiling

Helm-Estabrooks (1986) reported several cases of adults who acquired disfluent speech associated with other neuropathologies. One 48-year-old man became disfluent and developed memory loss following brain anoxia during open heart surgery. Another man, with adolescent onset of seizures, developed transient disfluency following an overdose of dilantin. A 16-year-old male developed severe disfluency and dysarthria following surgery to the right thalamus. Another man (a 30-year-old electrician) experienced transient disfluency of about 6 weeks in duration following inhalation of toxic fumes. Byrne, Byrne, and Zibin (1993) described a man who at 25 years of age acquired speech disfluency ("transient neurogenic stuttering") as a result of impairment of brain function secondary to chronic starvation. Statements of symptoms included "dysfluency . . . finishing sentences," "repetitions of syllables," "difficulty with both functors and substantives," "difficulties when pronouncing small words," and "repetition did not improve his performance in these areas" (p. 512). After he received a well-balanced diet during 2 weeks of hospitalization, all symptoms of speech disfluency disappeared.

Familiarity with neurogenic acquired stuttering is essential, lest we assume erroneously that all disfluency is stuttering. It is beyond the scope of our purposes to review thoroughly assessment and treatment methods for such disfluency. An overview of defining characteristics will suffice. Various lists of characteristics attempt to distinguish neurogenic acquired stuttering from psychogenic acquired stuttering and developmental stuttering. Canter (1971) noted the following characteristics of "neurogenic stuttering": (a) repetitions and prolongations on final as well as initial and medial syllables, (b) phonemic foci of disfluency that differ from those of developmental stuttering, (c) disfluency unrelated to grammatical function (function and content words may be equally troublesome), (d) no direct relationship between propositionality (linguistic complexity) and disfluency (self-formulated speech may be easier than automatic speech), (e) no adaptation effect (fluency does not improve with repeated readings of a passage), (f) absence of marked anxiety despite observed annoyance, and (g) no secondary features (facial tension, eye blinking, fist clenching). Similarly, Helm-Estabrooks (1999) listed the following characteristics: (a) disfluencies on grammatical (function) words nearly as frequent as on substantive (content) words; (b) annoyance without anxiety; (c) repetitions, prolongations, and blocks on more than just initial syllables of words and utterances, (d) no secondary symptoms (facial grimacing, eye blinking, or fist clenching) associated with the disfluency, (e) no adaptation effect, and (f) consistency of stuttering across different speech tasks.

Despite the consistency of such criteria over three decades, Van Borsel (1997) cautioned, "Clinical symptomatology does not enable one to safely distinguish neurogenic stuttering from developmental stuttering" (p. 21). Furthermore, as noted earlier, prediction with absolute consistency across symptoms in neurogenic acquired stuttering is imprecise at best, given the multidimensionality of the disorder (Helm-Estabrooks, 1999). More recently, Jokel, De Nil, and Sharpe (2007) presented the characteristics (i.e., speech, language, cognitive, psychosocial, and medical) of 12 patients, all of whom demonstrated neurogenic acquired stuttering, 6 following stroke and 6 following head injury. Jokel et al. mentioned the following challenges to the aforementioned characteristics: Stuttering was observed overwhelmingly on content words, self-perceived communication attitudes were negative and suggested anxiety about the disfluency, disfluencies occurred overwhelmingly on initial sounds (final sounds/syllables were disfluent only in the TBI group), secondary behaviors were observed but often not recognized by the patients, adaptation was observed (i.e., 3/6 of the patients with stroke and 2/6 of the patients with TBI), and disfluencies occurred in all speech tasks but were condition dependent. That is, the speaking tasks in decreasing order of observed disfluency were reading, conversation, and then monologue. Automatic speech, usually fluent among people with developmental stuttering, did not result in significantly improved fluency, particularly among people with TBI. Jokel et al. concurred with Helm-Estabrooks (1999) that neurogenic stuttering represents a heterogeneous phenomenon and that differential diagnosis is not always straightforward.

The significance of word-final disfluencies has been of ongoing interest (Humphrey & Van Borsel, 2001; Van Borsel, Van Coster, & Van Lierde, 1996). In this section, we have learned that repetition and prolongation of final, as well as initial and medial, syllables can be an indication of neurogenic acquired stuttering (Canter, 1971; Jokel et al., 2007). Van Borsel et al. (1996) reported on a 9-year-old boy who, at 3 years 10 months old, incurred a head injury resulting in unconsciousness. At 9 years old, the diagnostic evaluation revealed final part-word repetitions during conversation, monologue, and monologue with masking. These disfluencies occurred frequently, accounting for 19% of all the child's disfluencies and second only to whole-word repetitions. Part-word final repetitions contained only one or two units of repetition. In polysyllabic words, the entire final syllable was repeated (e.g., *diamanten ten*); in monosyllabic words, the final consonant or cluster of the syllable and the preceding vowel were repeated (e.g., *noemt oemt*). Final part-word repetitions occurred exclusively on lexical words and most often on the last word in a phrase or sentence. This was in contrast to initial part-word repetitions, which occurred predominantly on function words and never on the last word of a phrase or sentence. Van Borsel et al. (1996) challenged Canter's (1971) assertion as unsubstantiated that repetitions and prolongations of final consonants are typical of neurogenic acquired stuttering. Their case supports a neurological basis, however, in that there was no family history of developmental stuttering, no secondary symptoms, and no enhancement of fluency from auditory masking. Also, there was more disfluency during monologue with masking than during monologue alone, disfluencies occurred on lexical words (word-final repetitions) and function words (initial part-word and word repetitions), and two left-hemisphere subcortical lesions were found on the MRI. While these symptoms are characteristic of a child with focal brain damage (Van Borsel et al., 1996), word-final disfluencies are not the exclusive domain of neurogenic acquired stuttering. Indeed, Humphrey and Van Borsel (2001) chronicled the literature identifying word-final disfluencies in people with neurogenic acquired stuttering and others with developmental stuttering (see also McAllister & Kingston, 2005, who reviewed two case studies of school-age children, neither of whom stuttered or evidenced neuropathology, who demonstrated final part-word repetitions). Humphrey and Van Borsel concluded that word-final repetitions and prolongations may be less common among the population of people with neurogenic acquired stuttering than previously thought. They reviewed word-final disfluencies in four studies of people with neurogenic acquired stuttering and eight studies of people with developmental stuttering. Humphrey and Van Borsel indicated, "Because word-final dysfluencies have occurred independently in some cases, and have co-occurred with typical stuttering in other cases, it is possible that they are separate but related phenomena. The dysfluencies of the neurogenic stuttering patients have been attributed to their brain damage. Given the small number of reports, it is remarkable that word-final dysfluencies are noted in both neurogenic and developmental cases." At the very least, word-final disfluencies should garner close attention and be scrutinized for differential diagnosis and clinical implications.

In preparation for making intervention-related decisions, Helm-Estabrooks (1999) advised clinicians to obtain a thorough case history and to administer standardized tests to identify SAAND and any other coexisting language, memory, attention, or cognitive deficits. Related activities include repeated readings of a phonetically balanced (i.e., standardized) passage, automatized recitations, singing of familiar songs, and conversational analysis. Helm-Estabrooks (1999, p. 261) suggested that the clinician attend to the following questions: "Does stuttering present a communication handicap?" "Is the individual motivated to work on this problem?" If the patient is otherwise a potential candidate for intervention, then the clinician must ask, "Does the patient have a rapidly progressing neurological disorder?" Helm-Estabrooks advised clinicians to weigh the relative significance of the stuttering in light a degenerative or progressive disorder. If the patient's remaining lifespan is short, perhaps a form of drug therapy might be advised over traditional speech therapy. In any case, selection of patients for various types of intervention must take into account the patient's health status, the etiology of stuttering, its neurological correlates, its persistence, and the presence of concomitant disorders. Once selected for treatment, the patient needs to be as active as possible in setting goals and all subsequent phases of intervention. Treatment might take a variety of forms, including auditory masking and delayed auditory feedback (DAF, discussed in Chapter 7), biofeedback and relaxation, speech pacing, transcutaneous nerve stimulation, thalamic stimulation, pharmacological agents, and surgical intervention.

Another challenging distinction must be highlighted. Clinical experience and related literature have shown that many of the symptoms of apraxia of speech in adults (Daly, 2006; Darley, Aronson, & Brown, 1975) and developmental apraxia of speech (DAS), also referred to as *suspected childhood apraxia of speech* (sCAS) (ASHA, 2007a, 2007b; Hall, 2007), resemble the symptoms of developmental stuttering and particularly cluttering. Darley et al. described the following symptoms of apraxia resulting from left cerebral hemisphere damage: (a) variable and inconsistent articulation errors, (b) struggle behaviors to position articulators correctly, (c) groping to achieve correct oral posture and correct sequence of postures for word production, (d) difficulty making initial sounds, and (e) effortful attempts to correct speech production errors. Daly (2006) noted that for both people with apraxia and those with developmental stuttering, speaking becomes increasingly difficult with greater task complexity (e.g., polysyllabic words are produced less accurately than monosyllabic words). Similarly, for both groups of people, effortful struggle often accompanies attempts to correct postures and movement sequences, some words are avoided, and prosody is disrupted. Daly (2006) also noted that people with apraxia and those who clutter demonstrate involuntary motor planning disruption with significant articulation problems where speech production errors are not bound to specific sounds or blends. Dworkin (as cited in Daly, 2006) described developmental apraxia of speech as an expression of muscle weakness without identified neuropathology or hard neurological evidence, with the following characteristics: (a) inconsistent and imprecise articulation errors, (b) the most difficulty with initial sounds and clusters, (c) disfluencies and hesitations, (d) groping and false starts, (e) perseveration of automatic speech, (f) voice arrests and loudness outbursts, and (g) improvement with repetition. Daly (2006) emphasized the diagnostic value of engaging the client in repetition of multisyllabic words, diadochokinetic tasks, and word-lengthening activities (e.g., zip, zipper, zippering). Daly (2006) noted the following characteristics of developmental apraxia of speech and indicated those often seen among people who clutter (C) and those with developmental stuttering (S) as well: multiple repetitions (C, S), motor discoordination (C, less frequent with S), articulation errors (C), impaired language (C), delayed speech (C), awareness of the problem (S), poor concentration (C), written language disorder (C), soft neurological signs (C, less frequent with S), and resistance to treatment (C).

Other similarities and differences between neurogenic acquired stuttering and developmental stuttering abound. People with aphasia or apraxia tend to repeat incorrect sounds and words, but these repetitions stop once the phonemically correct target or close approximation is achieved. In comparison, people who stutter repeat sounds that are correctly articulated except for their frequency of occurrence (Culatta & Goldberg, 1995; Rosenbek, 1984). People with aphasia who experience dysnomia or people with dementia may demonstrate disfluencies in the form of interjections, pauses, and circumlocutions while searching for the correct word, but these disfluencies cease once the target word is accessed. In contrast, people who stutter demonstrate disfluencies that may appear similar, but they report being keenly aware of the word they are trying to say before, during, and after the word is spoken (Culatta & Goldberg, 1995). Whereas the onset of neurogenic acquired stuttering often is abrupt (recall the discussion of gradual onset, disappearance, reappearance, and worsening of disfluency with subsequent interruption of neurological function), the onset of stuttering has been reported both as gradual in developmental profiles (Bloodstein, 1960a, 1960b; Van Riper, 1982) and as abrupt in longitudinal investigations (Yairi & Ambrose, 2005). Neurogenic acquired stuttering also differs in its immunity to behavioral manipulation and lack of developmental history, which often relates to a client's self-image. About such distinctions and relating to a client's self-image, Rosenbek (1984) stated, "Disfluencies beginning after a long period of normal speech–language use may well be different from the disfluencies beginning in childhood, if for no other reason than that the adult may react differently to their appearance" (p. 46).

Understanding and distinguishing between neurogenic acquired stuttering, developmental stuttering, cluttering, and other fluency disorders is essential to preventing misdiagnosis (Culatta & Leeper, 1987, 1988, 1989–1990; Helm-Estabrooks, 1986, 1993, 1999), which has been responsible for too many people with neurological impairments unnecessarily experiencing emotional trauma, frustration, guilt, and failure when attempting to modify their speech with inappropriate stuttering therapy techniques (Culatta & Goldberg, 1995). Again, not all speech disfluency is stuttering.

Psychogenic Acquired Stuttering

Another late-onset fluency disorder is psychogenic acquired stuttering. Although less is known about this disorder than developmental stuttering, cluttering, and neurogenic acquired stuttering, the literature contains a number of reports of stuttering that began in adulthood in association with psychological disturbance or reaction to emotionally traumatic events (Arnold, 1965; Attanasio, 1987a; Deal, 1982; Deal & Doro, 1987). In each of these cases, the client had neither a history of developmental stuttering nor any positive indication of neuropathology. The onset of the speech disruption usually was sudden, but occasionally gradual, progressive, and episodic. For example, clients have been reported to experience the onset of psychogenic acquired stuttering following combat fatigue during World War II (Peacher & Harris, 1946), a direct missile attack to a ship during the Korean conflict (Dempsey & Granich, 1978), anxiety attacks (Culatta & Goldberg, 1995; Wallen, 1961), suicide attempts (Deal, 1982), a traumatic business experience (Weiner, 1981), sexual abuse (Mahr & Leith, 1992), and marital separation and divorce (Attanasio, 1987a). In some cases, the presence of psychopathology was determined (Clifford, Aronson, & Peterson, cited in Roth, Aronson, & Davis, 1989; see also M. D. Cox, 1986). Emotionally based speech disfluency has been referred to as *hysterical stuttering* (Arnold, 1965; Bluemel, 1935; Deal & Doro, 1987; F. H. Silverman, 2004), neurotic stuttering (Haynes, Pindzola, & Emerick, 1992), psychogenic stuttering (Baumgartner, 1999; Manning, 2010; Roth et al., 1989), and psychogenic acquired stuttering (Guitar, 2006; F. H. Silverman, 2004). Freund (1966) documented the historical use of such terms as *expectancy neurosis, compulsive neurosis, anxiety hysteria, lalophobia, phonophobia, paralalia syllabaris, pregenital conversion neurosis,* and *socio-affective dysphasia,* among others.

Deal (1982) described the following as characteristics of psychogenic acquired stuttering:

1. sudden onset
2. onset temporally close to an event reflective of extreme psychological stress
3. repetition of initial or stressed syllables
4. no observed reduction in disfluency with choral reading, white noise, delayed auditory feedback, singing, and different communication situations
5. no conditions in which fluency is observed
6. indifferent attitude toward stuttering (also referred to as *"la belle indifférence"* in the psychiatric literature)
7. no secondary symptoms
8. no change in disfluency during mimed reading aloud

Similarly, Mahr and Leith (1992) identified the following characteristics of psychogenic acquired stuttering:

1. a change in speech pattern resembling stuttering
2. onset of symptoms directly related to psychological factors of emotional conflict or secondary gain
3. absence of evidence suggesting organic etiology
4. a presenting history of previous mental health issues
5. atypical disfluency symptoms (e.g., no islands of fluency, no secondary symptoms)
6. *la belle indifférence*
7. bizarre interpersonal interactions

De Nil et al. (2007) recommended that clinicians address two essential diagnostic questions: Is the stuttering developmental or acquired, and, if acquired, is the stuttering neurogenic or psychogenic? They acknowledged, albeit cautiously, that the absence of a distinct neurological event preceding the onset of stuttering often is a differential diagnostic indicator of psychogenic stuttering. However, they noted that the absence of a neurological event does not eradicate the possibility that the stuttering is neurogenic in nature (i.e., the neuropathology can be identified subsequent to onset of stuttering). Also, the presence of an identified neuropathology does not necessarily exclude the possibility that the stuttering is psychogenic in nature (i.e., one who incurs neuropathology or a brain trauma may have a significant psychosocial reaction, taking the form of psychogenic acquired stuttering).

Also addressing differential diagnosis, Roth et al. (1989) noted that onset of stuttering in adults can have different, if not mixed, etiologies (e.g., purely neurogenic, purely psychogenic, psychogenic with psychogenically based neurogenic symptoms, psychogenic with coexisting but unrelated neuropathology, psychogenic as a reaction to the neuropathology). Roth et al. (1989) summarized the records of 12 patients evaluated and treated for psychogenic acquired stuttering:

- For 11 patients, stuttering was the primary complaint. Symptoms included rapid and multiple sound repetitions, prolongations, blocks, glottal spasms, speech interruptions with inhalatory breaks, rapid panting, tremor-like speech, and reduced speech rate. Repetitions, prolongations, and blocks were frequent, occurring at the beginning or middle of nearly every word. Symptom type and severity varied across patients but were fairly static for each individual patient.

- All patients had other complaints that raised suspicion of neuropathology (e.g., headache, numbness, tingling, clumsiness or weakness, breathing difficulty or chest pain, trembling or seizure-like behavior, disturbance of memory or thinking), necessitating differential diagnosis.

- Half of the patients demonstrated secondary features, including contractions of the face, neck, trunk, and extremities, grimaces, eye blinks or squints, lip purses, raised eyebrows, extraneous head movements, and clenched jaw; half of the patients did not demonstrate secondary features.

- For 10 patients, psychological disturbance occurred close in time to the onset of the acquired psychogenic stuttering (e.g., death in the family, family illness, unjust accusations of wrongdoing, work and family instability, disturbed interpersonal relationships, failing marriages, unemployment, family tragedies); psychological history was equivocal for 2 patients.

- Of the 10 patients for whom *Minnesota Multiphasic Personality Inventory–Second Edition* (MMPI-2; Butcher, Dahlstrom, Graham, Tellegen, & Kaemmer, 1989) data were available, "nine of the profiles were classified as abnormal, giving evidence of mildly to markedly severe disturbance in psychologic functioning" (p. 637).

Recovery data were available for 11 patients; all responded well to speech therapy and "demonstrated the capacity for normal speech" (p. 637). Roth et al. (1989) concluded that the patients in this study demonstrated "psychogenic stuttering" on the basis of the following: (a) no related neurological findings, (b) disturbed life histories and stressful events near the onset of stuttering, (c) abnormal results on psychiatric measures and the MMPI-2, and (d) normal speech in response to psychotherapy or short-term speech therapy (e.g., easy onset, bouncing). Long-term follow-up data were not collected.

Baumgartner (1999) similarly emphasized the importance of differential diagnosis to determine if stuttering is organic (neurogenic), psychogenic, or idiopathic (developmental). He emphasized that psychogenic acquired stuttering may be accompanied by demonstrable neuropathology; thus "neither suspicion nor presence of neuropathology is sufficient to place any acquired speech disorder, including stuttering, into the neurogenic category" (p. 271). He cautioned that "the presence of neuropathology does not mean the patient's stuttering is neurogenic, and the presence of psychopathology may not mean it is psychogenic. Neurogenic and psychogenic disorders often coexist and the presence of one does not render a patient immune to the other" (p. 276). Recommended evaluation components include the following: (a) case history information (e.g., onset pattern, surrounding circumstances, observed changes in fluency, situational variability, impact on life, and history of previous stuttering including nature and extent of recovery—strict definitions of psychogenic acquired stuttering exclude cases in which childhood stuttering resolved but then reappeared under conditions of stress; Guitar, 2006), (b) motor speech examination to rule out motor speech disorders (e.g., apraxia, Parkinson's disease; Duffy, 2005), (c) traditional fluency enhancing conditions (e.g., choral reading, speaking in time to rhythm, masking noise, delayed auditory feedback, and repeated readings), and (d) trial therapy within a counseling relationship. About differential diagnosis of a patient's response to fluency enhancing conditions, Baumgartner advised,

> Improved fluency during these tasks is not necessarily incompatible with psychogenicity, even though a clear pattern of improved fluency when demands on the speech control system are decreased is, by itself, more consistent with neurogenic than psychogenic stuttering. . . . There is, however, a pattern of performance on such tasks that is highly suggestive of psychogenicity—increasingly dysfluent speech as task difficulty is reduced. Therefore, if the clinician decides to utilize these additional tasks, improved fluency is of only limited value, but an increase in dysfluencies and/or struggle behavior is strongly suggestive of psychogenicity. (p. 275)

Baumgartner (1999) also advised that psychogenic acquired stuttering typically responds rapidly and dramatically to direct therapy conducted during the initial evaluation and that such "symptom reversibility" (p. 275) is evidence in support of psychogenic etiology. He indicated that dramatic improvement in fluency or return to normal speech, particularly during the patient's expression of emotionally sensitive material, should be viewed as a diagnostic indicator of psychogenic acquired stuttering.

Baumgartner (1999) summarized that psychogenic acquired stuttering often occurs before age 60, is not a transient disorder (i.e., may be present from days to years), is similarly prevalent in both males and females, and does not seem to be related to education or handedness. By itself, symptom variability does not distinguish neurogenic from psychogenic acquired stuttering; some variability is observed in both. However, stuttering that is highly intermittent or unpredictable (varying with the situation, person, or time of day) or that differs greatly between reading and conversation is not consistent with neurogenic acquired stuttering. The adaptation effect rarely is seen in either neurogenic or psychogenic acquired stuttering. Psychogenicity should be suspected if stuttering worsens during procedures to assess the adaptation effect. Similarly, psychogenicity should be suspected if stuttering worsens with easier tasks or if stuttering is unchanged during portions of the motor speech examination (e.g., conversation vs. vowel prolongation). F. H. Silverman (2004) described psychogenic acquired stuttering in similar terms:

> A typical patient who has this disorder is an adult, with no previous history of stuttering, who suddenly begins to stutter after (or while) experiencing a great deal of psychological stress and who has no neurological condition that could account for the behavior. Furthermore, the patient's disfluency may not vary on a situational basis, and he or she may not exhibit any behavior that indicates a desire to avoid it. (p. 64)

As noted, one of the hallmarks of psychogenic acquired stuttering is symptom reversibility (complete or near complete resolution of symptoms) as a consequence of trial management during the evaluation or early treatment. For people whose symptoms are not as remediable, combining speech therapy with psychotherapy is advisable, and longer speech intervention may be indicated. Baumgartner (1999) emphasized the importance of establishing an open and accepting atmosphere for treatment in which the clinician explains the diagnostic findings and shares the positive observation that psychogenic acquired stuttering is not organically based. The patient's understanding of this observation is essential in order to eliminate any barrier that might be perceived as interfering with more fluent and relaxed speech. Many of the treatments used for developmental stuttering can be used for psychogenic acquired stuttering (Baumgartner, 1999; Duffy, 2005; Guitar, 2006; Roth et al., 1989). These include a prolonged fluency shaping approach (Guitar, 2006; see Chapter 7), easy onsets with light contacts and gentle repetitions (Roth et al., 1989), diminishing extraneous motor behaviors and excessive tensions (Baumgartner, 1999), and a seven-step graduated sequence to reduce tension and change repetitive disfluencies into more natural-sounding prolongations (Duffy, 2005).

From my own clinical experience: An adolescent male presented with stuttering of sudden onset and a functional falsetto voice shortly after moving to a new high school. When neurological (including hormonal) evaluation failed to reveal any abnormality, speech intervention consisted of identifying the communication characteristics of others and comparing and contrasting those with his own. All the while, the informal clinical interaction was positive in nature, with an emphasis on pointing out all of the young man's talents and the absence of any organic pathology. Within 3 weeks of initiation of treatment, the client indicated that he "discovered" he could speak fluently and in a voice quality more in keeping with his age and gender. The client and I agreed that it would be advisable for him to elect this option on a regular basis for personal, social, educational, and vocational reasons. Remarkably, he seemed to be able to do so with ease. Treatment was reduced and ultimately eliminated, with follow-through for 1 year, until his graduation from high school. I understand from his guidance counselor that the client's improved speech patterns were maintained. The ease of symptom reversibility was indeed noteworthy.

Recalling this case and reviewing other cases of psychogenic acquired stuttering reported in this section (Baumgartner, 1999; Culatta & Goldberg, 1995; Deal, 1982; Dempsey & Granich, 1978; Duffy, 2005; Guitar, 2006; Mahr & Leith, 1992; Peacher & Harris, 1946; Roth et al., 1989; Wallen, 1961; Weiner, 1981), I am reminded of Dworkin et al.'s (2002) puzzlement over the remarkable improvement of a 39-year-old man who became severely disfluent after a motor vehicle accident in which he did not incur serious injury (i.e., neurology and psychiatry evaluations revealed no organic etiology). Disfluency was characterized by multiple repetitions and blocks, especially on initial sounds and syllables, on 45% of all syllables with a speech rate of 69 syllables per minute. Traditional fluency enhancing conditions (e.g., singing, recitation of memorized passages, whispered speech) failed to lessen the disfluency. During hospitalization, speech therapy proved unsuccessful and was discontinued in favor of a nontraditional approach (i.e., one treatment of laryngeal anesthetization via a transcutaneous lidocaine injection). The patient improved dramatically within 15 minutes of the procedure (i.e., disfluency reduced to 5% and rate increased to 82 syllables per minute). At 1 month and 18 months posttreatment, disfluent moments were nonexistent and speaking rate was at normal level. The authors reported, "The only unequivocal fact is that the patient attained and maintained normal fluency after a single therapy session of short duration. The intriguing question is 'What might be an explanation for the attainment of the fluent behavior?'" (p. 216). Finally, they confessed, "It appears from the results obtained that we have a solution in search of an explanation" (p. 222). We are reminded of Flower's (1985) timeless toast to our profession, "To bewilderment" (see Chapter 2), and acknowledge that the most perplexing conditions provide the best window to study and understand human phenomena.

Malingering

Seery (2005) noted that malingering, or feigning, "occurs when a person is faking symptoms of illness or incapacity, usually for the purposes of personal gain" (p. 284). Similarly, F. H. Silverman (2004) indicated that "malingering should always be considered a possibility if a client is likely to benefit in some way from this diagnosis [stuttering]" (p. 18). Silverman explained that the benefit might take the form of financial compensation from a person who is claimed to be the cause of the stuttering, eligibility for financial aid (e.g., vocational rehabilitation), or special consideration for hiring because of the exceptionality. Certainly, as reviewed in Chapter 2, faking a fluency disorder could also be a way to discredit a witness if that witness reported the crime to have been committed by a fluent speaker. Recall also from Chapter 2 how what is known about the nature, variability, and predictability of stuttering and people who stutter was used for forensic verification of whether two different people really had a fluency disorder or whether they were malingering (Bloodstein, 1988; Shirkey, 1987).

Other instances of malingering have occasionally dotted the literature. Lew (1995) reported that he was a political prisoner in China during 1989 because of anti-government activity at Tiananmen Square in Beijing. Self-described as a "stutterer," he deliberately planned to worsen his stuttering in order to reduce the impact of the police interrogation. Under pressure, however, Lew found that his fluency naturally disintegrated. This experience, he reported, helped convince the police that because of his stuttering, he would not have been sponsored as a spokesperson by an "anti-revolutionary organization," which led to his ultimate release from captivity. Lew recalled, "My stuttering helped me to be released. It not only helped me. It saved me. . . . My stuttering saved my life" (p. 5). Culatta and Goldberg (1995) reported on a 20-year-old man who admittedly malingered stuttering to maintain his deferment from military service, thus avoiding service in Vietnam. He reportedly intended to maintain this behavior until "after the war is over or until I am too old to go" (p. 40).

As noted earlier, Bloodstein (1988) and Shirkey (1987) characterized as insufficient our current methods for verifying stuttering in a person who is suspected of malingering and recommended that future research address this area. Nearly 20 years later, F. H. Silverman (2004) concurred, stating, "Unfortunately, there are no established guidelines for determining whether a person is malingering a fluency disorder" (p. 18). The challenges inherent in detecting malingering are heightened considerably when the person who is suspected has read the stuttering literature and is knowledgeable about the conditions under which stuttering varies. Shirkey suggested that diagnostic procedures for forensic verification include speech assessment under varying conditions, covert audio recordings, polygraph testing (lie detector), independent testimony from people who have observed the suspect's communication patterns, school and medical records, data regarding speech characteristics, and observation of speech in conditions that usually yield fluency. Similarly, Bloodstein (1988) recommended collection of an extensive case history, repeated oral readings (i.e., for anticipation/expectancy, adaptation, consistency, stuttering loci on content vs. function words), and speaking in fluency inducing conditions. In addition to the diagnostic procedures already recommended, F. H. Silverman (2004) suggested that assessing the client's age at onset, symptomatology, and phenomenology yields findings that are consistent or inconsistent with the nature of stuttering. If the findings are not consistent with what is known about stuttering, diagnosis of stuttering cannot be confirmed. If the findings are consistent with what is known about stuttering, Silverman proposed two possibilities: (a) The client has the disorder and is a person who stutters, or (b) the client has read enough about the disorder to simulate it. In the event that the client has read about the disorder, he recommended asking the client what he or she has read. If the client claims to lack knowledge from reading or other sources, he recommended that the clinician express concern about some aspect of a symptom observed by the clinician that seemed inconsistent with stuttering. If the client reacts by defending the symptom, the client's claim to be lacking of knowledge is undermined. Such inconsistency or falseness of the client's claim, despite being elicited somewhat indirectly, could impugn the integrity of the client's other behaviors or claims related to stuttering.

More recently, Seery (2005) created an excellent assessment protocol for forensic verification of stuttering. Acknowledging the challenges incurred with detection of malingered stuttering, Seery indicated that even in the most severe cases, judgments as to the veracity of someone's stuttering cannot be interpreted with certainty. She stated, "A professional opinion would be limited to an estimate of the probability of stuttering given the individual's speech characteristics and pattern of stuttering (if there was one), both present and past" (p. 288). Furthermore, she distinguished between degrees and types of malingering, noting, "Pure malingering is when all of an individual's symptoms are falsified. Partial malingering is when existing symptoms are exaggerated. Another form of malingering occurs when someone denies existing problems or symptoms" (p. 285). Indeed, objective evidence is essential. Seery faced such challenges when called upon to verify the presence of a fluency disorder in a man in his late 30s who had been accused of armed robbery at a gas station. Witnesses reportedly heard the man say fluently, "Lady, give me the money or I'll shoot." However, when incarcerated, he reported that he had stuttered all his life and presented an initial impression of severe stuttering. Seery collected four main categories of data: (a) speech samples (spontaneous and a series of oral readings), (b) speech samples from other speaking conditions (choral reading; imitation of words, phrases, and sentences; whispered, shouted, and lipped speech; automatic speech tasks; and therapeutic probes), (c) communication attitudes (interview and communication attitudes inventory), and (d) case history and background information (interview with the defendant, self-report of stuttering variability, inmate records, health/medical records, and reports of outside informants). Results supporting the differential diagnosis of developmental stuttering and truthful disclosure included early age of stuttering onset (preschool), evidence of core disfluency types, sound/syllable repetitions consisting of multiple iterations, typical descriptions of personal experiences with stuttering, location of stuttering on initial sounds of words and on expected grammatical structures of speech, typical affective reactions to speech and stuttering on relevant attitude inventories (e.g., Modified Erickson Scale of Communication Attitudes; G. Andrews & Cutler, 1974), and mention of stuttering in jail records from a previous arrest when the veracity of his stuttering was not suspect. Despite being diagnosed as a person with developmental stuttering, the client also demonstrated characteristics of partial malingering (e.g., uncharacteristic absence of variability in stuttering, a request to do the finger-tapping section again when confronted about the absence of variability, a disjunct between his claims of no stuttering variability throughout his life and others' reports of periods of fluency). Ultimately, the differential diagnosis could not be used to rule out the possibility that the defendant could have been fluent at the time of the crime. The case never went to trial and the defendant submitted a guilty plea prior to the scheduled court date in order to receive a lighter sentence. In addition to Seery's work on forensic verification of stuttering, she classified the characteristics of developmental stuttering, neurogenic acquired stuttering, psychogenic acquired stuttering, and malingering (see Table 4.1); this comparison can be helpful in the process of differential diagnosis.

Table 4.1 Comparison of Characteristics of Developmental Stuttering, Neurogenic Acquired Stuttering, Psychogenic Acquired Stuttering, and Malingering

Characteristic	Developmental stuttering	Neurogenic stuttering	Psychogenic stuttering	Malingering
Time of onset	Childhood	Adulthood (after adolescence)	Adulthood (after adolescence)	May report any age[a]
Type of onset	May be gradual or sudden	Usually sudden	Usually sudden	May be reported as gradual or sudden
Circumstances at onset	Variety of situations	Neurological impairment	Psychoemotional distress	Variety of situations[a]
Frequency of stuttering	Ranges from mild to severe; overall percentage rarely above 45% (Riley, 1994)	Ranges from mild to severe	Ranges from mild to severe	May tend to stutter too much[a] (i.e., in excess of very severe stuttering)
Types of stuttering behavior	Variety of disfluency types; usually core disfluencies near onset	Variety of disfluency types	Variety of disfluency types, syllable repetitions common	Variety of disfluency types; however, these may be atypical and/or too stereotyped[a]
Secondary or concomitant behaviors	Secondary behaviors present; difficulty with eye contact is common	Secondary characteristics not common; for example, maintains normal eye contact	Secondary behaviors not common; for example, maintains normal eye contact; may display bizarre behaviors unrelated to speech	May not have secondary behaviors or any difficulty with eye contact[a]
Word or utterance location of stuttering	Word-initial and utterance-initial locations; stuttering on last syllables or words is rare	Not mainly at initiation; stutters throughout an utterance	Not mainly at initiation; stutters throughout an utterance	Not mainly at initiation; may stutter throughout words and utterances[a]
Content/function word locations of stuttering	Proportionately more stuttering on content versus function words	No pattern of stuttering location related to content/function words	No pattern of stuttering location related to content/function words	No pattern of location related to content/function words[a]
Adaptation effect	Adaptation may or may not occur	No adaptation effect	No adaptation effect	No adaptation effect[a]

Consistency effect	Consistency effect likely	Unknown; no research found	Unknown; no research found	May not show consistency effect[a]
Variability of stuttering	Stuttering tends to be variable across situations	Less variable across situations	Less variable across situations; may have isolated experiences of spontaneously fluent speech	May stutter too constantly across situations[a]
Easier speech tasks	Stuttering usually improves	Stuttering may or may not improve	Stuttering may or may not improve, may even worsen	Stuttering is not apt to improve[a]
Response to fluency-inducing conditions (e.g., unison)	Usually improves or eliminates stuttering	May or may not improve	May or may not improve; fluency may return during psychosocial interaction (e.g., as circumstances surrounding onset are discussed)	May stutter or report to stutter without improvement in all these conditions[a]
Emotional response to stuttering	Attitudes of anxiousness or avoidance related to speech and stuttering	Feels annoyed, but not anxious or fearful about stuttering	Often indifferent toward stuttering; not in all cases, however	May not have emotional reactions to speaking and/or stuttering[a]
Experiences with listeners	Past experiences usually include listener harassment (e.g., laughing, teasing)	Usually has not felt harassed by listeners, but may be annoyed	Usually has not felt harassed by listeners, but may be annoyed	May not describe experiences of unwanted listener reactions[a]

Note. From "Differential Diagnosis of Stuttering for Forensic Purposes," by C. H. Seery, 2005, *American Journal of Speech–Language Pathology*, 14, p. 287. Copyright 2005 by the American Speech-Language-Hearing Association. Reprinted with permission.

[a]Does not apply if the malingering individual has enough knowledge of the characteristic to imitate it.

Tourette Syndrome

Tourette syndrome is a neurological disorder that is seen in every race, culture, and stratum of society (Sacks, 1995). The earliest descriptions of people barking, twitching, grimacing, gesturing strangely, and cursing involuntarily were recorded nearly 2,000 years ago by Aretaeus of Cappadocia. In 1825, Dr. Jean Marc Gaspard Itard, a French physician, reported the case of a French noblewoman, the Marquise de Dampierre, who demonstrated abrupt and involuntary body movements, barking, and cursing. Sixty years later, Gilles de la Tourette, the French neurologist after whom the disorder is named, made reference to Dr. Itard's case report and described in the medical literature eight additional such cases. These cases all had tics, some with involuntary repetition of others' words (*echolalia*) and gestures (*echopraxia*), and involuntary cursing (*coprolalia*). Until the 1970s, Tourette syndrome was thought to be rare. Today, however, prevalence estimates range from 1/100 for milder cases to 1/1,000 for more severe cases (Tourette Syndrome Association, 2006), with symptoms characterized by chronic tics (repetitive, rapid, sudden, involuntary movements or utterances) thought to be caused by abnormal metabolism of dopamine, a neurotransmitter. Over 100,000 people in the United States alone have this disorder, which indicates genetic predisposition (Colligan, 1989; Donaher, 2006; Tourette Syndrome Association, 2005). Males are three to four times more likely to be affected than females (Van Borsel, 2006; Van Borsel & Tetnowski, 2007). Approximately one third of patients with Tourette syndrome also stutter (Comings, 1995; De Nil & Sandor, 2008; Vinnard, 1990b).

Characteristics of this disorder have been described frequently (Bruun & Bruun, 1994; Colligan, 1989; Comings, 1995; Kwak & Jankovic, 2002; Lohr & Wisniewski, 1987; Scahill, Lynch, & Ort, 1995; Wand, Matazow, Shady, Furer, & Staley, 1993) and include the following:

1. Both multiple motor tics and one or more vocal (i.e., phonic) tics are observed.
2. Tics occur nearly daily, usually in bouts, persisting for at least 1 year with no tic-free period of more than 3 months.
3. Tics can be voluntarily suppressed for periods of minutes to hours.
4. Anatomic location, number, frequency, complexity, and severity of the tics vary over time.
5. Onset is usually before 18 years of age.
6. Occurrence is not limited to periods of drug abuse or central nervous system disease.
7. Marked distress or impairment in social, occupational, or other areas of functioning is observed.

Colligan (1989) presented a particularly useful guide—the Teacher's Checklist on Tourette Syndrome: Range of Symptoms (see Figure 4.3). This checklist distinguishes between motor and phonic symptoms. Motor symptoms are classified either as simple motor tics (fast, darting, and meaningless) or as complex motor tics (slower, more purposeful), and phonic symptoms are classified either as simple phonic tics (fast, meaningless sounds) or as complex phonic tics (words, phrases, and statements).

Various other problems may be associated with Tourette syndrome, including attention-deficit disorder (poor attention and concentration, distractibility, impulsivity), hyperactivity (fidgety, ceaseless movement), emotional disorder, obsessive–compulsive disorder (often indistinguishable from complex motor tics), and conduct disorder (short temper, unprovoked attacks of rage, opposition, lying, stealing, starting fires). Other co-existing problems may include learning disabilities, dyslexia, depression, mania, sleep disorders, and both stuttering and cluttering (Bruun & Bruun, 1994; Colligan, 1989; Comings, 1995; Donaher, 2006; Pauls, Leckman, & Cohen, 1993). While there is no

Instructions: Mark an X on the symptoms you have observed. This is not a diagnosis. This is simply an observation of symptoms for referral purposes.

Motor Symptoms		
Simple Motor Tics: fast, darting, meaningless	17. Kissing	
	18. Pinching	
1. Eye blinking	19. Writing, over and over, same word or letter	
2. Grimacing	20. Pulling back on pencil while writing	
3. Nose twitching	21. Tearing paper or books	
4. Lip pouting	**Phonic Symptoms**	
5. Shoulder shrugs		
6. Arm jerks	**Simple Phonic Tics: fast, meaningless sounds**	
7. Head jerks		
8. Abdominal tensing	1. Whistling	
9. Kicks	2. Coughing	
10. Finger movements	3. Sniffling	
11. Jaw snaps	4. Spitting	
12. Tooth clicking	5. Screeching	
13. Frowning	6. Barking	
14. Tensing parts of body	7. Grunting	
15. Rapid jerking of any part of body	8. Gurgling	
Complex Motor Tics: slower, purposeful	9. Clacking	
	10. Hawking	
1. Hopping	11. Hissing	
2. Clapping	12. Sucking	
3. Touching objects (or others, or self)	13. Uh-uh, eee, ah-uh, and other sounds	
4. Throwing	**Complex Phonic Tics: words, phrases, statements**	
5. Arranging		
6. Gyrating and bending	Shut up, stop that! Oh, I've got it! Right! How about it? (others)	
7. "Dystonic postures"		
8. Biting mouth, lip, arm (circle which)	Rituals: counting, repeating a phrase until it is "just right"	
9. Headbanging		
10. Thrusting arms	Coprolalia: obscene and aggressive words and statements (these may be obscured to sound like the letters fff or sss)	
11. Striking out		
12. Picking scabs		
13. Writhing movements	Palilalia: repeating one's own words	
14. Rolling eyes to ceiling	Echolalia: repeating words of others	
15. Holding funny expressions		
16. Sticking out the tongue		

Problems with hyperactivity? _____ Short attention span? _____ On medication for hyperactivity? _____

| Date | Student's Name | Nurse's/Teacher's Signature |

*A signature provides more accountability in providing the list of symptoms observed.

Figure 4.3. Teacher's Checklist on Tourette Syndrome: Range of Symptoms. *Note.* From "Recognizing Tourette Syndrome in the Classroom," by N. Colligan, December 1989, *School Nurse,* p. 3, Copyright 1989 by the Tourette Syndrome Association. Reprinted with permission.

cure for Tourette syndrome, intervention most often is neuropharmacological. Intervention agents have included haloperidol (Haldol), pimodize (Orap), fluphenazine (Prolixin), risperidone (Risperdal), clonidine (Catapres), clonidine patch (Catapres patch), clonazepam (Klonopin), and guanfacine (Tenex) (Erenberg, 2003). When there is more than one symptom to treat, multiple medications have been used simultaneously. This intervention is called *targeted combined pharmacotherapy*. For example, a person may be prescribed Haldol (haloperidol) to control the tics and Prozac (fluoxetine) to control obsessive–compulsive behaviors and related emotional problems. Another example is the combination of Catapres (clonidine) and Dexedrine (dextroamphetamine) to reduce tics and symptoms of attention-deficit/hyperactivity disorder (ADHD). Similarly, some of the medications prescribed to reduce the tics in Tourette syndrome are also used to treat other conditions. For example, Catapres (clonidine) is used to treat high blood pressure; Klonopin (clonazepam) is used to treat seizures. Sometimes the medications interact negatively, however. Some of the more common medications that are used effectively to treat ADHD, such as Ritalin (methylphenidate), Adderall (mixed amphetamine), and Dexedrine (dextroamphetamine), may cause increases in tics in some patients with Tourette syndrome. While these medications have been used successfully by individuals with Tourette syndrome, a trial stimulant medication may prove helpful when taken by individuals who have Tourette syndrome and significant ADHD symptoms (Erenberg, 2003).

Of continuing research interest are the differential effects of haloperidol on Tourette syndrome and stuttering (Brady, 1991; Ludlow & Braun, 1993; Quinn & Peachey, 1973; Tapia, 1969; Vinnard, 1990b; Wells & Malcolm, 1971). Finding the right medication and the right dosage can be difficult. Usually medication is started at a low dosage and gradually increased. During this time, the attending physician monitors symptom improvement and side effects (e.g., sedation, depression, restlessness, weight gain, fatigue, school phobia, liver and cardiac toxicity). In one of Sacks' (1985) graphic case presentations, "Witty Ticcy Ray," Ray discussed his experience with Tourette syndrome in the third person and questioned if there would be anything left of himself if the tics could be taken away. Prone to "ticcy witticisms and witty ticcisms" (p. 93), Ray discussed the tics as a gift as well as curse, yet expressed being unable to imagine life without Tourette syndrome, and doubted if he would care for life in that event. Experiencing great success with Haldol for lowering the incidence of tics, Ray discussed the experience of Tourette syndrome and the side effects of Haldol:

> Having Tourette's is wild, like being drunk all the while. Being on haldol is dull, makes one square and sober, and neither state is really free. . . . You "normals," who have the right transmitters in the right places at the right times in your brains, have all the feelings, all styles, available all the time—gravity, levity, whatever is appropriate. WE Touretters don't: We are forced into levity by our Tourette's and forced into gravity when we take haldol. *You* are free, you have a natural balance: We must make the best of an artificial balance. (Sacks, 1985, p. 96)

Other treatments for Tourette syndrome have included relaxation techniques, biofeedback, psychotherapy, and behavior modification (Bruun & Bruun, 1994; Colligan, 1989; Tolchard, 1995; Tourette Syndrome Association, 2006). Injection of botulinum toxin (Botox) is occasionally used to control tics that are isolated to a body region (focal tics) such as the eyes, neck, and vocal cords (Kwak & Jankovic, 2002).

Excellent personal accounts are available about well-known people who have a history of Tourette syndrome, such as Mahmoud Abdul-Rauf, formerly Chris Jackson, Denver Nuggets basketball guard; Jim Eisenreich, Philadelphia Phillies baseball outfielder; and Samuel Johnson, English author and lexicographer known for *A Dictionary of the English Language*, published in 1755, among others. Some speculate that Wolfgang Amadeus Mozart had Tourette syndrome (S. Palmer, 2007). Few accounts provide as clear a window to understanding Tourette syndrome as that of Oliver Sacks, a neurologist of international fame. Observing that people with Tourette syndrome come from all walks of life and have been successful writers, mathematicians, musicians, actors, disc jockeys, construction workers, social workers, mechanics, athletes, and physicians, Sacks (1995) described Tourette syndrome as representing an "it" apart from oneself; that "it" takes the forms of explicit impulsions and compulsions, as follows:

> One is driven to do this, to do that, against one's own will, or in deference to the alien will of the "it." There may be a conflict, a compromise, a collusion between these wills. . . . But the relation of disease and self, "it" and "I," can be particularly complex in Tourette's, especially if it has been present from early childhood, growing up with the self, intertwining itself in every possible way. The Tourette's and the self shape themselves each to the other, come more and more to complement each other, until finally, like a long-married couple, they become a single, compound being. (p. 78)

Sacks (1995) described both the unique professional skills and complex motor and phonic tics of Dr. Carl Bennett, an expert surgeon. When Dr. Bennett's surgical skill was consuming his absolute and complete concentration, it was flawless, and he was without tics for procedures of several hours. Dr. Bennett had a rule that when doing surgery, he was never to be interrupted. Sacks (1995) stated, "Such keen, fierce attention to every detail, such constant looking below the surface, such examination and analysis, are characteristic of the restless, questioning Tourette mind. It is, so to speak, the other side of its obsessive and perseverative tendencies, its disposition to reiterate, to touch again and again" (p. 80). With similar precision, Sacks described Dr. Bennett's tics, which were characterized by constant touching and centering of his eyeglasses and moustache, realigning of his hands and knees, darting of his hands and feet, abrupt touching of others, and sudden high-pitched barks and vocalizations, including the name of a former girlfriend, a tic described as *enshrinement* (i.e., the interplay between life and tics, the process by which the former is incorporated permanently into the latter). Sacks noted that some people with Tourette syndrome have flinging tics, "sudden, seemingly motiveless urges or compulsions to throw objects." He stated, "There may be a very brief premonition—enough, in one case, to yell a warning 'Duck!'—before a dinner plate, a bottle of wine, or whatever is flung convulsively across the room" (p. 83). Dr. Bennett described his own experience with Tourette syndrome as follows:

> Tourette's comes from deep down in the nervous system and the unconscious. It taps into the oldest, strongest feelings we have. Tourette's is like an epilepsy in the subcortex; when it takes over, there's just a thin line of control, a thin line of cortex, between you and it, between you and that raging storm, the blind force of the subcortex. One can see the charming things, the funny things, the creative side of Tourette's, but there's also that dark side. You have to fight it all your life. (Sacks, 1995, p. 100)

Others have described their personal experience with Tourette syndrome. Nick van Bloss, an award winning pianist, described in an interview (S. Palmer, 2007) how his tics seem to have a life of their own, a life he must resist and control at all times:

> Tourette's is me, it defines me. . . . It's a double-edged sword, because it's painful to control and it's painful to tic. If I let go and tic as I want to if I am on my own, it's exhausting. It's like doing aerobic activity all the time. . . . Day-to-day, I'm living life to the Tourette's rhythm. It dictates what it wants, when it wants. (p. 58)

He also noted that when he is fully concentrating on his music, the tics disappear. With the slightest distraction, however, the tics return and again must be controlled. Recalling an international piano competition in Spain where he played flawlessly until being distracted by the bright spotlights, van Bloss (2006) wrote,

> I was through to the third round and I was playing marvelously. But suddenly I was aware of all the lights on me, and I felt the tic energy coming. I wanted to jerk my head and to tense my arms, and you can't do that and coordinate a musical passage. I was fumbling around on the piano, panicking. I could feel something that I had never felt when I played the piano. My hands flew up and stayed flexed. And my head spun round. I remember I froze, because it was the last thing I had expected and the most unwelcome. I heard a gasp through the auditorium—it was very dramatic—and I just stood up and walked off. (p. 61)

Previously, the piano had been van Bloss' safe haven, the one place he felt confident and without affliction. His unfortunate experience in Spain led him to conclude, "'OK, Tourette's, you win.' It was the dirtiest trick I think a neurological complaint could play" (p. 61). That was the end of van Bloss' musical career, recalled in his autobiography, *Busy Body: My Life with Tourette's Syndrome* (2006).

Another instructionally valuable and graphic personal presentation is the videocassette *John's Not Mad: Tourette's Syndrome* (British Broadcasting Corporation, 1989). This 30-minute presentation follows John Davidson, a 16-year-old with Tourette syndrome, through one typical day in his life in Galashiels, Scotland. The film reveals both the motor and phonic tics through which Tourette syndrome expresses itself and the deleterious impact it has on him, his family, his classmates and teachers, and his community. Dr. Oliver Sacks provides excellent commentary about the neurology, psychology, and involuntariness of the disorder. A subsequent documentary (*The Boy Can't Help It: Living with Tourette's Syndrome*, British Broadcasting Corporation, 2002) follows John's personal and professional development to age 31, presents his mature assessment of the disorder and its implications, and compares his present symptoms and experiences to those of 15 years earlier. Other excellent personal accounts are available. In one such account, Krah (2002) likened the tics she experiences from Tourette syndrome to the Whac-A-Mole game at an amusement park. She stated, "You hold the weapon in your hand, ready to strike at whatever pops up. By the time you whack at it, three more pop up. As soon as they disappear, the first one reappears, sometimes with more force than before. It's frustrating, to say the least" (p. 5). Numerous informative materials are available from the Tourette Syndrome Association (see the Appendix for contact information).

Adductor Spasmodic Dysphonia

Spasmodic dysphonia (also referred to as *spastic dysphonia*) is characterized by spasms of the adductor laryngeal muscles, resulting in sounds that intermittently are strained and strangled. This voice condition has been referred to as "stammering of the vocal cords" and "laryngeal stuttering" (Aronson, 1973; Aronson & Bless, 2009; Boone, McFarland, Von Berg, & Zraick, 2010; Nicolosi et al., 2004). In some ways, the symptomatology of spasmodic dysphonia and stuttering is similar. Both are intermittent disruptions in the control of the speech (particularly laryngeal) musculature, the severity of which depends on similar situational factors, including the perception held by the speaker toward the listener and the significance of the communicative act. People with spasmodic dysphonia speak normally when reading in chorus; singing; repeating a memorized verse; and speaking to children, animals, and when alone, and they demonstrate an adaptation effect (the number of strained, strangled syllables decreases upon repeated readings of the same passage). There also is debate over whether the causes of spasmodic dysphonia are neurological, psychological, or both. Proponents of neurological causality argue that it is the result of a degenerative process in the central nervous system, supporting this notion by observing that some speakers demonstrate neuropathology; proponents of psychological causality state that it is related to psychological trauma, supporting their argument by observing that speakers with this condition can speak normally at times. The age of onset and frequency of occurrence of spasmodic dysphonia and stuttering are different, however. While in most cases stuttering begins during early childhood, spasmodic dysphonia begins during middle age. And while stuttering is more frequently seen in males than in females, spasmodic dysphonia occurs more frequently among females (F. H. Silverman, 2004). A recent study of 168 patients with spasmodic dysphonia revealed that age of onset ranged from 13 to 71 years, with an average age of 45 years; 79% of the patients with spasmodic dysphonia were female and 21% were male (Fogle, 2008; Schweinfurth, Billante, & Courey, 2002). Another clear difference is the response to traditional treatment. Most individuals with spasmodic dysphonia do not respond well to voice therapy approaches alone. Most success is achieved when a medical–surgical approach (i.e., injection of botulinum toxin, or Botox, into one vocal fold to create a temporary weakness in the fold, thus reducing laryngeal tension) is used in combination with voice therapy (M. L. Andrews, 2006; Fogle, 2008). On the other hand, people who stutter do not respond well to the same medical–surgical approach. Manning (2010) reviewed the scant literature on this topic, reporting at least short-term benefit of Botox injections for people who stutter (Brin, Stewart, Blitzer, & Diamond, 1994; Ludlow, 1990), which did indeed increase the airflow and facilitate fluency. However, Manning (2010) also highlighted a study (Stager & Ludlow, 1994) that reported 19 adults with chronic stuttering who failed to benefit from Botox injections. Manning (2010) argued that the use of Botox injection as an intervention for stuttering is contraindicated. While increased laryngeal tension often is associated with stuttering, there is no support for the frequently held misperception that excess laryngeal tension plays a primary role in causing stuttering.

Acquired Disfluency Following Laryngectomy

F. H. Silverman (2004) summarized the literature related to stuttering following laryngectomy and indicated that (a) some people who stutter continue to do so after relearning to speak using esophageal speech or an electrolarynx, (b) it is not unusual for laryngectomized patients to be highly disfluent at the early stages of relearning speech, and (c) there is some evidence that stuttering may be acquired following laryngectomy. The few case reports available in the professional literature (Freeman & Rosenfield, 1982; Rosenfield & Freeman, 1983) suggest that acquired disfluency of a lasting nature following laryngectomy is a relatively rare phenomenon.

Linguistic Disfluency

The existence of a relationship between language delay or disorder and stuttering is documented, yet not clearly understood (Bloodstein & Bernstein Ratner, 2008; Culatta & Leeper, 1989–1990; L. A. Nelson, 2002; Wall & Myers, 1995; R. V. Watkins, 2005; Yairi, Watkins, Ambrose, & Paden, 2001). Various accounts have noted an increase in disfluency with the initiation of language treatment and emerging language skills, and a decrease in disfluency with the development of linguistic sophistication (Colburn & Mysak, 1982a, 1982b; D. E. Hall, Wray, & Conti, 1986; P. K. Hall, 1977; Wexler, 1982).

This is not terribly dissimilar from the observed co-occurrence between phonological errors and those in other aspects of language (lexical, syntactic, semantic, and pragmatic). Fey (1986) reported that improvements from language intervention often effect positive changes in phonology, and improvements in phonological intervention often effect positive changes in language. These overlaps between different aspects of communication should not be surprising, since their distinction is in the mind of the observer; the child's communication skills represent a multidimensional outcome of an integrated system. The form of disfluency reflective of linguistic emergence is somewhat different from that of stuttering. The former demonstrates primarily part-word repetitions, prolongations, and disrhythmic phonation (D. E. Hall et al., 1986; P. K. Hall, 1977). Why disfluency increases with the child's attempt to use new linguistic processes is unclear, but might be explained on the basis any number of the theories discussed in the previous chapter.

Karniol (1992) presented a striking case report of a bilingual child who began to stutter in both languages at age 25 months, the point of transition into grammatical sentence construction. When the stuttering became severe, the parents responded to the child's request to drop the nondominant language (English), whereupon the child became a nonstuttering monolingual (Hebrew) speaker. When the nondominant language was reintroduced at 39 months, no stuttering returned. Karniol proposed stuttering as a function of syntactic overload. Others have suggested that syntax is a determinant of stuttering (Bernstein Ratner & Benitez, 1985; Colburn & Mysak, 1982a, 1982b). The individual's communication competence must be understood in light of strengths and both primary and secondary exceptionalities, and clinicians must not assume that all disfluency is stuttering. D. E. Hall et al. (1986) indicated that initial increase in disfluency among children with language delay who enter treatment is not reflective of stuttering, but the result of challenge to the child's communication system imposed by new linguistic rules. Culatta and Goldberg (1995) proposed that the method of identifying the disfluencies of children with language impairments has a major impact on treatment.

I maintain that as clinicians, we must recognize the child's communication system as uniquely organized and integrated, and be mindful that gains in one area of communication ultimately impact and result in gains in others. This observation provides a challenge for insightful differential diagnosis and an opportunity for systematic planning of individualized communication intervention, both of which are addressed in greater detail in Unit III (Chapters 8, 9, and 10). In the next chapter, we will discuss several multicultural aspects of stuttering, including the relatedness between stuttering and bilingualism, assessment of stuttering in familiar and unfamiliar languages, and speech–language pathologists' training and confidence in serving clients from culturally and linguistically diverse populations.

Normal Developmental Disfluency

Often mistaken as abnormal, disfluency is a normal occurrence reflecting developmental stages of language learning and communication development. Children who are developing communication skills typically will be their most disfluent between the ages of 2.5 and 4 years. These disfluencies often are characterized by effortless and rhythmic repetition of whole words and phrases, gentle sound prolongations, and occasional sound interjections. Parents and other care providers, as well as other people within the child's communication system, need to be informed that such disfluencies reflect a temporary and developmental stage, necessary for the establishment of communication proficiency (Ainsworth & Fraser, 2008; Gordon & Luper, 1992a, 1992b; Pindzola & White,

1986; Starkweather, 1987, 2002a, 2002b; Van Riper, 1982; Walle, 1976). Distinguishing between disfluencies that are normal and a necessary part of communication and those that represent the danger of incipient stuttering is a critical skill for speech–language pathologists. This will be addressed further in Chapter 8.

Other Forms of Disfluency That Resemble Stuttering

Disfluency in Manual Communication

Some people present a communication disorder so severe that their speech is not of functional utility. Many such people use manual communication (finger spelling or sign language) in combination with their speech (as an augmentative communication system) or as a replacement for their speech (as an alternative communication system). Simultaneously using speech and manual communication is referred to as "total" communication or "SimCom" (Snyder, 2006). As noted in Chapter 2, there are relatively few publications (e.g., Liles, Lerman, Christensen, & St. Ledger, 1992; B. M. Montgomery & Fitch, 1988; F. H. Silverman & Silverman, 1971) that document disfluencies in manual communication, such as repetitions or hesitations of signs and initial letters in finger spelling, and involuntary interjections and extraneous hand and finger movements. When manual communication was used to augment speech, manual disfluencies such as part-word repetitions, word repetitions, and prolongations sometimes were accompanied by speech disfluencies and at other times were not.

Snyder (2006) chronicled the scant literature addressing the coexistence of stuttering and sign language. This literature detailed stuttering and secondary manifestations in a child with congenital deafness (Voelker & Voelker, 1937) and surveyed oral schools for the deaf. The surveys found that 55 out of 13,691 (0.4%) students (Backus, 1938) and 42 out of 14,458 (0.3%) students (Harms & Malone, 1939) reportedly stuttered verbally or in sign.

Indeed, disfluency in manual communication that might be compared to stuttering during oral speech appears to be a relatively rare phenomenon. F. H. Silverman and Silverman (1971) reported that of the 78 responses received from teachers of deaf children at residential schools, 13 reported "stutter-like behavior in manual communication of the deaf" (p. 45). Of those, stuttered signing appeared more frequently during finger spelling, revealing repetition of a sign or initial letters of finger spelling and involuntary interjections of extra movements and hesitations in finger spelling. These symptoms were observed in SimCom as well. B. M. Montgomery and Fitch (1988) identified only 12 cases out of 9,930 students with hearing impairments who stuttered. Three of the 12 stuttered only during speech, 6 only during manual communication, and 3 during Sim-Com (i.e., in both speech and manual communication). Manual disfluencies included effortless repetition of signs and initial letters in finger spelling, and blocking on sign productions. Disfluencies during SimCom included those observed during speech and sign, namely repetition of initial syllables (spoken) and letters (signed) and repetition of words and phrases, blocks on words, and prolongation of sounds and signs. Liles et al. (1992) detailed the behaviors of a young male with a cognitive disability who demonstrated repetitions, prolongations, and blocks in speech and SimCom. Snyder (2006) reported on his own disfluency, during both speech and SimCom, noting, "Quite simply, when my mouth was stuttering, my hands would cease signing and patiently wait for the (oral) stuttered moment to pass." Questioning whether his signing was stuttered or whether the manual disruptions in his signing were symptomatic or secondary to stuttered speech, Snyder successfully trained his hands to continue signing, independent of any stuttered speech. He noted, "As my speech broke down, my signing would continue. However, this independent functionality was limited to the difficulty of producing two asynchronous expressive communications at once. When my two asynchronous expressive communication signals within SimCom get over a phrase apart, I have to stop altogether and restart synchronously."

These findings indicate that a stuttered sign phenomenon exists and is more prevalent in SimCom (Snyder, 2006). A collaborative venture (Snyder, 2006; Whitebread, 2004), notwithstanding significant methodological limitations, revealed the following potential characteristics of stuttered sign: (a) inconsistent interruptions in sign and finger spelling, (b) stuttered symptoms (most often at the initiation of a gesture), (c) hesitation of sign movement, (d) repetition of sign movement while keeping the original hand shape, (e) exaggerated or prolonged signs, (f) unusual body movements unrelated to linguistic communication, (g) poor fluidity of the sign, and (h) inappropriate muscular tension in the arm and hand associated with the sign.

The stuttered sign phenomenon has been interpreted in various ways. Van Riper (1982) indicated that "perhaps, in their manual communication, some deaf individuals show behaviors equivalent to stuttering" (p. 47). F. H. Silverman (2004) hypothesized, "Certainly, conditions that result in neurogenic acquired stuttering and psychogenic acquired stuttering could as easily affect the musculature of the upper extremities as that of the mouth" (p. 17). Silverman suggested that theoretical explanations for stuttering, such as anticipatory-struggle behavior or demands exceeding capacities, might also explain disfluency in manual communication. Snyder (2006) addressed the question of how stuttered sign is related to stuttered speech, and whether both are independent expressions of a more central malfunction in expressive communication:

> If we are to believe that stuttered sign is a reality, then it could be suggested that stuttering (in all its expressive modalities) may be a symptomatic compensatory response to processing errors at the central level. These processing errors may represent limitations or malfunctions in the formulation, processing, or execution of expressive output or communication. Stated differently, stuttering behaviors may represent a natural bodily response attempting to self-correct or bypass neural processing errors in expressive output or communication occurring at a central level.

Disfluency While Playing a Wind Instrument

There are even fewer published accounts of disfluent-like behavior occurring while playing a wind instrument. Those reported involved the trumpet (Van Riper, 1973), the flute (F. H. Silverman & Bohlman, 1988), the French horn (Meltzer, 1992; Macauley & Steckol, 2004), and the trombone (Packman & Onslow, 1999). A woman described her stuttering-like disfluency on the flute:

> I experienced something rather unique—i.e., stuttering on the flute. Whenever I would start to play my throat would tense, my facial muscles would freeze, and my whole body would stiffen. It would take me 15–30 seconds to start a piece of music. Once I had gotten past the first note, I would be able to play the rest of the piece without any type of blocking. (F. H. Silverman & Bohlman, 1988, pp. 427–428)

Similarly, Meltzer (1992) described stuttering-like disfluency on the French horn as "a blocking of the flow of sound as a result of closure and tightening in the throat and a breakdown in coordination of tonguing movements. The frequency of occurrence varied, increasing under conditions of fatigue, stress, anticipation, speed, and the need to maintain a high standard of performance" (p. 260).

Packman and Onslow (1999) described stuttering-like behavior on the trombone as a "delay in the onset of the note, a 'false start' at the onset of the note, or a brief prolongation of sound at very low amplitude at onset before the note achieved its full amplitude" (p. 296). The client described the problem as follows: "I take a breath and go to breathe out but it would be like everything would lock up; and it's the same kind of feeling as when I'm stuttering. As anyone who's done it knows, it's almost like you lose control" (pp. 295–296). Packman and Onslow reported that the client anticipated where and when the problem would occur (i.e., at the start of a phrase), that the problem was worse when he felt tense, and that the problem on the trombone often co-occurred with increases in stuttering.

Macauley and Steckol (2004) reported an instance of stuttering-like disfluency on the French horn. It was not clear, however, if the horn player, a graduate student, also was a person who stutters. The student described the problem as existing "when the vocal tract and respiratory system lock up and become so tense that the note won't come out" (p. 8) and the emotions as, "you become increasingly frustrated and ashamed and begin to fear certain notes and avoid solo pieces" (p. 8). The authors noted the following similarities between stuttering and "musical stuttering": primary features (noted above) and secondary features (e.g., facial grimacing and blinking when the problem occurs), the anticipation effect (predicting on which notes, songs, and solos blocks will occur), fluency inducing conditions (e.g., the affected musician will be more fluent when playing in unison with another musician), and development of fear and shame. Macauley and Steckol observed,

> The student put his horn to his mouth, took in a deep breath, and as he went to release the air, his throat tightened, his neck muscles tensed up, his chin began to tremor, and his embouchure (lip configuration for playing the horn) became so tight that no air could exit the vocal tract and no note was produced. He moved the horn off his lips, took a deep breath, and tried again. This time the same terrible blocking behavior occurred, but he closed his eyes tightly, nodded his head, and was able to get out a "blat" sound. (p. 18)

Four of the musicians on whom the reports focused also stuttered (Meltzer, 1992; Packman & Onslow, 1999; F. H. Silverman & Bohlman, 1988; Van Riper, 1973). Insufficient data were reported to determine if the horn player reported by Macauley and Steckol (2004) stuttered. F. H. Silverman (2004) hypothesized that because playing a wind instrument requires use of the same muscle groups as does connected speech (respiratory, laryngeal, and oropharyngeal), the cause or causes of stuttering might also interfere with playing a wind instrument. F. H. Silverman (2004) cautioned that both the prevalence of such a disorder and the likelihood that a person who does not stutter might develop it remain uncertain. Similarly, Packman and Onslow (1999) indicated that any functional relationship between difficulty in playing a wind instrument and stuttering is speculative. Nevertheless, Packman and Onslow noted that both "consist of failure to initiate sound appropriately" (p. 297) and have motoric similarities:

> Both activities integrate highly complex, skilled, and over-learned behavioral routines involving coordination of breathing and movements of the articulators. They both achieve acoustic targets by the voluntary regulation of air pressures and flows which, in turn, involves complex and varying interactions of inspiratory and expiratory muscles at different lung volumes. (p. 297)

As we close this chapter, what is apparent is not only how much we have learned about human communication and its disorders, but also how much we yet need to learn. Indeed, fluency disorders are bewildering. One disorder can have so many different expressions; different disorders can have expressions that, on the surface, appear so similar. We are ready for the challenges of differential diagnosis and treatment, topics that will be addressed shortly.

Chapter Summary

Not all disfluency is stuttering. Clinicians must be able to distinguish between stuttering and other fluency disorders. Those reviewed here include cluttering, neurogenic acquired stuttering (associated with stroke, traumatic brain injury, extrapyramidal disease, dementia and tumor, drug usage, AIDS, and other neuropathologies), psychogenic acquired stuttering, malingering, Tourette syndrome, adductor spasmodic dysphonia, acquired stuttering following laryngectomy, linguistic disfluency, and normal developmental disfluency, as well as disfluency in manual communication and disfluency while playing a wind instrument. Guidelines for differential diagnosis, case descriptions, and personal accounts were provided for each disorder. Making differential diagnostic distinctions presents a unique opportunity for understanding how each client's communication system is uniquely organized and integrated, which is necessary for individualized and effective communication intervention. Such differential diagnosis and effective intervention require thorough knowledge of speech fluency and its disorders, extensive observation of people with and without fluency disorders, and ongoing experience with people of all ages with diverse fluency disorders, gained through the academic, clinical, and supervisory processes.

Chapter Four Study Questions

1. This chapter addressed fluency disorders other than stuttering. Why is it important to differentiate between stuttering and other fluency disorders? What are the similarities and differences between the disorders in terms of behavioral, cognitive, and affective considerations? How might treatment considerations differ for each disorder?

2. How would you distinguish between a person who clutters, a person who stutters, a person who clutters and stutters, and a person who stutters and has other concomitant challenges?

3. How would you distinguish between a person with neurogenic acquired stuttering and a person with psychogenic acquired stuttering? What might be the characteristics of a person who has evidence of both?

4. What differences might be observed in verbal and nonverbal behaviors and expressed attitudes between people who stutter and those who are malingering? Why might a person malinger, and how would you distinguish between stuttering and malingering?

5. What significance is there in word-final disfluencies? Are they a differential diagnostic indicator of neurogenic acquired stuttering? Do they rule out developmental stuttering?

6. Why might a person who stutters demonstrate disfluency while playing a wind instrument? What are the neural and motor substrates of both? How are the disorders and the substrates alike? How are they different?

7. Stuttering and other fluency disorders are puzzling. What can we learn about human communication, its disorders, and, indeed, ourselves from such a challenging pursuit? What do we know? What do we yet need to know? How is an understanding of both (i.e., what is known and not known) essential to assessment and treatment of people with communication disorders?

Unit II

Central Intervention Assumptions

Chapter Five

Personal Constructs and Family Systems

Intrafamily Considerations

Build therefore your own world. As fast as you conform your life to the pure idea in your mind, that will unfold its great proportions. A correspondent revolution in things will attend the influx of the spirit. (Emerson, 1836)

Identifying and describing the concepts that form the core of our working assumptions in clinical intervention is more than an academic exercise. Doing so explains, if not justifies, what we do with people who stutter. Why do we need to explain or justify what we do? Because all of us, by virtue of making a professional commitment to understanding stuttering and people who stutter, have sworn an oath to do our utmost to facilitate positive change in someone's communication world (ASHA, 2007d, 2010). Our methods are based on systematic application of knowledge to the clinical process within an explicit and coherent theoretical context (ASHA, 2004a, 2005b; J. R. Johnston, 1983). No less critical is our sincere belief in our clients and their potential for communication growth and change, and in ourselves as professional facilitators of this change process (Daly, 1988). Too often, I have heard clinicians justify what they are doing clinically by saying, "That's how I was trained." Such thinking falls short of our ethical, legal, and social obligation to people who stutter (Messick, 1980). Furthermore, it fails to reflect the excitement within the challenge and privilege facing us in communicating with and coming to understand the world of another person.

In this chapter, we will establish the following:

- ▨ Stuttering is a personal construct. Stuttering-related thoughts, feelings, and behaviors reflect in part the consequences of active and alternative choices.

- ▨ Stuttering and other communication disorders exist and must be addressed within a family context. The experiences of and changes in a person who stutters trigger compensatory changes in family members and significant others.

Personal Construct Theory

Personal Constructs Defined

That all people, including people who stutter, have alternative choices is a basic postulate to effective treatment—and to healthy living. This premise is also central to personal construct theory (G. A. Kelly, 1955a, 1955b). The philosophical assumption underlying personal construct theory is "constructive alternativism":

> We assume that all of our present interpretations of the universe are subject to revision or replacement. . . . We take the stand that there are always some alternative constructions available to choose among in dealing with the world. No one needs to paint himself into a corner; no one needs to be completely hemmed in by circumstances; no one needs to be the victim of his biography. (G. A. Kelly, 1955a, p. 15)

This highly optimistic view assumes that we have the ability to change every aspect of our feelings, thoughts, and behaviors. We are highly adaptable because we have individually created an interwoven network of personal constructs—viewpoints of reality based upon past experience in life situations. Because life experiences are varied, typically we bring many personal constructs to bear on our interpretation of the world in which we live.

Defining constructs, G. A. Kelly (1955a) noted, "Man looks at his world through transparent patterns or templets [*sic*] which he creates and then attempts to fit over the realities of which the world is composed" (pp. 8–9). He elaborated:

> Man creates his own ways of seeing the world in which he lives; the world does not create them for him. . . . Each individual man formulates in his own way constructs through which he views the world of events. As a scientist, man seeks to predict, and thus control, the course of events. It follows, then, that the constructs which he formulates are intended to aid him in his predictive efforts. (G. A. Kelly, 1955a, p. 12)

The primary purpose of constructs is prediction of the future. According to this theory, we actively try to anticipate what may happen in the future and develop plans to cope effectively given a variety of outcomes. People are not passive participants in unveiling the future. Rather, we plan long-term goals and prepare in advance for the challenges that inevitably arise in pursuit of these goals. Personal construct systems should always be evolving, ever changing in light of new information and experiences.

Personal Constructs Applied to Intervention

Personal construct theory relates directly to our clinical interactions with people who stutter. In this theory, the client's personal experience and understanding of the social world, particularly the clinician–client relationship, are critical to the change process. According to Botterill and Cook (1987), personal construct theory

> holds that if therapists are to play a significant part in the exploration of another person's construct system there must be trust, empathic understanding and genuine respect between client and clinician. Effective help only occurs when the therapist is able to see events through the eyes of her client. This understanding will in turn lead to changes in the way the client construes his therapist. We feel that this level of mutual understanding is a prerequisite for effective therapy. (p. 149)

More recently, in an article titled "How Can You Understand? You Don't Stutter!" Manning (2004) underscored the importance of the clinician understanding the client's communication experience from the client's perspective. This understanding facilitates clients' adjustment to the new role of a fluent speaker through a narrative approach in which clients deconstruct their stuttering-dominated personal narrative and reconstruct an alternative narrative that is more compatible with being a fluent speaker (DiLollo, Neimeyer, & Manning, 2002). In one study, people who stutter were found to have more difficulty integrating their experiences meaningfully in a fluent speaking role than in a stuttering role; the reverse was found for fluent speakers (DiLollo, Manning, & Neimeyer, 2003; see also Plexico, Manning, & Levitt, 2009a, 2009b). These studies suggest that the internalized construct of a person who stutters needs to be assessed and monitored for change over time to ensure that the dominant, internalized role shifts in ways that are consistent with speech fluency, rather than maintaining the familiar role of stuttering and thus courting relapse.

Personal construct theory is based on the fundamental postulate of constructive alternativism, which posits that "a person's processes are psychologically channelized by the ways in which he anticipates events" (Kelly, 1955b, p. 561). This fundamental postulate was elaborated into 11 corollaries (G. A. Kelly, 1955b, pp. 561–562), several of which are noted below with an application to the clinical process with people who stutter.

- ⌨ "Construction Corollary: A person anticipates events by construing their replications." This means that we anticipate our future on the basis of our past. A 55-year-old client cannot envision what it might be like to talk fluently because stuttering is all he has ever known. People who stutter anticipate the words on which and situations within which they will stutter. Clients' motivation in treatment will continue only if they have experienced, and thereby can anticipate, success in treatment and related activities. A clinician's attitude toward stuttering therapy, and thereby the likelihood of a client's success (Daly, 1988), will be affected by the clinician's relative success in treatment with previous clients.

- ⌨ "Dichotomy Corollary: A person's construction system is composed of a finite number of dichotomous constructs." In other words, people view the world in terms of opposites. The common conceptualization of people as "stutterers" or "fluent speakers" embodies a dichotomous construct that obscures the reality that fluency is a continuous variable and that people who stutter (and their clinicians) are a heterogeneous population. Dichotomous categories must be reinterpreted (first *for* the client, then *with* the client, and eventually *by* the client) so as to identify and monitor changes that occur in fluency-related thoughts, feelings, and behaviors, in addition to constructive changes within family systems and interdisciplinary teams.

- ⌨ "Choice Corollary: A person chooses for himself that alternative in a dichotomized construct through which he anticipates the greater possibility for extension and definition of his system." This means that all people have and make choices, either implicitly or explicitly. Both stuttered speech and fluent speech are the consequences of what someone does, feels, and thinks. Once provided ownership of stuttered and fluent speech as realistic options within clinical and extraclinical settings, the person who stutters may choose, with guidance, accordingly. That moment of choice, once experienced by the person who stutters, is communicatively empowering.

- ⌨ "Experience Corollary: A person's construction system varies as he successively construes the replications of events." Building on the construction corollary, this means that both our anticipation of events and our view of the world evolve on the basis of past and particularly repeated experiences. This is how stuttering gains habit strength. "I have always stuttered. I stutter. Therefore, I will stutter." However, this same corollary can be used by clinicians to break the habit strength of stuttering by creating an opportunity for the client to build a foundation of successful fluency experiences on the basis of which the client begins to anticipate future fluency success. In other words, by creating opportunities for the client to achieve fluency success (a primary objective in effective treatment and a primary role of the clinician), the client becomes compelled to revise his anticipation of his communication future on the basis of personal experience. Indeed, success begets success. From the client's perspective, there is nothing more motivating than fluency success itself.

📖 "Individuality Corollary: Persons differ from each other in their constructions of events." This means that people are likely to hold vastly different interpretations of the same observed event. Indeed, the distinction between an event and its multiple interpretations is a hallmark of science. Because all people who stutter are different in how they construe (interpret) and predict their communication and their world, treatment must be tailored to fit each individual. Also, this corollary may explain why clinicians may hold different assessments and treatment recommendations for the same client. The uniqueness that defines all members within the interdisciplinary team—people who stutter, families, clinicians, educators, and allied human service and medical professionals—is diversity at its best and at the heart of multicultural appreciation (see Chapter 6).

📖 "Commonality Corollary: To the extent that one person employs a construction of experience which is similar to that employed by another, his psychological processes are similar to those of the other person." This argues for the client and clinician to create and use opportunities to shift perspective so as to consider other points of view—that is, for the client to see through the eyes of (experience the construct systems of) fluent speakers, and the clinician to see through the eyes of the client and all members of the family system and the interdisciplinary team.

📖 "Sociality Corollary: To the extent that one person construes the construction processes of another he may play a role in a social process involving the other person." This is an extension of the commonality corollary. People often do share common perceptions of the same experience. Examples might include the camaraderie noted at conventions held by self-help and mutual aid groups for people who stutter, or the sense of inclusion experienced by members of a group sharing a cultural identity. Others, however, can also come to see as others do by shifting perspective. To the extent that we can share the perspective of another person, we can begin to understand and participate within his or her reality. Such shifting of perspective is difficult yet essential for effective change (for learning, growth, transfer, and maintenance) and, as I will note later, perhaps is the essence of shared respect for individuals and groups representing all people, the heart of diversity and multicultural sensitivity.

All people, including people who stutter and clinicians, come to view their world and themselves on the basis of unique systems of personal constructs that develop from previous experience. These systems help us anticipate and respond to, if not shape, future events. When explicitly aware of our client's personal constructs, we can use this awareness to effect positive and proactive change in his communication skills and the way he views himself as a communicator. When aware of our own personal constructs regarding our role as a clinician and as a facilitator of change, we can plan for and effect growth in our own professional development. When only implicitly aware or relatively unaware of our constructs, we inevitably maintain the status quo and inadvertently dilute any effort to effect change. We do not have to stick with the past. If we become aware that our interpretation of past events, and thereby anticipation of future events, is incorrect or undesirable, we can revise our construct system to achieve outcomes that did not seem possible previously (such as speaking with greater fluency, using self-corrections more often, using fluency facilitating controls in outside settings, and participating as a communicator in unlimited ways and settings for untold purposes).

Personal construct theory indicates that people have choices—an active, deliberate, and conscious process—and that "all of our present interpretations of the universe are subject to revision and replacement" (G. A. Kelly, 1955a, p. 15). The ways we view and interpret the world, the words we use to discuss our personal constructs, and the areas within which we envision change are idiosyncratic and, perhaps, the very essence of constructive alternativism. The clinician, therefore, must gain an appreciation of the client's system of personal constructs in order to understand the client's conception of himself as a person and as a communicator within a social world, vision for targeted change, and portrait of presenting abilities and challenges. Furthermore, the clinician must determine the relative coherence among these three components. In other words, the clinician must shift perspective so as to see the client's world as the client sees it (Shapiro, 1987, 1994a, 1994b, 1995, 2002a, 2002b, 2002c, 2004a, 2004b, 2004c, 2004d, 2004e, 2004f, 2004g, 2005, 2006, 2007a, 2007b, 2008; Shapiro & Moses, 1989, 2005) and must assess whether the client's personal constructs accommodate or inadvertently hinder the desired change. Fransella (1972) noted that people who stutter ultimately choose to stutter because this role is the most familiar and predictable based on acquired experience. Making the transition from disfluency to fluency presents a difficult challenge of internal adjustments to one's system of personal constructs, a far greater challenge than simply bringing overt disfluent behaviors under control. This distinction explains why the long-term transfer and maintenance of feelings, thoughts, and behaviors that are characteristic of fluency prove to be so difficult. In Fransella's (1972) words, "The road from stuttering to fluency is paved by reconstructions" (p. 70).

⌕ Case Example ⌕

Consider the following example. Some years ago, I conducted the diagnostic evaluation of a 32-year-old woman who described herself as a "stutterer" and who reported feelings of insecurity and embarrassment related to her stuttering and particular concern regarding the listener's first impression of her as a communicator. After a thorough evaluation, I was left utterly unable to detect any overt behavior that might resemble stuttering. In fact, she was both skillful at communication and eloquent as a communicator. Nevertheless, the woman was visibly anxious that she might stutter and appeared shamed at the slightest twinge of normal disfluency. To me, she was an excellent illustration of an "interiorized stutterer" (Douglass & Quarrington, 1952) and a good reminder that even though the clinician might perceive an individual's stuttering as mild or nonexistent, that perception is not necessarily shared. Recall that the very same event, disfluency in this case, might generate vastly different interpretations (seeming normal to one person but communicatively handicapping to another). Bloodstein (1993) noted that "some of the most severe problems are presented by people who seem to talk with perfectly normal fluency" (p. 4).

In this case, it became clear that the woman's personal construct of herself as a communicator was inhibiting her recognition of her own communicative and interpersonal strengths, thus confining her perceived potential in other areas. For example, she had completed an associate's degree from a 2-year college and was working as a clerical assistant in a dentist's office. While she longed to pursue her education, she felt that ultimately she would be unsuccessful because of her perceived communication disorder. Her communication treatment involved providing an opportunity for her to identify and better understand her own system of personal constructs and to determine whether these were appropriate for her based upon past experience and, thereby, projected future experience. She was regularly involved in making and analyzing audio and video recordings and comparing her assessment with conversational partners' assessment of her communication skills. In short order, the mismatch between her perception and that of her listeners became evident to her. This procedure, recently described as integrating self-attribution (what the person who stutters thinks about herself) with social attribution (what others think about the person who stutters) (Daniels & Gabel, 2004), was successful in helping her to identify and shift her own perspective about herself as a communicator on the basis of concrete data and a steadily growing foundation of communication success. I followed this woman's progress for 10 years posttreatment. Several years ago, I learned that she had completed dental school and was successful in her practice of dentistry. ⌕

Summary and Extension—Personal Construct Theory

G. A. Kelly's (1955a, 1955b) personal construct theory indicates that all people, on the basis of past experience, construct systems to help anticipate and cope with life events. This is particularly true in the case of coping with personal difficulties, including stuttering. This theory has direct application to personal change and reconstruction, which are core elements of effective treatment. It has two key concepts. First, the client is actively involved in all aspects of the treatment process, including identifying, reassessing, and revising (as appropriate) his own system of personal constructs. Second, the client has choices to make among alternatives and is responsible for his own actions. Within limits, fluency and disfluency are alternative choices representing bipolar components within a personal construct. Both fluency and disfluency represent the composite outcome of feelings, thoughts, and behaviors of a person who stutters.

Botterill and Cook (1987) discussed three treatment stages of problem solving leading to the client's ability to see alternatives in situations (*circumspection*), arrive at a choice of action from among these alternatives (*preemption*), and ultimately bring a situation under control (*control*). They emphasized that the relative success of the chosen strategy is less important than the resulting refinement of the individual's construct system. Change must be initiated by the client, in terms of both its construction and its action. The clinician serves as a facilitator, all the while transferring responsibility for treatment design, implementation, evaluation, and follow-up to the client. As will be seen later, I maintain that the process of transferring fluency skills to extraclinical settings starts at the beginning, not the end, of treatment and is supported throughout the treatment process. Botterill and Cook offered this insight:

> It is our role as therapists to help clients explore their construct systems and appreciate how construct systems provide both the basis of current functioning and the vehicle for future change. . . . For many clients the chance to reconstrue themselves and their communication difficulties can at the very least make the problem more acceptable. For others such basic reconstruction is the prelude to more comprehensive change in many areas of social functioning including speech fluency. We do not suggest that all there is to the treatment of stuttering is a period of personal reconstruction; but equally we are convinced that it takes more than motor speech training to achieve lasting change in the treatment of dysfluency. (p. 165)

The implications of personal construct theory on assessment and treatment of stuttering are profound. Intervention methods are outlined in Chapters 8, 9, and 10, but a few illustrations of the significance of personal construct theory are in order. Often a client's stuttering is what the client and clinician notice most. Therefore, many clinicians focus initially on heightening the client's awareness of his stuttering and eliminating the stuttering. Indeed this is in contrast to what I recommend. Early in the first chapter, I pointed out that calculations of disfluency fail to highlight the majority of words that are spoken fluently and the islands of fluency between stuttered words. I continue my challenge of traditional intervention approaches by asking why, when many, if not most, of the client's words are spoken fluently, do clinicians elect to begin by focusing on the disfluency? As noted, personal construct theory indicates that we predict the future on the basis of our past. Many people who stutter reflect, "I have always stuttered. I am stuttering now. Likely, I . . . [will stutter]." In other words, without intervention, the client realistically anticipates fluency failure on the basis of an amassed foundation of fluency failure. Telling the client that he can be fluent or should be fluent is not enough. The client will believe what he experiences directly, not what we tell him. Indeed, nothing is more motivating than success itself. From my perspective, it is a clinician's responsibility to construct *for* the client (and eventually *with* the client and ultimately *by* the client) speaking opportunities that result in fluency success. The successes experienced directly by the client must be so frequent, consistent, and salient that the client becomes compelled to reconsider his anticipation of his communication future. We begin to construct an alternative foundation, one of fluency success, which provides a contrasting perspective on which the client can anticipate the future. The shift in the client's perspective is gradual, leading to an "aha" moment. Surely, the client's experiences speak louder than the clinician's words. How we construct those positive, successful speaking experiences will be the focus of subsequent chapters. The clinician's role is to construct opportunities that enable, if not compel, the client to reconsider and revise the way he anticipates his communication future, not on the basis of the clinician's words, but rather on the basis of successful experiences being accumulated by the client. There is no replacement for success; success begets success.

We now move from the individual to the family. We will see that experiences and changes in a person who stutters trigger compensatory changes in family members and significant others. Stuttering and other communication disorders exist and must be addressed within a family context.

Family Systems Theory

Family systems theory posits that the family, with few exceptions, is the most powerful emotional unit to which we ever belong, and it continues to affect the course and outcome of our lives (E. A. Carter & Orfanidis, 1996; Holland, 2007; Shames, 2006; Walsh, 2006). Members of the family unit or communication system are interdependent; thus, experiences or changes of one member trigger compensatory changes in other members. This primary impact makes the family unit our greatest potential resource for clinical intervention (Bowen, 1996; Corey, 2005; Whitaker, 1996). One part of the family cannot be understood in isolation from the other members of the system (J. R. Andrews & Andrews, 2000; Epstein & Bishop, 1981; Turnbull, Turnbull, Erwin, & Soodak, 2006; Walsh, 2006). Luterman (2008) underscored that a communication disorder always exists within a family context because, at its essence, communication only occurs within the milieu of a relationship. When there is a communication disorder, everyone in the family is affected by it, and it therefore becomes the responsibility of the speech–language pathologist and the audiologist to work with the needs of all members of the family:

> The basic notion underlying all family therapy is that the family is a system in which all of the components are interdependent. Every family member affects every other component of the family; for the family therapist, there is no such thing as individual therapy—any time a change occurs in one member of the family, everybody in the family is impacted. (p. 147)

Luterman (2008) further noted, "As we mature as a profession and throw off our technician shackles, we are recognizing the need to work at a family level. To do this successfully, we need to understand how the family system functions and the various roles that significant family members play" (p. 150).

A Paradigm Shift

While clinicians traditionally have tried to involve family members in the intervention process, such attempts have been based on a linear treatment model, in which an individual is the center of the treatment process (J. R. Andrews & Andrews, 2000). Mothers, and occasionally other family members, are directed by the speech–language patholo-gist to engage in treatment-related activity in settings outside of the treatment room. Under this arrangement, the most significant changes are viewed as occurring in the treatment session; family cooperation and understanding are seen as supplementary. Changing this conception of treatment, which is so deeply rooted in the behavioral tradition, necessitates a paradigm shift, a new construct or way of looking at the clinical world. We must move from a linear model to a more systemic one. This shift involves moving from a monocular perspective to a polyocular one, moving from a focus on labeling to one of understanding, and changing the focus of our attention away from discrete behaviors toward the systems in which those behaviors function (J. R. Andrews & Andrews, 2000).

Shifting from Monocular to Polyocular Perspectives

From a monocular perspective, a single interpretation is a desired goal. From a polyocu-lar perspective, different interpretations of the same event are not only accepted but also invited and nurtured. Such a perspective is consistent with the importance of being able to shift perspective, distinguishing an event from its multiple potential interpretations, and the notion of personal construct theory, where we actively choose a perspective from multiple alternatives. J. R. Andrews and Andrews (1990) provided the following example:

> One of the language delayed children that we treated was seen as stubborn by his mother, mechanically gifted by his father, cute by his grandfather, autistic by a school psycholo-gist, retarded by his teacher, and language impaired by a speech–language pathologist. Each of these views, though different, was correct from the perspective of the person expressing a "truth." Many factors, of course, influenced each view including the profes-sional, personal, and family relationship of each person to the child. The clinician must honestly view all these perspectives as accurate when considered from the point of view of the person expressing the opinion. (pp. 7–8)

A corollary to adopting a polyocular view is accepting different interpretations of an event as potentially equally correct. For example, parents with different parenting styles (such as orderly and structured vs. playful, relaxed, and spontaneous) will need to recognize and use the benefits of both styles, lest the difference become a source of tension. Likewise, clinicians must be aware of the significance of differing perspectives on a clinical matter, even though such perspectives often are not in agreement with our own. The importance of being able to shift perspective cannot be overstated (Shapiro & Moses, 2005).

Shifting from Labeling to Understanding

A second required shift involves moving from labeling behaviors to identifying interac-tive patterns and understanding the relevance of a problem within a meaningful com-municative context. Too often, labels applied to behavior fall short of conveying an understanding of the nature of one's communication strengths and challenges within meaningful social contexts. A corollary related to identifying communicative relevance is moving from a focus on problems to one on finding solutions. For example, rather than focusing initially on disfluent behavior, as most people who stutter have come to expect, the speech–language therapist should first identify, study, and understand the nature of the client's fluency and create opportunities for him to experience fluency success— in other words, provide guidance for the person who stutters to do more of what he is already doing that is conducive to fluency. Identifying what the person who stutters is doing that facilitates fluency, as well as helping him to increase what he already is doing, is significantly different from initially identifying what he is doing wrong and directing him not to do what he is currently doing. The former empowers a person who stutters to realize that he is capable of fluency, is an active and vital member of the change process, and already possesses target behaviors that need to be demonstrated even more frequently; the latter conveys the contrary, that he needs to rebuild his speech patterns under the control of the clinician, who is the primary member of the treatment team. Simply put, how many of us would continue to be motivated when what we are doing wrong (i.e., the problem, disfluent speech behavior) receives primary focus? This process "gets old" in a hurry, and we wonder why clients' cooperation and attendance slack off. I find that focusing on what the client already is doing right and providing guidance in how to do more of what he is already doing correctly "hooks" people who stutter and their families into a positive process that is motivating, rewarding, and solution-focused.

Shifting from Behaviors to Systems

A third shift involves moving from a focus on discrete behaviors to a focus on transformations within an integrated communication system. Improvements in language functioning effect changes in phonology (Paden, 2005; R. V. Watkins, 2005); changes in fluency often effect changes in self-concept, personal hygiene, academic performance, professional aspirations, and so on. Too often, behaviors are identified with an emphasis on communication *dis*order rather than on dis*order*. We are then surprised by related yet unplanned improvements beyond the target behaviors. Such surprise reveals that the clinician's intervention posture is typically reactive. As clinicians, we need to be more proactive, understanding communication-related changes that occur within a communication system, which enables us not only to handle and nurture them but also to plan systematically for them. The clinician can help the client and his family to become aware for the first time of new choices—personal outlooks on oneself, relationships, personal and professional options, and feelings of confusion and insecurity experienced by family members who need role clarification and support, such as spouses, parents, significant others, and teachers. We must plan for dynamic changes and system transformations, only some of which can be predicted. Nevertheless, while facilitating the processes of change, self-actualization, and growth, we can expect the unexpected, learn from previous and present experience, and recognize the uniqueness of each person who stutters within a family system.

Family-Based Treatment—Families and Professionals as Partners

In family-based treatment, the entire family is involved in all aspects of assessment and treatment. Such involvement requires understanding by the clinician of the nature and dynamics of the individual family. Turnbull and Turnbull (1990) discussed the "special partnership" between families, people with exceptionalities, and professionals as follows:

> We address the family in all its diversity: size, cultural background, geographic location, values, interaction styles, met and unmet needs, and the changing characteristics of a given family over time. By addressing the family as a system, we are not bounded by a focus on one family member, typically the person with an exceptionality. Indeed, we seek to show the complex interrelatedness of all members in a family and the importance of adopting a comprehensive view of professional interventions. We stress that each family must maintain its own critical balance, its unique center of gravity in order to allow any professional intervention to be beneficial to a family member or to the entire family. We encourage professional support of families. (pp. viii–ix)

Family members become equal partners with the professional members of the treatment team. Counseling is the medium for discussing aspects of family interactive patterns that facilitate or inhibit the targeted changes, which are jointly determined. Throughout the literature on family therapy, different principles guide the practice of intervention within a systems perspective. J. R. Andrews and Andrews (2000, pp. 11–15) have applied the following overlapping principles from family therapy (Epstein & Bishop, 1981) to family-based treatment in communication disorders:

- "One part of the family cannot be understood in isolation from the rest of the system." The behavior of each family member is understood more completely when interpreted within the context of family beliefs, patterns, and customs. This is surely applicable to the observation, assessment, and treatment of the behavior of a person who stutters.

- "The parts of a family are interrelated; change in one part influences change in other parts of the system." When one member of a family stutters, all other members are affected by it and the treatment process.

- "Transactional patterns of the family shape the behavior of family members." A fluency disorder frequently is embedded in the family pattern of interaction.

- "A family's structure, organization, and developmental stage are important factors in determining the behavior of family members." Understanding that every family develops and adopts certain roles over time is critical to involving the family meaningfully in treatment-related activities.

An obvious question might be, "Why should a family systems approach be taken seriously by clinicians working with people who stutter?" Or, by implication, "Isn't working exclusively with the person who stutters a more direct and time-efficient approach?" In response, I want to share a few observations illustrating that in a family systems approach, we clinicians have an opportunity to participate actively in and model the very behaviors we hope to nurture in the families of our clients who stutter. Then, I want to provide some representative data that support such methods.

Family-Based Treatment—Modeling Characteristics of Optimal Families

Luterman (2008) noted that when clinicians approach intervention from a family therapy perspective, "we in effect become a member of the family" (p. 159):

> Our job as professionals in working with persons with communicative disorders is to help the family become optimal, or as close to it as possible. We can teach parents, mainly by modeling, how to manage conflict, how to communicate openly and honestly with their children, and how to display their affection and caring for their children. In effect, what we must do is parent the parents, which creates for them in our relationship an optimal family. The parents then can take from our optimal clinical family the information and skills necessary for their own home situation. (p. 176)

Indicating that we are to demonstrate what we intend for our clients and their families, Luterman (2008, pp. 159–161) summarized the characteristics of optimal families. He noted that optimal families produce well-functioning individuals, both with and without exceptionality:

- "Communication among all family members is clear and direct." Communication is explicit, contains content and feeling, and is balanced by empathy and humor.

- "Roles and responsibilities are clearly delineated, overlapping, and flexible." Boundaries within and across family subsystems (e.g., parent–parent, parent–child, child–child) are clear, allowing for parental authority balanced with open communication. Roles and responsibilities change and are renegotiated to maintain a well-functioning unit.

⌕ "The family members accept limits for the resolution of conflict." Conflict is viewed as normal and healthy, resulting in growth and change. Resolution of conflict is fair, taking individual needs into account, allowing everyone to "win" in part of the solution. Clinicians' modeling of conflict resolution for families is essential.

⌕ "Intimacy is prevalent and is a function of frequent, equal-powered transactions." Caring and affection, in observable or more subtle ways, are communicated and received while respecting the need for space and distance. "Optimal families are cohesive without being enmeshed."

⌕ "A healthy balance exists between change and the maintenance of stability." Some change is predictable and some is not (e.g., who will stutter; see Yairi & Ambrose, 2005). The balance between accommodating change and maintaining stability (i.e., homeostasis) is accomplished by open, clear communication and role flexibility so others can help when demands increase on family time, mutual caring, and effective conflict resolution.

Family-Based Treatment—Modeling Characteristics of Successful Families

Families that are successful in coping with the changes and challenges required when a member has an exceptionality demonstrate other, related characteristics. Luterman (2008) reviewed a number of such characteristics (pp. 176–180), which again should be nurtured and modeled by the clinician:

⌕ "A successful family is one that feels empowered." People who stutter and their families need to feel that they own (have participated in the development of) the intervention strategy and that what they can do will make a positive difference. Professionals must not present a bleak picture, taking away the spark of hope. For this reason, I recommend focusing initially on what the person who stutters can, rather than cannot, do and helping him to do more of what he already is doing that is conducive to fluency; this includes nurturing feelings associated with fluency control. When experiencing success, one is motivated and wants to do more. As noted previously, success begets success. Ownership and success are empowering.

⌕ "In successful families the self-esteem, especially of the mother, is high." Related to empowerment, parents, spouses, and other family members need to be and to feel needed, involved, and successful. These experiences replace the need for denial as a coping strategy.

⌕ "In successful families there is a feeling that the burden is shared." Members of the family and occasionally friends share tasks and/or emotional support related to the intervention process. Luterman indicated that to prevent parents from becoming overwhelmed with feelings of total responsibility, he tells them: "This business is really in thirds—one third is your responsibility, one third is mine as a professional, and one third is the child's. You just be sure that you do your third, I'll do my third, and both of us will see that the child does his third" (p. 178).

⌕ Successful families need to make philosophical sense of the situation." When bad or challenging things happen, many people ask, "Why me?" Successful families have an answer, whatever it might be (such as biological, theological, or philosophical). Not having an answer breeds unproductive bitterness, negativity, and anger. Successful families come to see that growth results from challenge and stress.

Luterman (2008) conveyed his personal experience from sharing his wife's struggle with multiple sclerosis and his professional experience from working with families of people with hearing impairments:

For me there has always been growth in stress. I am pushed by the stress to develop more capacity in order to reduce the stress. I generally give to life what life demands. When life demands more, I am forced to expand. That increased capacity is my growth. I see this happening in all the families I have worked with. Although I can empathize and perhaps sympathize with the pain involved, I know that if they can just hang in, they will learn and grow. They have a powerful teacher in the disorder, and we as professionals must allow the process of growth to take place. We can facilitate the growth by not overhelping and by at all times respecting the dignity and the capacity of our clients to grow. Very often we have to let go of our preconceived notions. (pp. 179–180)

Family-Based Treatment and Heightened Effectiveness

A growing body of efficacy data supports a family systems approach to intervention. A reading of the literature on family systems across disciplines indicates that positive treatment outcomes for an individual with an exceptionality, defined in terms that are unique to that exceptionality, are related to the emotional and communicative health of the family members and their respective involvement in and commitment to the treatment process. This has been shown over and over (Cool, 2005; Elders, 2006; S. D. Klein & Schive, 2001; Millard, Nicholas, & Cook, 2008; Portnuff, 2006; Reinhardt, 2005; Russo, 2005; Venable, 2006; Westling & Fox, 2009; Yaruss, Coleman, & Hammer, 2006). After 40 years as an audiologist, Luterman (2008) concluded that if you take good care of the parents, the children will do well. Similarly, with chronically ill patients, if you take good care of the spouse and other family members, the identified patient also will do well. He noted that failure to deal with family needs invariably limits therapeutic effectiveness.

First-person accounts by families that have experienced a member's developmental disability across the lifespan powerfully convey the varied resources of family strength that were used for cognitive coping—for constructively approaching challenging situations in ways that enhanced self-esteem, feelings of control, and a sense of meaning (S. D. Klein & Schive, 2001; J. B. Schulz, 2008; Turnbull et al., 1993). Such methods enabled families to interpret the experience of having a member with a disability as an opportunity rather than a tragedy, to find positive benefit from the experience, and to enhance family well-being.

Rivara et al. (1993) studied changes in children's functioning in the year following traumatic brain injury and reported the following:

> A strong overall preinjury family functioning score, a high level of family cohesion, positive family relationships, and a low level of control (family hierarchy and rules that are rigid) are predictive of good child adaptive functioning, social competence and global functioning 1 year following TBI. (p. 1052)

Within this context, Rivara et al. (1993) reviewed studies of childhood chronic illness indicating that level of family functioning and extent of illness significantly predicted (was directly, positively correlated with) subsequent physiological, psychological, and social wellness of children with disorders of psychological adjustment, childhood diabetes, severe juvenile rheumatoid arthritis, and congenital or acquired limb deficiencies.

Similarly, Luterman (2008) summarized studies indicating that level of family empathy and positive treatment involvement contributed to (again, directly, positively correlated with) (a) the recovery rate of people who have incurred a stroke, (b) gains in academic achievement with children who have learning disabilities, (c) the success of young children using augmentative and alternative communications programs, and (d) the outcome of children with cystic fibrosis.

Zarski, DePompei, and Zook (1988) supported the importance of understanding family functioning when assessing a family's adaptation to a major stressor—in particular, a head injury to a family member:

Families that adjust successfully to the trauma reorganize by changing their power structure, role relationships, and relationship rules in response to the situational stress. In addition, emotional bonding, boundaries, coalitions, and decision-making factors are utilized in ways that focus on the head-injured member's normalcy rather than the symptomatology. In contrast, as families struggle to cope with the many social, physical, cognitive, linguistic, and emotional changes that accompany head injury, some families respond to the theme of loss by focusing on the limitations of the head-injured member, thereby organizing around the dysfunction. . . . These families are unprepared to deal with these changes and use denial as a major block to family reintegration. . . . The more severe the denial, the higher the risk the family will enter a severe crisis stage, further jeopardizing the recovery process. (pp. 38–39)

Taken together, these and other studies argue for the importance of assessing and understanding the family's strengths, needs, and level of functioning as factors in the intervention process. Furthermore, problems experienced by families when a member has an illness or exceptionality often are more closely related to their own resources, coping styles, and organization than to the member's limitations.

Family-Based Treatment and Fluency Disorders

The literature directly related to a family systems approach in working with people who stutter is limited (Cook & Botterill, 2005; Millard et al., 2008; Yaruss et al., 2006; see also Rollin, 2000). Empirical support appears to be borrowed from allied disciplines. Here, we review several family-based approaches and studies.

Rustin (1987) presented a program to treat disfluency in young children through active parental involvement. Making the point that stuttering is highly context sensitive, Rustin noted that the most significant context for the child is the family, and that the school setting is nearly as critical. Emphasizing that clinicians should focus on the family and social contexts of early stuttering, Rustin stated,

> If the problem of speech dysfluency is the result of an interaction between child and environment then intervention must be targeted at both; too often we "treat" the problem from only one perspective. To include any contextual intervention it is vital to involve the family. . . . The family is seen as the main focus for early intervention with the young dysfluent child. At the simplest level family participation involves parental training in the techniques of improving motor speech fluency. At the social level it means studying family dynamics with a view to promoting changes in the family systems which are likely to lead to further fluency development. (pp. 167–168)

Rustin and Purser (1991) reported preliminary findings from a survey of parents addressing the developmental history and family circumstances of children who stutter. Among many interesting findings on the 209 children sampled (163 boys and 46 girls—mean chronological age, 8.4 years; mean age at onset, 3 years 6 months), they reported the following:

- ⬚ Fifty-two percent of the boys and 36% of the girls were prone to "inconsolable temper tantrums" (p. 11).
- ⬚ There was a relationship between birth order in the family and stuttering—of the children sampled, all of whom stutter, (a) most were the youngest (34% boys, 36% girls) or oldest (40% boys, 32% girls), (b) fewer were only children (16% boys, 25% girls), and (c) fewest were middle children (10% boys, 7% girls).
- ⬚ Only 42% of the parents of the boys and 50% of the parents of the girls who stutter reported their marital relationship as "good," with the remainder characterizing it as "not completely satisfactory with the atmosphere at home often being uncertain and volatile" (p. 14) or offered responses that could not be classified.

Rustin and Purser (1991) concluded:

> It seems to us that even these broad findings do illustrate the need for a careful and systematic appraisal of the family dynamics as well as focusing on problems that the child experiences in conjunction with disfluency. . . . Understanding the contexts in which fluency problems arise, both in terms of the individual child and the family system in which that child is developing, offers considerable scope for more effective intervention. (p. 16)

Traditionally, it has not been uncommon for parents to play an important role in the treatment of children who stutter (Association Parole Bégaiement, 2005; Bezemer, Bouwen, & Winkelman, 2006; Bloom & Cooperman, 1999; Breitenfeldt & Lorenz, 1989; Conture, 2001; Gottwald, 1999, 2010; Gottwald & Hall, 2003; Gregory, 2003; D. G. Hill, 2003; Kully & Langevin, 1999; Kully, Langevin, & Lomheim, 2007; Langevin et al., 2006; C. S. Montgomery, 2006; Onslow & Packman, 1999; Onslow et al., 2003; Simon, 1999). What is increasing, however, is the focus on parents and family as equal partners in the treatment process. For example, Yaruss et al. (2006) designed a family-focused treatment for preschool children (i.e., between 2 and 6 years of age) who stutter that addresses communication behaviors and attitudes that children and their parents may encounter as a reaction to the stuttering experience. Both parent-focused and child-focused strategies are aimed at helping children to improve speech fluency, develop and maintain healthy communication attitudes, and achieve effective communication skills. The parent-focused treatment (parent–child training program) is a systematic treatment of short duration, is individualized to the unique needs of each family, and is intended to modify the parents' communication patterns as necessary (e.g., easy talking model, increased pause time, reduced demands, reflecting or rephrasing). The child-focused treatment (direct treatment) is intended to modify the child's communication behaviors as necessary (e.g., speech modification, stuttering modification, communication skills, concomitant disorders). Both the parent-focused and child-focused treatment are intended to build understanding and acceptance of stuttering (through parent counseling, education about stuttering and speaking, identification of stressors, focus on communication wellness, desensitization, and more). Preliminary evaluation of 17 children revealed that all children achieved improved fluency at the conclusion of treatment and at long-term follow-up. Additional follow-up for fluency maintenance, effective communication skills, and healthy communication attitudes is ongoing.

Cook and Botterill (2005) designed a family-based approach to therapy with primary-school children at the Michael Palin Centre for Stammering Children in London, England. Anchored in behavioral methodology, family systems theory, personal construct psychology, cognitive theory, and solution-focused therapy, the intervention is structured in small steps to achieve success, includes family and other significant others within the therapy process, identifies and works with the child's view of the world and the stuttering experience, integrates the affective and cognitive elements with the behavioral aspects of treatment, and considers the strengths and skills that the client and family bring to therapy, identifying potential solutions that already are within their repertoire. Both individual and group sessions comprise the therapy; individual sessions are family meetings with both the parents and the child, where possible. The parents learn about the stuttering intervention techniques and their constructive role in supporting the child's progress outside of therapy. These roles include letting go and relaxing (i.e., reinforcing the growth of the child's communication independence) as the child increasingly owns and accepts responsibility for the stuttering, communicates more confidently and effectively, and problem-solves and negotiates. Preliminary quantitative and qualitative outcome measures, including parental ratings, revealed reduced stuttering severity and, concomitantly, reduced parental concern and increased confidence regarding the management experience.

Another intervention program at the Michael Palin Centre for Stammering Children and related in principle to Cook and Botterill (2005) is Parent–Child Interaction Therapy (PCIT; Botterill & Kelman, 2010; Millard, Nicholas, & Cook, 2008; Rustin, Botterill, & Kelman, 1996). Designed to "empower parents to manage their child's stuttering and increase their confidence in their own skills as well as seeking to increase fluency in the child" (Millard et al., 2008, p. 638), PCIT begins with a detailed assessment, followed by six weekly sessions of clinic-based therapy and a 6-week period of home consolidation. The assessment entails both an evaluation of the child and collection of a case history, in which parent participation is essential. After review of the assessment results, the first treatment session is designed to negotiate a "special time," a 5-minute playtime that each parent has individually with the child three to five times per week. These special times, during which parents practice the interaction targets in a relaxed setting, are considered to be the foundation of the program and are conducted throughout the treatment process. Parents maintain written records of these interactions and receive feedback at the start of each subsequent session. In Sessions 2 through 6, the special time is reviewed, parent–child interaction is video-recorded and critiqued by each parent, interaction targets are selected by the parents, and proposed changes are discussed. Behavioral treatment (to be reviewed in Chapter 7) addresses explicit behaviors of the child in small steps; tangible rewards and verbal praise are used. Interaction strategies emphasize the positive aspects of the child's and parents' behavior within a collaborative context. In the 6-week home consolidation period, the parents continue the special time at home and implement the management strategies used in the clinic. Parents email their feedback to the clinician weekly during this generalization period, and the clinician emails reactions and feedback to the parent. Outcome measures revealed that four of the six children (aged 3 years 3 months to 4 years 10 months) significantly reduced stuttering (i.e., up to 1 year post-therapy compared to baseline) by the end of the therapy phase.

One unique program that not only emphasizes the importance of the parent's role in the stuttering intervention process but also identifies the parent as the primary agent of change is the Lidcombe Program (Bernstein Ratner & Guitar, 2006; Harrison & Onslow, 2010; Harrison et al., 2007; Onslow et al., 2003), mentioned here because of its utilization of the family structure as the context for treatment and change, not for its family systems implications. Indeed, Harrison et al. noted, "The Lidcombe Program is a direct treatment for stuttering in preschool children. That is, treatment is focused on children's speech and not on family relationships, parenting styles, or children's temperaments" (p. 56). During weekly visits to the speech clinic, clinicians train parents to deliver treatment during daily conversations and measure children's stuttering severity in everyday settings. Clinicians also monitor treatment and stuttering severity during clinic visits and adjust parents' behavior so as to be consistent with the program. The program has two stages. In the first stage, the goal is to eliminate or reduce the child's stuttering to a low level; the goal of the second stage is to maintain that reduction. Clinic visits occur regularly during the first stage and are decreased in frequency during the second stage. The two essential responses recorded from the child's spontaneous production are stutter-free speech and unambiguous stuttering. Two other responses, self-evaluation of stutter-free speech and self-correction of stuttering, are encouraged but not considered essential components in treatment. When the child demonstrates stutter-free speech, parents are trained to comment (i.e., to offer a "parental verbal contingency") with either acknowledgment (e.g., "Those words were smooth") or praise ("Wow, good smooth talking"). A third contingency for stutter-free speech is to ask children to self-evaluate their speech (e.g., "Was that smooth?" or "Were there any bumps there?"). When the child demonstrates unambiguous stuttering, the parents either acknowledge ("That was a bump there") or ask the child to self-correct ("Can you say 'orange' again smoothly?"). Onslow et al. noted, "To guarantee that the treatment is a positive experience for the child, a rule of thumb in the Lidcombe Program is that there should be at least five times the amount of acknowledgment and praise for stutter-free speech as there is for acknowledgement and asking for self-correction of stuttering" (p. 6). For regular monitoring of the child's response to treatment, parents collect two speech measures from outside settings (i.e., perceptual severity scaling of the child's stuttering and a stutter-count measure), while the clinician measures the percentage of syllables stuttered during clinic visits. Perceptual scaling by parents is a measure of severity rating (i.e., 1 = *no stuttering*, 2 = *extremely mild stuttering*, 10 = *extremely severe stuttering*); the stutter-count measure computes the stutters per minute of speaking time. Clinicians verify reliability of the parents' severity ratings by having them assign a rating to a sample of the child's speech and then having them rate the same speech sample a few weeks later (i.e., satisfactory reliability is indicated if first and second scalings differ by no more than one scale value). Regular discussions between clinicians and parents address their respective speech measures, in addition to types of stutters observed, validity of the samples, stuttering severity, and comparisons of speech measures with those discussed in previous sessions.

The clinical protocol for the Lidcombe Program has two stages. During the initial Stage 1 visits, the clinician teaches the parent how to apply contingencies to target responses only in conversations that are structured to facilitate stutter-free speech. As the child's severity ratings decrease, conversations become more unstructured and the parent learns how to conduct them in daily activities, usually for 10 or 15 minutes once or twice daily. Aspects of conversational structure being controlled by the parent include relative familiarity with objects and materials being used for interaction, complexity of linguistic cues (e.g., sentence completion, binary choice questions, modeling), and other components of conversation (e.g., motoric, linguistic, pragmatic), in addition to the location, timing, and choice of topic and stimulus materials. As Stage 1 continues, the child's stutter-free utterances become longer and more frequent, and stuttering severity becomes less variable and, ultimately, reduced. Contingent stimulation for the child's spontaneous self-evaluation of stutter-free speech is introduced (e.g., "Was that smooth?") as treatment moves from structured to unstructured conversations. Children spontaneously begin to self-correct their stuttering as treatment becomes increasingly unstructured. To prevent the child's excessive focus on his stuttering, self-correction of stuttering is not taught to the child. After spontaneous self-correction, however, the parent or clinician offers specific praise (e.g., "Well done, you fixed your bumpy word"). As severity ratings of the child's stuttering decrease, an increase of stutter-free utterances is observed. Weekly clinic visits and daily treatments within Stage 1 continue until three criteria are met (i.e., less than 1.0% stuttered syllables within the clinic, weekly severity ratings average less than 2.0 outside the clinic and no more than three scores of 2.0 or higher in any week, and less than 1.5 stutters per minute of speaking time outside the clinic).

In Stage 2 of the Lidcombe Program, the parents withdraw treatment gradually, ensuring that the same level of stutter-free speech is maintained as during the end of Stage 1. A series of 30-minute clinic visits of decreasing frequency are held, again ensuring maintenance of the aforementioned criteria during conversations with the child, both inside (with the parent and clinician) and outside (with the parent) the clinic. Webber and Onslow (2003) determined that half of the children will not meet the criteria during a Stage 2 clinic visit. When this occurs in early Stage 2, the child may continue on the same step until criteria are met. When this occurs in later Stage 2, the child may be moved to an earlier step until criteria are met or the parents and clinician decide to move the child back to Stage 1. The expected outcome of the Lidcombe Program is consistent, effortless, stutter-free speech by the end of Stage 2. Anecdotal evidence from parents indicates that children become more confident and active conversational participants. Harrison et al. (2007) presented a series of case studies supporting such parental reports and reviewed quantitative evidence indicating the Lidcombe Program's effectiveness in achieving fluency improvements beyond what would be expected from natural recovery (Harris et al., 2002; M. Jones et al., 2000; Rousseau, Packman, Onslow, Harrison, & Jones, 2007). Harrison et al. also reviewed evidence attesting to the Lidcombe Program's safety as an intervention, compliance of participating families and clients, and preliminary effectiveness; positive response of clients to the treatment within a reasonable period of time; and positive response of clients to the treatment within the context of randomized controlled trials (see Jones et al., 2005). Finally, Harrison et al. referred to the Lidcombe Program as "the first empirically developed treatment for early stuttering" and recommended further efficacy studies.

Franken et al. (2005) compared the Lidcombe Program and a program following a demands and capacities model (as reviewed in Chapter 3). In demands and capacities, stuttering is assumed to occur when demands on fluency exceed the child's capacity for fluency. Both demands and capacities include motor, emotional, linguistic, and cognitive correlates. Treatment, therefore, is designed to decrease demands until increased capacity is achieved in these four aspects of development. Parents are directed to speak more simply and slowly, yet naturally, to reduce demands on the child's speech motor behavior. Franken et al. randomly assigned 30 children to one of the two treatments and obtained stuttering frequency and severity ratings immediately before and 12 weeks after treatment. Findings revealed no significant differences between the two forms of treatment or in the level of cooperation or satisfaction of the parents.

Franken et al. (2005) suggested that the Lidcombe Program and the demands and capacities treatments "are equally effective because of procedures common to both treatments (e.g., daily extra time with the undivided attention of a parent)" (p. 197). As we seek to understand the nature and influence of individual treatment components, among those warranting additional attention are the factors commonly referred to "demands" and "capacities." Packman, Onslow, and Attanasio (2004) cautioned that these terms cannot be defined operationally, cannot be measured, and, therefore, cannot serve as a foundation for measurable, evidence-based treatment (see also Onslow, 2004). Packman et al. (2004) noted, however, that the concept of "demands" is embedded in the Lidcombe Program:

> The Lidcombe Program, for example, clearly imposes demands on the child to speak without stuttering. Indeed, that is the essence of treatment. The parent draws the child's attention to stuttering in everyday speaking situations, conveys to the child that he or she should try to speak without stuttering, and reinforces stutter-free speech when the child produces it. (p. 72)

What remains unclear is the operational definition of "demands" and "capacities," as used by proponents of both the Lidcombe Program and demands and capacities treatments. Some years ago when I visited the Australian Stuttering Research Center in Sydney, Australia, I had the opportunity to observe delivery of the Lidcombe Program by master clinicians. I must confess that the first time I saw a parent and a clinician identify and bring to the preschool child's attention instances of the child's stuttering, I thought I would fall over. "This is not the way it is supposed to be done," I thought. Soon thereafter, I was better able to observe not only what was being done, but how it was being done. None of the preschoolers even winced. Play and joy filled the intervention rooms. Soon I realized that the delivery of feedback to the child could not have been more gentle by the parent or the clinician, who was training the parent. Indeed we must consider not only what intervention is being used, but how it is being delivered. These very factors must be analyzed and understood within the context of any treatment comparison and evidence-based inquiries. I have since received professional training in delivery of the Lidcombe Program in order to build my own clinical repertoire and understanding.

Many other treatment programs incorporate parents and other family members into the treatment process; however, the rationale is more practical (to facilitate development and maintenance of fluency) than conceptual (based in family systems principles) in nature. Nevertheless, the importance of approaching stuttering intervention from a family systems perspective cannot be overstated. Empirical support for this perspective has come more from allied disciplines than from communication disorders. In order to understand more fully the manner in which a family affects and is affected by a member who stutters, we need to understand the nature of that family from a systems framework. Because families are becoming increasingly diverse, as will be noted, each family must be treated as unique, and our approach to working with families must be individualized. To build this understanding, we focus next on the nature and dynamics of the family unit.

Family Diversity

Turnbull et al. (2006) indicated that traditional, somewhat nostalgic associations with the word *family* (e.g., father as breadwinner, mother at home, two or three children, all under the same roof) are not only outdated; it is unlikely that such a reality of the American family ever existed. Attempts to characterize families in general terms are futile because they are so diverse. In actuality, many people today are delaying marriage or living alone. The vast majority of married women between 18 and 34 years of age with or without children are employed outside the home. The divorce rate has topped 55%, and 20% of families with children under 18 are headed by a single parent. Beyond demographics, families differ in religion, ethnicity, education, socioeconomic status, location, values, beliefs, and family and social structure, among other ways. Each family is unique. Turnbull et al. (2006) conceptualized family systems as dynamic composites of family characteristics, interactions, and functions that develop and change over the lifespan. We will look briefly at some of their ideas to help us understand the reciprocal interactions between people who stutter and their families.

Family Characteristics

Turnbull et al. (2006) noted that the following variables influence the impact of an exceptionality on the family: characteristics of the exceptionality, characteristics of the family, personal characteristics, and special challenges.

Characteristics of the Exceptionality

First, the characteristics of the exceptionality itself affect the family's reactions, although Turnbull et al. (2006) stressed that "there is no clear-cut evidence that the particular nature of the disability alone can predict how parents, siblings, or extended family will respond and adapt to the disability" (p. 20). Turnbull also emphasized that "if you assume that a disability invariably burdens a family, you would be wrong" (p. 20). While research is needed to determine the impact of stuttering on the family system, it is clear that the nature of the exceptionality presents each family with unique challenges, special needs, and positive contributions. Given these caveats about one-size-fits-all assumptions regarding how exceptionality might affect the family system, the clinician must approach the topic with an open mind.

Characteristics of the Family

Second, characteristics of the family affect its reactions to the exceptionality. These characteristics include the family's size and form, cultural background, socioeconomic status, and geographic location. The clinician must become aware of the presence, nature, and number of children, parents, stepparents, and extended family, among other significant people. Turnbull et al. (2006) indicated the increased likelihood that clinicians will encounter families of more than two parents due to remarriage of one or both parents from the original family. The resulting blended family presents an array of family variations and emotional situations. Turnbull et al. warned against prejudgment and stereotyping, noting that the home atmosphere, quality of the family's interactions, and family's perception of itself affect the quality of family life, regardless of whether the family is nuclear, remarried, adoptive, or foster.

The individual family's cultural background often influences its rituals, traditions, and foods, in addition to its perspectives and values, which influence the members' attitudes and reactions to an exceptionality. Another factor potentially influencing a family's reactions is socioeconomic status (SES), including income, level of education, occupation, and implied social status. While higher socioeconomic status often translates to greater access to and knowledge about available services, these resources do not necessarily imply better coping skills. Families of lower socioeconomic status might have large families and broad social support networks that can be valuable resources. Related to socioeconomic status are values that impact a family's attitude toward exceptionality. For example, Turnbull et al. (2006) reported that higher socioeconomic status often relates to more achievement orientation and control of one's environment, both of which might result in greater disappointment by parents toward their aspirations for a child with an exceptionality. On the other hand, families of lower socioeconomic status might regard family solidarity and happiness as more important than achievement and control, perhaps resulting in greater acceptance and nurturing.

Again, prejudgments must not be made. Every family is unique. I remember very clearly a 3-year-old girl who stuttered with whom I worked for nearly a year before the father was transferred by his work to a city over 200 miles away. This family of few financial means did everything imaginable to be actively involved in all aspects of the intervention process, in addition to traveling the distance in an unreliable vehicle, arranging for housing with relatives, and caring for other pressing concerns. At one point the family moved locally in order to receive treatment, which resulted in either temporary separation from or extensive commutes for the father. While I was utterly moved by this family's commitment to one another and to its continuing and abiding faith (never once did I hear a complaint or unkind word), I was nevertheless uncomfortable with being responsible for the family being apart and incurring additional burden. This arrangement was alleviated when we investigated together similar and affordable intervention services in the family's new city, supplemented by ongoing indirect and less frequent direct intervention from me. This anecdote also conveys another factor—geographic location—that influences availability and affordability of services, either of which can influence a family's attitude toward the exceptionality. All people within families present both needs and positive contributions. We must work with each family individually and learn with and from them.

Personal Characteristics

Personal characteristics, including tolerance to stress, coping styles, and intellectual capacity, among others, affect a family's reactions to stuttering. These characteristics might be strengths or limitations for the individual family and will affect the clinician's approach to the family. Turnbull et al. (2006) discussed various methods for coping, or reducing feelings of stress, including *passive appraisal* (setting aside your worries), *reframing* (changing how you think about a situation in order to emphasize its positive aspects over its negative ones), *spiritual support* (deriving comfort and guidance from your spiritual beliefs), *social support* (receiving practical and emotional assistance from your friends and family members), and *professional support* (receiving assistance from human service professionals and agencies).

Turnbull and colleagues (1993) presented a series of moving essays conveying how individuals and families cope with exceptional circumstances. In one of these essays, J. B. Schulz (1993) defined cognitive coping as "the process of restructuring stressful events in positive ways" (p. 31) and indicated that her family openly discusses stressful issues and uses coping strategies including family support, previous successful experience with coping, and humor. Schulz raised important questions that might be considered by service providers, including whether cognitive coping strategies can be taught to families and people with exceptionalities to help them solve their own problems. Clinicians must be aware of the coping strategies being used so that intervention and recommendations are appropriate to the individual family. Schulz (2008) conveyed in loving terms the importance of coping strategies and positive human capacities (e.g., love, courage, persistence, resilience, hope, faith, humor) that enabled one family to be willing and able to learn and grow for over 50 years with a family member with special needs.

Another personal variable is the intellectual capacity of the family members, including the person who stutters. In other words, the extent to which people understand and can be helped to understand what is happening will affect their attitudes toward stuttering and the intervention process, and will affect how they are included as active participants.

I remember a boy of 4 years with whom I worked because of his stuttering. Recognizing the young mother's significant cognitive limitations, I included her in the intervention process but to a different extent and in a different way than I would other parents who were more cognitively able. Specifically, she was taught how to take conversational turns with her son. This was the only expectation placed upon her. Working with her was a good reminder of what we will discuss in Unit III about how to prepare parents and others to participate meaningfully in the intervention process. Such preparation, or teaching, involves no fewer than three distinct steps: telling, showing, and then directly coaching what you expect. Unfortunately, this mother's limitations were neither recognized nor accounted for by other service providers. When her son became absent from treatment for an extended time, I investigated and learned that the boy was in the hospital. I learned that he first became ill when the mother bathed him in a partially frozen creek. This was not uncommon, because the home had no indoor plumbing. The boy's illness persisted, and the caseworker urged the mother to bring the boy for medical attention. Following directions as she interpreted them, the mother filled the boy's prescription and fed him the entire bottle at one sitting. The instructions were printed on the bottle, but she was unable to read them. Thus, all persons can and should be involved in the intervention process, but the nature of involvement must take into account a variety of personal strengths and limitations. This requires that clinicians come to know their clients and their families.

Special Challenges

Finally, some families find themselves facing special challenges that might affect not only reactions toward the exceptionality but also the family's willingness to participate in and contribute to intervention programs. Such situations include families who live in poverty or are homeless, in rural areas, in homes where abuse or neglect occurs, or where one or more members are ill, disabled, involved in substance abuse, or imprisoned. Too often, professionals assume that parents who do not participate in the intervention process care less about their children than those who do. Another interpretation, often verified if given the opportunity, is that for some people, the more basic needs of their children, such as food, shelter, and health, take precedence, leaving few available resources in terms of time, money, and physical and emotional energy to address the child's communication needs.

I remember interviewing a mother who referred to me her 9-year-old son because of stuttering. The mother was 34 years old, was African American, and took the day off work to travel 120 miles for the evaluation. At first, her manner was at best guarded and her communication style was passive. She responded briefly to questions asked of her, offered little elaboration, and did not initiate topics for discussion when invited to do so or when provided silence. What I most recall was that when we were seated, she demonstrated no direct eye contact, a forward slouching posture, and constantly fidgeting hands. This woman was tense. The evaluation proceeded, after which I conferenced with her again to describe my observations and evaluation. As usual, I began by highlighting the aspects of the interaction I observed between the woman and her son that were particularly facilitative of fluency and gentle, uninterrupted conversational turn-taking. I also expressed my sincere appreciation to her for doing all she had to in order to be present for the evaluation. As the summary continued, I noticed that she began to participate more in the conversation, asking questions, seeking clarification, and initiating topics. Her posture became more inviting, and when she offered me her eye contact, I noticed that her eyes were reddening. What followed would best be described as a conversationally and emotionally cathartic experience for this woman. The following statement was taken from among the many significant feelings and observations she shared:

> You are the first professional who has made me feel that I am worth a damn. Most of the others think that because I am on Welfare that I am not a good mother. I love my boy. He's all I got. I would do anything for him. But I got to work. All the others tell me what I do wrong, tell what I should do. They don't know me. They don't want to know me. They judge me. I know it. You tell me I do something right. That is everything.

Families who live in rural areas often report feelings of loneliness and social isolation, particularly with respect to having others with whom to discuss feelings and experiences related to stuttering. Also, those in rural areas might incur geographic, in addition to financial, limitations in accessing services. Unique challenges are experienced by families in which abusive situations exist and when other members, including parents, are ill or disabled. These and other such situations already described are reminders of the importance of individualizing treatment with families and working from a team approach, a topic to be explored later in this chapter.

Family Interactions

In addition to being keenly aware of family characteristics, clinicians must become knowledgeable about the unique patterns of interaction within each family. Events affecting any one member can impact all family members and others within the communication system. J. B. Schulz (1993), referring to family members as "heroes in disguise," added that "in family system theory, we frequently state that what happens to a person with a disability happens to the entire family. What we fail to mention is that what happens to the family also happens to the person with a disability" (p. 31). Turnbull et al. (2006) discussed four family subsystems that must be recognized and understood. These are the *marital subsystem* (interactions between husband and wife or same-sex partners), *parental subsystem* (interactions among parents and their children), *sibling subsystem* (interactions among the children in a family), and *extended family subsystem* (interactions among members of the nuclear family, relatives, and others who are regarded as relatives, e.g., friends, neighbors, and professionals). In regard to extended family subsystems, note that in Native American families (Turnbull, Turnbull, & Wehmeyer, 2007) and African families (Mandela, 1995), distinctions between degrees of relation are typically not made. Mandela noted,

> In African culture, the sons and daughters of one's aunts or uncles are considered brothers and sisters, not cousins. We do not make the same distinction among relations practiced by whites. We have no half brothers or half sisters. My mother's sister is my mother; my uncle's son is my brother; my brother's child is my son, my daughter. (p. 8)

Within each of these subsystems, the impact of a family member with an exceptionality is experienced in many different ways. Thoughts, feelings, and behaviors all are affected. Such an experience can have a positive, bonding impact within the interactions, or can have a negative, interpersonally destructive impact within the family. Again, without prejudgment, the clinician must assess the impact of the stuttering and tailor the intervention and the respective participation of the family members accordingly. Before discussing the interaction between family patterns and the change process, I will introduce the concepts of family cohesion and adaptability as aspects of family interaction. Both these constructs should be viewed as points on a continuum rather than as representing a family typology.

Family Cohesion

Elements of interaction, including cohesion and adaptability, are used to help understand the ways people within a family interact. Turnbull et al. (2006) noted that "family cohesion refers to family members' close emotional bonding with each other and to the level of independence they feel within the family system" (p. 43). Cohesion within interpersonal relationships is characterized as falling along a continuum from *high enmeshment* on one end and *high disengagement* on the other (Epstein & Baucom, 2002; Gladding, 2007; Luterman, 2008; M. P. Nichols, 2004; Turnbull et al., 2006; Walsh, 2003, 2006). Both enmeshment and disengagement define the relative degree to which boundaries are open versus closed for relationships within and across the interpersonal subsystems described. High enmeshment means that boundaries between family subsystems are not well defined; thus relationships often are characterized by overinvolvement, overprotection, and insulation from demands requiring independence or risk taking. Most decisions and activities are family focused, allowing little privacy for individual family members. In such families, one often finds the stuttering to be the center of the family's existence, the focal point around which most activity and interactions are based; this style of interaction can isolate the family from contact with others.

In contrast to highly enmeshed families are those described as disengaged. Highly disengaged families maintain strict boundaries between family subsystems. The family may deny the existence of the stuttering, thus withholding emotional support and friendship from the member who stutters and who may experience loneliness. Such families are characterized by little involvement among its members, few shared interests, extensive privacy, more time apart than together, and independent rather than joint decision making. Most healthy families experience a balance between enmeshment and disengagement, clearly understanding family limits and boundaries, and thus inviting close bonding and nurturing independence and autonomy. As noted earlier, clinicians need to be aware of the level of cohesion within and between family subsystems in order to tailor intervention and recommendations that are sensitive and responsive to each family.

Family Adaptability

Another variable for clinicians to consider is *family adaptability*, the ability to change or adjust in response to stresses. Just as individuals need to have an awareness of their personal constructs in order to gain active control over the alternative choices they are facing, so families need to understand their view of a problem to accommodate change when appropriate. Families that are unwilling or unable to change are considered *rigid*; those that are always changing without a sense of structure or plan are considered *chaotic*. Just as healthy families have struck a balance between enmeshment and disengagement, so too do healthy families fall between the extremes of rigidity and chaos. Families that are rigid experience high control and structure, strict rules and role definitions, and little sharing or negotiation. The intervention process from a systems perspective requires that family members actively participate and support the person who stutters. This expectation often proves problematic with rigid families. While structure varies with each individual family, as noted, there are still some in which the mother is expected to meet the child's ever-changing academic, social, extracurricular, and developmental needs. In such families where roles are firmly and inflexibly established, the mother may feel overly burdened and stressed by addressing alone the added accommodations required when a child stutters. Without shared family ownership of the challenges presented by a person who stutters and the resulting intervention plan, the potential effectiveness of intervention is significantly reduced. Furthermore, the reality of stuttering and the intervention may be denied, if not rejected, by the other family members, causing further conflict.

Chaotic families, by contrast, are relatively unstructured and their interactions are guided by few rules, which are rarely enforced and frequently change. People outside of the family can no more count on commitments made by the family than the members can themselves. Often there is no family leadership, which results in little control, endless discussion and negotiation, unclear family role distinctions, and little concern for future planning. All families experience temporary periods of rigidity and chaos during particularly stressful life events. Most families fall somewhere between the two polar opposites. Only when such extremes become a family's mode of operation does a problem arise for working with its members in a program of fluency intervention. In any case, intervention and related recommendations must reflect and be responsive to the uniqueness of each family system and its members.

Family Patterns and Change

Family interactions tend to be highly reciprocal, patterned, and repetitive (E. A. Carter & Orfanidis, 1996). As noted, a systems perspective assumes the interactions are indeed systemic (circular) rather than linear (J. R. Andrews & Andrews, 2000). In other words, it is of limited utility for family members (or a clinician) to look exclusively for direct cause-and-effect relationships. For example, while it might be tempting blame someone for a family member's worsening stuttering, doing so falls short of identifying interactive and perpetuating patterns and tracing their flow. Carter and Orfanidis noted that all family patterns, once established, are perpetuated by everyone involved in them. Nevertheless, when stress enters into any of the two-person subsystems (parent–parent, parent–child, child–child), a pattern of scapegoating, or *triangulation*, frequently is observed. This means that the two people experiencing a problem come to focus on a third person (or thing, or external issue) in order to divert anxiety in the relationship. This pattern is dysfunctional in that it offers stabilization by diversion, thus perpetuating the problem rather than working toward resolution or change. Luterman (2008) noted that a child is often triangulated into a marital conflict and that the child's symptoms, whatever they might be, serve to distract the parents from their other problems. The cost to the child is significant. If the child's symptoms are removed or alleviated, the family's homeostasis, or conditions operating to promote status quo functioning, would be threatened. Therefore, family members experience conflict—they alleviate the child's symptoms (gain) at the expense of the parent's shared focus (cost), or maintain the child's symptoms (cost) to promote apparent harmony among the parents (gain). In any case, this zero sum conflict (if one gains, the other loses) exacts a mighty toll on the child, who already is experiencing significant demands and therefore is likely to be functioning under reduced capacity.

Hartman and Laird (1983) described the potential benefits and drawbacks of change within a family as creating a paradox:

> Change can be frightening. In some families, any change is perceived as an enemy which must be warded off—a threat to coherence, stability, or even continued existence. . . . Families over a period of time propagate rules and patterns of behavior which gain certain coherence and which serve to preserve the family. "Symptoms" or problematic behaviors are often an essential, indeed key part, of the family's effort to maintain itself. . . . The symptom should be understood, then, not as a problem but rather as a solution to another more grievous or threatening problem, one which might expose a feared secret, threaten the family with dissolution, or otherwise shake its very foundations. Such a family is in a paradoxical situation in the sense that they want the disturbing symptom to change but they do not want, or rather are afraid for, the family itself to change. Yet one cannot happen without the other. (pp. 326–327)

Others have documented marital partners in conflict who triangulated a family member, frequently a child, with exceptionalities ranging from psychiatric disturbance (Satir, 1983), psychosomatic illness (e.g., asthma, anorexia, diabetes), dependence, depression, academic failure, sexual promiscuity (Hartman & Laird, 1983), and stuttering (Rollin, 2000). All recommended that intervention occur at the level of the family rather than the individual. Hartman and Laird noted that the family unit is both a resource of and target for change that must be understood within the context of its own unique ecological environment (the complex interrelationships among physical, social, psychological, and cultural forces). Luterman (2008) reminded us that many of the families with whom we work are stressed because they include a person with a communication disorder, but they are not necessarily dysfunctional. Clinicians must be aware of and sensitive to issues and concepts related to family interaction, including the subsystems and relative cohesion and adaptability of the members.

Turnbull et al. (2006) indicated that family interactions are influenced by available resources, characteristics of the exceptionality, values, and ethnic background. The nature of the subsystems and the respective interactions change as a family moves through the life cycle. Clinicians are reminded that intervention with people who stutter should not be approached in isolation, or from what has been referred to as a linear perspective. My own observations, however, unfortunately suggest that this is often the case. Luterman (2008) concluded as follows:

> The family is a system in which all of the components are interdependent. Every family member affects every other component of the family; for the family therapist, there is no such thing as individual therapy—any time a change occurs in one member of the family, everybody in the family is impacted. Working in individual therapy with an identified patient in a dysfunctional family burdens the individual to become a change agent for the family. This is often too difficult a task for the patient, especially if the patient is a child. Family therapists find it much more efficacious to work at the systems level; in fact, many family therapists refuse to work with individuals. (p. 147)

Family Functions

Sometimes in our interactions with people who stutter and their families, we clinicians inadvertently assume that the family's sole function is to participate in our intervention plan. As a consequence, we experience a measure of discouragement in what appears to be our clients' failure to recognize the source and degree of inspiration from which the plan was derived. I am not making light of the fact that a high level of sincere motivation and commitment from both the client and clinician is essential to the clinical process. However, I do want to underscore that clinicians' expectations must be tempered by an understanding of the different and at times conflicting functions of our clients and their families that might occasionally interfere with participation in intervention. Family functions are interdependent and occasionally pose conflicting demands. These functions fall into eight broad categories: economic, daily care, recreation, socialization, self-esteem, affection, educational/vocational, and spiritual (Turnbull et al., 2006). While these and other functions are distinct, any one dimension of family functioning often impacts other dimensions.

For example, it is easy to see how economic constraints can limit resources and outlets for recreation, socialization, and education. Family tension can be increased by financial pressure, thus negatively impacting the affection offered to others, particularly those who, because of stuttering or another exceptionality, might pose an additional financial burden. Turnbull et al. (2006) pointed out that "some families have increased consumptive demands and decreased productive capacities, also known as lost opportunities, because of their children's disabilities" (p. 59). Furthermore, "Family resources vary tremendously, and finances affect how families respond to the challenges of their children's exceptionality. You should not assume that families who cannot spend at the level you want them to are less committed to their children than more affluent families" (p. 58).

I am reminded of a man in his 50s who, with absolute support and participation of his family, demonstrated a model commitment to the treatment process. During one of our many conversations, he discussed the actual cost incurred by his family for the treatment process. The direct cost of treatment was only the beginning. The time he took off from work to attend treatment had a significant financial impact because he was paid on an hourly basis. When it was possible for him to make up the hours, he was paid at the regular rate, rather than for overtime. His wife, an active and regular participant in the treatment process, also needed to adjust her work schedule, which required administrative approval although it presented no additional financial burden. He pointed out that the long drive necessitated additional car repairs, which to him seemed minor in the long run. While the man's tone was positive and did not present even the shadow of a complaint, this discussion was a good reminder for me of the commitment offered by this man and his family. One day during treatment, the man indicated that he would be absent for one session the following month. He explained that he and his family had planned an important social and recreational activity that would be fairly expensive, and when combined with treatment would create a financial hardship for that month. How easy it would have been for me or any other clinician to misinterpret this honest expression as an indication of the client's waning commitment for treatment. Rather, I chose to express appreciation for his candor, particularly in light of his resolute participation in the treatment process, and to honor the importance of the social event to him and his family.

I have said that we must value people who stutter as members of a family system, all of whose functions, including, but not limited to, fluency intervention, must be acknowledged and respected. In this case, I arranged to waive the fee for treatment during that particular week so that the client could engage in both important activities. While the suggestion of this arrangement startled the client and caused visible reactions of embarrassment, conducting the session as planned and at no cost sent a powerful message regarding the degree to which he and his family were valued as people and active participants in family functioning, including the treatment process. My intention here is not to recommend my decision for other clinicians, to discuss the implications of fees for service, or to debate the sincerity of the client's candor. We clinicians, when designing and implementing treatment, must value people who stutter as functioning in capacities beyond those that we directly observe. That value must be appreciated implicitly and acknowledged explicitly.

Another reminder is that for all of us, including people who stutter, there are just so many hours in a day. Clinicians need to be mindful of the many and often conflicting demands upon our clients as participants in different family functions. Treatment-related activities must be planned *with*, rather than *for*, our clients with an appreciation of the many demands upon them. Believe me; I am not reluctant to hold people who stutter to their treatment obligations, albeit within a positive framework. However, a client's occasional lack of follow-through might well reflect bona fide demands, not lack of commitment to treatment.

I once worked with a 35-year-old man who was in a failing marriage. While he was in fluency treatment, his marriage dissolved and he gained sole custody of his two sons, then aged 7 and 9 years. To make ends meet, this man worked three jobs and was a full-time college student pursuing a career in computer programming. While his parents helped occasionally with childcare, the demands of daily living combined with economic hardship were keen. This man, in my estimation, was responsible to a fault. Assignments were always jointly designed and completed satisfactorily. Independently, he initiated and designed a personalized evaluation system to critique his extraclinical speech-related activities, which were recorded frequently each day in a pocket journal. Treatment was canceled frequently, however, due to the demands related to his family obligations, including children's illness, teacher conferences, and doctor's appointments, among others. One time, he called to explain that he had just pulled out of his garage on the way to treatment when his old truck caught fire. The firefighters were extinguishing the blaze as we spoke. Surely, these frequent interruptions reduced treatment progress. We discussed this and other issues of treatment continuity and transfer and compensated as much as possible through tailored home assignments. Some clinicians would have terminated his enrollment because of breach of attendance. I chose not to. I believed that he demonstrated absolute commitment and responsibility to all of his obligations and family functions, including fluency intervention. As he progressed through treatment, which was protracted and adjusted frequently to meet his unique needs, he gained control of his fluency and other aspects of his life. He is a successful father, college graduate, computer programmer, respected citizen, and yes, fluent speaker. I admire his dedication and his personal constructs, which helped him to maintain strength and perseverance through adversity. He recently shared with me his excitement over having met a wonderful woman. My classes have been inspired and moved to tears on more than one occasion when he and his sons have shared their experiences and their appreciation for the support and understanding they feel they received during the treatment process.

Once again, we need to remind ourselves that we all, clients and clinicians, are members of family systems and experience interdependent functions and occasionally conflicting demands. When we work with people who stutter, we are challenged not to become narrowly focused in our efforts or judgmental in our interpretations. The mother of a 15-year-old boy who stutters, actively participating in the treatment process, realized that she, not the clinician, had become too narrowly focused on problems that commanded her immediate attention. The mother's words might remind clinicians of the importance of viewing people who stutter as able members of a family and communication system and of incorporating that view into the treatment process. Her words, taken from a letter to the clinician, follow:

> Observing you with my son helped me understand the "magic" of your success with him. You are so interested in who he is and who he is becoming, in his goals, in what is important to him. You are excited by his interests. Your genuine acceptance and approval of him is very inspiring to him. You honor the adolescent struggle of forging a separate identity. Listening to you rekindled that awareness in me. You reminded me to celebrate this "rite of passage." I am ashamed that I allow the urgent, daily life to overshadow these more important things. Thank you for helping me to refocus on this awesome developmental process.

Family Life Cycle

Describing the family life cycle, McGoldrick and Carter (2003; see also B. Carter & McGoldrick, 2005, p. 1) referred to the family as "a system moving through time" (p. 376). It is within this cycle that the family is viewed as the major context for the development of its members. Each family frames and approaches challenges within the contexts of past and present experiences in addressing challenges and problems, and the future toward which the family is moving. The experience of stuttering and its influence on members of the family system can be viewed as one such challenge. McGoldrick and Carter indicated that distinct phases in the developmental cycle can be identified and predicted. An understanding of the family life cycle is essential for dealing with people who stutter, all of whom are members of, influence, and are influenced by their respective family units.

Family Roles Affect Fluency Treatment

Some may ask why an understanding of a family's life cycle is important to working with people who stutter. As noted, anything happening to one person affects and is affected by other members of the family system. For this reason alone, it is foolhardy to direct our clinical efforts to the person who stutters without consideration of the others with whom this person communicates regularly. The needs of all involved must be taken into account for treatment to be effective and generalizable.

For example, when adjusting the clinical activities for home programming with a man who stutters and his wife, both of whom were in their 50s, I deliberately asked how the fluency changes were being addressed by the couple. The man said things were fine. The woman expressed uncertainty as to the limits of her responsibility. He was to talk with her as part of his assignments to report fluent words and experiences of self-correction, and she was to feel comfortable providing positive feedback when she heard him use his fluency controls. She was not expected, however, to correct him with respect to the nature of their relationship as husband and wife, and not to assume that she was the clinician in absentia. Furthermore, we had discussed that he needed to handle increasing amounts of responsibility for fluency independence and guard against building dependence on the clinician, his wife, or anyone else. Although the respective involvement of each was a topic of weekly discussion, followed by modeling and feedback, both had come to assume that she was to correct him when he failed to use his fluency controls. Both expressed feelings that she was letting him down when she did not correct him or keep him on task. The subsequent discussion was essential to restate and redemonstrate the roles of each, and particularly to provide her with an opportunity to continue to feel needed and appreciated in ways other than as his spokesperson. Without such regular discussion and attention to the needs of both parties, her involvement would likely have become an irritant and an inhibitor, rather than a facilitator, of treatment.

Family Stress Affects Fluency Treatment

Another reason that we need to understand the family life cycle is to recognize stressful experiences for what they are and how they may affect a person's fluency and the treatment process. Stress experienced within a family often occurs around transition points in the life cycle, frequently disrupting the cycle or producing symptoms of dysfunction (B. Carter & McGoldrick, 2005; McGoldrick & Carter, 2003). Stuttering can be one such symptom of stress or disruption (Rollin, 2000). Stress increases the demand on a person, which can limit one's capacity for fluency and other aspects of coping. For these reasons, we need to know what stages a family might be experiencing to better understand the effect of potentially stressful events. One's readiness for treatment, too, will in part depend on the stage within the life cycle being experienced by the person who stutters and the family.

For example, given the assumptions underlying the theory of stuttering as resulting from multifactorial causes, parents of a preschool child who is beginning to stutter often are directed to adjust the demanding family functions to accommodate the requirements of treatment (such as time for participating in treatment, home activities, financial cost, and rescheduling of other activities). Likewise, if one of the parents requests fluency intervention for himself or herself, a realistic question will involve the extent to which the family can accommodate the requirements of treatment. I have worked with a number of young parents who have demonstrated to themselves the ability to speak fluently, but because of conflicting demands (a newly born infant, recovery of mother, work demands, and others) were unable to put themselves and their management of speech fluency as a priority. The relative priority of the fluency treatment within the existing demands on the person and the family will impact a clinician's decision regarding the appropriateness of the timing for intervention and the viability of the person as a candidate for intervention. Perkins (2000, 2006) spoke of clients' opting for disfluency over fluency because the constant cost, measured in the effort expended to maintain fluency, proved too high.

Families as Portraits of Development and Change

In each family, there are distinct developmental stages during which each member is engaged in fairly predictable tasks related to his or her period in life. Such tasks are influenced by factors already discussed, including family characteristics (size, membership, ethnicity, values, special challenges, and faith, among others), interactions within and between family subsystems, and diverse and at times conflicting family functions and individual commitments. Turnbull et al. (2006) pointed out that all life-cycle interpretations are culturally and historically specific, generalized representations of family change, and therefore unique to each family. Common family changes are experienced as its members are born, grow up, leave home, develop long-term relationships, retire, and die. Consequently, the characteristics and functions of the family and its members also change developmentally with such transitions and idiosyncratic variation.

Different authors have presented varying representations of the family life cycle. When becoming familiar with and thinking about such models, clinicians should consider the reciprocal interaction between the family's stage and its experiences related to the person who stutters. McGoldrick and Carter (1982) presented what they considered to be the usual (i.e., statistically predictable) family life cycle in middle-class America in the last quarter of the 20th century, and noted that such realities are changing. These changes were precipitated by lower birth rates, longer life expectancy, and increasing divorce and remarriage rates. Whereas childrearing once occupied adults for their entire active life span, it now consumes less than half the time span prior to old age. Conceptualizations of family, therefore, are changing because they are no longer organized primarily around this activity and because both men and women are considering more varied personal and professional options. Indeed, McGoldrick and Carter (2003) more recently advised,

> It is time for us as professionals to give up our attachments to the old ideals and put a more positive conceptual frame around what is: two-paycheck marriages; permanent "single-parent" households; unmarried, remarried, and gay and lesbian couples and families; single-parent adoptions; and women of all ages alone. It is past time to stop thinking of transitional crises as permanent traumas, and to drop from our vocabulary words and phrases that link us to the norms and prejudices of the past: "children of divorce," "out-of-wedlock child," "fatherless home," "working mother," and the like. (p. 381)

As with classification schemes in general, conceptualizations of the family life cycle in terms of predictable developmental sequences or stages provide a context for comparison in order to identify the uniqueness of each family's development, and they should not be used to pigeonhole families. The importance of recognizing the uniqueness of each family was highlighted by McGoldrick and Carter (2003):

> Families comprise persons who have a shared history and a shared future. They encompass the entire emotional system of at least three and frequently four or even five generations, held together by blood, legal, and/or historical ties. Relationships with parents, siblings, and other family members go through transitions as they move along the life cycle. Boundaries shift, psychological distance among members changes, and roles within and between subsystems are constantly being redefined. (p. 376)

Bearing these cautions in mind, and cognizant of the dynamic changes occurring in the "American family" in this first quarter of the 21st century, B. Carter and McGoldrick (2005) described the family life cycle as a sequence of six stages, with particular emphasis on the emotional network and transitions within the family, as follows:

- ⚏ The unattached young adult, who is between family systems, is in the process of separating from parents, which requires differentiating self from family, developing peer relationships, and securing and maintaining a job.

- ⚏ The newly married couple, which has joined families through marriage, is establishing a commitment to a new system. This requires formation of a marital family system and realignment of relationships with extended families and friends.

- ⚏ The family with young children, which is in the process of accepting new members into the system, must adjust the marital system to make room for the child or children, take on new parenting roles, and realign relationships with extended family to include parenting and grandparenting roles.

- ⚏ The family with adolescents, which is increasing the flexibility of family boundaries to accommodate children's independence, must adjust the parent–child relationship, refocus on midlife marital and career issues, and begin to focus on concerns of older age.

- ⚏ The family that is launching children and moving on must accept a multitude of exits from and entries into the family system. At the same time, the partners must renegotiate the marital system as a dyad, nurture adult relationships with grown children, realign relationships to include in-laws and grandchildren, and deal with failing health of parents (i.e., grandparents).

⌗ The family in later life must accept the shifting of generational roles. This requires maintaining one's own and the couple's functioning and interests during physiological decline, exploring new family and social role options, supporting the more central role for the middle generation, making room in the system for the needs and wisdom of the older generation, preparing for and dealing with loss of spouse, siblings, and peers, and preparing for one's own death. This is the period of life review and integration.

Turnbull et al. (2006) identified four life-cycle stages of family development, emphasizing the potential impact that an exceptionality of one member may have on the family unit. A summary of their thoughts follows:

⌗ *Birth and early childhood (ages 0–5 years)*: The parents have had some experience integrating their own values and responding to each other's needs and now are challenged to nurture the child's needs without forgetting their own. Also, this stage is often when the exceptionality is identified, when families are in first contact with educational and allied health professionals, and when expectations are established or revised for the children. Families and providers of early intervention should celebrate the child's positive contributions and abilities. The need for a positive outlook is particularly relevant to developmental stuttering.

⌗ *School age (ages 6–12 years)*: Upon entry into school, children broaden social horizons and establish friendships. Parents begin a long process of letting go, turning over responsibility for their child to others. Children with exceptionalities often move from noncategorical to categorical intervention, where clinical labels are applied. They are apt to encounter their first experience of social stigma for being different. A positive approach contributes to the family–professional partnership.

⌗ *Adolescence (ages 12–21 years)*: This stage is characterized by stressful changes, both physical and psychological. Coinciding with puberty are a variety of challenging tasks, including development of self-identity, development of positive body image, adjustment to sexual maturation, emotional independence from parents, and development of mature social relationships. Parents often find this period stressful because their authority is challenged by their child's growing independence and because they begin to face issues of midlife; for example, their own perceived attractiveness and youthfulness begin to decline at the very time their children are becoming attractive adults. Adolescents who stutter must balance the implications of social stigma with the development of self-advocacy skills.

⌗ *Adulthood (ages 21+ years)*: There are many cultural variations for when and how adulthood is attained. Generally, however, this means the acquisition of greater independence and responsibility. In the last quarter of the 20th century for middle-class America, this has meant finding employment and moving away from the parents' home. Not all families separate emotionally or geographically.

Summary—Family-Based Treatment

Many models exist to represent the family life cycle. They attempt to reflect the ongoing and developmental process of change within families. At each developmental stage and particularly at points of transition, changes occur within families' interactions and approach to life. Clinicians working with people who stutter must address their needs from a family systems perspective. One member of a family cannot be understood in isolation from the rest of the system. A family's structure, organization, and interactional patterns are among the factors that determine the behavior of the person who stutters and that of the other members. Therefore, changes in the behavior of one member of a family affect and are affected by the behavior of the other members of the family. For these and other reasons, clinicians must be aware of such factors when approaching the challenges of fluency intervention. Turnbull et al. (2006) pointed out that under the best of circumstances, life transitions within families are difficult. This difficulty is compounded when a family member has an exceptionality. Turnbull and Turnbull (1990) offered valuable insights for clinicians working from a family systems perspective with a person who has an exceptionality:

1. Every family brings a different set of characteristics, values, and styles to their experience with exceptionality; thus, you will need to individualize your approach to working with families.

2. Families have an interactional style that dictates the way the members fall into subsystems as well as their preferred levels of closeness and flexibility. To be effective, you will find it helpful to encourage balance and to adapt interventions according to family needs and preferences.

3. Families have a variety of coping skills that enable them to meet their tangible and intangible needs. Respect each family's priorities and encourage the family to attend to the different needs of all its members.

4. Families change over time; therefore, families will need you to help them meet the needs of different developmental stages and also to ease the stress of transition from one stage to another. (p. 141)

Chapter Summary

This chapter reviewed central and guiding intervention assumptions from intrafamily perspectives. Specifically, we addressed personal constructs and family systems. An understanding of personal construct theory and its relevance to intervention reveals that stuttering-related thoughts, feelings, and behavior reflect in part the consequence of active and alternative choices. All people, including those who stutter and their clinicians, develop a perspective about the world and themselves based on previous experiences. These systems of personal constructs help us anticipate and respond to, if not shape, future events. When we are explicitly aware of our client's personal constructs, we are better able to effect positive and proactive changes in his communication skills and how he views himself as a communicator. When we are explicitly aware of our own personal constructs regarding our role as a clinician and as a facilitator of change, we can make necessary adjustments to meet our clients' objectives while planning for and effecting growth in our own professional development. Personal construct theory tells us that we do not need to stick with the past or maintain the status quo. By becoming aware of our assumptions, and thereby our interpretation of past events, clients and clinicians can evaluate the appropriateness of the constructs that they have formed. If the constructs are found to be incorrect, inappropriate, or undesirable, we can consciously revise them to achieve the outcomes that were not or did not seem possible previously (such as speaking with greater fluency, using self-corrections more often, or considering the client's point of view). Personal construct theory holds that all people have choices and that "all of our present interpretations of the universe are subject to revision and replacement" (G. A. Kelly, 1955a, p. 15). This constructive freedom, combined with personal responsibility, is at the heart of "constructive alternativism." Clinicians must shift perspective so as to see and understand the client's world as the client sees it.

In practical terms, personal construct theory means that we interpret our present and predict our future on the basis of our past (e.g., people who stutter anticipate fluency failure on the basis of an amassed foundation of fluency failure). Therefore, it is the clinician's responsibility to construct *for* the client (and eventually *with* the client and ultimately *by* the client) speaking opportunities that result in fluency success. The successes experienced directly by the client must be so frequent, consistent, and salient that the client becomes compelled to reconsider how he anticipates his communication future.

He begins to construct an alternative foundation, one of fluency success. The client's experiences speak louder than the clinician's words. When the client discovers that it is inappropriate to anticipate fluency failure from a foundation of fluency success, he revises his personal construct on the basis of his own experiences. How we construct those positive, successful speaking experiences will be the focus of subsequent chapters.

This chapter also addressed family systems theory, which emphasizes that the changes in or experiences of one member trigger compensatory changes in other members. Thus, one part of the family cannot be understood in isolation from the other members of the system. Clinicians must understand and work with the families of their clients who stutter. Doing so requires that clinicians shift from a monocular to a polyocular perspective (from holding one perspective as correct to viewing different interpretations of the same event as potentially equally correct), from labeling to understanding (moving from labeling behaviors to identifying interactive patterns and finding solutions), and from behaviors to systems (moving from a focus on causes and effects to transformations within an integrated communication system). Family-based treatment requires that families and professionals interact as partners, and that clinicians understand, model, and nurture the characteristics of optimal and successful families. Various studies were reviewed that empirically support the efficacy of family-based treatment. In order to understand how a family affects and is affected by a member who stutters, the nature and dynamics of the family unit must be addressed, including family diversity, characteristics, interaction, functions, and life cycle. Several examples of family-based treatment for fluency disorders, built on the foundation of family systems principles, were reviewed (Botterill & Kelman, 2010; Cook & Botterill, 2005; Millard et al., 2008; Yaruss et al., 2006). Other programs that utilize the family structure as the context for treatment and change, emphasizing the importance of the parent's role in stuttering intervention, albeit not based on family systems principles, were reviewed as well (i.e., Lidcombe Program; see Bernstein Ratner & Guitar, 2006; Harrison & Onslow, 2010; Harrison et al., 2007; Onslow et al., 2003). Proponents of all programs of stuttering intervention, including those based upon the demands and capacities model and the Lidcombe Program, must work toward collecting efficacy data to establish effectiveness, to analyze the influence of the individual treatment components, and to ensure selection of a treatment that is most appropriate for each individual family (Franken et al., 2005).

Chapter Five Study Questions

1. Understanding our own and our client's personal constructs is essential for providing effective intervention. How might a client's or clinician's personal constructs impact the assessment and treatment processes? What can be done to maximize a positive treatment outcome?

2. Constructive alternativism invites constructive freedom combined with personal responsibility. What is the relevance of constructive alternativism to assessing and treating people who stutter, predicting treatment outcome, and working with families? What is the relevance of constructive alternativism to engaging in professional preparation (the academic, clinical, and supervisory processes), maintaining professional growth, and engaging in lifelong learning?

3. A family systems approach to intervention emphasizes the importance of working with families, rather than just with individuals who stutter. Indeed, clinicians' interpersonal (i.e., counseling) skills are critical for effective intervention. How will you

as a clinician remain within the limits of your professional training and competence? What challenges do you feel are within the boundaries of your training? Which exceed the limits of your training? How will you recognize the difference and what will you do should you find yourself expected to perform outside these limits? What other challenges do you feel you will encounter from a family systems perspective? What are the similarities and differences between a family systems approach and more traditional forms of intervention? In what ways might working from a family systems approach facilitate interdisciplinary forms of intervention?

4. We have emphasized the importance of understanding the nature and dynamics of families. How does an understanding of the family life cycle affect you personally and professionally? How has your understanding developed over time? How will your understanding continue to develop? In what ways might this understanding impact your work with clients who stutter and their families?

5. How do you define "family"? How do you describe the "American family"? How have conceptions of the "American family" changed over time, and how are those changes relevant to the way we approach assessment and intervention?

6. Intervention is affected by many different variables. One such variable is setting. How might different treatment settings (school, university, private clinic, hospital, or day care, among others) influence your potential application of personal construct theory and family systems theory? What about the impact of other variables (e.g., status, power, degree, professional training, gender, age, cultural differences)?

7. Franken et al. (2005) discussed the importance of selecting a stuttering intervention program that is most appropriate for the uniqueness of each individual family. What factors would you consider in selecting a stuttering intervention program for a person who stutters and his family? What factors would lead you to select a treatment based upon the demands and capacities model? What factors would lead you to select the Lidcombe Program? What factors would help you distinguish between the two types of programs (you might want to take a sneak peek at Chapter 7)?

8. The title of an article written by Manning (2004) is "How Can You Understand? You Don't Stutter!" How does one gain an understanding of stuttering? Does a person who stutters necessarily have a better understanding of stuttering than a person who does not stutter? Why or why not? What are the implications of personal construct theory and family systems theory on understanding stuttering and people who stutter? In what ways might efficacy data reflect an understanding of the stuttering experience? In what ways might efficacy data constrain an understanding of the stuttering experience? What do you wish you knew about stuttering and people who stutter? What do you wish people who stutter knew? How can we facilitate that knowledge? How has your understanding of stuttering developed over time? In what ways do you expect your understanding to continue to develop?

9. Go out into the community with one of your classmates or colleagues so that each of you can take a turn as a person who stutters. At no time should you reveal that you really speak normally. After the experience, consider your physical, cognitive, and affective reactions, those of your colleague, and those you perceive were experienced by your conversational partner. What insights did you gain from this experience about communication, stuttering, people who stutter, and yourself?

Chapter Six

Interdisciplinary Teaming and Multicultural Awareness
Extrafamily Considerations

Let us remember one thing about the soul. It is like a wild animal: tough, self-sufficient, resilient, but also exceedingly shy. Let us remember that if we go crashing through the woods, screaming and yelling for the soul to come out, it will evade us all day and all night. We cannot beat the bushes and yell at each other if we expect this precious inwardness to emerge. But if you are willing to go into the woods and sit quietly at the base of a tree, that wild animal will, after a few hours, reveal itself to you. (P. J. Palmer, 1997, p. 9)

The present chapter addresses interdisciplinary teaming and multicultural awareness, both of which are critical to effective and responsive intervention with people who stutter. Within this chapter, we will discuss the following:

- Interdisciplinary practice provides for collaborative opportunities to work with and learn from people who stutter, family members, and allied professionals while ensuring the highest quality of service delivery.
- Multicultural education invites clinicians to appreciate human diversity in all of its forms and to resolve to approach each person, including those who stutter and their family members, as individuals who are blessed with similarities and differences.

Interdisciplinary Practice

The concept of interdisciplinary practice, or collective collaboration, among allied professionals is not new. Our enthusiasm for this process, our expectation for people with exceptionalities and their families to participate actively in this process, and our concern over the paucity of efficacy data to validate the process, however, are relatively recent (Caldwell, Atwal, Copp, Brett-Richards, & Coleman, 2006; Franks et al., 2007; E. J. Shapiro & Dempsey, 2008). Interdisciplinary team intervention has been described as both "family-centered" and "community-based" (Rokusek, 1995, p. 1). Interdisciplinary teams involve a "partnership [that] requires a shift from valuing the individual to valuing the individual within the family within the community" (Sokoly & Dokecki, 1992, p. 24). This partnership, which includes people who stutter, their families, allied professionals, paraprofessionals, and community resources, among others, assumes a balance of shared responsibility for individually tailored and effective intervention.

Interdisciplinary Practice Defined

As with most other concepts within the human service professions, there are at least as many definitions for interdisciplinary practice as there are practitioners. One of the most succinct is "involving, or joining, two or more disciplines" (Thyer & Kropf, 1995, p. i). Rokusek (1995) indicated that interdisciplinary practice involves "individuals coming together to identify the course of action that is most effective and reasonable for the challenge(s) presented. It means equal input and respect from all persons to reach a goal—or scores of goals" (p. 1). Rokusek also stated,

> Interdisciplinary practice is the ability to practice one's own profession while linking into the work of others. Interdisciplinary practice requires knowledge and skill that differentiates one's work from that of others within a single frame of reference. Consumers/patients gain from the numerous advantages of interdependent practice in that various (and often numerous) needs are met, continuity of service is likely, and professionals/practitioners are open to several approaches and options. (p. 4)

Ogletree, Saddler, and Bowers (1995) defined interdisciplinary practice as "collaborative goal-setting from a 'whole-person' perspective . . . [that] depends on the integrated efforts of numerous team members, each of whom brings unique contributions to the assessment and treatment of persons with disabilities" (p. 220). Others have emphasized key elements of interdisciplinary practice, such as collaboration ("direct interaction between at least two coequal parties voluntarily engaged in shared decision making as they work toward a common goal"; Friend & Cook, 2010, p. 7) and communication ("continuous integrative communication and accommodation"; Franks et al., 2007, p. 170). While terms used to refer to interdisciplinary practice vary, most capture the concept of collaboration of diverse members, each of whom shares valuable expertise, thus ensuring that multiple perspectives are considered during the assessment and intervention processes. The participants necessarily include the person who stutters, family or significant others, and professional and paraprofessional practitioners. Ferguson (2008) and Hinckley (2008) reviewed the importance of individual and shared narratives in collaboration and interdisciplinary practice. While sharing insights about observed behaviors, practitioners should retain rather than abandon their professional identity as experts in their respective area of specialized knowledge. For example, the speech–language pathologist will be viewed as the expert in communication disorders who is receptive to related or contrasting views about communication from others outside of the discipline, just as the classroom teacher is the expert in academic design who is open to feedback or suggestions about curricular planning. Such a depiction is one of colleagueship, where each participant is viewed as a valued contributor who flexibly gives, receives, and shares, always with the communicative interests of the person who stutters and the family in mind.

Case Example

Consider the following case example. Ginny was a junior in high school when she came to my attention. She presented several learning disabilities, including receptive and expressive language deficits, in addition to noticeable stuttering. Her academic performance had plateaued and she was presently failing. She expressed frustration with the school experience, feeling unable to understand and master the curriculum (which was increasingly challenging conceptually), unable to communicate in classroom and social settings because of her stuttering and subsequent embarrassment, and discouraged about her inactive social life. Because of her home situation, Ginny worked in the afternoon and evening to contribute money to her family. For these and other reasons, she said that she was considering dropping out of school.

The interdisciplinary team meetings included Ginny and her mother, several classroom teachers, the learning disabilities specialist, the guidance counselor, and me (speech–language pathologist). The team realized the urgent need for effective and integrated intervention if Ginny was to succeed and stay in school. Each member shared insights reflecting respective expertise. The communication intervention plan involved identifying areas in which Ginny experienced academic success and using them within a communication context, with particular emphasis on conceptual processing, problem solving, and transfer and maintenance of speech fluency skills. From this positive foundation, and with the full support and understanding of all team members, I served as a resource providing additional curricular support in challenging academic content areas, with the foci noted above. The positive, successful context in which Ginny and I designed opportunities for her to experience and acknowledge her own success, combined with an integrated approach in which communication skills were viewed as pivotal to all other areas of learning, resulted in dramatic changes in Ginny's performance and her expressed attitudes about herself as a person and as a communicator. Some of the activities included subvocally repeating verbal instructions and taking telegraphic notes so as to retain information for subsequent recall and processing; improving money-changing, check-writing, and financial-balancing skills; relating the content of one class to that of others; and finding daily application for apparently unrelated class content.

Significant and continuing improvements were observed during the ensuing year and a half in classroom participation, performance on examinations, standardized testing of language-related conceptual processing, and, most noticeably, conversational speech fluency. Ginny now expressed feelings of success and pride. Secondary improvements were observed in her personal hygiene and grooming, posture, and positive and inviting manner of interpersonal communication. Ginny graduated high school and completed a degree at a technical college. Indeed, this story illustrates the importance of interdisciplinary teaming and the impact of success across a person's communication and life skills.

Background and Justification for Interdisciplinary Teaming

Rokusek (1995) reviewed the history of interdisciplinary teaming under various labels in medicine, education, and social service from 1920 to 1995; Franks et al. (2007) reviewed the evolution of interdisciplinary teams to the present date. An interest in interdisciplinary teams emerged during World War II, when many rehabilitation centers representing different disciplines were established across the United States.

Several key events stimulated the development of collaborative models of service delivery, including interdisciplinary teams (Kauffman & Hallahan, 2005; Villa & Thousand, 2005). These included, first, the passage of P.L. 94-142 (Education for All

Handicapped Children Act) in 1975. In 1986, an amendment (P.L. 99-457) to this act stipulated that the Individualized Education Program (IEP) is a legal document and must be developed in collaboration with the child's parents or legal guardians. The parents, who ultimately had the power to approve or reject the IEP, became recognized as legal partners in the design of goals and procedures. In 1990, P.L. 94-142 was reauthorized as the Individuals with Disabilities Education Act (IDEA); it was amended in 1997 (IDEA Amendments of 1997) and again reauthorized in 2004 as the Individuals with Disabilities Education Improvement Act (IDEIA, often referred to as IDEA). In 2001, the No Child Left Behind Act (NCLB) strengthened public expectations for high standards and accountability for teaching and learning in the schools, equal opportunity to learn, and achievement of each individual's performance potential, regardless of the presence or absence of a disability. Second, collaborative models of service delivery emerged from the field of early intervention, which, during the 1980s, addressed "transdisciplinary" service programs. More will be said about such programs shortly. Suffice it to say now that the term *transdisciplinary* signifies actual crossover in roles assumed by allied professionals and family members. In this way, the different team members participate in one another's goals and procedures and learn treatment techniques from one another. Third, collaborative models of assessment and intervention emerged from the recent interest in "whole language." This concept assumes a linguistic foundation underlying the development of oral language and literacy, both of which are predicated on the individual's active construction of meaning. Other catalysts for interdisciplinary practice could be identified, including the civil rights movement, the deinstitutionalization movement, and the education reform movement of the late 1960s and early 1970s (Kauffman & Hallahan, 2005), as well as paradigm shifts regarding how and where people with disabilities should be served (i.e., addressing functional needs in naturalistic settings), demographic shifts toward increasingly older populations, and trends toward movement of people with special needs into community-based programs (Rokusek, 1995).

Individual professionals and service providers, while retaining professional identity and being valued for unique areas of expertise, are no longer viewed as possessing all of the knowledge and skills necessary for intervention planning or for meeting the diverse needs of people with exceptionalities to live integrated, independent, productive lives within communities (Ogletree, 1999; Rokusek, 1995). In addition to the allied educational and medical team members noted previously, some argue that team size and makeup should be dictated by the needs and desires of the person being served, opening potential membership to such diverse persons as community planners, clergy, architects, engineers, attorneys, chamber of commerce representatives, business managers, fund-raisers, police officers, hospital aides, multiskilled technicians, human resource leaders, and city housing, labor, and transportation representatives (Rokusek, 1995). The emergence of an interdisciplinary perspective has helped bring the strengths and needs of people with exceptionalities into focus. People who stutter and their families stand to benefit from these advances.

Models of Team Practice

When designing intervention with people who stutter, clinicians must be aware of different treatment models. Ogletree and Daniels (1995) presented a concise discussion of four different models (*unidisciplinary*, *multidisciplinary*, *interdisciplinary*, and *transdisciplinary*):

> The unidisciplinary model is best characterized by independent service provision. Although popular, unidisciplinary services are limited by a lack of interprofessional collaboration (i.e., interaction). As a result, treatments may not be "cutting edge" and are

often poorly coordinated. . . . Unlike unidisciplinary services, the remaining models allow for some degree of collaboration. In a multidisciplinary model, professionals provide services independently, yet have a formal means of collaboration (e.g., staffings). An interdisciplinary model, while allowing independent functioning, emphasizes a greater degree of interaction between professionals, typically resulting in joint decision making regarding treatment goals and strategies. Finally, a transdisciplinary model incorporates the concept of professional role release where disciplines share roles and responsibilities. (p. 231)

Rokusek (1995) elaborated these models and indicated that professionals need to feel comfortable in a unidisciplinary (also called an intradisciplinary) setting before they can be comfortable in more collaborative environments. A multidisciplinary model, from a traditional medical setting, identifies a team leader or chair who is ultimately responsible for the direction and final decision making of the group. The focus is on providing input to the team leader, who assimilates and directs the outcome or recommendations. Interdisciplinary teaming, also called interprofessional teaming, assumes that each member is an equal in all decision making and consensus building; the work relationship is interdependent. Transdisciplinary teaming, derived from interdisciplinary practice, addresses collectively a specific need and brings in other team members as necessary. Transdisciplinary teaming again assumes equal team membership and a high level of discipline comfort but also emphasizes cross-discipline understanding, thus permitting role release. Various authors have elaborated these and other concepts related to models of treatment or team practice (e.g., Caldwell et al., 2006; Franks et al., 2007; Friend & Cook, 2010; Ogletree, Fischer, & Schulz, 1999; Stoneman & Malone, 1995). Ogletree and Daniels (1995) acknowledged that a variety of factors impact decisions regarding appropriate treatment models, including family needs and both availability and attitudes of professionals. While collaborative models appear more consistent with public legislation such as IDEA, they may not be preferred by families, or they may not be possible because of unavailability of practitioners in certain regions or inflexibility of some professionals to adjust their style of service delivery.

Conceptual Foundation and Necessary Competencies for Interdisciplinary Practice

Rokusek (1995) and Stoneman and Malone (1995) addressed reasons why practitioners should take interdisciplinary practice seriously and defined the necessary competencies for such collaboration. In my estimation, both of these foci are significant for clinicians who design intervention with people who stutter.

Conceptual Foundation

The conceptual foundation for interdisciplinary practice is first and foremost a commitment to the welfare of a person with an exceptionality. The foundation also reflects a commitment to one's own individual discipline and to the value of related human service disciplines. Similarly, Rokusek (1995) indicated that the conceptual foundation of interdisciplinary practice is primarily "a commitment to one's individual discipline or experiential background, to recognizing the value of others' disciplines and backgrounds, and to integrating the work of others with one's own" (p. 6). She indicated that this premise leads to at least four significant conceptual derivatives:

- an ability to look at the "whole" in the delivery of services that focus on a consumer in holistic fashion while operating in numerous personal and professional environments
- recognition of the interdependency of disciplinary practice and other environmental input from paraprofessionals, families and consumers

▦ respect for the expertise of all disciplinary professionals, paraprofessionals, families and consumers

▦ recognition of the ultimate benefit to consumers and their families through increased knowledge and skills and cross-disciplined assessment, problem-solving, intervention, prevention, and short- and long-term planning. (p. 6)

Similarly, Stoneman and Malone (1995) indicated that current changes in the design and delivery of services for people with disabilities reflect a "conceptual revolution" (p. 236). "Professionals who work with individuals with disabilities have been challenged to set aside their belief that determining the best interests of their constituents is solely within their jurisdiction" (p. 234). Adopting and implementing interdisciplinary considerations, Stoneman and Malone noted a number of conceptual underpinnings:

▦ *Shift to a support paradigm.* Shifting to a support paradigm requires focusing on community partnerships, including the community member with an exceptionality (i.e., interdependence), and moving from interdisciplinary teams that are professionally dominated to those that include family, friends, and community members.

▦ *Self-advocacy.* People with exceptionalities are demonstrating that through organized political action, they can effect changes in laws, regulations, and practices that impact their lives (e.g., Stuttering Foundation of America, National Stuttering Association, International Stuttering Association, and other organizations that advocate for people who stutter by fostering interpersonal and international understanding and acceptance, eliminating discrimination, and expanding opportunities).

▦ *Person-centered approaches.* The person with an exceptionality explores what he wants for his life (i.e., whole-life planning), and the clinician and other team members engage in joint problem solving to help realize these dreams (e.g., to be able say what is on one's mind without fear of ridicule).

▦ *Natural and informal supports.* People who care about the person with an exceptionality are identified (friends, family members, neighbors, and community members) and engaged in intervention. For example, a best friend might assist a child with transference of fluency to the classroom, or a spouse might offer praise when the person who stutters demonstrates gentle contacts when ordering in the restaurant.

▦ *Family-focused, family-driven supports.* The family is viewed as central in the lives of all people. Viewed as advocates for the person with an exceptionality, families need to be involved in all aspects of the intervention process, leading to feelings of empowerment and shared ownership of the process and its outcome.

▦ *Full community inclusion and inclusive education.* Inclusion refers to the idea that the person with an exceptionality participates in all aspects of community life and is educated in regular education classrooms with peers who do not have exceptionalities. Inclusion has been the primary focus of several pieces of federal legislation (IDEA, NCLB, and the American with Disabilities Amendments Act of 2008); even so, these concepts continue to stimulate heated debate (see Villa & Thousand, 2005; Kauffman & Hallahan, 2005).

▦ *Blurring of professional roles and turf.* The focus shifts from professional domains to the multifaceted needs of the person being served.

▦ *Cost containment.* Interdisciplinary teams are potentially expensive. Stoneman and Malone (1995) noted, "Human need is increasing, but fiscal resources to support that need are finite" (p. 239), arguing that use of interdisciplinary teams within a support model decreases the cost for most people but increases the cost for some. The need for efficacy data is critical.

▦ *Accountability.* Stoneman and Malone (1995) stated that "theoretically, and intuitively, interdisciplinary teams provide a relatively good fit with holistic models of human development" (p. 239). However, "few, if any, published studies exist which document that interdisciplinary teams are better than other modes of service delivery" (p. 239). Again, the need for efficacy data is critical.

Necessary Competencies

Rokusek (1995) indicated that dominance, control, superiority, and extreme individualism are not compatible with interdisciplinary practice. Rather, all members of interdisciplinary teams must share the ability to

- understand a common professional language
- decrease control of all work boundaries
- understand the delivery system(s) available and remain open to all available resources
- communicate openly and effectively to peers and others in and outside of the professional work environment
- integrate their professional abilities and unique personal qualities into the team, and recognize the specialized culture, values, traditions, knowledge, training, personal emotions, and experiences that the other members bring to the team
- work well in teams and contribute towards consensus building. (pp. 5–6)

To these vital requirements, I would add that clinicians must have an understanding of and sensitivity toward the people and interpersonal dynamics within the family system, as described in Chapter 5.

Similarly, Stoneman and Malone (1995) addressed the competencies that are required to be an effective team member. In doing so, they recalled Garner, Uhl, and Cox's (1992) "10 Cs," which might be viewed as individual members' skills or team characteristics, as follows: communication, cooperation, collaboration, confronting problems, compromise, consensus decision making, coordination, consistency, caring, and commitment. Stoneman and Malone noted that additional competencies for interdisciplinary team practice include the following:

- *Relinquishing professional power.* The person with the exceptionality is a key member of the team; thus, negotiating, rather than imposing our professional will, is essential. "Respecting the family's right to self-determination, while acknowledging that families do not always make the best choices for the family member with a disability, requires a difficult blend of compromise and advocacy" (p. 241).

- *Shared dreaming.* The ability to dream with another person and to enable that person to imagine, sometimes for the first time, and to realize goals that he may never have imagined possible indeed is a professional competency. Stoneman and Malone warned that "the gift of dreaming has been extinguished in all too many professionals" (p. 241). Rather than engaging in dreams of fantasy, dreams or visions should be reality based. Recall Daly's (1988) reminder of the importance of the clinician truly believing in the client's potential. This cannot be overstated.

- *Holistic thinking.* The ability to think holistically enables a clinician to shift from "fixing" the person who stutters (addressing disfluent speech only) to accentuating, better understanding, and facilitating the fluency already demonstrated by that person. As noted earlier, the person who stutters is viewed as one with many abilities rather than as a "stutterer." Fluency is viewed as the root of dis*fluency*.

- *Community-building skills.* In order to facilitate interaction between the person who stutters and opportunities within the community, clinicians must be comfortable with advocacy and leadership skills, coalition building, conflict resolution, resource management, and negotiation strategies.

- *Building systems of natural and informal supports.* The concept of natural supports was reviewed earlier as part of the conceptual foundation of interdisciplinary teaming. Here, building such supports is viewed as a necessary competency for collaborative clinicians. Those competencies noted for community-building skills are relevant here as well.

- *Providing supports to people where they are.* Both assessment and treatment with people who stutter must reflect ecological contexts (i.e., settings that directly resemble where they need to use, and therefore improve, their speech fluency skills). This means that intervention must not be limited to clinical settings and must facilitate transfer to optimally meaningful communication contexts from the earliest contact.

⬚ *Taking responsibility for finding solutions.* Clinicians have a responsibility to see to it that after getting to know, listening to, gaining trust from, dreaming with, and thereby building a meaningful relationship with a person who stutters, they carry out intervention plans to the point of solution. Too often in a traditional diagnostic model, clinicians design plans for someone else to carry out, and never know if the plans were implemented.

⬚ *Creativity in problem solving.* As people who stutter actively design and achieve their own communication life goals, new challenges are encountered. Many years ago, a wise couple told me that meaningful challenges take a long time to accomplish, and those that are seemingly impossible take a bit longer. So it is for people who stutter. Valuable problem-solving skills include listening, facilitating, identifying and administering supports and resources, and achieving solutions (see Moses & Shapiro, 1996; Shapiro & Moses, 2005; Shapiro, Ogletree, & Brotherton, 2002, for discussion of constructivist concepts applied to creative problem solving). Our intervention, problem solving, and solutions are both constructed and conducted *with*, rather than *for*, people who stutter.

Summary—Interdisciplinary Practice

Interdisciplinary team practice involves a process of collective collaboration. Being both family centered and community based, interdisciplinary practice is an outgrowth of the idea that people who stutter are viewed as able individuals who actively interpret and make decisions about their communication and the world, based on their personal constructs and as interactive members within family systems. Thus, interdisciplinary teams are partnerships involving people who stutter, their families, allied professionals, paraprofessionals, and community resources in shared responsibility for designing and implementing individually tailored and effective intervention. Interdisciplinary practice is an appropriate mechanism for clinical intervention with people who stutter.

Multicultural Awareness

A Context for Multicultural Appreciation

Human beings have a remarkable capacity for richness and variation in communication behavior, interpersonal dynamics, and conceptual interpretation. It is little wonder that understanding communication and its disorders, particularly intervention with people who stutter, is no small undertaking. Each person, including those who stutter, usually experiences a sense of belonging to a family. Families may identify with some larger group within society, and that larger group may identify with a still larger group. For example, ethnicity and religion often influence our daily lives, including the foods we eat, our rituals, and our traditions (Turnbull et al., 2006). These aspects of our cultural heritage shape our values and perspectives on the world, including our attitudes toward communication and its disorders.

Battle (2002b) emphasized that speech, language, and communication are embedded in culture. In order to communicate successfully with a client, clinicians must be familiar with that individual's personal history and understand how historical, geographic, social, and political factors, among others, both bind that individual to a group and distinguish that individual from the group. Too often, race, ethnicity, and culture are interpreted erroneously as synonymous terms. Battle (2002a, 2002c) noted that *race* is a statement about biological and anatomical attributes and functions (e.g., skin color, facial features, hair texture) that are passed genetically from generation to generation. Two people may be of the same biological race but may differ vastly in their cultural identity, personal history, and view of the world. Indeed, race is an entirely physical phenomenon determined by heredity. *Ethnicity* is determined by heritage and refers to belonging to groups that share unique social and cultural traditions. Battle (2002a) stated, "Ethnicity is not passed genetically from generation to generation. Rather, ethnicity is constructed and reconstructed in response to particular historical circumstances and changes" (p. 4). Often united by aspirations of political self-determination, individuals of a given ethnicity identify themselves with patterns of family life, language, recreation, and religion. *Culture* is about the behaviors, beliefs, and values of a group of people who are brought together by their commonality. Battle (2002a) indicated that culture can be distinguished by explicit and implicit behaviors. *Explicit cultural behaviors* are those that are visible and thus identify members as a group. Such behaviors include dress, language and speaking patterns, food preferences, customs, and lifestyles. *Implicit cultural behaviors* are less visible but no less significant in contributing to the essence of the person with whom we communicate. Implicit cultural behaviors are associated with age, gender roles within the family, child-rearing practices, socioeconomic status, educational values, religious and spiritual beliefs, fears and attitudes, perceptions of what is considered disabling, and exposure to and adoption of other cultural ways. Ethnicity and culture are not mutually exclusive. *Multiculturalism* refers to a society containing diverse races, ethnicities, and cultures with varied religions, languages, customs, traditions, and values. Battle (2002a) underscored that multiculturalism is a mosaic of individuals (of differing socioeconomic class, gender, sexual orientation, and ability level) that work together to form a rich whole, where each individual has both a group identity and an individual identify and is respected and valued for his or her contribution to the community.

As clinicians, we must see through the eyes of the people we serve. "Any attempt to generalize statements or attributes to all members of an identified group fails to recognize individual differences in life history, personal experiences, personal values, or personal beliefs" (Battle, 2002c, p. xv). Battle further noted, "Understanding of individuals within a culture implies a fully developed sense of the complex web of meanings, perceptions, actions, symbols, and adaptations that make individuals and cultural groups who they are" (p. xvi). And: "Because culture permeates every dimension of communication, the culturally competent clinician understands that most, if not all, truths are merely perceptions of truth viewed through the prism of culture" (Battle, 2002c, p. xviii). Battle also indicated that our challenge as clinicians is to recognize both the similarities among racial and ethnic groups and the individual differences within any group and among its individual members.

We cannot study or understand communication and its disorders without reference to the cultural, historical, and societal bases of communication. For example, the conversational partners that people choose, what they talk about, when and where they talk, and even what constitutes meaningful communication and what represents a communication disorder must be interpreted and understood within a cultural context. One must understand the salient cultural values, perceptions, attitudes, and history of a group in order to draw conclusions about the communication competence of a particular person within that group. The speech–language pathologist, when assessing a client's speech fluency, must be mindful that cultural factors may impact the client's willingness to initiate conversation, to discuss feelings, to have or maintain eye contact, or even to speak with a particular conversational partner. Clinicians must be knowledgeable about and sensitive to the cultural heritage of those with whom they interact and must realize that culture influences how each person views the world.

If heightened multicultural knowledge, awareness, and sensitivities are positive attributes of clinicians working with people who stutter, we must at the same time be careful not to assume that each individual member of a particular cultural group shares the same values and beliefs as the group (Bunning, 2004; Ferguson, 2008; P. M. Roberts & Shenker, 2007; Turnbull et al., 2006; Westby, 2000). Doing so inadvertently promotes cultural stereotypes, the antithesis of multicultural appreciation (Cole, 1989; Cooper & Cooper, 1993). People differ. In fact, working with families of diverse cultural backgrounds has taught me that different members of the same family may hold differing values and beliefs. I am reminded of a young woman from a traditional Greek Orthodox family who, as part of her fluency treatment, discussed the challenges she experienced in having parents who are immigrants and whose expectations of her are different from those she holds for herself. Some of the differences involved career ambition (she wanted to practice medicine), dress (she wanted to wear more contemporary clothing), and social etiquette (her parents were horrified that she would call a man to initiate a social engagement).

Many of our students at Western Carolina University, where I teach, are among the first generation in their family to pursue a college degree. This is not an uncommon experience for the adult children of families from mountainous regions in rural Appalachia. These students bring with them all of the experiences, needs, and fears, combined with the hopes and dreams, of those who have broken the traditional family mold. Many years ago, a television advertisement pictured a man with Native American features enthusiastically eating a sandwich made with rye bread. The caption boasted, "You don't have to be Jewish to love Levi's [Jewish rye bread]." Multicultural education leads clinicians to appreciate human diversity in all of its forms and to resolve to approach each person, including those who stutter and their families, as individuals who are blessed with similarities and differences.

Background Related to Multicultural Awareness

In 1944, Wendell Johnson claimed that the Hopi people, a Native American tribe in the American Southwest, did not demonstrate stuttering behavior because they did not have a label for stuttering. This claim was challenged repeatedly (Van Riper, 1982; Zimmermann, Liljeblad, Frank, & Cleeland, 1983). Nevertheless, Johnson's assertion has been recalled frequently to support the need for understanding cultural considerations in communication and its disorders. Taylor (1986) noted that prior to a debate between John Michel and himself at the 1968 ASHA Convention in Denver, minimal interest existed within the professions of speech pathology and audiology regarding the unique clinical needs of culturally and linguistically diverse clients. This meeting resulted in greater attention to issues of cultural relevance and spawned various professional developments. These included formation of the ASHA Black Caucus, which expressed the concern that speech pathologists were viewing the language differences among African Americans from a pathology perspective (referring a disproportionate number of African American children for communication intervention); the Black Caucus urged ASHA to require coursework in sociolinguistics and Black history, to stimulate training and research opportunities in these areas, and to develop legal and legislative safeguards.

Since that time, significant developments have resulted in major improvement in the assessment of speech and language disorders in culturally diverse populations (S. Adler, 1993; Screen & Anderson, 1994). ASHA has enforced its policies opposing discrimination and promoting affirmative action and cultural diversity (ASHA, 1991; Cole, 1992). These policies determine acceptable locations for national meetings, define ethical conduct and clinical practice, affect appointments to committees and boards, identify topics and faculty for educational programming, and generate an assortment of official position statements, guidelines, and definitions regarding multicultural issues. These and other activities reflective of ASHA's ongoing commitment to multicultural concerns and heightened understanding and acceptance among the general membership culminated in 1991 with a published plan, "Multicultural Action Agenda 2000" (ASHA, 1991). This plan specified objectives to be completed by 2000 that would increase the proportion of people who identify with federally designated racial and ethnic minority groups in ASHA's general membership, leadership roles, and national office staff and managerial positions. ASHA advised its members of their responsibility to upgrade their own knowledge and skills to better understand and serve multicultural populations. This advice was essential, given the significant shortage of professionals within ASHA who were qualified to work with people who identify themselves with ethnic or racial minority groups. In 1993, Taylor reported that approximately 75% of the speech–language pathologists certified by ASHA stated that they did not have sufficient knowledge or competence to provide clinical services to bilingual or non-standard-English-speaking clients. Similarly, B. A. Johnson and Mata-Pistokache (1996) noted that 91% of certified speech–language pathologists reported having received no training in minority-language populations in preprofessional or graduate training and that only 8% of the applicants for the Certificate of Clinical Competence in Speech–Language Pathology had elected to take a course on multicultural communication. With "Multicultural Action Agenda 2000," ASHA took an important step toward ensuring that its programs related to cultural diversity would be maintained; that educational opportunities would be sponsored; that multicultural understanding and commitment would be interwoven with certification and accreditation requirements; and that its governmental, legislative, and public relation efforts would be consistent with its policies.

Since 2000, other significant developments have occurred. At their heart, these developments recognize the challenge faced by allied human service disciplines (e.g., speech–language pathology and audiology) to prepare a largely White, English-speaking workforce to deliver professional services to a culturally diverse population (Stockman, Boult, & Robinson, 2008). Such developments include required instruction on multicultural and multilingual issues for clinical certification of speech–language pathologists and audiologists and for accreditation of professional preparation programs (ASHA, 2009a, 2009b, 2009c). Also, all graduates of professional education programs in communication sciences and disorders must demonstrate knowledge and skills acquisition (ASHA, 2009a) related to multicultural and multilingual issues. In 2004, ASHA's Multicultural Issues Board (ASHA, 2004b) articulated specific areas of knowledge and skills needed by speech–language pathologists and audiologists to provide culturally and linguistically appropriate services. This document should be required reading for all service providers, as it is invaluable for program assessment and strategic planning and for individual self-study and self-guided improvement. The knowledge and skills areas addressed include cultural competence; language competencies for the clinician; and identification, assessment, and treatment of language, articulation and phonology, voice and fluency, swallowing, and hearing and balance disorders. The document also provides a wealth of references and related terminology.

In 2005, ASHA's Working Group on Quality Indicators (ASHA, 2005c) presented factors that reflect currency, appropriateness, and effectiveness of service delivery in audiology and speech–language pathology. These quality indicators address diagnostic and treatment practices that are individualized to meet specific needs of persons served, including cultural and language background, in addition to age and developmental status, gender, cognitive ability, learning style, impairments, activity limitations, participation restrictions, environmental challenges, family and caregiver needs, and related regulations and policies (i.e., federal, state, local). Other indicators address professional ethics, stating that services and employment practices cannot discriminate on the basis of race or ethnicity, gender, age, religion, national origin, sexual orientation, impairment, or activity limitation. Also in 2005, ASHA's Board of Ethics (ASHA, 2005a) addressed issues related to cultural competence. The central tenet of the Code of Ethics (ASHA, 2010), specifically Principle of Ethics I, is to hold paramount the welfare of the people we serve. Also, we are bound to provide all services competently and to use every resource, including referral when appropriate, to ensure the highest quality (Principle of Ethics I, Rules A and B). Furthermore, we are cautioned to engage in service only within the scope of our competence, considering our level of education, training, and experience (Principle of Ethics II, Rule B). This means that we cannot provide services without appropriate knowledge and skills. Yet, when we do not feel culturally competent or adequately trained (e.g., when there are cultural or linguistic differences between the clinician and client that could affect service delivery), are we absolved of our professional responsibility? ASHA responds with a resounding "No." ASHA reminds us that we cannot discriminate in the delivery of professional services (Principle of Ethics I, Rule C) or in our relationships with colleagues, students, and members of allied professions (Principle of Ethics IV, Rule K) and directs us to continue in lifelong learning (Principle of Ethics II, Rule C). These reminders and mandates are intended to commit us to develop the knowledge and skills required to provide culturally and linguistically appropriate services rather than to justify not providing those services.

Other ethical implications are these: We cannot delegate tasks that are beyond the competence of the designee and, when we do delegate tasks, we are obligated to provide adequate supervision (Principle of Ethics I, Rules E, F, and G). This issue becomes complex when the certified individual does not speak the language being used and the assistant or interpreter is not appropriately trained. The quality of service and supervision cannot be compromised; responsibility for the client's welfare is paramount. ASHA (2005a) states that a frequently occurring situation such as this does not negate the responsibility of the certified individual to understand the issues relevant to cultural and linguistic diversity (e.g., second language acquisition, dialectal differences, bilingualism). Rather, the certified individual remains responsible for the quality of the assessment and treatment provided and received.

To understand the significance of ASHA's and its members' commitment to cultural competence in all aspects of clinical education, service delivery, and research, clinicians need to appreciate the magnitude of demographic changes taking place in the United States. Various authors (ASHA, 2004b, 2004c, 2005a, 2005c; Battle, 2002a, 2002b, 2002c; Stockman et al., 2008) have cited the 2000 U.S. census (U.S. Census Bureau, 2000) in order to characterize this change. As of 2000, the reported population of the United States (284,460,799) comprised the following: White (of British or European ancestry), 68.4%; African American, 12.2%; Hispanic (Cuban, Mexican, Puerto Rican, Other), 12.4%; Native American or Eskimo, 0.87%; Asian and Pacific Islander, 3.7%; and Multiracial, 2.4%. Because the structure of the census was revised in 2000, allowing people for the first time to identify themselves as multiracial, comparison between the 1990 and 2000 census data should be made cautiously (Battle, 2002a). Nevertheless, these data reveal that between 1990 and 2000, the population of the United States increased 13.2%. The growth in the population of each composite group was as follows: White, 3.4%; African American, 15.6%; Hispanic, 57.9%; Native American and Eskimo, 26.4%; and Asian and Pacific Islander, 46.3%. Estimates indicate that between 1995 and 2020, the population of the United States will increase by 8.5%. Projected growth in the population of each composite group is as follows: White, 2.4%; African American, 11.9%; Hispanic, 26.4%; Native American and Eskimo, 13.1%; and Asian and Pacific

Islander, 26.4% (Battle, 2002a). At this rate, many large cities are now more than 50% "minority" and, by 2056, White Americans will be a minority group (Westby, 2000). The 2000 census data reveal that 31.6% of the U.S. population was other than White; 68.4% of the population was White. Yet only 7% of the total ASHA membership are from a racial or ethnic minority background and fewer than 6% of the ASHA members identify themselves as bilingual or multilingual (ASHA, 2004b, 2004c). Note also that neither the census data nor the ASHA demographics questionnaires include categories such as sexual orientation or disabilities and that both questionnaires rely on voluntary reporting (Battle, 2005).

Thus, while ASHA is committed to building a membership base that more realistically reflects the constituent population being served and to enabling its membership to provide culturally competent services (ASHA, 2009c), we still have much work to do. New and seasoned professionals alike must take seriously the challenge to become culturally competent in all aspects of our professions, including our purpose and scope of services, service delivery, program operations, program evaluation and performance improvement, and ethics and management of professional issues, in all work settings (school based, health care, and private practice) (ASHA, 2005c). Our country is becoming increasingly diverse, both culturally and linguistically. Speech–language pathologists are being called upon, more than ever before, to work with people from a variety of cultures having different cultural behaviors, learning and interpersonal styles, social beliefs, and worldviews. The responsibility to acquire and maintain the knowledge and skills needed to provide culturally and linguistically appropriate services is ours. There is a plethora of educational opportunities for achieving improved cultural literacy. These include continuing education, professional education, materials, conferences and workshops, and ASHA resources such as the Multicultural Issues Board, the Office of Multicultural Affairs, the Board of Ethics, and Special Interest Division 14 on Communication Disorders and Sciences in Culturally and Linguistically Diverse Populations. It is incumbent upon each and every professional in our field to access these learning opportunities and thereby become competent to serve our richly diverse client population.

Multicultural Considerations for Research on Stuttering

Clearly, stuttering is a universal phenomenon (Bloodstein & Bernstein Ratner, 2008; Van Riper, 1982), but there are few data regarding the influence of cultural factors on the nature of stuttering. Cooper and Cooper (1993) asserted that this dearth of knowledge has resulted from researchers isolating independent variables by keeping their research populations homogeneous. As a consequence, we know relatively little about fluency-related characteristics of minority groups and culturally diverse populations. This knowledge base has improved somewhat in recent years, as researchers have explored the role of (a) culturally based considerations in regard to people who stutter and their families within specific racial, ethnic, and cultural groups (Cooper & Cooper, 1993; Daniels, Hagstrom, & Gabel, 2006; Higdon, 2002; Jewett, 2003; Jewett, Gallagher, & Taggart, 2002; Klompas & Ross, 2004; Langevin et al., 2006; Molt, 2005; Novak, 2002a, 2002b; Robinson & Crowe, 1998; Robinson, Davis, & Crowe, 2000; Panagiotopoulos, 2001; Shapiro et al., 2000, 2001, 2004); (b) attitudes in different countries about stuttering (St. Louis, 2005; St. Louis et al., 2009); and (c) procedures and implications for researching culturally diverse groups (Cartwright, Daniels, & Zhang, 2008; Finn & Cordes, 1997; Huer & Saenz, 2003).

One area of research over the last decade is stuttering and bilingualism (P. M. Roberts & Shenker, 2007; Shenker, 2004; Van Borsel & de Britto Pereira, 2005; Van Borsel,

Maes, & Foulon, 2001) and related issues of language development, delay, and disorder (Glennen, 2002, 2007, 2008; Glennen & Masters, 2002; Paul, 2007; Roseberry-McKibbin, 2007). Van Borsel et al. (2001) noted that stuttering is probably more prevalent in bilinguals than in monolinguals (notwithstanding lack of empirical replication; see Au-Yeung, Howell, Davis, Charles, & Sackin, 2000; P. M. Roberts & Shenker, 2007). It seems, at least in some cases, that bilingualism is a contributing factor to the development of stuttering, but other environmental factors may play a role as well (e.g., being placed in a new situation, being exposed to mixed linguistic input). Stuttering can affect one or both languages. When stuttering occurs in both languages, both may be equally affected, but the dominant pattern is that the languages are affected unequally. Factors determining which language is more affected include language ability and psychosocial and cultural factors; linguistic factors may influence the distribution of disfluencies. Diagnostically, it is important but challenging to distinguish between stuttering and disfluencies that are attributable to limited language proficiency. Van Borsel et al. noted that diagnostic indicators for stuttering include disfluencies occurring in both languages, secondary behaviors and related negative feelings or attitudes, and a family history of stuttering. Indirect therapy approaches for bilingual children who are beginning to stutter include temporarily eliminating one language or, if this is not possible, limiting the interaction with each conversational partner to only one language ("the principle of one person, one language"; p. 200).

The interaction between stuttering and bilingualism raises a number of questions that are yet to be answered by research, including whether or not deferring bilingualism prevents stuttering and whether or not bilingual children who stutter have any less favorable treatment prognosis than monolingual children who stutter. Van Borsel et al. (2001) advised, for both diagnostic and treatment purposes, obtaining the assistance of a native speaker if the clinician has not mastered the language used by the client. Van Borsel et al. also indicated the need for clinical research to determine the prevalence of stuttering, its manifestations, and therapy outcomes among bilingual people who stutter. Noting that the divergence in research findings may be attributable to the heterogeneity of the population of bilinguals who stutter, Van Borsel et al. stated, "No two bilinguals are alike" (p. 201). The discussion of evidence-based practice in Chapter 2 invites us to consider the extent to which we may be homogenizing a heterogeneous population for the sake of control and replication in clinical research (see also Cooper & Cooper, 1993).

Another obstacle in our knowledge of cultural variations in fluency disorders is the continuing lack of universally accepted or standard definitions for key terms (e.g., *fluency, disfluency, stuttering, stammering*), particularly in studies from other than White, English-speaking Western cultures. This problem with definitions, reviewed more thoroughly in Chapter 1, significantly limits the potential for comparison and generalization of results across studies. More recently, however, researchers have used more robust designs and more reliable terms and definitions to address fluency disorders in minority populations and in cross-cultural investigations. Nevertheless, none of these challenges will be resolved easily. As reviewed in Chapter 2, early studies of prevalence in other cultures, albeit with significant methodological limitations, suggest that in some countries, stuttering prevalence is lower than that found in the United States, England, and other countries representative of European culture; in others, prevalence seems to be greater. Various researchers have speculated on these findings. Leith (1986) stated,

> The sociocultural variables we consider when appraising cultural influences would be the cultural value placed on such attributes as competitiveness and achievement, childrearing practices as related to the amount of pressure put on the child, attitudes toward language and expressive behaviors, and the treatment of defective or handicapped

individuals in the culture. Cultures that have all or most of these characteristics have a higher incidence of stuttering, since they are "stress cultures" or "tough" cultures. Cultures that have few if any of these characteristics have a lower incidence of stuttering, since they are not "stress cultures"; they are "easy" cultures. (p. 13)

Cooper and Cooper (1993) challenged such interpretations of varied prevalence, stating, "As fetchingly simplistic and patently plausible as these recurrent speculations might appear, neither the prevalence data nor any significant body of data pertaining to the etiology of stuttering support them" (p. 197). Cooper and Cooper (1993) also questioned the usefulness of dividing the world into two types of societies, cautioned those who might allow preconceived notions about stuttering to limit their interpretations of what they observe, and concluded that "the frequency of fluency disorders does vary from one culture to another, but the universality of the problem tells us that fluency disorders are not simply the result of cultural considerations" (p. 197).

Relatedly, cultural values affect a community's assumptions about the etiology of stuttering, the extent to which stuttering and people who stutter are accepted within a community, and how the community conceptualizes the treatment of stuttering (Bloodstein & Bernstein Ratner, 2008; Shapiro et al., 2000, 2001, 2004; St. Louis, 2005, 2006; St. Louis et al., 2009). These and other foci invite continued research related to stuttering and multicultural considerations.

Multicultural Considerations for Intervention

When striving to understand the cultural influences on people who stutter, clinicians must be mindful to approach each person and his family as an individual entity unto itself, without preconceived notions or stereotypical assumptions about the family's general cultural group. P. M. Roberts and Shenker (2007) described the challenge faced by clinicians:

> The clinician must walk a fine line: on the one hand being aware of the potential impact of macro- and microcultural factors, while on the other hand remembering that each client comes to us with his or her own individual values and views, not as a representative of any particular group. Also, it is important not to overstate the importance of cultural factors. (p. 188)

P. M. Roberts and Shenker (2007) also indicated the importance of avoiding potentially offensive or perplexing questions, such as, "How is stuttering seen in your culture?" Rather, they recommended a series of questions that should precede asking about the feelings that stuttering elicits in the child or in the family: "What do you think caused the stuttering?" "What strategies have you tried so far to reduce or manage the stuttering?" They noted that these questions are appropriate not only for bilingual clients who stutter but also for all culturally and linguistically diverse clients. I might add that these questions often are appropriate for all clients who stutter and their families because such questions lead to dialogue or observations that inform the clinician about the influence of culture on an individual client's and family's communication experience. This informed dialogue and observation yield a more authentic cultural representation than artificial questions that imply cultural stereotypes or pigeonholing.

Leith (1986) advised clinicians to become aware of a variety of factors that might have precipitated or might be perpetuating the stuttering. These include the family's child-rearing and discipline practices, reactions to stuttering, and cultural factors that might interfere with fluency facilitation. These will be addressed separately.

First, while different families demonstrate different child-rearing practices and interpersonal styles with their children, concern arises when a child stutters and the family is oriented more toward adult needs and values than toward those of the child. In such families, "children are to be seen and not heard." Potentially, this puts significant pressure on the child who wishes to speak or needs to speak with an adult. The child feels that he is intruding in an adult world and anticipates scolding for such interference, regardless of the importance of what is to be said. Leith (1986) indicated that the content and function of such infrequent interactions are noteworthy as well, typically taking the form of commands, instructions, or reprimands from the adult to the child, and the briefest responses from the child to the adult—and these only when directed or invited. Likewise, the family's performance expectations for the child in different domains can pressure the child and thus may contribute to the development or maintenance of stuttering. In any case, the absence of easy dialogue or presence of high expectations for the child's performance may contribute to stuttering and may interfere with treatment progress.

Second, Leith (1986) pointed out that people's reactions to stuttering may reflect cultural beliefs. For example, if the cultural group believes that stuttering is due to factors such as the child being possessed or under the spell of an evil eye, the child might be penalized by negative reactions and be made aware of his being possessed or under a spell. He and his family might experience shame and might explore cultural treatments such as ritualistic dances, prayers, and folk remedies. People from other cultures might respond with ridicule, assuming that the child who stutters is being foolish, or react with anger, assuming volitional stuttering. Leith noted that American people who stutter may experience a double jeopardy—a fairly predictable reaction from their own cultural group and a more unpredictable reaction from the general culture. The familial lineage, whether traced through patriarchal or matriarchal lines, will also influence attitudes toward stuttering. In a patriarchal society, where the male is the dominant figure, stuttering in a boy is considered grievous because of its projected influence on his role in society. Stuttering in a girl is less serious, but noteworthy, in its impact on marriageability. In a matriarchal society, however, stuttering in a girl is more serious because it will impact not only marriageability but also the woman's later role in society.

Third, there are special cultural influences, including the role that verbal communication plays in a particular culture and the diverse roles that different members fill in that culture. Leith (1986) presented an enlightening assortment of scenarios from his clinical experience clearly indicating that an interaction within the clinical context may be interpreted very differently, and misinterpreted, from different cultural orientations. We discussed earlier the importance of distinguishing between an event and its multiple interpretations (Shapiro & Moses, 2005). Acknowledging and interpreting an event from multiple perspectives is critical for clinicians working with people who stutter so that they can better understand the participants and nurture the clinical process. The events Leith described, each of which caused the client discomfort, address a variety of cultural factors. For example, the clinician might interpret client lateness as a sign of disrespect or lack of commitment to the treatment process, whereas such lateness might reflect a different conceptualization of time or other demands on the family's time (e.g., an inflexible work schedule). The following summaries of the clinical situations described by Leith present the typical clinician interpretation of and response to the client's behavior along with an alternative, more culturally sensitive interpretation, and then a recommendation for how to deal with the situation:

> ⊞ Family arrives late for their scheduled appointment and is admonished by the clinician. Family is irresponsible and unmotivated versus family's culture is not time oriented. Recommendation: Clinician might schedule this family earlier to allow for late arrival.

> ⊞ Clinician who is feeling time pressure begins an interview by asking parents questions about the child's development and is met with resistance on the part of the parents.

Clinician uses clinical time efficiently versus clinician rudely discusses business before an appropriate period of social interaction. Recommendation: Value people and build interpersonal rapport first.

⟐ Clinician directs questions to the mother; she does not respond, but defers to the father. Mother is conversationally passive and uninvolved versus in this patriarchal family, the father speaks for the family and the wife does not speak when the husband is present. Recommendation: Address both parents and allow them to decide who will respond; address individual parents in separate settings.

⟐ Having determined that the father speaks for the family, clinician directs questions to him, but the father seems awkward and responds tentatively. Father becomes inexplicably upset at questions versus father is not accustomed to a female (i.e., clinician) being in authority and questioning his responses. Recommendation: Share purposes and accept tentative responses.

⟐ Clinician interviews parents about communication-related family matters, and parents seem unresponsive and closed off. Parents are inexplicably silent and agitated versus family matters are private and not to be shared with strangers. Recommendation: Plan treatment based on general information as opposed to asking what might be considered questions that are too intimate.

⟐ Clinician repeatedly praises child and child's behavior to the mother, who responds with suspicion. Mother is inexplicably uncomfortable hearing compliments versus mother believes clinician might abduct the child or cast the evil eye (a powerful spell) on the child. Recommendation: Be positive but not to excess; see how the parent responds.

⟐ Family refuses to allow a male clinician to escort a female child away from her parents to the clinical room. Family has trouble with separation versus culture does not allow a female child to be alone with a male stranger. Recommendation: Allow parent to accompany child or assign a female clinician.

⟐ Clinician pats child on head and parents react negatively. Clinician offered nonverbal form of reward versus clinician broke a religious rule that the hair is sacred and not to be touched by a stranger. Recommendation: Know the family before using touch as a nonverbal form of reward or affection.

⟐ Client does not stutter openly as directed by clinician. Client is not committed to treatment process versus culture highly regards speech; thus disfluency invites ridicule by others. Recommendation: Use a more fluency-oriented program.

⟐ Client refuses to maintain eye contact with the clinician as prompted by clinician. Client does not follow instructions versus client's culture views direct eye contact as a sign of hostile or sexually aggressive behavior and lowering the eyes as a sign of respect. Recommendation: Interpret apparent resistance from multiple perspectives.

⟐ Clinician offers a gesture of positive reinforcement by forming a circle with tip of thumb touching index finger, after which client falls silent. Clinician's gesture is a form of nonverbal praise versus the gesture is interpreted as an obscenity in the client's culture. Recommendation: Use verbal forms of feedback.

⟐ Client does not observe or perform deliberate repetition of a disfluency on a word containing *th*. Client is noncompliant versus client is reluctant to expose the tongue, which is considered impolite. Recommendation: Modify behavior so that tongue is barely visible between the teeth.

⟐ Child has not performed transfer activities at home. Client is noncompliant versus client's home is not child oriented, and speech initiation by child is penalized. Recommendation: Interpret apparent resistance from multiple perspectives.

⟐ Child refuses to engage in dialogue with clinician. Child is conversationally passive versus child is taught not to speak with strangers (this cultural lesson might also interfere with extraclinical transfer activities). Recommendation: Interpret resistance from multiple perspectives.

⊞ Child has not completed assignments or maintained fluency. Child is uncooperative versus child is punished at home for using new speech (i.e., parents believe that stuttering is punishment for sin and that stuttering will disappear when they atone; reducing stuttering by treatment interferes with their belief and reduces their punishment). Recommendation: Invite and understand client's and family's causal assumptions about stuttering and expectations for treatment.

It is both impossible and undesirable to anticipate all of the potential exchanges we might have with our clients who stutter and their families, particularly those whose cultural framework is different from our own. As always, clinicians need to be both sensitive to and accepting of differences that exist within such an increasingly pluralistic society. Every interaction is an opportunity to learn about others and ourselves. To increase the likelihood of constructive interactions and effective communication, clinicians are advised to remember the importance of considering all exchanges from multiple perspectives, particularly those contrasting with their own, and to remain flexible. Differences provide a source of richness and an opportunity to appreciate human diversity. Differences are to be not tolerated but, rather, invited and nurtured (Shapiro, 1987, 1994a, 1994b; Shapiro et al., 2000, 2001, 2004). Cole (1989) pointed out that *E Pluribus Unum* ("From many, one") describes the homogenization of the U.S. population that has occurred since the day the Declaration of Independence was signed, stating,

> Although this motto may still represent our common belief in democratic ideals, it has a less noble meaning when considering the diversity of the people who inhabit this land. The dramatic demographic shift that is jolting this nation makes E PLURIBUS PLURIBUS (From Many, Many) a more accurate motto. (p. 65)

Cultural Sensitivity and the Clinical Process

An awareness of cultural patterns heightens sensitivity toward and appreciation of differences among all people. Yet we must remain mindful to guard against generalizations, which form the core of stereotypes (Cooper & Cooper, 1993; see also Battle, 2002b; Centeno, Anderson, & Obler, 2007; Culatta & Goldberg, 1995; Langdon, 2008; Lynch & Hanson, 1997; Nellum Davis, Gentry, & Hubbard-Wiley, 2002; Paul, 2007; Roseberry-McKibbin, 2007; Turnbull et al., 2006; for discussions addressing the challenges in providing valid and reliable assessment and treatment with people who have culturally or linguistically diverse backgrounds, see ASHA, 2004b, 2004c, 2005a, 2005c; Bernstein Ratner, 2004b; Ferguson, 2008; Hammer, Detwiler, Detwiler, Blood, & Qualls, 2004; Hinckley, 2008; Hirschberg & Hirschberg, 2007; Isaac, 2002; Jeffreys, 2006; McLeod, 2007; Paul, 2007; P. M. Roberts & Shenker, 2007; Robinson & Crowe, 2000; Shenker, 2004; Strauss, 2008; Van Borsel & de Britto Pereira, 2005; Westby, 2000). This section provides a number of recommendations, some specific, some general, that might be useful for working with people from different cultures who stutter. The recommendations are not intended to be all-inclusive or necessarily applicable to all people with diverse backgrounds. Rather, they are intended to help us remember to guard against preconceptions; to address all people, including members of the same family, as individuals; and to invite and nurture our understanding and acceptance of different behaviors and beliefs as opportunities to learn about ourselves, our clients, and our world.

Clinicians should be aware that there is no standard cultural group (Leith, 1986). Any group is made of subcultures, depending on degree of assimilation, socioeconomic level, geographic location, educational level, and other factors. Cultural variation often exists across members of the same family. An awareness of this variation should help prevent cultural stereotyping. Similarly, Culatta and Goldberg (1995) advised clinicians to determine the client's macroculture and microculture. Macroculture consists of the values that bind a population together as a whole and on which most political and social institutions of a country are based. For example, the macroculture of the United States values occupation, education, and financial worth; work and achievement; access to the comforts of living; cleanliness; and self-governance and humanitarianism. Microculture represents the individual's interpretation of values, speech and linguistic patterns, learning styles, and behavioral patterns based on variables such as ethnicity or national origin, religion, gender, age, exceptionality, geographic region, and class. Culatta and Goldberg indicated that for most people in the United States, cultural identification involves a blending of different microcultures.

Leith (1986) advised clinicians to determine the cultural group's and the client's own beliefs about and assumptions regarding a number of factors that might influence the assessment and treatment processes:

- *Privacy about family and personal lives.* Families demonstrate different degrees of willingness and comfort to discuss personal matters.

- *Protectiveness toward the children.* Parents and children demonstrate different levels of comfort in regard to the children communicating with adults outside of the family.

- *Appropriate level of speaking loudness.* Some clients may appear shy but in actuality are reluctant to speak or be spoken to in a loud (impolite) voice.

- *Attitudes toward stuttering and people who stutter.* Attitudes toward stuttering influence receptivity toward treatment programs and should be a factor in treatment design.

- *Roles of male and female children and adults.* Gender roles might impact who provides information for the family, the reluctance of males to acknowledge fear, and reactions toward female clinicians and others in a helping role. Also, if a family is not child oriented, efforts to seek parental cooperation in home programming may fail.

- *Communication with people from other cultures.* In some cultures, females do not interact with people from other cultures, which would result in difficulty for the clinician in conducting home visits and establishing home programming.

- *Interpretation of eye contact, touch, and gestures.* The clinician should be cautious about initiating eye contact, touch, and gestures because such behaviors might be misunderstood by clients.

- *Reluctance to sign forms.* In some cultures, families may be reluctant to sign documents, because doing so is seen as bringing embarrassment or shame to the family.

- *Status accrued for oral ability.* If oral ability is accorded high status, a person who stutters may feel a keen social stigma, and common treatment procedures such as voluntary stuttering or discussion of feelings may be both stressful and distasteful.

- *Views about etiology.* If a family views stuttering as a curse or a God-given condition, treatment will need to account for such beliefs. Otherwise, clinicians might inadvertently challenge clients to decide between the clinician's advice and personal beliefs.

- *Stuttering in native language.* Stuttering in a child's native language may contraindicate teaching English as a second language until stuttering is resolved. Communicative stress is a factor in the development and maintenance of stuttering.

Battle (2002c, pp. xviii–xx) offered a number of related suggestions for working with people from diverse cultures:

- Consider one's own personal and cultural beliefs, attitudes, and values and be aware of how they contribute to the cross-cultural interaction.

- Use the name of the culture or geographic group that is assigned by its members. This helps recognize the heterogeneity among groups and shows respect for the individual. Also, it is better to use a more specific term rather than a more general one. For example, use *Colombian* to refer to a person from Colombia, not *Hispanic* or *Latino*; use *Japanese* for a person from Japan, not *Asian*; use *Nigerian* for a person from Nigeria, not *African*. Using the names assigned by the members of a group often reduces uncertainty about using terms such as *Black* or *African American*, *Latino* or *Hispanic*, *Asian* or *Oriental*, *American Indian* or *Native American*, and *White* or *Caucasian*.

⬚ Use accurate and appropriately descriptive terms to refer to a person's race or ethnicity. For example, use *African American* rather than *minority*; use *Hispanic* rather than *bilingual*.

⬚ Be aware of the inaccurate, albeit common, assumption that most or all members of a racial or ethnic group are the same. We must acknowledge intragroup variation, even intrafamily variation, based on gender, age, socioeconomic status, education, sexual orientation, and geographic and life history, among other factors. Battle advised not to assume that all African Americans speak African American English, that all White Americans speak standard English, or that all Asian Americans or Latinos share the same beliefs or cultural patterns.

⬚ Avoid pejorative terms that assume European Americans are the standard (such as *culturally deprived*, *at-risk*, *culturally disadvantaged*) and qualifiers that reinforce racial or ethnic stereotypes (e.g., *Indian giver*, *black sheep*, *articulate Black student*, *white lie*, *Chinese fire drill*, *Chinese auction*, and *yellow journalism*). These terms and qualifiers have racist and ethnocentric connotations.

⬚ Be aware of possible nonverbal sources of cultural conflict and miscommunication (e.g., role of touch during conversation, spatial distance, appropriate topics for conversation, social rituals, and styles of greeting behavior) and verbal ones (beginning the professional agenda immediately vs. establishing social and interpersonal rapport).

Multicultural education provides an opportunity to reflect on our own awareness of and sensitivity to that which we consider to be different. Indeed, such reflection is essential for becoming aware of our own thoughts and attitudes about human diversity; that awareness is necessary for considering a variety of alternative approaches (e.g., to accept, reject, or revise our current way of thinking and acting). I invite you to join me and others in such reflection. For example, Brawner (2005) revised her own interpretation of human diversity, originally as an expression of differences, to the removal of boundaries in order to learn from others. She stated,

> Diversity can be a removal of boundaries and allowing oneself to step outside of these boundaries in order to learn about the ideas of others. . . . Being able to accept and recognize that everyone has *something* to share and releasing one's own mental barriers to being receptive may be at the heart of diversity. This, in turn, may be the driving force in one's outlook on life and the way issues and problems are approached. Diversity is less about learning every single "different" thing about something or someone but more about an expansion of our minds in looking at things from multiple perspectives. The concept of diversity opens possibilities and solutions. To address the topic of diversity is to reduce misunderstanding and increase awareness and sensitivity. (pp. 8–9)

Caruso (2002) noted, "It does seem as though societal attitudes have not advanced at the same pace as treatments or therapies" (p. 4). Also, he expressed concern that our professions' heightened objectivity may inadvertently lead to reduced "humanness" in how we approach and conduct our work in communication sciences and disorders. Imploring us not to depersonalize our interactions with real people, Caruso reflected on human diversity as follows:

> Yes, we are diverse in our makeup. People come in all shapes, sizes, and colors, as well as with varying ranges of abilities and skills. But in spite of these observable differences, we have much in common. . . . In spite of how we sound or move, how old we look, what color we are, or differences among us regarding issues of gender and sexual orientation, we have this in common: *We all want to feel cared for, we all want to be treated with respect, and we all want to have our dignity maintained.* (p. 4)

Explicit and implicit cultural behaviors (Battle, 2002a) invite clinicians to consider whether we, as one people, are more similar than we are different (Shapiro et al., 2000, 2001, 2004; see also Hirschberg & Hirschberg, 2007). Such searching questions are hardly new; they are timeless. They invite us to visit, revisit, and celebrate both our uniqueness and our commonality. That, at its essence, is human diversity. Carl Sandburg (1955), one of America's finest writers, editors, and poets, proclaimed,

> There is only one man in the world
> and his name is All Men.
> There is only one woman in the world
> and her name is All Women.
> There is only one child in the world
> and the child's name is All Children. (p. 3)

Summary—Multicultural Awareness

Multicultural education invites clinicians to appreciate human diversity in all of its forms and to resolve to approach all people, including those who stutter and their family members, as individuals. As clinicians, we need to be knowledgeable about and sensitive to the cultural heritage of those with whom we interact and realize the influence that culture has on how each of us views and reacts within our own communicative worlds. At the same time, however, we must not assume that all members of any particular group share the same values and beliefs held by the group as a whole. In other words, in our sincere efforts to better understand, accept, and accommodate our clients and their families, we must be mindful to prevent cultural stereotyping. This section reviewed the background to our professions' appreciation of multiculturalism and multicultural literacy, and discussed multicultural considerations that influence research on stuttering and the clinical process with people who stutter and their families. Related recommendations for clinicians were offered as a reminder and facilitator to invite and nurture our understanding and acceptance of different behaviors and beliefs as opportunities to learn about ourselves, our clients, and our world.

Chapter Summary

This chapter explored the extrafamily considerations of interdisciplinary teaming and multicultural awareness, which must be taken into account as we develop intervention plans with people who stutter.

Interdisciplinary teaming provides for collaborative opportunities to work with and learn from people who stutter, family members, and allied professions while ensuring the highest quality of service delivery. Such collaboration requires objective consideration of multiple and diverse perspectives regarding all aspects of case management. A number of significant events served as catalysts to the emergence of collaborative models of service delivery. These events include the passage of IDEA, which stipulated that the Individualized Education Program is a legal document and must be developed in collaboration with the child's parents or legal guardians, and legislation mandating that the opportunity to learn and achieve one's potential is a protected right for all people (No Child Left Behind, the Americans with Disabilities Amendments Act), as well as the emergence of early intervention transdisciplinary programs in the 1980s and interest in the concept of whole-language intervention. Other significant events that paved the way to collaborative models of service delivery include the civil rights, deinstitutionalization, and education reform movements; paradigm shifts in how and where people with disabilities should be served; demographic shifts toward increasingly older populations; and trends toward movement of people with special needs into community-based programs.

The foundation of interdisciplinary practice is a commitment to the welfare of the person and family being served (ASHA, 2010) and to one's own discipline and related disciplines. The conceptual underpinnings necessary for adopting and implementing interdisciplinary practice include shifting to a support paradigm, self-advocacy, person-centered approaches, natural and informal supports, family-focused and family-driven supports, full community inclusion and inclusive education, blurring of professional roles and turf, cost containment, and accountability. Members of interdisciplinary teams must share the ability to understand a common professional language; decrease control of work boundaries; understand delivery systems and remain open to available resources; communicate openly and effectively to peers and others; integrate professional abilities and unique personal qualities into the team and recognize the specialized culture, values, traditions, knowledge, training, personal emotions, and experiences that the other members bring to the team; and work well in teams and contribute toward consensus building. Related competencies were reviewed.

Multicultural awareness invites clinicians to appreciate human diversity in all of its forms and to resolve to approach each person, including those who stutter and their family members, as individuals with similarities and differences. While clinicians must be aware of differences in race, ethnicity, and culture, they must also be careful not to allow this awareness to lead inadvertently to stereotypes about racial, ethnic, or cultural groups. Despite the continuing growth of racial, ethnic, cultural, and linguistic diversity in the United States, few professionals are qualified to work with people who identify themselves with specific ethnic or racial groups. Prevalence and incidence of stuttering appear to differ among different cultural populations, suggesting that cultural factors may precipitate or perpetuate stuttering. Such factors include child-rearing practices, assumptions about and reactions to stuttering, and the roles that communication and family play in the culture.

Cultural factors that may influence the assessment and treatment processes include privacy about family and personal lives; protectiveness toward the children; appropriate level of speaking loudness; attitudes toward stuttering and people who stutter; roles of male and female children and adults; communication with people from other cultures; interpretation of eye contact, touch, gestures, and other nonverbal behaviors; reluctance to sign forms; status accrued for oral ability; views about etiology; and stuttering in native language. Quality indicators for clinical service include diagnostic and treatment practices that are individualized to meet specific needs of persons served, such as cultural and language background, in addition to age and developmental status, gender, cognitive ability, learning style, impairments, activity limitations, participation restrictions, environmental challenges, family and caregiver needs, and related regulations and policies. The ASHA Code of Ethics (ASHA, 2010) mandates clinicians to be competent to serve all people with communication disorders, including those with diverse languages and cultures. Battle (2002c) suggested that professionals working with people whose culture is different from their own should use the name of the culture as assigned by its members, use accurate and appropriately descriptive terms to refer to race or ethnicity, be aware of the inaccurate assumption that most or all members of a racial or ethnic group are the same, avoid pejorative terms that assume that European Americans are the standard and qualifiers that reinforce racial or ethnic stereotypes, and be sensitive to nonverbal and verbal sources of cultural conflict and miscommunication. Clinical competence requires that clinicians consider their own assumptions about human diversity, multiculturalism, and how similarities and difference among all people reflect on themselves and the human condition.

Chapter Six Study Questions

1. Rokusek (1995) stated that professionals need to feel comfortable in a unidisciplinary setting before they can function effectively in more collaborative environments. What implications does this statement hold for professional preparation?

2. Some models of interdisciplinary practice advocate role release among professionals, while others suggest that professionals retain their identity as experts in their respective area of specialized knowledge. How does each philosophy impact the effectiveness of the assessment and treatment processes? As a clinician, which do you feel more comfortable with and why? What factors would indicate one intervention approach over another?

3. Interdisciplinary practice implies sharing and exchanging of information and skills for the sake of providing clinical services of the highest quality. How could such an arrangement impact and be impacted by confidentiality? What should be shared and what should not? What should you do if the information that the client or family provided to you confidentially could be of use to other professionals serving the same people? What is confidentiality and what are its limits?

4. Ferguson (2008) and Hinckley (2008) reviewed the importance of individual and shared narratives that comprise collaboration and interdisciplinary practice. In what ways do narratives contribute to the clinical process? Whose narrative would you find most helpful? What would you do if the narratives of different participants are in conflict with each other? What would you do if someone's narrative conflicted with your own? In what ways does understanding and managing narratives facilitate versus inhibit the process of collective collaboration?

5. Stoneman and Malone (1995) and Garner et al. (1992) reviewed necessary competencies to be an effective team member. Which competencies do you feel to be most important and why? Which do you feel to be least important and why? Which of these competencies do you already possess? Which do you need to develop? How will you develop and maintain these competencies over the course of your career?

6. Clinicians must be sensitive to cultural differences that might influence assessment and treatment. However, might a clinician's professional values or judgment be compromised when accommodating a client's cultural differences? For example, if a client's culture does not allow a female child to be alone with a male who is not a family member, is it appropriate to assign a female clinician when a male clinician is qualified to provide the treatment? In a university training setting, when might the missions of service delivery and clinical instruction be in conflict?

7. We have reviewed intrafamily (personal constructs and family systems) and extrafamily (interdisciplinary teaming and multicultural awareness) intervention considerations. How does the concept of diversity relate to both intrafamily and extrafamily considerations? How do these areas of diversity relate to assessment and treatment with people who stutter and their families?

8. This chapter began with a quotation by Parker Palmer (1997), author of "The Grace of Great Things." He likened the human soul to a wild animal. How do his insights and advice relate to your understanding of intrafamily and extrafamily considerations, and how do these relationships inform the intervention process and your own professional development?

9. Cooper and Cooper (1993) expressed concern that conscientious researchers have successfully isolated independent variables by keeping their research populations

homogeneous (i.e., they have excluded culturally divergent participants). Van Borsel et al. (2001) expressed concern about the heterogeneity of the bilingual population in controlled research. The consequence of these concerns is that we know relatively little about the fluency-related characteristics of members of diverse cultures. In clinical research, are we homogenizing a heterogeneous population for the sake of control and replication? What do you recommend for future research? How can we best apply the rules of science and evidence-based practice to understanding the prevalence of stuttering, its manifestations, and therapy outcomes among multicultural populations?

10. The chapter ended with an invitation to reflect on your own thoughts and attitudes about human diversity (Brawner, 2005; Caruso, 2002; Sandburg, 1955). What does diversity and multiculturalism mean to you? In what ways do your thoughts impact your actions? In what ways do your actions reflect your thoughts? To what degree is there a consistency between your thoughts and your actions? How might your thoughts about diversity affect your role as a clinician with people who stutter and their families? Does being open to diversity require an acceptance of closed-mindedness? How might adopting a practice of seeking multiple perspectives contribute to diversity? How might Parker Palmer's (1997) conceptualization of the human soul inform your clinical practice?

Chapter Seven

Stuttering Modification and Fluency Shaping

Psychotherapeutic Considerations

*Many clinicians believe they need to use one approach or the other
[i.e., stuttering modification or fluency shaping] because the two approaches appear to be incompatible, even though choosing one over the
other may be difficult or confusing. Fortunately, the two approaches need
not be antagonistic. In fact, techniques based on one approach can be
helpful to clinicians using the other approach. (Guitar, 1998, p. 137)*

Stuttering modification and fluency shaping are endpoints of a psychotherapeutic continuum. Understanding these two points, and particularly the continuum that lies between them, is useful for distinguishing the many treatments available and currently
being used with people who stutter. The primary purpose of presenting the continuum,
however, is to provide a theoretical framework for tailoring the design of treatment for
each individual who stutters. The design of effective treatment is not arbitrary; rather,
it is systematic and based on coherent, psychotherapeutic decision rules, in addition to
the intrafamily and extrafamily considerations already reviewed. In this chapter, we will
compare and contrast stuttering modification and fluency shaping approaches, emphasizing the following points:

- Understanding the principles and procedures underlying stuttering modification and fluency shaping and familiarity with exemplar treatments enable clinicians to tailor intervention for each person who stutters.
- Differential diagnostic criteria relating to how a person who stutters confronts his feelings
  about himself and about communication guide the design of individualized treatment.

General Definitions

Stuttering modification therapy (Guitar, 1998; Guitar & Peters, 2008) refers to a category
of intervention approaches used *with* people who stutter. These approaches assume that

stuttering results from avoiding or struggling with disfluency, avoiding feared words, and avoiding feared situations. The intervention process seeks to reduce speech-related avoidance behaviors, fears, and negative attitudes, while modifying the form of stuttering. Guitar (1998) and Guitar and Peters (2008) explained that this can be accomplished by different methods, including reducing the struggle behavior, smoothing out the form of stuttering, and reducing the tension and rate of stuttering by stuttering in a more relaxed and deliberate way. Such techniques are used to help a person who demonstrates advanced stuttering to stutter in a more fluent manner. Gregory (1979) noted that these techniques help people "stutter more fluently" (p. 2). Similarly, Curlee and Perkins (1984) characterized these techniques as "those that manage stuttering" (p. iii). Taken together, stuttering modification approaches help the person who stutters to stutter more fluently (i.e., with less effort, struggle, and abnormality). Gregory (1979, 2003) emphasized that the person who stutters must make his speech behavior the object of study, become familiar with it, and gradually modify his stuttering by thinking about, identifying, and practicing methods of stuttering more easily. By allowing the stuttering to occur so as to study and modify the behavior, the person who stutters changes his speech-related behaviors, feelings, and attitudes, thus reducing his avoidance behavior.

One of the best-known exemplars of stuttering modification therapy is Van Riper's (1973) treatment for the "confirmed stutterer" (p. 203), referred to as MIDVAS (Motivation, Identification, Desensitization, Variation, Approximation, Stabilization) (Van Riper, 1972, 1973). Other approaches that are reflective of stuttering modification include, but are not limited to, those of Bloodstein (1975), Breitenfeldt and Lorenz (1989), Conture (2001), Dell (2008), Luper and Mulder (1964), Manning (2010), Sheehan (1970), and Williams (1957, 1971, 1979, 2003, 2004, 2006).

On the other end of the continuum is *fluency shaping therapy* (Guitar, 1998; Guitar & Peters, 2008). This category refers to intervention approaches used *for* people who stutter, and assumes that stuttering is learned. Therefore, intervention is based on principles of behavior modification (i.e. operant conditioning and programming). Unlike stuttering modification, where the goal of treatment is to modify stuttering into an easier, gentler form, fluency shaping first seeks to establish fluent speech by eliminating stuttering in a controlled stimulus environment. The fluent response is reinforced (positively and/or negatively) and stuttering behavior is punished. Through successive approximation, fluency is gradually modified to approximate normal-sounding conversational speech in a controlled clinical setting. Then, efforts are directed to generalize the fluent speech to the person's natural speaking environments. Gregory (1979) characterized such treatments as those that direct the person who stutters to "speak more fluently" (p. 5). Likewise, Curlee and Perkins (1984) categorized these treatments as "those that manage fluency" (p. iii). Taken together, fluency shaping techniques increase the length and complexity of the fluent responses of a person who stutters, first in the treatment setting and then in extraclinical settings, ultimately so as to replace the stuttering behavior with fluency.

Programmed Conditioning for Fluency (Ryan & Van Kirk, 1971), also referred to as the *Monterey Fluency Program* (Ryan & Van Kirk, 1978) and *Programmed Therapy for Stuttering in Children and Adults* (Ryan, 1974, 2001), represents a well-known example of fluency shaping therapy. In the original form of this treatment (Ryan, 1974), fluency is established in one of four programs. One program is referred to as GILCU (Gradual Increase in Length and Complexity of Utterance), in which the client is directed to talk slowly and to generate a fluent (not stuttered, by definition in this case) single-word response. The response is gradually increased to two, three, and so on to six words before a sentence becomes the target response. Another establishment program is delayed auditory feedback (DAF). The client uses headphones to hear his speech in 50-millisecond decrements of delay from 250 to 0 milliseconds. This delayed auditory feedback helps the person who stutters to speak in a slow, prolonged, nonstuttered manner. The third establishment program (programmed traditional) shapes a fluent response first by identifying stuttered words and then by using cancellations, pull-outs, and preparatory sets (terms borrowed from Van Riper, 1973, which will be discussed later in this chapter). The last establishment program (punishment) reduces the frequency of stuttering by presenting aversive events. In the more recent version, Ryan (2001) embedded punishment (i.e., aversive consequences for stuttering) into GILCU and DAF-prolongation, thereby deleting programmed traditional and punishment from the treatment. Other proponents of fluency shaping treatment include, but are not limited to, Boberg (1981, 2006); Boberg and Kully (1985, 1994); Costello (1980, 1983); Goldiamond (1965); Harrison et al. (2007); Ingham (1999); Kully and Langevin (1999); Kully et al. (2007); Onslow et al. (2003); Perkins (1973a, 1973b); Perkins, Rudas, Johnson, Michael, and Curlee (1974); Runyan and Runyan (2007, 2010); Shames and Florance (1980); Shine (1980, 1984); R. L. Webster (1979); and Wingate (1969, 1976).

One form of fluency shaping intervention, electronic devices utilizing altered auditory feedback (AAF), has recently been the subject of increased empirical and commercial interest (Lincoln, Packman, & Onslow, 2006). *Altered auditory feedback* refers to changing the speech signal electronically so that speakers perceive their voice differently than they ordinarily would. Such alteration has taken the forms of delayed auditory feedback (DAF, referred to earlier), masking auditory feedback (MAF), and frequency-altered feedback (FAF). The underlying logic is consistent with the observation that stuttering frequency significantly decreases in response to altered auditory feedback (Goldiamond, 1965). Delayed auditory feedback increases the time it takes for the speech signal to be heard by the speaker; masking auditory feedback sends a white noise (i.e., triggered by vibration of the vocal cords) to the ears of the speaker so he cannot hear himself while speaking; frequency-altered feedback changes the pitch of the speech signal heard by the speaker so it is perceived either as higher or lower than it actually is. Interest in masking auditory feedback has waned as a result of studies indicating that delayed auditory feedback and frequency-altered feedback are more effective than masking in reducing stuttering. Also, masking auditory feedback created the practical limitation of being unable to hear any other auditory signals (i.e., including conversational partners and environmental sounds) if they occurred while the person with such feedback was speaking. The devices incorporating delayed auditory feedback and frequency-altered feedback have become increasingly miniaturized and consist of a signal processor, headphones, and a microphone. Bluetooth technology has eliminated the need for most wires. The SpeechEasy (Kalinowski & Saltuklaroglu, 2006) is among the most technologically sophisticated, offering digital signal processing of both delayed auditory feedback and frequency-altered feedback by inconspicuous devices that fit completely in the ear canals. Numerous altered auditory feedback devices are commercially available, have been found to reduce stuttering in structured settings, and are in need of validation through empirical efficacy investigations, particularly in conversational contexts. One recent investigation of the SpeechEasy (Pollard, Ellis, Finan, & Ramig, 2009) revealed a significant reduction of stuttering immediately after the device was fitted, relatively more stuttering reduction during oral reading than during conversation, and elimination of the treatment effect (i.e., return of stuttering) after 4 months. Lincoln et al. (2006) presented an excellent review of commercially available altered auditory feedback devices and related empirical investigations; other sources are available as well (see, e.g., Armson & Kiefte, 2008; Howell, Sackin, & Williams, 1999; Natke, Grosser,

& Kalveram, 2001; O'Donnell, Armson, & Kiefte, 2008; Ramig, Ellis, & Polland, 2010; Stuart, Kalinowski, Rastatter, Saltuklaroglu, & Dayalu, 2004).

Significant Differences Between Stuttering Modification and Fluency Shaping

Stuttering modification and fluency shaping can be further distinguished on the basis of behavioral treatment goals, affective treatment goals, procedures, and structure (Guitar, 1998; Guitar & Peters, 2008). These distinctions are represented in Table 7.1.

Behavioral Treatment Goals

Three different behavioral treatment goals for people who stutter have been outlined (Guitar, 1998; Guitar & Peters, 2008). The optimal goal is *spontaneous speech fluency*, which is characteristic of the "normal" speaker. Neither tension nor struggle behavior is observed; speech is characterized by ongoing smoothness. Repetitions and prolongations are easy, are nearly effortless, and occur only occasionally. The rate and rhythm are even, regular, and not noticed by the speaker. The relative effort is minor; thus the speaker attends to the thoughts and ideas being conveyed and exchanged rather than to the speech itself.

In cases where the goal of spontaneous speech fluency is not possible, the goal of *controlled fluency* is pursued. The smoothness (continuity) of speech in controlled fluency is similar to that of spontaneous fluency. However, in order to maintain controlled fluency, the person who stutters must monitor and adjust his speech to maintain natural-sounding speech. Guitar (1998) indicated that this might be achieved in various ways, including making a fluency adjustment before (preparatory set) or during (pull-out) a disfluent word, reducing rate of speech, softening articulatory contacts, prolonging syllables, and responding to auditory and proprioceptive feedback. These adjustments might be slightly noticeable to an astute listener. By attending to and adjusting speech rate and rhythm, a person who achieves controlled fluency expends greater effort in order to achieve nearly normal-sounding speech smoothness. Distinguishing spontaneous from controlled fluency, Guitar and Peters (2008) indicated that the former "is the fluency of the normal speaker" (p. 3), while in the latter, "the speaker must attend to his manner of speaking to maintain relatively normal sounding fluency" (p. 4).

The third and least preferred goal is *acceptable stuttering*, in which the speaker demonstrates noticeable disfluency that is of relatively low severity. The speaker also demonstrates and reports feeling relative comfort in his role as a communicator despite his stuttering. As with controlled fluency, the person who demonstrates acceptable stuttering monitors his speech and makes adjustments to maintain a reduced or acceptable level of stuttering. However, with acceptable stuttering, all dimensions of fluency (rate, rhythm, continuity, and effort) are affected and potentially noticeable to conversational partners.

All clinicians, regardless of whether they practice stuttering modification, fluency shaping, or a combination, work toward the ultimate goal of spontaneous fluency. Clinical research indicates that this objective becomes increasingly difficult as stuttering advances through the lifespan. If spontaneous fluency proves unattainable as a realistic objective, then clinicians of both theoretical orientations would treat controlled fluency as the next best objective. If both spontaneous fluency and controlled fluency prove unattainable, the stuttering modification clinician then would turn to acceptable stuttering as the most appropriate treatment goal. For a fluency shaping clinician, however,

Table 7.1 Distinctions Between Stuttering Modification (SM) and Fluency Shaping (FS)

Premise

SM: Stuttering results from avoiding or struggling with disfluencies, fears, and negative attitudes.

FS: Stuttering is learned.

Behavioral Treatment Goals

SM: In decreasing order of desirability, goals include spontaneous fluency, controlled fluency, and acceptable stuttering.

FS: Spontaneous fluency and controlled fluency are the only acceptable goals. Any evidence of noticeable stuttering is regarded as a program failure.

Affective Treatment Goals

SM: Fears and avoidances related to stuttering are reduced by identifying, studying, and understanding thoughts, feelings, and attitudes about communication and oneself as a communicator. Positive social and vocational adjustments are targeted directly.

FS: No attempt is made to reduce communication-related fears and avoidances or impact the attitudes of the person who stutters. As a result of improved fluency, however, fears often reduce and positive social and vocational adjustments occur indirectly.

Procedures

SM: Much attention is given to reducing speech fears and avoidance behaviors. The client is taught to be more fluent by various techniques to modify stuttering. Fluency is maintained by reduction of fears and avoidance behaviors.

FS: Little attention is given to reduction of speech fears and avoidance behaviors. The client is "programmed" for stutter-free speech via specific contingencies. Fluency is maintained by modifying the manner of speaking and, if necessary, reinstatement of fluency by repeating sections of the original program.

Structure

SM: A less structured format (such as a teaching or counseling interaction) is used.

FS: The format is highly structured (which is typical of behavioral conditioning and programming).

Note. From *Stuttering: An Integration of Contemporary Therapies* (Publication 16, 4th ed., pp. 1–58), by B. Guitar and T. J. Peters, 2008, Memphis, TN: Stuttering Foundation of America. Copyright 2008 by the Stuttering Foundation of America. Adapted with permission.

---

any form of noticeable stuttering is regarded as evidence of a program failure. Therefore, acceptable stuttering typically is not a viable treatment objective for fluency shaping clinicians.

Affective Treatment Goals

Stuttering modification and fluency shaping also differ in terms of their respective affective treatment goals—the extent to which and the ways in which treatment addresses the communication-related feelings and attitudes of the person who stutters. Stuttering modification emphasizes the importance of identifying, studying, and understanding the feelings and attitudes of the person who stutters, thereby reducing the fears and avoidances related to stuttering. People who stutter are encouraged to seek out and systematically master speaking situations that were formerly avoided. Through desensitization and strategically designed successes, the person who stutters develops communication competence and confidence, thereby achieving a more positive attitude toward his speech, the process of communication, and himself as a communicator. Furthermore, stuttering modification attempts to impact the overall adjustment of the person who stutters, thus facilitating development of his social and vocational skills.

Fluency shaping, on the other hand, does not attempt to reduce the communication-related fears and avoidances or otherwise impact the attitudes of the person who stutters. As a consequence of fluency success from programmed treatment, however, fears are often reduced and attitudes are improved, albeit indirectly. Likewise, while fluency shaping does not attempt to impact the social or vocational adjustment of the person who stutters, such changes may occur as a by-product of programmed treatment.

Treatment Procedures

Both stuttering modification and fluency shaping help the person who stutters achieve an initial measure of fluency by using deliberate and controlled techniques. These might include speaking with an even rate (i.e., perceived as slower) and gentle onset (prolonged, nearly effortless initiation) with or without use of a delayed auditory feedback device, engaging in choral reading, or shadowing the speech of the clinician. After initial fluency is established, however, stuttering modification and fluency shaping methods differ with respect to how later objectives (such as spontaneous or controlled fluency) are achieved.

Stuttering modification seeks to facilitate fluency by reducing communication-related fears, avoidances, and negative attitudes, seeking adjustments in such internal dimensions as a consequence of improved fluency. Once fluency is established, people who stutter are encouraged to combat the natural tendency to avoid feared words and situations. They are guided in how to approach such feared contexts by using techniques for controlling and canceling instances of stuttering. Furthermore, since the morale and self-esteem of people who stutter are considered to be critical factors in the maintenance of fluency, stuttering modification seeks to monitor and enhance, if appropriate, the social and emotional adjustment of such persons. Guitar (1998) indicated that relapse into periods of uncontrolled stuttering is a significant issue, particularly for people whose stuttering has advanced into adulthood. To reduce the likelihood of such occurrences, Guitar and Peters (2008) recommended that stuttering modification clinicians urge clients to combat the tendency to avoid words or situations, keep speech fears at a minimum level, master stuttering modification skills, and become their own clinician and thereby assume responsibility for their own therapy. Other strategies to facilitate transfer of fluency skills and minimize the likelihood of relapse that I will address include beginning transfer activities from the very first contact with the client, identifying and modifying as necessary one's personal construct, working within family systems and interdisciplinary contexts, and preparing for relapse so as to minimize its negative effects. Stuttering modification, therefore, tends to consider the person who stutters in dynamic totality.

Fluency shaping, by contrast, addresses directly observable speech behavior on the reasoning that stuttering is acquired through conditioning principles. Therefore, fluency (stutter-free speech) is established in a controlled stimulus environment and maintained by the use of techniques such as slowing speech rate and monitoring the ease of speech onset. Often such techniques are found in behaviorally (operantly) designed programs that seek to instate or reinstate fluency through sequenced steps in which the response expectation is prescribed and increased systematically. Should relapse occur, the client is recycled through the earlier steps in the program, which enabled him to achieve his fluency prior to relapse. Guitar and Peters (2008) indicated that within fluency shaping, the manner of speaking is modified rather than the moment of stuttering.

Treatment Structure

Stuttering modification treatment is typically conducted within a teaching or counseling context in which dialogue between the clinician and client is the medium of exchange. The interaction, while systematically planned, is relatively unstructured, with the clinician and client interacting as equal participants, each with dynamic roles and contributions to the treatment process.

Fluency shaping treatment is a highly structured approach in which stimuli, responses, and subsequent events are preprogrammed. Guitar (1998) noted that "specific responses from the client are targeted, and specific reactions to these responses are required from the clinician" (p. 146).

Advantages and Disadvantages

Stuttering modification techniques directly address the communication-related feelings and attitudes of people who stutter in addition to their speech behaviors. Furthermore, as noted, the person who stutters is an active participant in all aspects of the treatment process, requiring interpersonal, problem-solving, and professional skills on the part of the clinician. Some may interpret as a disadvantage the fact that the actual change in speech behavior takes relatively longer in stuttering modification (compared to fluency shaping) because of the nature and context of the change. However, this observation is counterbalanced by the advantage that change occurs not only to speech behavior, but also to feelings and attitudes, thus facilitating the maintenance and transfer of fluency over time and communicative settings. In other words, stuttering modification tends to result in slower observable fluency change but is more effective in reducing speech fears and reversing negative attitudes while strengthening generalization of the speech behaviors. Guitar and Peters (2008) pointed out that stuttering modification is a dynamic process in which the person who stutters is not directed to speak in an abnormal pattern (as in fluency shaping), but is expected and supported to confront his communication-related fears and avoidances (unlike fluency shaping). While clinicians find stuttering modification to be less structured and often more conversationally inviting than fluency shaping, such a dynamic, interactive clinical context requires more advanced professional skills on the part of the clinician. These abilities include providing emotional support, engaging in clinical problem solving, and responding to clients' individual differences, some of which prove troublesome for beginning clinicians. These and other clinician competencies will be addressed in the chapters to follow, particularly in Chapter 11.

Fluency shaping techniques, on the other hand, target speech behaviors only. The person who stutters is more passively involved in a relatively highly structured program designed and directed by the clinician. Observed behavior change occurs relatively rapidly. Balancing this potential advantage, however, is that maintenance and transfer of the fluency skills are usually not as promising as in stuttering modification. Guitar and Peters (2008) indicated that fluency shaping procedures tend to engage the client in an abnormal or artificial pattern of speaking in order to achieve stutter-free speech. Highly prescribed, the procedures tend to be less motivating, if not boring. Many commercially available fluency shaping programs direct both the clinician and client through a clinical script, indicating what to do and when to do it. Clients do not directly confront speaking-related fears or avoidances. The delivery of services requires less advanced professional skills, less clinical insight, and less clinical sensitivity.

Differential Diagnostic Indicators for Treatment Design

As noted earlier, the purpose of reviewing stuttering modification and fluency shaping is to establish a theoretical framework for individualizing treatment for people who stutter. The most effective treatment for an individual typically falls somewhere between the anchor points of stuttering modification and fluency shaping. It is incumbent, therefore, on clinicians to know how to combine stuttering modification and fluency shaping. Both schools of thought have merit when applied judiciously. Neither is appropriate for all people who stutter.

Guitar and Peters (2008) reported that stuttering modification and fluency shaping treatments are most distinct when designed for adults who stutter (those of or beyond the high school years), less distinct for children in elementary school (particularly among the lower age range), and least distinct for preschool children. The impact of a person's history and emotional reaction to stuttering is more pronounced as he accumulates experience with stuttering. For reasons of illustration, this discussion focuses on the differential diagnostic indicators for the design of treatment for adults who stutter.

We will discuss later (in Chapters 8 and 9) how treatment is modified for individuals who have less experience stuttering. Guitar and Peters (2008) noted that as a person continues to stutter, overt speech behavior often becomes more severe and related feelings and attitudes become more handicapping. With respect to planning treatment, they commented, "In reality, the six or seven year old is often more like the preschool stutterer. The twelve year old stutterer, on the other hand, can be more like the high school stutterer" (p. 46). Therefore, the factors guiding the design of treatment extend beyond one's chronological age and severity of overt symptomatology. Specifically, one of the most deciding factors in the design of treatment is the extent to which a person tends to conceal stuttering or avoid communicative situations that incline him to stutter. These factors relate to how the person who stutters confronts his feelings about himself as a person and as a communicator.

Guitar and Peters (2008) noted that a stuttering modification approach is neither indicated nor contraindicated by the severity of stuttering:

> This approach works as well with mild as with severe stutterers. The important thing to consider is how much the stutterer avoids or hides his stuttering. If he spends considerable energy disguising his stuttering, he is more likely to profit from stuttering modification therapy. (p. 24)

Stuttering modification is also indicated when a person experiences a personal penalty for stuttering. Such penalties may take the form of feeling poorly about oneself as a communicator, feeling that others are not accepting of oneself because of the stuttering, or feeling that stuttering interferes with one's life dreams or future ambitions. As will be seen, the extent to which a person may perceive a personal penalty can be determined from the diagnostic process, from trial management within and subsequent to the diagnostic interview, and from informal, unstructured (conversationally based), and more standardized (attitude questionnaires) assessment of feelings and attitudes. Another indication for stuttering modification is when the person demonstrates a more positive response to stuttering modification trial management. This means that the person responds positively to opportunities to discuss the nature of observed fluency and disfluency, to practice ways of stuttering more easily, and to address feelings and attitudes about himself as a communicator. This person may express discomfort with the communicative artificiality of fluency shaping techniques. In other words, an intervention approach more in the direction of stuttering modification is indicated for a person who

- ⌇ hides or disguises his stuttering,
- ⌇ avoids speaking,
- ⌇ perceives personal penalty as a consequence of stuttering,
- ⌇ feels badly about himself as a communicator, and
- ⌇ demonstrates a more positive response to stuttering modification trial management.

A candidate for fluency shaping, on the other hand, is more likely to demonstrate a positive self-image as a communicator (Guitar & Peters, 2008). This person's stuttering does not seem to be maintained by negative emotions. Thus, the person is talkative whether or not he stutters severely. Although the stuttering may be experienced as an annoyance and even as an impediment to his life, this person nevertheless remains positive, does not feel that the stuttering is a significant handicap, and feels accepted by family, friends, and associates despite his stuttering. Also, a person for whom fluency shaping is indicated does not attempt to conceal his stuttering or avoid speaking situations. His stuttering, therefore, is easily observable. A positive response to fluency shaping trial management is observed, and the candidate expresses acceptance of the prolonged speech pattern often characteristic of fluency shaping. In fact, he may express relief to have gained increased conversational fluency by use of such methods. In summary, indications for fluency shaping include an individual who

- ⌇ stutters openly,
- ⌇ does not avoid speaking,
- ⌇ perceives annoyance or interference but no personal penalty from stuttering,
- ⌇ feels positive about himself as a communicator, and
- ⌇ demonstrates a positive response to fluency shaping trial management.

In reality, most people who stutter present indications for both stuttering modification and fluency shaping. Most forms of intervention, therefore, are combinations of these two approaches. Again, a challenge facing clinicians is knowing how to combine the approaches most effectively for each person who stutters. Guitar and Peters (2008) noted,

> In our experience, most clients will benefit from a combination of stuttering modification and fluency shaping approaches at some stage of their treatment. We believe this for the following reasons. We think that fluency shaping therapy is more efficient than stuttering modification therapy for changing speech patterns. We also think, however, that stuttering modification therapy is more effective in reducing speech fears and improving speech attitudes for those clients who need it. (p. 26)

Furthermore, candidates for a combined approach typically have some fear of stuttering, but not to the extent of internalizing deep hurt, rejection, and penalty. Variation in the frequency and severity of stuttering may be present. Similarly, evidence of occasional avoidance, including circumlocutions and stalling tactics, may be observed. Usually candidates for a combined approach have a somewhat positive response to both fluency shaping and stuttering modification trial management. In other words, the reduction in disfluency resulting from fluency shaping is as motivating to candidates as the opportunity to discuss and better understand the nature of their own fluency and disfluency, as well as related feelings. Therefore, an approach combining stuttering modification and fluency shaping is indicated for a person who

- ⊞ stutters openly, but may demonstrate some avoidance,
- ⊞ perceives some sense of personal penalty and negative feelings from stuttering, but not to an extreme or handicapping degree,
- ⊞ feels relatively positive about himself as a communicator, but desires personal change, and
- ⊞ demonstrates a positive response both to stuttering modification and fluency shaping trial management.

Most people who stutter demonstrate criteria, to a greater or lesser degree, for a combined approach of stuttering modification and fluency shaping. We might interpret combined approaches as those that are used both *with* and *for* people who stutter. Frequently, people whose stuttering is advanced indicate that stuttering influences many aspects of their life (e.g., how they define themselves as communicators and as people, educational and employment ambitions, social interactions; see Corcoran & Stewart, 1998; Craig et al., 2009; Crichton-Smith, 2002; Gabel et al., 2004; J. F. Klein & Hood, 2004; Klompas & Ross, 2004). Most people who stutter benefit from intervention designed to develop and use strategies (i.e., fluency facilitating controls) to stutter more easily on moments of stuttering by gaining control of relative effort, rhythm, rate, and continuity, while becoming more accepting of themselves as communicators and as persons by confronting and reducing negative feelings and attitudes. This book offers a method that combines stuttering modification and fluency shaping techniques to enable a person who stutters to achieve fluency freedom, to become an independent communicator, to feel positive about himself and his place in the world, to access and contribute to his community, and to return the favor to others who have not yet realized their own communicative dreams. Other approaches that are reflective of intervention combining stuttering modification and fluency shaping include, but are not limited to, Bloom and Cooperman (1999), Cooper and Cooper (2003), Daly (1988), Gregory (2003), Guitar (2006), C. S. Montgomery (2006), Starkweather and Given-Ackerman (1997), and Wall and Myers (1995).

As noted in Chapter 2, evidence-based practice is widely supported as consistent with our oath to client welfare (ASHA, 2010). Many practitioners, however, interpret evidence-based practice too narrowly (Fey & Justice, 2007). Some clinicians who want to adhere to evidence-based practice feel discouraged from using professional judgment gained from years of documented clinical success in favor of published randomized controlled trials; others appear dismissive toward clinicians who do not have or do not rely on published data despite reliable and valid accountability for changes in the affective, behavioral, and cognitive dimensions of the communication experience. This controversy is particularly relevant to the assessment of the merits of stuttering modification, fluency shaping, or a combined approach. Within the clinical literature, fluency shaping has been labeled as evidence based, while stuttering modification has been labeled as assertion based (Prins & Ingham, 2009; see also Blomgren, Roy, Callister, & Merrill, 2005; Onslow, 2003; Ryan, 2006). This distinction has resulted in a theoretical encampment of clinicians who argue for the data-driven accountability of fluency shaping and others who argue for the social and ecological validity of stuttering modification. As will be seen in Chapters 8, 9, and 10, the best of both worlds is not just possible but also essential.

Recently, Prins and Ingham (2009) asserted that from a historical perspective, both fluency shaping and stuttering modification are evidence based and conform to the definition of evidence-based practice ("the conscientious, explicit, and judicious use of current best evidence in making decisions about the care of individual patients . . . integrating individual clinical expertise with the best available external evidence from systematic research"; Sacket, Rosenberg, Gray, Haynes, & Richardson, 1996, p. 71). Prins and Ingham noted that fluency shaping seeks outcome evidence even as it has eschewed theory; stuttering modification is theory driven, even as it has eschewed outcome evidence. The different approaches ask different questions and, as consequence, use different procedures and seek different data. Fluency shaping asks what procedures reduce the frequency of stuttering events. The objective of fluency shaping is stutter-free, natural-sounding speech; procedures include carefully described and replicable steps, performance-contingent progress during treatment, and quantitative measurement of process and outcomes. Stuttering modification asks what procedures are justified by the nature of the stuttering event from affective, behavioral, and cognitive perspectives. The objective of stuttering modification is to reduce the defensive reaction to perceived fluency disruption; procedures include exploring, calming, and modifying such learned struggle and avoidance behaviors, thereby gaining voluntary control over the stuttering event, mastering the motor sequences, and achieving positive changes in attitudes and beliefs. These distinctions will be clearer after the review of exemplar treatments, reviewed below.

Prins and Ingham (2009) asserted that a treatment's long-term effectiveness (the most vexing challenge of every intervention) may have nothing to do with fluency shaping or stuttering modification. Rather, successful outcomes, which have been observed and documented for both approaches, may be a function of self-management, modeling, or other strategies yet to be identified. Indeed, much is to be learned about the components of intervention that prove to be most effective—with a particular individual, with that same individual at different times, and across individuals. In Chapters 8, 9, and 10, I contend that both a coherent theory and outcome evidence for affective, behavioral, and cognitive elements are essential, and offer an intervention approach that combines stuttering modification and fluency shaping.

Exemplar Stuttering Modification and Fluency Shaping Treatments

As we will see, stuttering modification and fluency shaping can—and should—be combined. In order to appreciate the relative strengths of these approaches, it is helpful to first look at each treatment modality separately. Here we review the stuttering modification treatment described by Charles Van Riper (1972, 1973) and the fluency shaping treatments described by Bruce Ryan (1974, 2001; Ryan & Van Kirk, 1971, 1978). Many other treatments could be discussed as well; interested clinicians are encouraged to explore these treatments (e.g., Bennett, 2006; Bloodstein & Bernstein Ratner, 2008; Conture & Curlee, 2007; Guitar, 2006). For purposes of illustration, the treatments summarized here will address intervention with young adults who demonstrate confirmed or advanced characteristics of stuttering.

Stuttering Modification: Van Riper

Van Riper (1972) indicated that two facts are important cornerstones in his form of treatment. Specifically, stuttering is intermittent, and the occurrence, frequency, and severity of stuttering vary systematically with the strength of certain specific, observable, and therefore manipulable factors:

> If we can focus our therapy on these factors so that those which make stuttering worse are weakened sufficiently and those which make for less stuttering are strengthened, the

frequency and severity of stuttering will decrease, and ultimately stuttering will disappear. (p. 283)

Van Riper underscored that like all other human behavior, stuttering obeys certain predictable patterns or laws. For example, conditions that tend to worsen stuttering include the following: penalty, frustration, anxiety, guilt, and hostility; situation fears based on previous stuttering in similar situations; word and phonetic fears based on previous stuttering on similar words and sounds; and greater real or perceived communication importance or meaningfulness of what is being said. Such predictability and individuality of the stuttering experience result in three principles that ground the intervention process: learning theory, servotheory, and psychotherapy (Van Riper, 1973).

With respect to learning theory, the person who stutters is guided to unlearn maladaptive responses to the fear and experience of fluency disruption and to learn new, more adaptive ones. Second, servotheory holds that speech is automatically controlled by feedback and that stuttering is a consequence of failure in the auditory processing system. Van Riper's treatment emphasizes monitoring speech by proprioception, essentially bypassing or reducing the reliance upon the auditory feedback system. Finally, Van Riper acknowledged that adolescents and adults who stutter often "come to us with intense fears, frustrations, and other emotional reactions due to their disrupted speech and feelings of deviance" (1973, p. 204). For this reason, the treatment is designed so that psychotherapy for secondary or expectancy type neurosis suffuses all interactions. When a more primary or central neurosis exists, a referral is made to an appropriate practitioner.

Diagnosis

The clinician should begin with a diagnostic evaluation to appraise the person and the presenting problem, a process of assessment that continues throughout treatment. Factors being assessed include overt (stuttering severity, nature of fluency) and covert (motivation, frustration, anxiety, guilt, shame, hostility, fears, ego strength) manifestations of communication. Van Riper (1973) recommended the following general procedures, to be carried out in an interview format:

- Discuss with the client an outline of the diagnostic process.
- Invite the client to describe the presenting problem, and verbalize the client's likely feelings.
- Engage the client in conversation and reading. Discuss with the client the observed stuttering behavior (e.g., comparison to client's usual speech, hierarchic sequences, and strategic function).
- Analyze core behaviors (e.g., speed, regularity, coarticulation of syllabic repetitions), noting the simultaneous and successive motor movements; how and where tremors begin and end; timing of respiration, phonation, and articulation; and other factors. Also analyze avoidance and release behaviors, noting variability and consistency.
- Analyze the client's fluent speech (e.g., rate, pitch, intensity, quality).
- Determine the client's prediction of stuttering, which can help in identifying phonemic or situation cues.
- Explore the onset and development of stuttering, penalties and rejections, possible profits and secondary gains, and emotionality.
- Explore attitudes and perceptions through formal and informal assessment.
- Determine the impact of communication stress (e.g., listener loss, interruptions, time pressure, speaking on the phone, speaking to a small group).

⊞ Conduct trial therapy and summarize impressions. The diagnostic session should end by instructing the client to prepare a thorough autobiography describing significant experiences that shaped him and people who influenced him.

The clinician must interpret the strength, frequency, and duration of the client's habits of avoidance and struggle, and differentially diagnose possible organicity and other types of disfluency. Van Riper (1973) cautioned that "we cannot rely solely on frequency counts of stutterings. The disorder is too variable, too influenced by too many external and internal stimuli. We cannot treat the stuttering alone. We must treat the stutterer" (p. 219). It is generally not possible in the initial evaluation to explore fully and in depth all of the client's communication strengths and limitations. Therefore, following establishment of initial impressions, the clinician must continue to question and learn about the client as a person and as a communicator throughout the treatment process.

Van Riper's treatment contains four sequential phases. The *identification phase* is intended for the person who stutters to explore, analyze, and classify overt behaviors and covert experiences characteristic of his stuttering. Second, the *desensitization phase* decreases speech anxieties and other related negative emotions, and "toughens" the person who stutters to the threat and experience of fluency failure. Third, the *modification phase* is intended first to vary and then to unlearn habitual avoidance and struggle responses, and then to learn to use counterconditioning in a new, more fluent and less abnormal way of stuttering. Finally, the *stabilization phase* is intended to help the person who stutters make the less abnormal, more fluent way of stuttering more automatic and to develop proprioceptive monitoring of his speech. Van Riper noted that his methods must not be seen as a static template to be applied to all people who stutter. Rather, he emphasized the importance of tailoring treatment to each client's special strengths and needs.

Within these four phases, there are a number of overlapping subphases referred to by the acronym MIDVAS (Van Riper, 1972, 1973), each letter of which stands for a phase of treatment in sequence. Treatment begins with *M*otivation, followed by *I*dentification, *D*esensitization, *V*ariation, *A*pproximation, and *S*tabilization. Treatment is cumulative and overlapping, so that each phase has a special emphasis based on all previous goals. The phases will be summarized briefly.

Motivation

According to Van Riper, no other phase in treatment is more important to success or failure than the assessment, understanding, and management of the client's motivation. In this phase, the clinician conveys her role as a companion and guide, one who is willing to share the burden of stuttering and who is both positive and optimistic about its management. Van Riper noted that "out of the therapist's faith can come the stutterer's hope" (1973, p. 230). The clinician demonstrates her genuine interest in the person who stutters. Verbally recognizing and identifying the components of the client's speech and the client's related feelings with complete acceptance, the clinician conveys support, permissiveness, and understanding. The clinician may replicate the stuttering in her own mouth. Doing so helps to initiate a close relationship and to extinguish, at least partially, the evil effects and hurt experienced from previous stuttering. Encouraging the client to express feelings about stuttering and himself as a communicator, the clinician tentatively verbalizes the client's feelings and invites correction.

From the clinician's patience, understanding, and acceptance, the client learns that he can share anxiety, guilt, and hostility, thus reducing through sharing the fears associated with stuttering. The client is helped to realize that his present speech possesses a degree of fluency and fluent, non-struggled stuttering. The clinician might adjust tentatively through modeling a characteristic or two of the client's stuttering. This builds an understanding that the client can speak more fluently and possesses certain abilities and choices (concepts that will be pivotal to the intervention methods presented in later chapters). He comes to see that the problem is his inefficient, learned coping reactions to the fear associated with stuttering. By learning to stutter more fluently and with less abnormality, the client is able to reduce both the severity and frequency of stuttering. The clinician provides a brief overview of treatment and discusses the importance of the client accepting responsibility as an active participant in all aspects, including setting goals and making and completing assignments. The client must understand and accept the "cost" of treatment (time, energy, and discipline) for its anticipated outcome (more fluent speech, less abnormal stuttering, more efficient coping reactions). Likewise, the clinician must appreciate that clients will not work with continued motivation and commitment without demonstration of a "payoff."

Van Riper indicated that people who stutter severely tend to have a more positive prognosis than those with milder stuttering because the former know that they have far to go and expect to work harder. Their expectations regarding the costs of treatment are more realistic, and their expected payoff is greater. It also is true, however, that those who stutter more severely may demonstrate decreased motivation at first, when they feel that they have progressed enough to communicate effectively. Waning motivation is often observed in the terminal stages of treatment, when the person who stutters is enjoying a degree of fluency that seems much improved over the original stuttering. Van Riper noted that management of motivation is a continual challenge because it wanes and waxes daily. This challenge is met by understanding and relating to the client's unique motives, establishing realistic objectives with the client, responding to the client's fears to reenter situations in which he may have been grievously wounded, respecting the cost-to-profit ratio, and providing undaunted support and commitment to the client. Reflecting the essence of motivation and its management with people who stutter, Van Riper (1973) noted, "Somehow we blow the trumpet that sends the stutterer forward into the battle for his freedom and somehow we get him to blow it himself. Faith is said to move mountains but it is the therapist's dedicated care and concern, if not love, that moves stutterers" (p. 243).

Identification

The basic goal in the identification phase is to engage the person who stutters in identifying and evaluating the unique factors that comprise his stuttering. Typically, this person is only globally aware of what he does when he speaks. Describing and dialoguing about what he does with respect to what he thinks he does within the context of the clinician's interest and freedom from punishment creates an opportunity for "unlearning, relearning, and new learning" (Van Riper, 1973, p. 245). Van Riper highlighted that within this phase, the valuable process of desensitization begins. He noted, "For once, the experience that he has always avoided is sought and desired. The untouchable can be touched" (p. 247). The major premise being addressed in this phase is that any learned habits are easier to change once they are made conscious. Habits persist when they are automatic and subconscious. Four critical areas are addressed in this phase: combating denial, discriminating behaviors and feelings so as to identify what exists and what needs to be changed, desensitizing through examining stuttering behaviors with the clinician, and providing the client with a role and responsibility in treatment (establishing the client as an active participant in the treatment process). These goals and objectives are accomplished through a variety of procedures, all of which facilitate identification. Overt behaviors are identified, including fluently spoken words, easy stutterings, and ultimately hard stuttering and avoidance behaviors.

Van Riper noted that at first, the person who stutters is not expected to modify his stuttering. "His role is that of a collector and cataloguer, not corrector or extinguisher. We want to know and we want him to know what he does when he says he stutters. We are defining and learning the problem" (1973, p. 249). Also defined are the precipitants of stuttering, including verbal, situational, and emotional cues; core behaviors; loci of tension; recoil behaviors; post-stuttering reactions; and feelings of frustration, shame, and hostility. A critical emphasis of this phase is on self-therapy. The person who stutters is encouraged to complete assignments, which are increasingly designed by him. These are specifically intended to ensure success and evoke reporting of experiences and feelings, both of which are rewarded. The person who stutters comes to seek speaking experiences rather than avoiding them. The identification experience often leads to sharing and exploring the client's feelings about himself:

> As hostility begins to pour forth, the therapist must expect to become the target of some of this long repressed aggression especially in those stutterers who have turned their hatred inward upon themselves because they couldn't project it outwardly for fear of being clobbered some more. We are not appalled when this happens. The therapist's receptacle should be large enough to receive such evil. Better to have it come out than to keep it within. Better to have it expressed in words rather than in stuttering behavior. Good therapists are self-flushing anyway. (Van Riper, 1973, pp. 264–265)

He noted also that the identification phase is one of exploration, which by itself often produces nearly immediate decreases in the amount and severity of stuttering, fear, and avoidance. Such reductions are temporary at best and not yet a direct objective of treatment. As with motivation, identification will continue throughout treatment.

Desensitization

The desensitization phase addresses stress. Unless reduced, stress maintains the avoidance and escape behaviors, which are noticeable characteristics in stuttering. This phase aims to reduce the speech-related anxieties and negative emotions held by the person who stutters so that he can learn new ways of coping with and responding to stuttering. The methods used are more direct than those in motivation and identification. Van Riper (1973) again emphasized the role of the clinician, who creates in the treatment room a "zone of safety and security, where basically the stuttering is felt with little frustration and where the listener is not punitive" (p. 268). At the same time, the clinician works to "toughen" the client to the factors that formerly resulted in disintegration and stuttering. A concomitant reduction in avoidance is important in order to begin to approach stuttering with the intention of modifying it (i.e., we cannot modify that which we avoid). As avoidances are reduced, the client's feelings of anger, fear, and hostility often surface and may be shared with, if not directed at, the clinician. The client's stuttering may become more severe, albeit temporarily. The clinician needs to verbalize her understanding and acceptance of the client's emotions and explain that the heightened disfluency reflects greater awareness of what needs to be changed.

Expressing both emotionality and greater disfluency in a benign, nurturing environment enables the person who stutters to prepare for the change process. Using different procedures and assignments, the clinician determines the client's stress tolerance, regulates the amount of stress, and again verbally acknowledges the amount of stress the client is feeling. One assignment is for the client and clinician to build a communicative situational stress hierarchy. Speaking contexts (involving situations, listeners, and others) that later become clinical tasks and assignments are progressively ordered from least to most challenging. The client will move up the hierarchy in the smallest possible steps to ensure success. The clinician will often model the task several times before the client attempts it. For example, the clinician might enter a store with the client and pseudostutter (i.e., fake stuttering) to a clerk. The clinician will convey that she is not upset; afterward, she will recall and discuss with the client what the clerk did and how the clinician and client honestly felt. That another person would be willing and able to undergo such an experience and remain integrated conveys a powerful message of support to the client. Activities such as these provide opportunities for the client to unlearn old reactions and learn new ones, all the while confronting stuttering (seeing, hearing, feeling, and identifying core behaviors, listener reactions, and related thoughts and feelings). Desensitization includes counterconditioning, or linking old stimuli with new reactions, involving assertiveness training (seeking out stuttering so that it can be modified) and disinhibition (reversing the habituated tendency to be on guard, always scanning speech for feared sounds or words, thus speaking tentatively as though expecting trauma). Desensitization also involves the following:

- *relaxation*—clinician-induced visualization promoting cognitive restructuring (Van Riper reported poor transfer of this technique to actual stuttering)

- *pseudostuttering*—volitional, intentional stuttering

- *adaptation*—collecting, logging, and analyzing stuttering (flooding the client with heightened awareness of stuttering so as to strengthen the approach gradient and decrease the avoidance gradient)

- *nonreinforcement*—repeating certain words on which the client stutters over and over until he says each of them fluently, and then continuing to say each word with increasing loudness

- *negative suggestion and flooding*—presenting the internalized fears of the client as a probability (e.g., "I bet you will stutter miserably on this next phone call")

- *response prevention*—the client deliberately stutters on nonfeared sounds of nonfeared words until the clinician signals to release

- *adaptation with negative suggestion*—verbalizing for the client feelings that he has reported during real fixations (e.g., "Oh no, I'm stuck again. I'm helpless!"), first during pseudostuttering and eventually during real stuttering

- *adaptation to stress*—flooding the client with communicatively stressful situations in which he must speak fluently, so that in comparison, his daily speaking challenges seem less onerous

- *eliminating other sources of anxiety*—helping the client resolve other conflicts (such as finding a job, passing a course, and other sources of stress) so that stuttering-related fears will decrease; Van Riper (1973) said the following about his life and the lives of other people who stutter:

  We who stutter must learn to live better lives than normal speakers if only so that we can keep from amplifying our stuttering fears. Even after we have learned to speak and stutter fluently, we cannot afford to let other sources of guilt, hostility, or anxiety convert themselves into precipitants of stuttering. Sad as the prospect may seem, we must deny ourselves the human privilege of wallowing in the muck of sin and folly. If we do, then we pay the price in fear and in stuttering. If there is any injustice involved in having to be a stutterer and to be fluent in spite of stuttering, it is in this denial of the right to live foolishly. This author has always resented this constraint. (p. 298)

- *reassurance*—providing realistic, positive support for the client's potential as a communicator; Van Riper (1973) noted about clients that "they know that they are no longer alone and this special kind of reassurance is one of the most potent attenuators of negative emotion ever invented" (p. 299)

- *anxiety reduction by modifying stuttering*—reducing the client's fears and negative emotions by helping him learn a new way of stuttering that will not evoke penalties and frustration

In the desensitization phase, the client thus develops greater resiliency. The client

> comes to us full of anxiety and shame, unable to confront his problem, disguising it, avoiding contact with it. Through a preliminary period of desensitization we calm him and gentle him enough so that he can do this new learning. And as he realizes he is coming to grips with his problem and making progress, his morale goes up and his fears go down. And so does his stuttering. (Van Riper, 1973, p. 299)

Variation/Modification

In the variation/modification phase, the person who stutters learns that it is possible to stutter and be more fluent (i.e., stutter more fluently). The purpose is to break up the client's old responses and to attach new responses to old cues. Much of the strength of the habitual compulsive reactions lies in their stereotype, or the consistency of their pattern. Varying these patterns weakens them. The variation phase typically is short in duration because it passes naturally into the next phase (approximation). Having already collected and identified many instances of easy, unforced stuttering, the client is encouraged to experiment with change, to realize that he has a range of responses from which he can choose. Van Riper proposed a wide range of behaviors for the client to vary. He cautioned, however, that the assignments by themselves have little value. "Only when shared with the therapist and when feelings are expressed and when rewards are appropriately timed, do the experiences they evoke have potency in modifying the attitudes and outward behavior of the stutterer" (1972, p. 327). The assignments and procedures in this phase address the following:

- *exploration of self*—recognizing the way a person characteristically behaves and identifying the idiosyncratic patterns of thinking, feeling, and acting, which comprise the person's way of living (e.g., patterns of sitting, walking, talking, eating, and reading; also dress, appearance, manners, and routines)

- *"rut breakers"*—deliberately varying the habitual patterns

- *role playing*—deliberately assuming a different role or the role of another person to facilitate variation of behavior

- *attitudinal change*—deliberately shifting from one mood of feeling to another (e.g., recognizing the influence of previous negative autosuggestion, a client first might express such thoughts aloud and then formulate alternative thoughts and memories)

- *varying the stuttering behaviors*—deliberately changing the form of the anticipatory behaviors—postponement and avoidance reactions (e.g., if the client prolongs *ah* or repeatedly interjects *well* before attempting a fluency modification, he might shorten or break up the *ah* into units or interject a different word or words)

- *varying the escape behaviors*—adjusting the behaviors that closely reflect feelings of blockage (such as sudden eye closings, abnormal mouth positions, jaw jerks, breathing abnormalities), behaviors that according to Van Riper are the most resistant to change (Van Riper suggested a modeling approach in which the clinician assumes the client's abnormal mouth postures and revises them before finishing the word, or stutters in unison, adopting the first part of the abnormality but then introducing a variation and asking the client to follow the model presented)

Approximation/Modification

Once the client can vary his reactions to the factors that typically make stuttering worse, he and the clinician embark on the approximation/modification phase, the objective of which is to learn new responses that will gradually diminish stuttering. The aim is to modify the form of stuttering so that fluency is reinforced and the appropriate motor sequence of the word is being approximated. The easy, more fluent form of stuttering, which has already been discovered occasionally and analyzed, will serve as the template. Van Riper emphasized the importance of clarifying the sequence of the motor model and heightening proprioceptive awareness through masking, delayed auditory feedback, and pantomiming, among other methods. Specific methods for approximating properly sequenced, more fluent speech include the following:

- ⬚ *Stuttering in unison*—The clinician stutters with the client, first duplicating the behavior, then easing out of the tremors, ceasing the struggle, and smoothly finishing the word. The clinician shares the client's initial behavior and then diverges. Modifications are made in small steps (e.g., first stutter with eyes open rather than closed, then with relaxed rather than tense lips) and with a manageable and deliberate degree of stress. Expression of feelings is encouraged. Mutual sharing, faith, and acceptance create a context for change and growth.

- ⬚ *Cancellation*—In cancellation, the client learns new responses to stimuli that trigger stuttering responses. The client stops immediately after a stuttered word has been completely uttered. After a deliberate pause for reposturing, he then says the word with the modification he has just learned. In other words, the modification is used *after* the word containing the disfluency has been spoken. Forward movement of communication stops once he stutters and continues only after he has used a more appropriate stuttering response. In this procedure, reinforcement shifts to the word finally spoken fluently, thus removing the reinforcement value of the old struggle behaviors.

- ⬚ *Pull-out*—Once the modifications have been practiced in unison with the clinician and in cancellation, the client incorporates them within the moment of stuttering (i.e., *during* the disfluency while it is occurring, without any pauses). This is called "pull-out." The modification is moved forward in time, from the period just following the stuttering to the moment of stuttering itself.

- ⬚ *Preparatory set*—With preparatory set, the modification is moved into the period of anticipation of stuttering. Typically, people who stutter know in advance the word and the location in a word where stuttering will occur and covertly rehearse before an anticipated instance of disfluency. Having used the modification after and during the actual stuttering, the client now is challenged to implement the modification *before* the stuttering occurs, during the stage of anticipatory rehearsal.

Cancellation, pull-out, and preparatory set are illustrated in Figure 7.1. Van Riper (1972) noted that as clients master the different techniques, both the severity and frequency of stuttering tend to decrease. Fears of words and then situations decrease as well. Self-confidence grows, as does tolerance of communicative stress.

Stabilization

By the time the client reaches the stabilization phase, he is using reliable fluency. He no longer responds to fluency challenge with helplessness and feels good about communication and himself as a communicator. Van Riper (1973) indicated that treatment is often terminated prematurely at this point. The stabilization phase is intended to help the client consolidate his gains, make his new form of more fluent speech and stuttering more automatic, heighten proprioceptive monitoring of his fluent speech, and adjust his self-concept and pragmatic skills to those of a fluent speaker. At this point, individual treatment decreases in favor of group treatment. Self-treatment is encouraged, in which the client is responsible for charting, logging, and analyzing behaviors, thoughts, and feelings. Specific procedures include the following:

- ⬚ *Fluency practice*—To remove any remaining gaps in the speech where disfluency used to occur and to heighten the feeling of fluency, the client is encouraged to shadow (use echo speech) or pantomime the speech of a fluent speaker on television or radio, repeat whole sentences in which he or another speaker demonstrated a disfluency, and self-talk when alone.

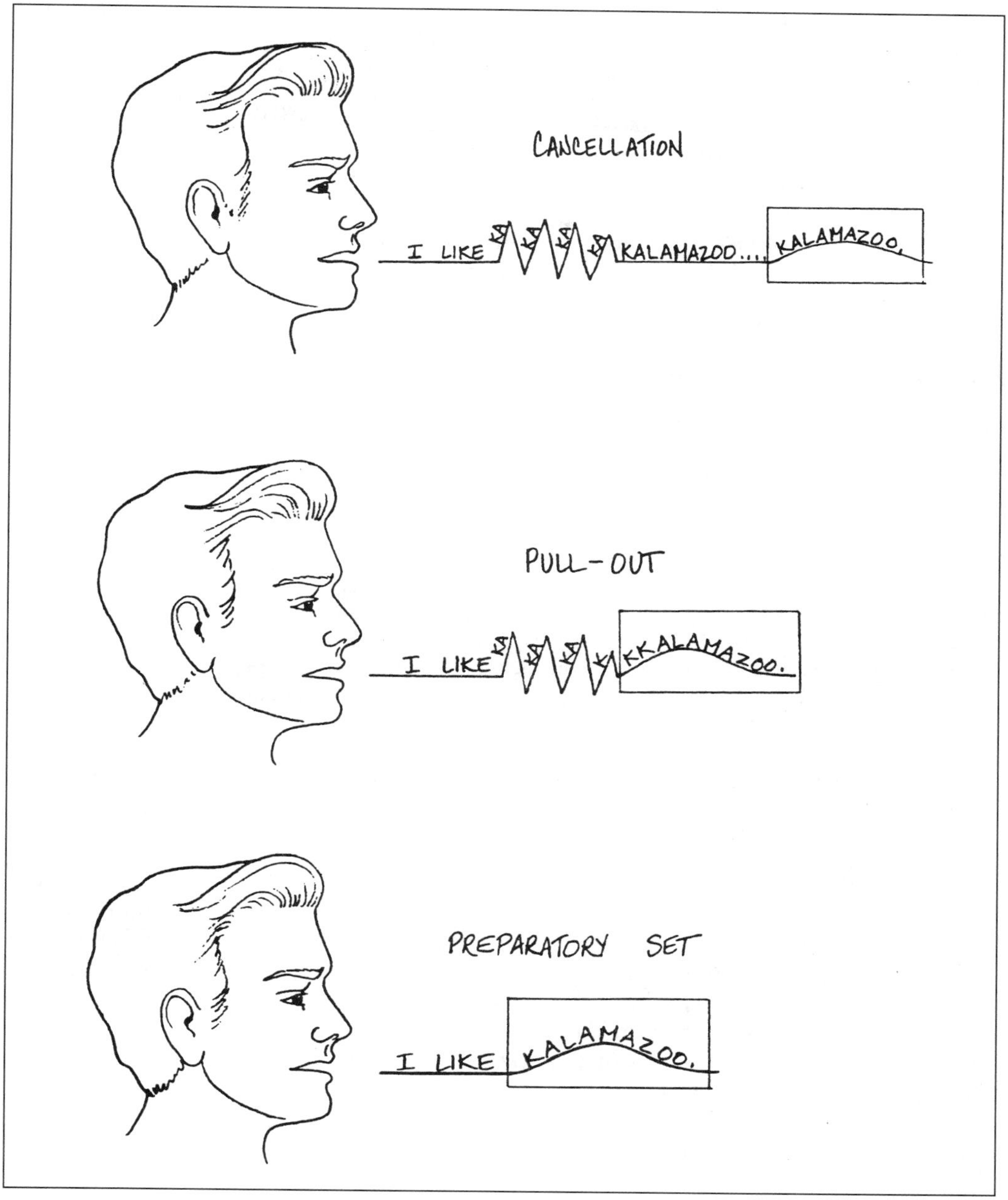

Figure 7.1. Stuttering modification techniques. *Note.* From *Stuttering: An Integrated Approach to Its Nature and Treatment* (2nd ed., p. 219), by B. Guitar, 1998, Baltimore: Williams & Wilkins. Copyright 1998 by Williams & Wilkins. Reprinted with permission.

⚇ *Faking*—To heighten control, the client is directed to fake easy, repetitive, or prolonged stuttering within fluent speech casually in certain daily situations. Also, the client fakes an occasional disfluency in the original form and follows it with a cancellation or pull-out. Although these procedures strengthen the fluency controls, most clients resist this phase of stabilization.

⚇ *Assessment*—The client must inventory his fluency-related behaviors, thoughts, and feelings on an ongoing, daily basis.

- *Resistance therapy*—To maintain the methods of fluent stuttering and fluent speaking within the context of varied communicative stresses, conditions are created in which pressures to stutter in the old way are strong and the client must do his utmost to resist them. By seeking out and entering situations that were feared in the past, the client strengthens the new behavioral responses to the old cues (i.e., to the old stimuli that resulted in responses of avoidance and struggle). Other forms of negative practice that foster resistance to old habits include teasing, interruption, and suggestion (during fluent speech in unison, the clinician stutters and the client is expected to remain fluent).

- *Termination of treatment*—Termination of treatment follows achievement of all objectives and reflects communication independence. Van Riper suggests that cases be followed for 2 years posttreatment.

Fluency Shaping: Ryan

Programmed Therapy for Stuttering in Children and Adults (Ryan, 2001), as well as *Programmed Conditioning for Fluency* (Ryan & Van Kirk, 1971) and the *Monterey Fluency Program* (Ryan & Van Kirk, 1978), are based on the principles of fluency shaping. Ryan (2001) articulated the premise of fluency intervention as follows:

> I still view stuttering as learned behavior, but I now believe there is a physiological basis to stuttering. . . . However, that new thinking has not changed the treatment much since we do not know exactly how this physiology operates nor how to change it except through behavioral technology. . . . My approach to treatment has been known alternatively as behavior modification or contingency management or operant conditioning or programmed instruction. . . . This system's most laudable characteristics are measurement, clear description, and organization of treatment steps (programming through establishment, transfer, and maintenance with follow-up), and attention to the importance of providing consequences to determine behavior. Some authorities may still view the installation of fluent speech as only one of the many goals for people who stutter, or it may be the single goal, as I believe. (pp. v–vi)

The treatment program, which assumes that "normal, fluent speech is a realistic goal for all people who stutter" (Ryan, 2001, p. 302), can be applied to children and adults who stutter, and requires an average of 20 hours of treatment to complete; it is outlined in Figure 7.2. If the answer to the question implied by the decision indicated in the diamond is "yes," go down to the next box and complete the activity as stated. If the answer to the implied question is "no," recycle back to the preceding activity. For example, after the fluency interview is completed, the implied question in the diamond is "Is the SW/M greater than 3.0?" If the answer is "yes," the clinician goes to the box below and administers the first criterion test. If the answer is "no," the clinician recycles back and readministers the fluency interview after waiting 3 months.

Fluency Interview

The prospective client first is given the fluency interview, which determines whether or not he is a candidate for the fluency program. Requiring about 20 minutes to administer, the interview yields a sample of talking in 10 speech categories: automatic (counting; saying the alphabet; reciting a poem, the pledge of allegiance, or a nursery rhyme; and singing), echoic (imitating words and sentences), reading (optional for children; reading selection should be at or below reading level), picture naming, speaking alone (clinician leaves room), monologue, responding to and asking questions, conversation, telephone (optional for children), and observation in another setting with another conversational partner. A stuttering rate (stuttered words per minute, or SW/M) is computed. A rate of more than 3.0 SW/M indicates that the person is a candidate for fluency training; a rate

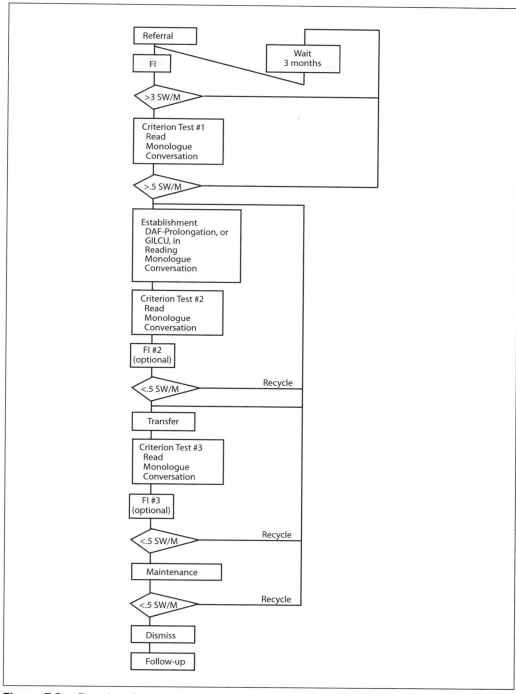

Figure 7.2.   Flowchart for establishment, transfer, maintenance, and follow-up. *Note.* From *Programmed Therapy for Stuttering in Children and Adults* (2nd ed., p. 90), by B. P. Ryan, 2001, Springfield, IL: Charles C Thomas. Copyright 2001 by Charles C Thomas. Reprinted with permission. *Note.* The text in the diamonds indicates decisions that need to be made on the basis of stated criteria; text in boxes indicates activities to be completed. FI = fluency interview; SW/M = stuttered words per minute; DAF = delayed auditory feedback; GILCU = gradual increase in length and complexity of utterance.

of less, with few exceptions, indicates that the person is not a candidate, pending the results of a reevaluation scheduled in 3 months. The fluency interview is audio-recorded for later analysis.

Counting, Charting, Timing

The program uses two different measurements. First, the *stuttering rate* (stuttered words/minute, SW/M) is figured by counting only the number of words that demonstrate whole-word repetition, part-word repetition, prolongation, or struggle. Each stuttered word is counted only once and only according to these four categories. The number of stuttered words is divided by the talk time (e.g., 15 stuttered words/5 minutes = 3 SW/M). Only the client's talking is timed. Second, the *base rate* (i.e., baseline; total words read or spoken) is computed in the same way, but only in the fluency interview and criterion tests. Both the stuttering rate (SW/M) and base rate (total words spoken/minute, WS/M; total words read/minute, WR/M) are charted for visual demonstration and evaluation of treatment.

Criterion Test

If the person is selected for treatment, he is given a criterion test consisting of 5 minutes each of reading, monologue, and conversation. The first criterion test provides his baseline, or pretreatment rate of stuttering. If his stuttering rate is more than 0.5 SW/M in any of the three modes (reading, monologue, or conversation), he is put through an establishment of fluency program in that mode or modes. The criterion test is a measure of stuttering rate (stuttered word output) and talking rate (total word output) before and after each of the three phases of therapy: establishment, transfer, and maintenance. The criterion test is the same each time it is given. Withholding reinforcement, the clinician directs the client to read, monologue, and converse for 5 minutes each. A stuttering rate of more than 0.5 SW/M indicates that the client needs training or recycling of training; less than 0.5 SW/M indicates that the client can advance to the next phase.

Establishment

Clinicians select from two different establishment programs, gradual increase in length and complexity of utterance (GILCU) and delayed auditory feedback (DAF), both of which are reportedly effective. The client is to complete each mode in the establishment phase, provided he demonstrates a stuttering rate of more than 0.5 SW/M and is capable of the requisite tasks (reading, monologue, and conversation). Reading is omitted for nonreaders. The target of both establishment programs is "normal, fluent speech (<2 SW/M) at normal speaking rates of circa 150 WS/M or 200 SPM (syllables per minute) with noted exceptions in DAF-Prolongation program and CT passing criteria of 0.5 SW/M" (Ryan, 2001, p. 89).

GILCU. With 54 steps, GILCU starts with reading a single word and works up to 5 minutes of fluent conversation in the clinic room. The minimum run time for this program is 1.8 hours (Ryan, 2001), and it requires no special equipment other than a stopwatch. The client is instructed to read fluently (i.e., verbal stimulus), is rewarded with "good," receives a token (for each fluent word, sentence, or designated duration of fluency), and is reinstructed to "Stop, speak fluently" contingent on each stuttered word. The target responses progress from reading one word fluently, to two words, three words, and so on, to six words (the criterion is a sequence of 10 consecutive productions with 0 SW/M at each step); reading fluently one sentence, two sentences, to four sentences (the criterion is a sequence of 5 consecutive productions with 0 SW/M at each step); reading fluently for 30 seconds to 5 minutes with 30-second increments (the criterion is 1 production with 0 SW/M at each step); and ultimately advancing to the next mode (i.e., monologue or conversation). In each subsequent mode, the same stimulus and response structure is followed (verbal instruction to engage in monologue or conversation, starting with fluent single words and working up to 5 fluent minutes in that mode). The client receives reinforcement (verbal, social, or redeemable tokens) for each novel fluent response. If the client persists on the same step for 20 minutes (i.e., the client's talk time only), the client is put on a branching program (Ryan & Van Kirk, 1978) designed for the clinician to model the correct response. If the client cannot produce correct responses, the clinician models them and gradually reduces the modeling through the branch steps until the client can produce the desired response without the model. Once the model is faded, the client returns to the establishment program. If the client cannot produce the response independently, Branch Index Step 245 is exercised, in which the clinician is directed to do anything reasonable to help the client pass that step, respond to the type of error, do special practice (i.e., whispering, singing, prolonging, loose contacts, sliding, talking softly, modeling), and break down the response unit into sounds or syllables. If all else is unsuccessful, the clinician is directed to consider using the DAF-prolongation program. If the client fails the post-establishment program criterion test (demonstrates a stuttering rate of more than 0.5 SW/M), he is recycled through the program in that mode or modes with a reduced criterion of performance, working back gradually to the expected criterion.

DAF-Prolongation. DAF-prolongation requires a delayed auditory feedback (DAF) device with at least six settings (i.e., 250, 200, 150, 100, 50, and 0 milliseconds of delayed auditory feedback) and requires a minimum of 1.8 hours for completion (Ryan, 2001). The clinician provides brief verbal instructions to speak slowly (i.e., stimulus), appropriate to each of the 27 steps within this program. The client's target response is "superfluent, slow, prolonged speech" (Ryan, 2001, p. 93) within the clinic room. This means that the client speaks slowly, prolonging each sound and word, thus eliminating juncture and significantly reducing inflection. Vocalization is continuous, articulation is deemphasized, sounds are of equal intensity, and pitch is monotone. Ryan provided the following examples: "Mmmmmmyyyyyynnnnnnaaaaaammmmmmiiiiiissssssss-Mmmmmmaaaaaarrrrrryyyyyy" (My name is Mary; 1974, p. 75); "IIIaaammmsssppp-eeeakiiinggggiiinnnpppaaattteeerrrnnn" (I am speaking in pattern; 2001, p. 103). The client first identifies stuttered words during reading, after which he is instructed to read slowly to accommodate the maximum DAF setting (250-millisecond delay). By following the intended prolonged speech pattern, the client is positively reinforced with "Good" and a token, if a token system is being used. If the client breaks the intended pattern and stutters, he is told, "Stop, use the slow, prolonged, fluent pattern" (Ryan, 2001, p. 94). Within each mode, the rate of prolonged speech (i.e., response) gradually increases by decreasing the amount of delay in five steps by 50-millisecond units (i.e., stimulus; 250-, 200-, 150-, 100-, 50-, 0-millisecond, or no delay). After the use of headphones has been faded, the client is taken off the DAF device. This same structure is used in the subsequent modes of monologue and conversation. The client should approximate a "normal" rate of speech, defined earlier as 150 words per minute (this is a departure from Ryan, 1974, and Ryan & Van Kirk, 1971, where normal rate of speech was defined as 120 words per minute in reading and 100 words spoken per minute in monologue and conversation). If the client persists on the same step for 20 minutes of training without reaching criterion, the client goes through a branching program similar to that described for GILCU. Essentially, the branching program takes the client back to a previous step with more reinforcement. In DAF-prolongation, a branch is a repeat of the first five steps in order to reteach "the pattern" and then to rerun the 1-, 2-, 3-, 4-, and then 5-minute step in the failed mode. When the client passes the branch steps, he returns to the regular program step. If he fails the branch steps, a special branch index (i.e., 245) similar to that described for GILCU is available. In it, the client is reinstructed and provided models for a smooth, prolonged speaking pattern. If even it proves unsuccessful, the clinician is advised to consider the GILCU program. If the client fails Criterion Test 2 (failing to achieve a stuttering rate of less than 0.5 SW/M), he is recycled through the program using every other step in that mode or modes, after which he is again given Criterion Test 2. A rate control program is available (Ryan & Van Kirk, 1978), if necessary, to speed up the rate to normal. About the DAF establishment program, Ryan (1974) commented,

> The client comes out of this program being able to prolong, count stuttered words, articulate more precisely, and be generally fluent although the client may feel dependent upon the machine. The clinician can help the client avoid addiction to or dependency on the machine by adhering to the rules of the program and getting the client through the steps as quickly as possible. . . . We view the DAF Program as one of the most powerful establishment programs available to us in operant stuttering therapy. Its effect is dramatic and quite consistent across clients. For best results, however, it should be used in a systematic, programmed manner. Simply exposing a client to brief, random periods on the DAF machine may not produce positive changes. (pp. 80, 82)

After reviewing over 40 years of related research, Ryan (2001) concluded,

> From my experience and research and from reading the literature, I can only conclude that PS (Prolonged Speech, i.e., DAF-Prolongation) with components that provide for a result of natural speech and/or speech at normal speaking rates, is a highly effective, repeatedly validated procedure for treating children, adolescents, and adults who stutter. The caveat is that appropriate transfer and maintenance procedures must also be employed following PS treatment to ensure that the fluent speech obtained from such PS establishment procedures continues. Additional clinical research is still necessary to continue to refine the PS procedures to improve their efficiency and effectiveness. (p. 111)

Transfer

Once fluent speech has been established in the treatment room, the goal of the transfer phase is to use this speech in a wide variety of settings and with many different people. This phase requires between 10 and 15 hours of treatment time (Ryan, 1974). Typically, transfer takes less time if the older children and adults have been engaged in regular home practice during the establishment phase. Most of the transfer steps target the response of fluent conversation, although some target fluent speech in large-group settings. As in the establishment program, the clinician instructs the client to speak slowly and fluently. A criterion of between 5 and 10 minutes of fluent speech (0 SW/M) is set for each step. Only social reinforcement is offered during the transfer phase, which contains 54 steps for adults and 17 steps for children. The clinician is with the client for all of the transfer steps, except for some at the home setting. The contexts targeted for transfer of fluent speech (Ryan, 2001) include the following:

- *physical settings*—increasing distance from the treatment room with the clinician present
- *audiences*—increasing the size of the audience in the treatment room from one to three conversational partners
- *home*—increasing the size of the family audience at home, first with and then without the clinician present, from one to six conversational partners
- *classroom*—increasing the size of the interactive group and the level of communicative demand with and then without the clinician present (moving from small- to large-group activity to giving a speech to the class)

- *telephone*—making phone calls, first in role play, then to a recorded message, then to conversational partners, while offering an increasing number of questions and statements and eventually of increasing duration

- *strangers (optional for children)*—conversing with increasing numbers of strangers in settings of increasing distance from the clinic

- *work*—conversing at work with the clinician, friends, coworkers, and people of increasing authority, in small and eventually large groups

- *residual*—addressing any remaining situations in which the client reports continuing difficulty

- *all day*—gradually extending the number of hours spent targeting fluent speech, based on a 16-hour day

These transfer contexts are adjusted to accommodate the individual (e.g., older adults do not interact in the classroom; children do not interact with strangers). Ryan (2001) recommended branching steps if a client fails to achieve 0 SW/M on the transfer phase for three sessions or 40 minutes on one step. Criterion Test 3 is given after completion of the transfer phase. Greater than 0.5 SW/M requires recycling through the transfer phase. Less than 0.5 SW/M allows for advancement to the maintenance phase.

Maintenance

The goal of the maintenance phase is fluent speech in a wide variety of settings and with many different people. However, the maintenance phase emphasizes the test of time (continuing to use fluent speech over years). Basically, this is done by fading the number of treatment activities until the client can direct the treatment or until he no longer needs it. The client engages in counting the number of stuttered words each day, home practice, and clinic contact for measurement and reinstruction. This phase provides for clinic rechecks, which are faded out over a 2-year period. Three-minute samples of reading, monologue, and conversation are collected at each recheck to evaluate fluency maintenance. A rate above 0.5 SW/M indicates the need for more training. The clinician inquires about fluency in other environments and identifies the need for additional training in situations that are reported as difficult, such as telephone calling or giving speeches. Maintenance rechecks are held once each week for 2 weeks after the third criterion test is passed, then held again in 1 month, 3 months, 6 months, and finally in 12 months. When the client can maintain less than 0.5 SW/M in each mode during the last scheduled rechecks, he is dismissed.

Postscript

Ryan (2001) is emphatic about the goal of treatment: "The goal for all people who stutter should be normally fluent speech not controlled stuttering" (pp. 301–302). And again: "Research has shown that normal, fluent speech is a realistic goal for all people who stutter. For the profession to accept or to continue to offer less (e.g., controlled stuttering) is unthinkable" (p. 302). Ryan (2001) reasserted and extended this point:

> Normal speech fluency (with no need to monitor) is a reasonable, achievable, primary, major goal and criterion for success of treatment for all persons who stutter, especially children, and is possible and desirable. Normal fluency may be operationally defined as speech with <2.0 %SW or 1.0 %SS composed of single part- or whole-word repetitions at 150 WS/M or 200 SPM. (p. 303)

> Each clinician or clinician-researcher should evaluate the stuttering treatment he or she is using to provide the efficacy data which could be compared to that collected by those of us practicing and reporting operant conditional treatment. . . . If those data are not comparable, that is, do not result in normally fluent speech or do not reduce stuttering to

less than 1.0 %SS, or 2.0 %SW at normal speaking rates maintained over at least 2 years within an average of 20 hr of treatment, the clinician should examine treatments to find one that does. (pp. 302–303)

However, we must guard against at least two unfortunate extensions of such thinking. The first is that people who cannot achieve, maintain, and transfer "normal speech fluency," despite doing their level best in all aspects of the stuttering treatment experience, have failed because they have not tried hard enough or demonstrated sufficient commitment. The second is that clinicians who stutter, by virtue of their stuttering, are not suited to serve people who stutter. Asserting this latter sentiment, Ryan (1974) suggested that a clinician running a successful operant speech fluency program that is helping clients achieve normal fluency also would want to achieve and model such fluency: "The clinician who stutters has the opportunity now, through operant speech fluency programs, to become fluent. The clinician may also choose to continue to stutter" (p. 159). Ryan (2003) again admonished clinicians who stutter, stating,

> It is their right to choose to continue to stutter. But, in light of all the present published treatment efficacy research over the past 30 years . . . it is a misguided, sad, unnecessary accomplishment and, in my opinion, professionally inappropriate. In my opinion, these people represent our profession's failures. (p. 36)

Ryan thus insists that we focus on our clients' fluency and that people who stutter, including clinicians, might do so in part as a consequence of having made a choice. These two points will be visited again as we address my suggestions for intervention methods that integrate stuttering modification and fluency shaping principles and as we discuss interpersonal and intrapersonal factors of effective clinicians.

Unequivocally, however, I do not agree that "normal fluency" is necessarily a realistic, achievable goal for all people who stutter or that clinicians, by virtue of their own stuttering, cannot be effective clinicians. Indeed, normal fluency is not realistic for some people who stutter, and there is no reason that clinicians who stutter cannot be among our profession's best. To say the least, I am concerned by assertions, under the guise, if not misuse, of evidence-based practice, that one size can fit or should ever fit all, or that data about human performance can be interpreted without an understanding of the human condition. Evidence-based practice is about objectively identifying, exploring, and documenting ways to enable people to achieve their communicative best. Much more will be said in the remaining chapters about helping both people who stutter and clinicians to achieve their full potential and about recognizing and celebrating that shared achievement. It is the birthright of all people to enjoy opportunities for achieving all that they are capable of; it is our obligation to return the favor by enabling those who have not yet had such good fortune to begin discovering and realizing their dreams.

Chapter Summary

This chapter examined psychotherapeutic considerations, the third and final set of central and guiding intervention assumptions addressed in Unit II. Stuttering modification and fluency shaping approaches, both of which are supported by evidence-based practice, were presented as endpoints of a psychotherapeutic continuum. A thorough understanding of these types of treatment, combined with consideration of intrafamily (personal constructs and family systems) and extrafamily (interdisciplinary teaming and multicultural awareness) factors, is necessary for designing effective intervention.

Stuttering modification approaches assume that stuttering results from avoiding or struggling with disfluency and avoiding feared words or situations. These approaches emphasize reduction of fears, negative attitudes, and avoidance behaviors while seeking to modify the form of stuttering. The client is directed in how to study his own communication behaviors, thus becoming familiar with and learning to modify his behavior, feelings, and attitudes. While spontaneous fluency is the ultimate behavioral treatment goal, controlled fluency and acceptable stuttering are considered appropriate goals if higher levels of fluency remain unattainable. Affective treatment goals include reducing the client's stuttering-related fears and avoidances, thereby helping him form a more positive view of himself as a communicator. The clinician offers guidance in how to approach feared words and situations and teaches the client techniques for controlling or canceling instances of stuttering. Treatment sessions are relatively unstructured, and the clinician and client interact as equal partners in the treatment process. Because stuttering modification techniques address behaviors, feelings, and attitudes, observed changes in speech behavior tend to take longer, but are transferred and maintained more readily. Stuttering modification intervention is typically indicated for persons who avoid speaking, hide or disguise their stuttering, feel poorly about themselves as communicators, perceive a personal penalty as a consequence of stuttering, and demonstrate a more positive response to stuttering modification trial management. Van Riper's program was discussed as an exemplar of stuttering modification. He recommended a thorough diagnosis of the fluency disorder and four sequential phases of treatment: identification, desensitization, modification, and stabilization. Within these four phases, a number of overlapping steps are represented by the acronym MIDVAS: motivation, identification, desensitization, variation/modification, approximation/modification, and stabilization.

Fluency shaping approaches assume that stuttering is learned and apply the principles of behavior modification to fluency treatment. Stuttering is first eliminated in a controlled stimulus environment through operant procedures; fluency is then generalized to more natural environments. Spontaneous fluency is the ultimate goal of fluency shaping approaches, although controlled fluency is considered acceptable if higher levels of fluency prove unattainable. Any form of noticeable stuttering, however, is considered to be evidence of program failure. While not addressing directly the feelings and attitudes of the individual client, improvement in these areas may be a by-product of improved fluency. Treatment sessions typically are highly structured and use programmed techniques to improve speech fluency. Behavioral change is relatively rapid; however, transfer and maintenance tend to be more difficult than in stuttering modification techniques. Fluency shaping treatment is usually indicated for persons who stutter openly, do not avoid speaking, perceive annoyance or interference but no personal penalty from stuttering, feel positive about themselves as communicators, and demonstrate a positive response to fluency shaping trial management. Ryan's *Programmed Therapy for Stuttering in Children and Adults* is based upon the principles of fluency shaping and consists of fluency interviews, criterion tests, and establishment, transfer, and maintenance programs, with the requisite counting, charting, timing, and follow-up. One subset of fluency shaping intervention utilizes electronic devices with altered auditory feedback.

In reality, most intervention can be designed by combining stuttering modification and fluency shaping principles, depending on the unique strengths and needs of the client. Combined stuttering modification and fluency shaping treatment is typically indicated for persons who stutter openly but may demonstrate some avoidance, perceive some sense of personal penalty and negative feelings from stuttering but not to an extreme or handicapping degree, feel relatively positive about themselves as communicators but wish for personal change, and demonstrate a positive response to both stuttering modification and fluency shaping trial management.

Chapter Seven Study Questions

1. This chapter reviewed psychotherapeutic considerations related to stuttering modification and fluency shaping. How do psychotherapeutic considerations relate to the intrafamily considerations (personal constructs and family systems) reviewed in Chapter 5 and the extrafamily considerations (interdisciplinary teaming and multicultural awareness) reviewed in Chapter 6?

2. This chapter familiarized you with the similarities of and differences between stuttering modification and fluency shaping. How do the premises and principles of stuttering modification relate to those of fluency shaping? How would you determine which type of treatment or combined treatment is "right" for a particular client? How might the client's needs vary so that one type of program would be appropriate at one time, and either another type or a different type of combined program would be appropriate at another?

3. After reviewing Chapter 2 and Prins and Ingham's (2009) assertions about evidence-based practice, what do you believe to be the implications of evidence-based practice on your selection, use, and documentation of one intervention approach over another (i.e., stuttering modification, fluency shaping, or combined)?

4. Given your understanding of the criteria for using stuttering modification, fluency shaping, or a combined approach, what would be your decision rules for using an electronic device with altered auditory feedback? For whom do you think such a device would be the intervention of choice; for whom would it be contraindicated? What does the literature tell us about the effectiveness and efficacy of electronic devices with altered auditory feedback? What implications are there from an evidence-based practice perspective for decisions to use or not use electronic devices?

5. Van Riper stated that people with more severe stuttering have a more positive prognosis than those with milder stuttering. The reasoning is that those who have more severe symptoms are willing to work harder because they expect greater improvement. In other words, those whose stuttering is more severe typically experience greater or more pronounced need. How might this information be useful clinically and how might it impact the clinical process?

6. Motivation is the first of Van Riper's phases in treatment. What does this imply about Van Riper's philosophy of treatment? How does such a philosophy compare and contrast to that of Ryan and to your own philosophy? What avenues are available for a clinician whose client or family is lacking in motivation? Why might a client be lacking in motivation? Does that mean that the client will not or cannot succeed? What should the clinician do?

7. Stuttering modification treatment approaches require more advanced clinical skills than do fluency shaping approaches, including the ability to provide emotional support, clinical problem solving, and responses to individual client differences. How might this observation be related to the structure or style of intervention designed and provided by clinicians? Considering avenues of professional preparation and lifelong learning, what are some ways in which clinicians might improve their skills in order to provide clients the most effective intervention possible?

8. Stuttering modification approaches directly address communication-related behaviors, thoughts, feelings, and attitudes. Fluency shaping approaches directly address behaviors only and interpret changes in the affective domain as a by-product of programmed treatment. Why might thoughts, feelings, and attitudes vary among people who stutter and others within their communication system? In working with these people, how would you ensure that your methods for addressing thoughts, feelings, and attitudes are within the domain of your training and ASHA's Scope of Practice?

How would you know if you were beginning to function outside of these boundaries? What would you do in that event?

9. We noted that for some people who stutter, spontaneous or controlled fluency is not a realistic or achievable goal. How should a clinician determine whether or not such a goal is realistic for a particular client? How do timing and each individual client's life circumstances impact his potential for fluency improvement? How can we explain clients who failed to make significant improvement during over 50 years of intermittent treatment and then achieve spontaneous or controlled fluency in treatment during their later or senior years?

10. What are your reactions to Ryan's (2003) statement that speech–language pathologists who continue to stutter and who work with people who stutter represent "a misguided, sad, unnecessary accomplishment," are "professionally inappropriate," and "represent our profession's failures"? What are your reactions to his statement that normal speech fluency (no need to monitor) is a "reasonable, achievable, primary, major goal and criterion for success of treatment with all persons who stutter, especially children, and is possible and desirable"? What evidence-based practice implications would argue for these statements? What evidence-based practice implications would argue against these statements?

Unit III

❖ ❖ ❖

Assessment and Treatment Strategies with People Who Stutter

A Life Span Perspective

Chapter Eight

Preschool Children
Assessment and Treatment

Over the years one of the questions that has haunted most responsible clinicians is "How do I tell if a person is 'really' stuttering or if he or she just has a great many normal disfluencies?" It's easy to become enmeshed in this trap. The trap is there only if clinicians turn their attention solely to the speaking behavior of the child and on the basis of it attempt to make a decision. . . . There is no person alive today who can describe exactly the point on the continuum of disfluency at which a child would fall from the category of "speaking normally" into that of "stuttering." (Williams, 1978, pp. 285–286)

Distinguishing between normal disfluencies and incipient stuttering is one of the most vexing challenges facing parents, teachers, and clinicians. We will see that making such a distinction involves both quantitative and qualitative considerations, which require both careful description and subsequent evaluation. Equally challenging is planning intervention for preschool children who are at risk for stuttering or who are beginning to stutter. Williams (1978) noted that *stuttering* is an evaluative word, not a descriptive one. Description requires observation, analysis, and reporting in molecular form. Because most children demonstrate disfluencies of repetition and prolongation and because children are remarkably heterogeneous, clinicians are often asked questions about a child's speech: "Is he normal?" "Is he stuttering?" Clinicians are also asked questions about a child's disfluency: "Is he doing too much of it?" Williams (1978) noted, "'Too much' is a floating cork on the continuum of disfluency" (p. 285).

Although our understanding of the onset and development of stuttering, and indeed the nature of stuttering in early childhood, has increased substantially as a consequence of longitudinal investigations, the following facts remain:

Preschool-age children . . . vary greatly in their stuttering and their reactions to it. Although they may exhibit very complex stuttering and be seriously affected by it, on the whole they constitute a significant portion of those individuals for whom the effects of

236

the disorder appear to be limited in several respects. Nevertheless, the majority of all cases of stuttering begin in preschool years, and the prevalence of the disorder in very young children is higher than in any other age group in the population at large. Critical developments in stuttering occur in childhood, and several major factors, such as growth of language and phonology skills, have their greatest impact during that period. (Yairi & Ambrose, 2005, p. 2)

In the first unit, we underscored that planning and conducting intervention with people who stutter require a broad understanding of stuttering, including its onset, development, nature, and etiology from past and present perspectives. We also established the importance of being able to distinguish stuttering from other fluency disorders. In the second unit, we discussed a variety of central and guiding assumptions (intrafamily, extrafamily, and psychotherapeutic considerations) that are essential for designing and implementing effective intervention. In the present unit, we are ready to apply the material presented so far and present specific assessment and treatment strategies from a life-span perspective with people who stutter. Each chapter concludes with a clinical portrait that spotlights an individual communicator and emphasizes the importance of the central and guiding assumptions. Using this format, we will address preschool children (Chapter 8), school-age children (Chapter 9), and adolescents, adults, and senior adults (Chapter 10). This order was selected for a variety of reasons. First and foremost, it is consistent with a life-span perspective. Second, notwithstanding the longitudinal findings that stuttering does not necessarily worsen over time during the preschool years (i.e., see Chapter 2; see also Yairi, 2004; Yairi & Ambrose, 2005), it still could be argued that "stuttering is constantly developing in complexity the longer the child lives and copes with the problem" (Williams, 1978, p. 285). Third, these groupings were chosen for instructional purposes. We will see that in reality, the procedures for a person in one group frequently overlap with those of another.

In this chapter, we will discuss how to structure the communication assessment of a preschool child and the family, what to look for, and how to design different methods for intervention with the child and significant others. In doing so, we will emphasize the following major points:

- There is a fine (sometimes invisible) line between normal disfluency and incipient stuttering. Identifying this line and making such a distinction requires analysis of the child's behaviors, thoughts, and feelings, and professional judgment on the part of the clinician.

- Intervention with preschool children and their families requires understanding of the communication environment, full support and involvement of all members within the communication system, and identification and elimination of potential precipitating and perpetuating factors.

General Precepts About Preschool Children

All people are different and present unique opportunities and challenges. Taking a bird's-eye perspective initially creates a general view of a territory. Moving in for a closer look brings uniqueness and individuality into focus. We will do this now with preschool children and subsequently with the other populations noted. The process of moving from a molar to a more molecular perspective will prepare us for the assessment and treatment decisions that lie ahead.

The following represent general considerations of preschool children as a group. As always, individual members often demonstrate different or contrasting patterns. Hence, preschool children, as do all groups of people, represent a heterogeneous category within which individual differences are valued and nurtured.

⬚ The preschool period is a time of intense development, both quantitatively and qualitatively (Yairi & Ambrose, 2005). Speech fluency and disfluency vary within and across children, as do their relative awareness of and observed frustration over such fluctuation (Ambrose & Yairi, 1994; Ezrati-Vinacour et al., 2001; Vanryckeghem et al., 2005). Maintaining the child's positive attitude toward communication is a critical factor in the prevention of stuttering.

⬚ Play and fun represent the language of childhood (Shapiro, 2002a, 2002b, 2002c, 2004a, 2004b, 2004d, 2004e, 2004f, 2004g, 2005, 2006, 2007a, 2007b, 2008). Too often, clinicians emphasize the medium of questions and questioning to the near exclusion of play, thus turning a potentially fun, interactive opportunity into an interrogation. More will be said later about stages of play. When in doubt, ask less and play and observe more.

⬚ Children vary in their apprehension of the clinical setting. Haynes and Pindzola (2008) noted that such fear results from one or more of the following: inadequate preparation for the assessment or treatment appointment; uncertainty over what will be done to or with the child by the clinician; traumatic memories of visits to dentists, physicians, and other professionals; contagious anxieties of parents; and stress and conflicts recalled from past listener reactions to speech impairments. Clinicians must be mindful of children's fears, thus giving them a responsible role and engaging them in the play interaction.

⬚ While vulnerable in their tendency to do whatever they are told, children are affectively insightful (Ezrati-Vinacour et al., 2001). Occasionally, children will mirror the clinician's (or other adults') emotions before either is keenly aware of them. This means that clinicians must be sincerely positive about working with young children (children rapidly perceive disinterest or lack of confidence), use absolute honesty in all interactions (always keep your promise for activities, rewards, and punishments), maintain appropriate complexity of language presented to children, and provide but limit choices offered to children (limit choices for which the alternatives conflict with the clinical goals). With respect to choices presented, for example, do not ask if the child would like to go with you, do this activity, or other such questions. Children invariably will say, "No." The questions imply that a promise will be kept. When the child's refusal, which was invited, is not accepted, the implied promise is broken. It is more effective to provide choices for which the alternatives are acceptable. The clinician might ask, "Do you want to play here or here?" or "Which do you want to do first, activity X or Y?"

⬚ People of all ages have a story to tell (Shapiro, 1995, 2000, 2002a, 2002b, 2002c, 2004a, 2004b, 2004c, 2004d, 2004e, 2004f, 2004g, 2005, 2006, 2007a, 2007b, 2008). Preschool children are no exception. While children may lack the relative cognitive insight to analyze a problem objectively (Haynes & Pindzola, 2008), children's and adults' stories differ more on the basis of subject matter than in the depth of feeling or inherent quality (E. Johnson, Sickels, & Sayers, 1970). Clinicians have the responsibility to create opportunities for children to tell their story and thereby the privilege to learn from them and to see again as children do.

Preassessment Procedures

Case History Form

When a preschool child is referred for a communication evaluation, a case history form is sent to the primary care provider (parents, relative, or guardian) in advance of the scheduled appointment. (As implied here and discussed in Chapter 5, the person or persons serving as the child's primary care provider may vary across families. While remaining sensitive to individual families, I use the term *parents* generically to refer to any person serving in this responsible role.) The information provided tells the clinician about the child's developmental and medical history; family structure; communication strengths and limitations; and onset, development, and current perceptions regarding the presenting communication problem. This information also gives the clinician an indication of questions that need to be asked during the parent interview and which previous service providers may need to be contacted for related information.

Each question paints a more complete and individual portrait of stuttering and may have prognostic significance on the basis of retrospective, cross-sectional, or longitudinal investigations. Such questions, which will be discussed in more detail later in the chapter, might include the following (Yairi & Ambrose, 2005, pp. 318–324):

- When did the child begin stuttering? As the interval since onset increases, likelihood of spontaneous recovery decreases, arguing for intervention over waiting.

- What were the initial signs or characteristics of stuttering at its onset? I ask the parents to describe and demonstrate what they recall and reflect on the child's speech characteristics and secondary behaviors, in addition to cognitive and affective reactions.

- How did it happen? Was the presentation sudden or gradual? How long did it take to be noticed? Was it an abrupt change or one over several days or weeks?

- What were the circumstances surrounding the onset? What was the child's physical or emotional health? What were the conditions and events in the child's personal life or family that might have triggered or complicated the stuttering?

- What other factors might have been involved? This question explores processes and behaviors such as accelerated or delayed language development, speech sound development, nutrition, and medical issues that might have been considered as unrelated.

- Who or what might be a contributor? This question explores the parents' perception of negative influences, family history of stuttering, and related trends toward recovery or persistence.

- How has the stuttering progressed? How has the stuttering developed or changed over time?

Responses and dialogue related to these and other questions inform the clinician about the parents' understanding of stuttering at its onset and in its present form in terms of description, frequency, relative severity, and developmental trends, in addition to familial patterns of recovery.

Audio or Video Recording

When possible, it is helpful to obtain an audio or video recording of the child interacting with his family or other members of the household. This recording serves a variety of functions. First, it reflects the communication and interpersonal dynamics of the members of the child's family. It also reveals the nature of the communication concern at the time it was expressed. This is particularly important when there is a lapse between the initial referral and the time of the evaluation (Yairi & Ambrose, 2005). We noted previously that speech fluency of preschool children generally fluctuates over time. Clinicians need to determine how representative the child's speech at the time of the evaluation is of his usual speaking behavior. The recording provides a point of comparison with the speech sampled during the evaluation. Finally, the recording provides a sample of the child's speech in a different setting and with different people compared to that collected at the evaluation.

Preliminary Phone Call

A phone call to the child's parents (i.e., primary care providers) before the evaluation enables the clinician to prepare the family for the evaluation process. The clinician can address the family's preliminary questions and help them prepare the child for the evaluation itself. This might involve conveying to the child what will transpire (e.g., the clinicians are friendly and fun people who want to talk and play with you) and encouraging him to bring several familiar items (such as toys, books, photographs, or other favorite objects) to share with the clinician. Not knowing what to expect and then encountering unfamiliar people in an unfamiliar setting at the evaluation can be potentially frightening for a young child. This fear can be prevented with relatively little effort. In my experience, preparing the family and the child for the evaluation truly has been "an ounce of prevention" resulting in "a pound of cure."

There is yet another benefit of a preliminary phone call to the family that cannot be minimized: The clinician conveys to the parents that she cares, that she is willing and able to help, and that the communicative welfare of the child and the family is important. These benefits are consistent with one of the clinician's major responsibilities as I see it—to help the person who stutters (or is at risk for stuttering) and the family feel realistically better and more optimistic about themselves as communicators and their communication world and future as a result of having interacted with the clinician. This results from serving as a readily available resource of positive support and knowledge, shared planning and helping to achieve fluency success, and conveying and demonstrating a sincere belief in the individual's and the family's potential for communication improvement (Daly, 1988). In other words, conveying by word and deed that the client and family have a comrade in you, the clinician, is a remarkably empowering experience for our clients. Creating such experiences is indeed our responsibility. The phone call is a relatively small effort that yields potentially large and unfolding benefits. In support of such efforts, Haynes and Pindzola (2008) noted that "the very first contact with a client—the manner in which he or she is treated during a clinical examination—is a crucial determining factor in response to therapy" (p. 35).

Assessment Procedures

General Considerations

The first face-to-face contact the clinician has with the family of the preschool child is often at the scheduled appointment for the diagnostic evaluation. The parent interview generally precedes a direct observation of parent–child interaction. These two components, however, occasionally are reversed as indicated by the needs of the child. When the child can be separated readily from the parent and when there is a clinician or other responsible adult to interact with the child during the interview, the parent interview typically is held first. When these two conditions are not present, then the parent–child interaction may be held first to facilitate separation, as will be seen. An important point, however, is that I tend not to have the preschool child present during the initial interview if possible because of two potentially conflicting needs: to talk absolutely candidly with the family members who are present and to prevent the child from becoming increasingly aware of, if not concerned about, the observed behaviors.

To achieve both of these ends, it is helpful for the child not to be present during the interview. Where separation remains impossible, however, I have held parent interviews in the same room with a child who is actively engaged with another child or adult or in play-based activities within view. This scenario is workable but not preferred, requiring creativity and flexibility, because both the parents and clinician must attend to the other interaction, thus taking at least some attention and energy away from the interview itself. Guitar (2006) cautioned, however, not to force the child to separate and emphasized that relative openness may reduce the fear of stuttering being internalized by both the child and the family. Guitar (2006) further advised that it is more important to afford the child a positive association with the treatment experience, even if we are unable to collect all the information we would like. If the child will not separate, Guitar suggested that the clinician talk with the parents about general things in one part of the room while the child plays with toys in another. A short while later, the clinician might suggest moving with the parent to an adjacent room with the doors open, leaving the child in view to play with the toys. Sometimes, if all must move together, the child will become bored and will gravitate back to the toys that are in sight in the original room. Guitar noted, and I concur, that children rarely have more than a momentary difficulty separating from the parents.

What follows are general guidelines for conducting a communication evaluation with a preschool child and the family. The proceedings should be video recorded for analysis and subsequent retrieval. Video recording equipment provides an excellent clinical tool and is increasingly available at low cost. I have often said that if I were dropped onto an inaccessible island and could bring with me only one diagnostic or clinical tool, I would choose a pocket-size video recording camera, which comes with a digital hard drive and monitor. Combined with a clinician's trained eyes and ears and an empathic heart, video equipment proves invaluable. Of use, but less preferred, is audio recording equipment, which cannot capture the visual aspect of communication and its disorders, specifically stuttering. The guidelines that follow should be adjusted as indicated by the child, family, clinician, and setting.

Parent Interview

Preparation

Based on the case history form, initial video or audio recording, and preliminary phone call, I develop questions and topics that I want to pursue. Typically, I outline for myself in telegraphic form information that I want to receive and provide. In addition, I write a reminder to myself to *listen*. I am convinced that one of the most important contributions a clinician can offer during the interview is a willingness and ability to listen. Haynes and Pindzola (2008) provided an excellent chapter on interviewing "do's and don'ts" and methods of improving interviewing skills. I recommend this chapter to all clinicians. In addition to many other valuable suggestions, they warn clinicians to avoid talking too much and providing information too soon. More will be said about this when we address clinician competencies (Chapter 11) and professional preparation and lifelong learning (Chapter 12).

Social Greeting

The initial interview is typically held with the child's parent or parents. Deliberately, I begin with a social comment and positive greeting. Too often, the communication problem, rather than the people with whom we are interacting, becomes the immediate focus. A social greeting enables clinicians and clients to begin the journey as coequal participants in a shared process and helps to establish a social and personal foundation. Before we can respect and respond to each other's role and responsibility as clients or clinicians within the clinical process, we first must value each other as people. The importance of establishing positive rapport cannot be overstated.

Questions and Dialogue

The parent interview consists of many direct and open-ended questions. Their purpose is not to limit the exchange, but rather to provide focus within a flexible, dynamic context. The exchange should be inquiring, supportive, and conversational. After the necessary permission forms are signed and after the clinician provides a general orientation as to the assessment process, various areas are probed.

Typically, the first questions I ask the parents are why they came to meet with us and what they hope to accomplish as a result of our meeting. Some parents are taken aback by such questions because they may have become accustomed to professionals' immediate focus on "the problem." The answers to these questions help provide me with an idea of what the parents perceive as their own and the child's needs and objectives, each of which I respond to deliberately before the conclusion of the evaluation. This is essential for at least two reasons. First, by inviting their objectives for the meeting, I am giving the parents an active role in the process from its outset. Furthermore, I do not want to presume that I understand their needs before I inquire about them. Surely, our training and experience help us predict commonalities among families of preschool children who are at risk for stuttering. However, let us not forget that all people and families are different. Asking what their needs are also helps to communicate our interest in understanding the child as an individual and the family as a unique communication system. Second, we should not assume that the parents are concerned about stuttering. Even if they are, we cannot assume that what the clinician means by "stuttering" is what the parents mean by "stuttering." I have worked with some parents who initially expressed concern over "stuttering," only to discover that their use of the term was a global reference to communication disorders (such as articulation, language, or other area of impairment).

Asking parents the questions noted earlier (why they came and what they hope to accomplish) provides an opportunity for them to begin to explain the nature of their concern. If they haven't already spoken about it, I ask them to discuss the nature of their concern. Whatever word or words they use to describe their concern (e.g., *stuttering, stammering, freezing,* or other terms), I ask them to elaborate on what they mean when they use that word. Generally I do not use the term *stuttering* until they do because, as noted earlier, the term is evaluative and is relatively useless without description and qualification. Once they have described their concern, I ask them to discuss, to the best of their memory, the onset and development of the problem they have just characterized. I am interested to know how, when, and by whom the problem was first noticed and how the speech patterns might have changed since the disfluency was first detected (e.g., amount and type of disfluency, remissions, or conditions of predictable fluency or disfluency). Were there any special events in the child's life (e.g., birth of a sibling, death of a relative, language or cognitive leaps, family tension) that coincided with the beginning of disfluency?

Once the parents have described the communication problem and the surrounding events further, I ask them to describe the family's typical daily routine. In doing so, I am looking for a description of the family structure and the family's typical communication interaction. This helps me begin to identify sources of potential communicative pressure at home (e.g., where the child might feel he needs to say things in a hurry so as not to be interrupted, where the child might be directed not to speak because of seemingly more important events), which will assist me in making specific recommendations later. Williams (1978) noted that it is essential to determine the general atmosphere of pace and tension within a family, which might contribute to the child's development of disfluency. It is equally important, he observed, to determine if the child receives special consideration when he is disfluent that he does not receive when he is fluent. For example, do the parents attend to what he says, limit interruptions, and excuse him for misbehaving only when he is disfluent? In either case (excessive rush and tension contributing to disfluency or overcompensation as a consequence of disfluency), disfluency is being inadvertently precipitated or perpetuated. More recently, the positive impact of parental adjustments (e.g., limiting interruption, normalizing speech rate and linguistic complexity, providing appropriate speech models) that lead to reduced stuttering has received renewed empirical and clinical support (Bernstein Ratner, 2004a; Onslow et al., 2003; Yaruss et al., 2006).

Other areas probed include observed patterns (e.g., specific words, situations, people, times of day, or activities) in which the speech fluency is noticeably better or worse. Additionally, how does the child react to the communication context when fluent and disfluent? How do the other family members react to the child when he is fluent and disfluent? What have the family members done to try to help the child when he is experiencing disfluency, and how has the child responded to such efforts? I inquire what the parents believe to be the cause of the disfluency. This helps me understand their causal assumptions, which may impact their participation in and confidence regarding the clinical process. Williams (1978) stressed the significance of the language used by the parents to describe why the child is disfluent. Specifically, do their words reflect a belief that the disfluency is a symptom of something wrong within the child, or a response by the child to environmental conditions? What is the parents' outlook on the child's communication future? Do they seem more concerned about how the child is functioning and reacting today, or are they more concerned about how the disfluency might impact his life as he gets older? Has the child received any previous communication assessments or intervention?

I ask about whether any other family members have experienced speech–language problems, the developmental course of such problems (i.e., recovery or persistence in the case of stuttering), and the nature and outcome of any treatment, all the while exploring feelings and welcoming questions. A significant area to address is any observed awareness or frustration on the part of the child in response to fluency breakdown. Particularly significant is how the awareness develops and moves from potential neutrality to negativity and frustration. The parent interview itself may take a variety of directions depending on the needs of the parents or child, information presently available, and causal assumptions held by and level of participation of the parents, among other factors.

During the parent interview and throughout the assessment process, many other areas are probed. The essential purpose is to gain an understanding of the child's and the family's communication past and present in order to begin to project to the future. Additional areas of inquiry might include birth and developmental history; speech–language, motor, and social development; family history and interactive patterns; social and emotional temperament; and situational hierarchies (Conture, 2001; Gregory, 2003; Guitar, 2006; Yairi & Ambrose, 2005).

Parent–Child Interaction

Valuable information is obtained from observing one or more parents interacting directly with the preschool child. In a university-based speech and hearing center, we observe this directly through a one-way observation window. Where such a facility is not available, the parents and child may interact while the clinician, in the same room, appears to be busily engaged in some other activity. All the while, however, she is listening intently to the interaction. When limitations preclude such an observation, the clinician may observe the parents and child before the assessment begins, perhaps in the waiting area or in the nearby hallway. In any case, observing the interaction provides a sample of the child's speech behavior with a familiar person (e.g., parents), which then can be compared with that collected with an unfamiliar person (e.g., clinician). Typically, the parents are the persons with whom the child feels most comfortable. Occasionally, however, the relationship between the child and the parents is strained, resulting in increased disfluency being observed in the child's speech.

It is instructive to observe how the child and parents interact with and react to each other. Garrard (1990–1991) presented a useful series of observation worksheets addressing nonvocal and vocal behaviors of the child and parents in addition to the language-facilitation strategies provided by the parents. Observed nonvocal child behaviors involve attention span, eye contact and joint focus with the conversation partner, receptive language, communication intentions, facial expressions, body movements, cooperative behavior, turn-taking, activity initiation, bids for attention, and social play, in addition to vocal behaviors collected during speech–language sampling (e.g., language fluency). Nonvocal parental behaviors include involving the child in play, rapport, warmth and approval, facial expressions, physical proximity, nonvocal responsiveness, pause time, power balance, following child's interests, and nonvocal reinforcement. Vocal parental behaviors include utterance length, appropriateness of prosody, speech clarity, expansions and extensions, topic comments and shifts, repetitions of child's utterance, reference training (e.g., verbalizing child actions and parent actions, labeling objects and events), verbal cues and prompts for child to take a vocal turn, praise, child content, acknowledgment of child interests, confirmation of child comment, chaining to child responses, questions, and types of responses to child's communicative attempts. Parental language facilitation strategies include natural, positive reinforcement to the child's response (verbal—"good," "great," "super"; physical—a smile, pat, hug, clap; or tangible—giving toy, drink, food); physical proximity (parent shares play in close proximity to child); imitations or repetitions of child's words or attempts; expansions and extensions (conversational chaining by adding semantic content to child's utterance); semantic appropriateness (content and vocabulary) for the child; verbal cues or prompts; pausing after conversational turns to encourage turn-taking; speech clarity (distinctness, loudness, pronunciation); and warm approval (affection and approval of child through facial or body expressions and confirming verbal responses). Aspects of vocal and nonvocal interaction influence the nature of the exchange between the child and his parents. Observing these and other factors will prove enlightening regarding how language is used and facilitated and how communication, including speech fluency, is nurtured.

I remember observing a conversational interaction between a father who was a minister and his son, who had just turned 3 years old. The father initiated and maintained a number of topics that were all within an abstract, conceptual domain. For example, he spoke of devotion, resurrection, faith, divinity, heaven, and damnation. The boy spoke very little and responded infrequently to the father's questions of increasing verbal and emotional intensity. When he did speak, the boy's speech was characterized by significantly disfluent speech. Before the end of the assessment, during the period of trial management (a period for using different treatment strategies to determine their relative effectiveness with the child), I explained, demonstrated, and then coached the father in how he might interact with his son about the very same topics while reducing the excessive demand being placed on the boy's developing language, speech fluency, and other aspects of communication. We began with having the boy draw his own picture of the Lord at home, which is called Heaven. An artist's representation of Jesus was used to make the boy's understanding of Jesus as the son of the Lord more concrete. Other concepts were discussed with direct connection to concrete objects, including birth, death, following rules, and being nice to other people.

Additionally, I illustrated for the father how he could encourage his son to become a more active participant in the conversation. We discussed different types of questions, turn-taking, modeling, and expansion, among other topics. The father indicated that he appreciated my acceptance of the content as important to his family and my willingness to help him convey it more understandably to his son. Over the course of working with the father on three separate occasions focusing on pragmatic language skills with his young son and after subsequent phone contact with the father, the boy's fluency improved significantly, as did the father's interactional skills with his son. The father relayed that what he learned in treatment also helped him interact more effectively with other young children in the Sunday School program. By directly observing the child interacting with the parent, the clinician gets an idea of the interaction styles, parity of turn-taking, and appropriateness of the language model presented to the child. Moreover, the clinician begins to determine how conducive the parent–child interaction is for facilitating the child's speech fluency. The clinician also learns about factors that might be addressed with the parents to help them know what they can do to reduce the child's speech disfluency and to facilitate fluency.

Child–Clinician Interaction

Typically, a clinician enters the assessment session and excuses the parents, who observe the remaining session if observation facilities are available. If a clinician interacted with the child during the parent interview, it is helpful if that same clinician enters the session now. Familiarity with the clinician from earlier play interaction often facilitates separation. After collecting a speech–language sample between the child and one clinician, it is useful to have a second clinician or other adult enter the assessment session. Doing so enables a comparison of the child's speech across different listener contexts and settings (at home via video recording, with the parents during the assessment, with one unfamiliar adult, with two or more unfamiliar adults). It is quite possible that limitations unique to the setting might preclude using a second clinician or other adult.

The child–clinician interaction enables the clinician to directly observe the child's fluency and disfluency and the extent to which both are modifiable. The interaction also results in a speech–language sample that is as broad based as possible, allowing for comparison within and between the various components (e.g., speech sample provided via video recording, parent–child interaction, and those discussed herein). In other words, I am looking to sample the child's speech fluency control across diverse speaking contexts that vary in degree of communicative challenge from least (e.g., uninterrupted conversation) to most (e.g., deliberate interruption and abrupt topic shifts). While the specific speaking tasks and their sequence may vary, typically they include a speech–language sample and structured activities with and without communicative pressure.

Speech–Language Sample Without Communicative Pressure

To gain rapport with the child, I begin with speech–language sampling without communicative pressure. Most clinicians are familiar with procedures for collecting a language sample with a child. In this case, the sample should be of no less than 5-minute duration of the child's talking (approximately 300 words), which might take 10 to 15 minutes of real time. Conture (1997, 2001) noted that the sample size should be sufficient to permit averaging across several 100-word samples. In most cases, a sample of 300 words or more is adequate and collected with ease. However, for a client who stutters severely, the length of time he would take to produce 300 words may be counterproductive to the goals of the evaluation. In such cases, a sample of between 50 and 100 words may be sufficient, being supplemented at the beginning of scheduled treatment by an additional sample from a larger corpus. The clinician attempts to be minimally directive, both playing and talking with the child and following the child's lead. Objects, toys, and pictures are introduced gradually, but only as needed. Too often, the objects inhibit rather than enhance the conversation between the child and the clinician. The clinician deliberately creates opportunities to converse about events past, present, and future and for the child to demonstrate language (syntactic, semantic, pragmatic, and phonologic) competence.

Excellent suggestions are available for facilitating spontaneous talking with young children (e.g., Fey, 1986; Garrard, 1990–1991; Haynes & Pindzola, 2008). Clinicians need to remember the "child" in childhood language, that play is a natural context for interacting with children, and that play and fun represent the language of childhood.

Occasionally, however, some children, particularly those who are reluctant to separate from their parents, will not talk with a clinician. Student clinicians have nightmares in anticipation of just such a situation. It is possible for a child to learn language with his mouth closed (refusing to speak) during language intervention, but a child's speech fluency cannot be determined under the same circumstances. All is not lost, however. Van Riper (1972) represented the interaction between a clinician and child as an evolving, developmental process from solo play, through tangential play and intersecting play, to cooperative play (see Figure 8.1). When a clinician understands the relative stages of play, performance expectations are adjusted accordingly and the child's needs remain the clinician's focus.

Van Riper (1972) noted that most adults, including parents, clinicians, and other authority figures, often attempt to get a child to speak by asking questions. Questions are demands, however, subordinating the child to the authority of the questioner, who is in control. Similarly, such question-asking techniques in the confines of the treatment room are on the low end of the continuum of communicative naturalness (Fey, 1986), lacking in ecological validity (Muma, 1978), and result in "impoverished samples" (Van Riper, 1972, p. 108). Furthermore, eliciting speech by questions resembles an interrogation more than a meaningful conversation. Van Riper (1972) suggested, particularly with reticent children,

> How then should one begin? We suggest that you simply greet the child, then do some simple *self-talk*, commenting on what you are doing, or perceiving, and with plenty of moments of comfortable silence interspersed, until you have him playing with his box of toys. And then, in the role of adult playmate, you can play with those in your box. Silently at first. No question. No demands. *Solo play!*
>
> Once the child is comfortable in this activity, you should begin to put some self-talk into your own solo play; first noises (those of trucks, animals, etc.), then single words, then short phrases and simple sentences. All of these refer to what you are experiencing at the moment. Usually the child will begin to follow suit. His noises, his self-talk, begin to flow. Next you should shift to contact play very gradually. Let your toy truck occasionally touch his fire-engine, or help him find a block, or put another one on his toppling pile, or straighten it up a bit so he can make it higher. When you feel the time is ripe in this *tangential contact play*, begin to accompany it with some noises or commentary, using *parallel talking*, telling him what he is doing, perceiving, or feeling, again making sure that you have more silence than speech.
>
> From tangential play, you can often proceed rapidly to *intersecting play* in which your activity becomes a part of his. (Let your truck go over the bridge he has built or feed your doll or toy dog a piece of the play fruit he has put on the playhouse table.) Verbalize what you are doing. Next, seek to achieve *cooperative play*, assisting him to do the things he is doing. (Have your truck bring to him the blocks he needs to build his tower.) Usually by this time the child is speaking very easily and often copiously, your own verbalizations being primarily confined to reflecting what he has said. From this point onward, the communication can proceed fairly normally and naturally. (pp. 109–110)

Clinicians are encouraged to apply their understanding of the stages of play to procedures that facilitate more spontaneous talking among reticent preschool children. The purpose is to reduce the communicative demand (pressure) placed upon the child while encouraging verbal exchange in a relatively natural context. I remember being invited to do a fluency evaluation of Dawn, a little girl who was 4 years old, at a local health department. I had noticed Dawn's tension as she eyed me, a bearded man wearing a tie.

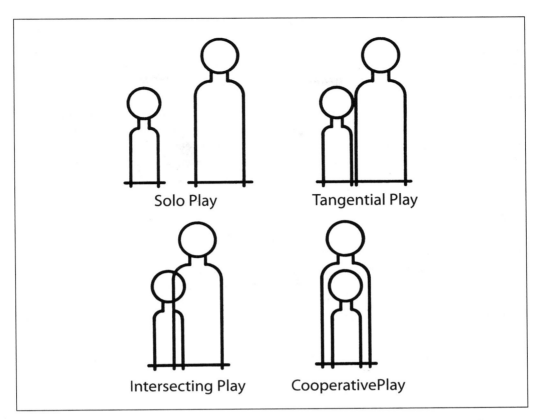

Figure 8.1.   Diagram of interaction between a clinician and child. *Note.* From *Speech Correction: Principles and Methods* (5th ed., p. 109), by C. Van Riper, 1972, Englewood Cliffs, NJ: Prentice Hall. Copyright 1972 by Allyn & Bacon/Pearson. Reprinted with permission.

Her parents were not present, and the nurse introduced me to her as *Doctor* Shapiro. At this, her tension immediately and visibly turned to panic as, no doubt, she imagined some kind of unpleasant medical procedure. Why else would the nurse have introduced me to her and then left so quickly? Well, the stages of play are useful for a reticent child, but not for one paralyzed with fear. I remember getting Dawn to the soda machine and learning by head nod that she liked orange soda. With permission, I bought the two of us orange sodas and walked out to the parking lot, where we sat on the curb and drank soda. I talked, relieving her fear by clarifying that I was not a medical doctor and that my sole purposes were to talk and play with her. While she seemed to believe me (her crying subsided enough to drink soda), she did not want to reenter the building with me, where previously she had been treated medically. So we sat on the curb and completed our evaluation as Dawn consumed her orange soda.

In addition to assessing the child's speech behavior, we need to assess the relative valence (positive, neutral, or negative) of his expressions of feelings and attitudes about communication and his communication skills. Most preschool children talk ceaselessly during all waking moments. Of particular concern, however, is when a preschool child develops an overall communication reticence, saying "I don't know," "I can't say that," or just "I can't." I remember another child, Andrew, who was 3 years 6 months old and who stuttered severely and only spoke when he concealed his face behind his hands, a book, paper, or other object. Assessing the feelings and attitudes of the preschooler without creating additional awareness or concern on the part of the child regarding the speech disfluency is indeed a challenge for clinicians. It is accomplished by asking the parents about the child's feelings and attitudes during the parent interview, by observing during the parent–child interaction, and by reviewing the audio or video recordings made before and during the assessment session. Significant indicators include the child's willingness to talk, amount of eye contact, facial expressions, and nonverbal body language (Guitar & Peters, 2008), all of which might be influenced by multicultural factors. Other indicators include overall degree of tension, speaking volume and rate, spontaneity of response, eye movement, voice quality and pitch, and relative increase or decrease in frequency of total disfluency or of any one disfluency type (Williams, 1978). Another method is probing by the clinician during the child–clinician interaction.

Some of the most useful and sensitive suggestions for talking with children about talking were presented by Williams (1971, 2003, 2004, 2006). Because these suggestions address school-age children, who experience stuttering differently from preschool children, further discussion is reserved for Chapter 9. Guitar (2006) noted that the feelings and attitudes of the preschool child about speech disfluency range from apparent unawareness of disfluency, to occasional awareness although rarely bothered, to awareness and frustration, to significant awareness combined with frustration and fear. Indeed children as young as 2 years 6 months old have demonstrated awareness and frustration related to their experience of speech disfluency (Ambrose & Yairi, 1994; Ezrati-Vinacour et al., 2001; Vanryckeghem et al., 2005; Yairi & Ambrose, 2005). If it is clear that the child is aware of or frustrated about his disfluency, then I will probe the child's feelings further, and my directness will be in proportion to the child's observed or expressed awareness.

For example, Tony was a 4-year-old boy who demonstrated noticeable disfluency with concomitant facial, neck, and body tension, yet no reluctance to initiate or respond to a conversational turn. I said to him, "You know, Tony, sometimes when I am tired or get in a hurry, it is a little hard for me to talk." After a brief silence, he offered, "You know, me too! Me too!" I followed up with, "How does that make you feel?" To this, he said, "It makes me feel embarrassed." We talked about his feelings, about how everyone is good at things and must work at others, and about how we feel when we try our best at things that are difficult for us that seem easy to others. Significantly, Tony related to and extended the probe I offered. He could have not responded during the silence (silence is an essential part of a probe); he could have denied it (offering expressions such as, "Not me. No. That never happens to me."); or he could have been noncommittal ("So?" or "Big deal."). But Tony's response left no doubt regarding his degree of awareness and developing frustration. On the basis of information available from the sources noted earlier and particularly from observing Tony's active participation as a conversational partner, it did not appear that fear or negativity had entered his view of himself as a communicator.

Guitar (2006) suggested other probes to determine a preschool child's awareness about disfluency. He suggested asking the child if he knows why he has come to see the clinicians, to which some children will be noncommittal, while others might respond forthrightly, "Because I don't talk right." Guitar viewed this interaction as a possible opportunity to discuss stuttering further and to convey to the child both that he is not alone and that others who also "get stuck on words" have been helped. He also suggested that it might help a child to talk about his stuttering by first telling him about another child who stutters—while using appropriate vocabulary ("getting stuck" or "having trouble on words"). If the child conveys disinterest in talking about stuttering, the clinician might drop the subject initially. Later, the clinician might insert some normal-sounding disfluencies into her own speech and first offer a self-comment that sometimes she has trouble getting words out, and later ask the child if he ever has trouble like this. Again, the clinician interprets the child's relative willingness to discuss stuttering and whether or not an opportunity exists to discuss it further. These and other procedures, according to Guitar (2006), are intended "(1) to see if he accepts himself and his disfluencies enough to discuss them and (2) to assure him that he is not alone with the problem and that his parents and I may be able to help him" (p. 233).

Structured Activities Without Communicative Pressure

Once I have a rich conversational speech–language sample, I engage the preschool child in several structured activities that yield elicited verbal responses for analysis. Some clinicians may prefer to begin with structured activities. Generally, I find beginning with conversational interaction to be more successful in building rapport with young children, however. Structured activities may include, but are not limited to, the following:

🔲 Discussing a current event (e.g., birthday, football game), holiday (e.g., Thanksgiving, Halloween), or possession (e.g., dog, bicycle). This can be done easily with the carrier phrase, "Tell me about X."

🔲 Explaining a familiar game (e.g., soccer) or activity (e.g., baking a cake, removing a tree with a backhoe, making honey). You might ask, "How do you [play soccer, make honey, etc.]?"

🔲 Asking questions designed to elicit responses on a continuum from shorter (e.g., "What is your name?" "How old are you?" "What is your favorite TV show?") to longer (e.g., "Why do you like that show?" "What do you do with your brothers?" "What's your dog like?").

🔲 Repeating words and sentences of varied length and complexity. The words and sentences are presented in random order, and the clinician is looking to see how increasing linguistic complexity and different phonemic sequences influence speech fluency. Words range from short and simple (e.g., *I, you, got, fish*) to longer and more complex (e.g., *airplane, cowboy, reported, conversation*). Sentences likewise vary from simple (e.g., "I like it," "That is my dog") to more complex (e.g., "Please sit in your seat," "We have two dogs and three cats at home"). As always, these may be adjusted based on the preschool child's age and communication competence.

Williams (1978) suggested other structured activities, such as naming objects (making one-word responses in naming objects on picture cards), making short phrase responses (responding to "What's going on in the picture?"), and telling a story about a picture (or series of pictures requiring a longer sequential response). As noted in Chapter 7, Ryan (1974, 2001) and Ryan and Van Kirk (1971, 1978) presented a comprehensive list of structured activities (i.e., fluency interview) for assessing preschool and young school-age children. These activities include automatic speech (counting, saying the alphabet, singing, reciting a poem), echoic speech (imitating words and sentences), reading (except for young preschool children), picture naming, speaking alone (clinician leaves the room), monologue, command speech (client directs the clinician), talking with gestures, talking with time pressure, talking with drawing, talking with phonemic difficulty (imitating complex words), responding to and asking questions, speaking on the telephone, engaging in conversational speech, and observing the child in a natural setting. The purpose of these activities is to provide the child ample and varied opportunities for structured speech so that the clinician can evaluate what factors tend to relate to fluctuations in speech fluency.

Speech–Language Sample and Structured Activities with Communicative Pressure

Once the speech–language sample and structured activities without communicative pressure are completed, components of both are expanded, now with communicative pressure. Communication pressure takes the form of different demands that deliberately challenge the child's ability to remain fluent. The purpose is to determine the relative impact of perceived communicative pressure (including time pressure, linguistic

ambiguity, violation of conversational or pragmatic rules) on speech fluency. For example, during conversation with the child, structured activities noted earlier, or other
related treatment tasks (games that are appropriate for the child, such as drawing, board
or card games, and puppet activities), the clinician might begin to

- ⌘ rush the activity (by significantly increasing her rate of speech, amount of hand movements and extraneous gestures, or speed of requesting answers),

- ⌘ interrupt the child (taking a conversational turn well before the child is about to complete
  his, or asking a question and then asking a new question before the child finishes answering the first question),

- ⌘ demonstrate loss of attention (while the child is relating an event, doing something else
  that indicates by her action that she is not attending to him), or

- ⌘ request that the child say something again (by saying, "I didn't understand that. Would
  you tell me again?") (Williams, 1978).

The clinician also might make abrupt topic shifts (by introducing a topic prematurely that is unrelated to the child's discussion), overstep the boundaries of the child's
linguistic competence (using vocabulary clearly not within the child's semantic repertoire), or introduce deliberate linguistic ambiguity (offering contradictions) or verbal
absurdity (such as, "What's this I hear about you sleeping in the garage?" or "How come
you make pizza in the bathtub?"). The clinician must remember to share with the parent her clinical rationale for imposing deliberate demands upon the child, particularly
when such procedures result in disfluency. Otherwise, the parent might interpret erroneously that the clinician is insensitive or unkind.

Trial Management

The preceding assessment activities enable the clinician to evaluate the child's speech
fluency so as to arrive at a diagnosis and to establish a baseline of the child's communication behavior, from which progress in treatment, if necessary, can be monitored
(Haynes & Pindzola, 2008). As will be seen, the process leading from assessment and
evaluation to diagnosis is ongoing and dynamic, not limited to a fixed time frame. Even
when treatment has begun, assessment continues and leads to a more precise or refined
diagnosis. From the assessment activities, the clinician decides whether or not she feels
that a more formal evaluation of articulation/phonology and language is necessary. If
the child has demonstrated repetition or prolongation of syllables or shows any evidence
of awareness of communication concern, frustration, or speech fluency–related communication reticence, the clinician should engage in a brief period of trial management
during the assessment session itself. Because the feelings and attitudes related to speech
fluency are typically just developing with preschool children, the distinction between
fluency shaping and stuttering modification treatment techniques is least clearly defined
(compared to that with school-age children and adults). The trial management techniques (different treatment activities to determine relative effectiveness with a particular child) performed during the assessment session and the child's response thereto help
the clinician to design appropriate intervention methods for the preschool child and to
offer specific recommendations.

Fluency Shaping

Fluency shaping techniques for trial management include having the child sing a short
song and recite a nursery rhyme in chorus with the clinician (both of which are essential
for differential diagnosis, as noted in Chapter 4); modeling and impersonating, through
puppetry and play, both turtle speech (slow and gentle) and rabbit speech (fast and

hard); modeling slow, relaxed, slightly prolonged speech (with slight prolongation on vowels and light articulatory contacts on consonants while maintaining naturalness in the suprasegmental aspects of speech); and perhaps moving from established fluency in monosyllabic words to polysyllabic words, then to phrases, and finally to sentences.

Stuttering Modification

Stuttering modification techniques include modeling slow, relaxed, prolonged speech; modeling easier versions of the child's stuttering; inserting instances of slight disfluency in the clinician's speech with a self-comment (e.g., "Gosh, that was a little hard") in the context of emotional neutrality, leading to interacting with the child about the clinician's disfluency (e.g., "Did you hear the word I just said that was a little hard? What did you think?"); and providing praise to the child for slow and gentle speech (e.g., "I love the way you said that. You said wwwell," modeling gentle production of "well").

Post-Assessment Procedures

A preliminary analysis of the speech sample is conducted before the post-assessment parent conference in order to present preliminary findings and recommendations. The analyses described later in this section, however, are performed after the assessment session in preparation for the diagnosis, detailed in the clinical summary report. The purposes of the speech analysis are to quantify (i.e., use precise numbers, tallies, summary statistics) and qualify (i.e., describe narrowly) the speech characteristics along the continuum from speech fluency to disfluency. Common errors are to assess the characteristics of disfluency only (while forgetting that the majority of speech of people who stutter is more fluent than not) and to assume that characteristics of speech disfluency are invariant and static. Rather, we must highlight both the fluency and disfluency characteristics in addition to the related feelings, thoughts, and attitudes.

Making a distinction between normal disfluency and incipient stuttering in the preschool child often proves challenging because multiple factors must be considered simultaneously (e.g., the frequency, type, and duration of disfluency; Gordon & Luper, 1992a, 1992b; Riley, 2009), and because, again, we are dealing with continuous, multidimensional variables rather than dichotomous, unidimensional ones. Who can distinguish the upper limits of normal disfluency from the lower limits of beginning stuttering? On the basis of behavioral analysis alone, this proves impossible. Our judgment is helped some by assessing the feelings, thoughts, and attitudes, as noted, and other factors such as feelings of internal control (Cooper & Cooper, 1995; Finn, 2007; Quesal, 2007; Yaruss & Quesal, 2006, 2008; Zebrowski, 2007). In the end, there continues to be a critical place for informed and sensitive professional judgment, the value of which cannot be replaced by any isolated assessment technique.

Zebrowski (1995) noted that to distinguish stuttering from normal disfluency, clinicians need to be familiar with the behaviors that are relevant to making this distinction; be able to observe, quantify, and qualify these behaviors; and integrate this information to judge the likelihood that a child is either stuttering or at risk for stuttering. More recently, Curlee (2007) noted that reliable identification of stuttering in early childhood requires identification of clusters of signs and symptoms that distinguish children who are stuttering from those who are not:

> These signs and symptoms include qualitative and quantitative features of a child's disfluent speech and his or her reactions to it, which vary widely among the clinical population. There is no single sign or symptom that must be present, except for stuttered speech, which distinguishes stuttering from the disfluencies of nonstuttering children. (p. 4)

Curlee (2007) indicated that thorough clinical evaluation of young children suspected of stuttering provides clinicians with information to support one of the following conclusions:

1. Few if any signs of childhood stuttering are present, and the child's spoken language is age-appropriate.

2. Inconsistent signs of childhood stuttering are present, making further observation and testing necessary.

3. Signs of childhood stuttering have been present less than 1 year, and few negative reactions to stuttering are apparent or have been reported by parents.

4. Signs of childhood stuttering are frequently present, as are one or more other speech–language problems.

5. Stuttering has been present consistently for a year or more without any signs of remission.

Therefore, in this section, we will look first at the behaviors that guide our professional judgment in distinguishing between normal disfluency and beginning stuttering. Then we will consider how we quantify and qualify such behaviors. Finally, we will deal with the processes of establishing a diagnosis and conducting the post-assessment parent conference.

Normal Disfluency, At-Risk Disfluency, and Incipient Stuttering

Clinicians often struggle with the distinction between normal disfluency and beginning stuttering and, therefore, must determine if the child is stuttering, at risk for stuttering, or normally disfluent (Curlee, 2007; Zebrowski, 1994, 1995). Children who stutter and those who do not demonstrate some similarity in types of speech disfluencies, but exhibit differences in the degree and relative frequency of disfluency (Bloodstein & Bernstein Ratner, 2008). All children produce all types of disfluency (including within-word and between-word disfluencies). As a group, however, children who stutter are generally more disfluent overall and tend to demonstrate more within-word disfluencies. In other words, while all children demonstrate whole-word and phrase repetitions, interjections, and revisions (between-word disfluencies), children who stutter tend to demonstrate more part-word (sound or syllable) repetitions and sound prolongations (within-word disfluencies).

Various observational guidelines are useful for distinguishing between normal disfluency and beginning stuttering. Listeners typically recognize to a high degree of reliability when the fluency seems awry (see Bloodstein & Bernstein Ratner, 2008, and Yairi & Ambrose, 2005, for reviews of this literature). However, parents and novice clinicians are not as sure about why they are coming to this conclusion or the characteristics upon which their conclusion is based. Guidelines, therefore, are useful for observation and accountability. One such guideline, represented in Table 8.1, that helps facilitate objective description was presented by Van Riper (1982), who noted that it is "tentative, incomplete, and unsubstantiated by research" (p. 24), as well as lacking in item weights. It is nevertheless useful for clinicians and for discussion with parents, teachers, and others. The first column contains 26 behavioral characteristics within seven categories: syllable repetitions, prolongations, gaps (silent pauses), phonation, articulation postures, reaction to stress, and evidence of awareness. Clinicians must be mindful, however, not to interpret the second two columns (Stuttering vs. Normal disfluency) as discrete variables. Indeed they are continuous variables and are presented in dichotomous columns only for instructional purposes. Assessment of stuttering cannot be made on the basis of frequency counts alone. Each variable presented, however, provides an area of focus inviting molecular analysis and quantification. From my own experience, children with normal disfluency tend to demonstrate relatively effortless, infrequent, and inconsistent

Table 8.1   Guidelines for Differentiating Normal From Abnormal Disfluency

Behavior	Stuttering	Normal disfluency
Syllable repetitions		
a. Frequency per word	More than two	Less than two
b. Frequency per 100 words	More than two	Less than two
c. Tempo	Faster than normal	Normal tempo
d. Regularity	Irregular	Regular
e. Schwa vowel	Often present	Absent or rare
f. Airflow	Often interrupted	Rarely interrupted
g. Vocal tension	Often apparent	Absent
Prolongations		
h. Duration	More than 1 second	Less than 1 second
i. Frequency	More than 1 per 100 words	Less than 1 per 100 words
j. Regularity	Uneven or interrupted	Smooth
k. Tension	Important when present	Absent
l. When voiced (sonant)	May show rise in pitch	No pitch rise
m. When unvoiced (surd)	Interrupted airflow	Airflow present
n. Termination	Sudden	Gradual
Gaps (silent pauses)		
o. Within the word boundary	May be present	Absent
p. Prior to speech attempt	Unusually long	Not marked
q. After the disfluency	May be present	Absent
Phonation		
r. Inflections	Restricted; monotone	Normal
s. Phonatory arrest	May be present	Absent
t. Vocal fry	May be present	Usually absent
Articulating postures		
u. Appropriateness	May be inappropriate	Appropriate
Reaction to stress		
v. Type	More broken words	Normal disfluencies
Evidence of awareness		
w. Phonemic consistency	May be present	Absent
x. Frustration	May be present	Absent
y. Postponements (stallers)	May be present	Absent
z. Eye contact	May waver	Normal

Note. From *The Nature of Stuttering* (2nd ed., p. 25), by C. Van Riper, 1982, Englewood Cliffs, NJ: Prentice Hall. Copyright 1982 by Allyn & Bacon/Pearson. Reprinted with permission.

syllable repetition (e.g., *me-mean*) and word repetition (e.g., *this this*) and occasional prolongation (e.g., *sssomething*). In addition, increases in both the qualitative (type) and quantitative (amount) characteristics of disfluency, and particularly any evidence of speech-related stress, awareness, or frustration, are indicators of concern. More detail will be provided in the next section.

Another guideline was presented by Pindzola (Pindzola & White, 1986) and is represented in Figure 8.2. Like that presented by Van Riper, it is useful for guiding description and accountability and for presenting visual representations to parents, teachers, and

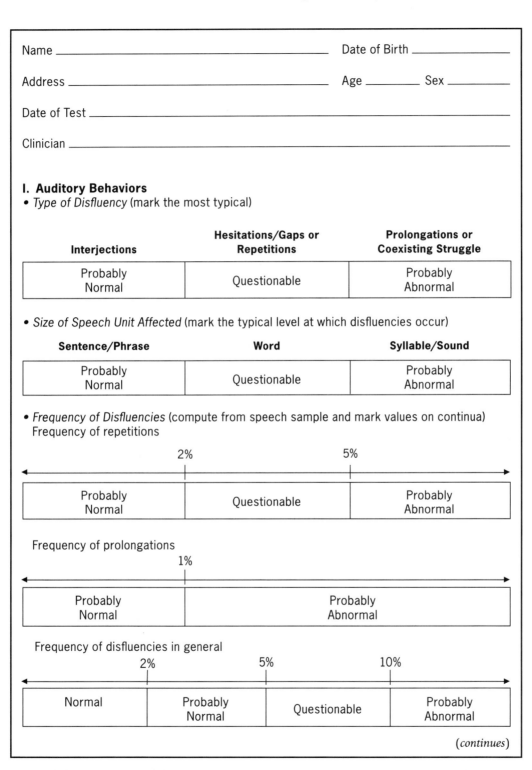

Name _____ Date of Birth _____

Address _____ Age _____ Sex _____

Date of Test _____

Clinician _____

I. Auditory Behaviors
• *Type of Disfluency* (mark the most typical)

Interjections	Hesitations/Gaps or Repetitions	Prolongations or Coexisting Struggle
Probably Normal	Questionable	Probably Abnormal

• *Size of Speech Unit Affected* (mark the typical level at which disfluencies occur)

Sentence/Phrase	Word	Syllable/Sound
Probably Normal	Questionable	Probably Abnormal

• *Frequency of Disfluencies* (compute from speech sample and mark values on continua)
Frequency of repetitions

2%   5%

Probably Normal	Questionable	Probably Abnormal

Frequency of prolongations

1%

Probably Normal	Probably Abnormal

Frequency of disfluencies in general

2%   5%   10%

Normal	Probably Normal	Questionable	Probably Abnormal

(*continues*)

Figure 8.2. Protocol for differentiating the incipient stutterer. *Note.* From "A Protocol for Differentiating the Incipient Stutterer," by R. H. Pindzola and D. T. White, 1986, *Language, Speech, and Hearing Services in Schools, 17*(1), pp. 12–15. Copyright 1986 by the American-Speech-Language-Hearing Association. Reprinted with permission.

- *Duration of Disfluencies*
  Typical number of reiterations of the repetition _____

Less than 2	2 to 5	More than 5
Probably Normal	Questionable	Probably Abnormal

Average duration of prolongations _____

Less than 1 second	1 or more seconds
Probably Normal	Probably Abnormal

- *Audible Effort* (mark those that apply)

Lack of the following items	Presence of the following items
Probably Normal	Probably Abnormal

hard glottal attacks _____   pitch rise _____

disrupted airflow _____   others: _____

vocal tension _____

- *Rhythm/Tempo/Speed of Disfluencies*

Slow/normal; evenly paced	Fast, perhaps irregular
Probably Normal	Probably Abnormal

- *Intrusion of Schwa Vowel During Repetitions*

Schwa not heard	Presence of Schwa
Probably Normal	Probably Abnormal

- *Audible Learned Behaviors* (mark those that apply)

Lack of the following items	Presence of the following items
Probably Normal	Probably Abnormal

word/phrase substitutions _____

circumlocutions _____

avoidance tactics (starters, postponers, and the like) _____

pitch rise _____

others: _____

(*continues*)

Figure 8.2.   (*continued*)

II. Visual Evidence (list behaviors observed)

• Facial Grimaces/Articulatory Posturing: _____

_____

• Head Movements: _____

_____

• Body Involvement: _____

_____

III. Historical/Psychological Indicators (comment on the following based on client and/or parent interviews, observations, and supplemental tests or questionnaires, if any)

• Awareness and Concern (of child; of parents): _____

_____

• Length of Time Fluency Problem Has Existed: _____

_____

• Consistent Versus Episodic Nature of Problem: _____

_____

• Reaction to Stress: _____

_____

• Phoneme/Word/Situation Fears and Avoidances: _____

_____

• Familial History: _____

_____

• Other Covert Factors: _____

_____

IV. Summary of Clinical Evidence and Impressions

_____

_____

_____

_____

_____

_____

_____

_____

Figure 8.2. (*continued*)

others. Pindzola presented eight categories of auditory behaviors (type of disfluency, size of speech unit affected, frequency of disfluencies, duration of disfluencies, audible effort, rhythm and speed of disfluencies, intrusion of schwa vowel during repetitions, and audible learned behaviors) and three categories of visual evidence (facial grimaces and articulatory postures, head movements, and body involvement). Visual evidence may be indicative of excessive speaking effort, awareness of a communication problem, adjustment to the disfluency, or relative severity. Seven historical and psychological indicators are then noted (awareness and concern, length of time fluency problem has existed, consistent vs. episodic nature of problem, reaction to stress, fears and avoidances, family history of stuttering, and other covert factors). Finally, clinical evidence and impressions are summarized.

Another guideline that I have found helpful, more for conveying basic information about the development of stuttering than for differential diagnosis, is one that is adapted from a video titled *Prevention of Stuttering [Part 1]: Identifying the Danger Signs* (Walle, 1976). This guideline contains less detail than the other protocols reviewed but is nonetheless useful in helping parents, family members, and others visualize fluency and disfluency along a continuum (see Figure 8.3).

The guidelines provided above emphasize the onset and development of stuttering on the basis of traditional developmental classifications from cross-sectional analysis. From Chapter 2, you will recall the somewhat contrastive portrait presented from longitudinal analysis (Yairi & Ambrose, 2005). It indicates that for some children, onset of stuttering can be sudden (between 1 and 3 days) or intermediate (between 1 and 2 weeks), within fairly stressful contexts (illness, upset, or fatigue), abrupt in its advanced presentation with physical concomitants, and subject to spontaneous or natural recovery without treatment. The Illinois stuttering research also indicated the significance of stuttering-like disfluencies (part-word repetitions, single-syllable word repetitions, and disrhythmic phonation) and other disfluencies (interjections such as *um* and *uh*, multisyllable word and phrase repetitions, and revisions and abandons) for predicting persistent stuttering. Children whose stuttering persisted tended to demonstrate a significantly higher number of stuttering-like disfluencies 6 months after onset (i.e., SLDs were not predictive before 6 months) and a higher number of other disfluencies (particularly interjections) 3 years after onset (ODs were not predictive before 3 years). This longitudinal portrait suggests that stuttering-like disfluencies should receive particular attention in assessment, follow-up, and prognosis (see Chapter 2).

Speech Analysis

Once we are familiar with the characteristics (including behaviors, thoughts, and feelings) that distinguish normal disfluency from beginning stuttering and predictors of stuttering that will naturally recover from that which will persist, we can begin to discuss how we analyze what we observe to help us reach a diagnosis and begin to plan treatment, if indicated. Parameters of speech fluency that are analyzed include, but are not limited to, the frequency of speech disfluency, type of disfluencies and proportion of each type, molecular description of disfluency (such as frequency and real time of units that occur in instances of repetition, prolongation, interjection, and other forms of disfluency), rate of speech, and other associated speech and nonspeech behaviors (Conture, 2001; Curlee, 2007; Gregory, 2003; Guitar, 2006; Quesal, 2007; Starkweather, 1993; Yaruss, 1998, 2000; Zebrowski, 1994, 1995).

Frequency of Speech Disfluency
Frequency of speech disfluency refers to the amount of disfluency, regardless of the individual types or relative severity, contained within the child's speech. This is a general

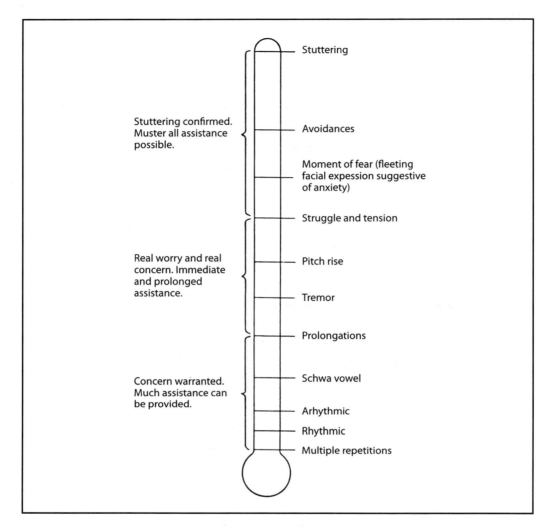

Figure 8.3. The danger signs of developing stuttering. *Note.* From *Prevention of Stuttering [Part 1]: Identifying the Danger Signs* [Videotape], by E. L. Walle, 1976, Memphis, TN: Stuttering Foundation of America. Copyright 1976 by the Stuttering Foundation of America. Reprinted with permission.

but important diagnostic measure that indicates the overall extent to which the disfluency disrupts the forward flow of speech. This measure is often used to document the broad effect that treatment has on a person's speech (Conture, 2001; Zebrowski, 1994, 1995). Frequency is reported as a percentage, usually as both an average and a range of disfluency, with the word or syllable as the unit of measure. When the word is the unit of measure, frequency of disfluency is computed by counting the total number of disfluent words (i.e., words that contain one or more form of disfluency) and dividing it by the total number of words spoken (both disfluent and fluent) within the sample collected. The resulting decimal is multiplied by 100 in order to convert to a percentage (in order to move the decimal point two places to the right). The syllable can also be used as the unit of measure. This is done by counting the total number of disfluent syllables, dividing it by the total number of syllables spoken (both disfluent and fluent), and then multiplying by 100. It is critical to use the same unit of measure over time so as to permit comparison for estimation of progress and change. We will assume for most clinical purposes, however, that the word is an adequate unit of measure. In simple form, the frequency of speech disfluency (*disfluency frequency index*, DFI) is computed as follows:

$$DFI = \frac{\text{total number of disfluent words}}{\text{total number of words spoken (disfluent + fluent)}} \times 100.$$

The speech sample being analyzed is typically of predetermined size or duration. For example, one could figure the number (percentage) of disfluent words in 100 words spoken, in the total number of words produced, or in 1 minute of conversational speech (Zebrowski, 1995). When reporting the frequency of disfluency as a percentage over 100 words spoken, the clinician should collect at least one 300-word sample and compute the average and range of disfluency produced (Conture, 2001; Zebrowski, 1994). For example, over a 300-word sample, a child might have had 10 disfluent words in the first 100 words spoken, 18 in the next 100, and 8 in the third 100, as follows:

$$\frac{10 + 18 + 8}{300} = \frac{36}{300} = .12 \times 100 = 12 \text{ stuttered words per 100 words spoken.}$$

This child demonstrated an average of 12 stuttered words per 100 words spoken (12%), averaged over a 300-word sample. Furthermore, he ranged from 8 to 18 disfluent words per 100 words spoken. Note that you can easily verify your mathematical accuracy. Calculate the *fluency frequency index* (FFI) by dividing the total number of fluent words by the total number of words (both fluent and disfluent) spoken, as follows:

$$FFI = \frac{\text{total number of fluent words}}{\text{total number of words spoken (fluent + disfluent)}} \times 100.$$

Adding the DFI and the FFI together should equal 100%. Using the illustration above, we can figure the FFI by dividing the number of fluent words (264) by the total number of words spoken (fluent, 264; disfluent, 36; total 300), as follows:

$$\frac{264}{300} = .88 \times 100 = 88 \text{ fluent words per 100 words spoken.}$$

In this case, 12 (12%) disfluent words per 100 words spoken plus 88 (88%) fluent words per 100 words spoken equals 100 (100%) of the words (disfluent + fluent) spoken.

Another way to calculate the DFI is to analyze a video-recorded random sample or samples from the child's conversation or other context. The DFI is computed in similar fashion. However, the total number of words is not predetermined and therefore must be calculated from transcription (Rustin, Botterill, & Kelman, 1996). The additional procedures involved tend to reduce the interrater reliability of this method of assessing the frequency of disfluency. However, while transcription is a time-consuming process, particularly for novice clinicians, it proves invaluable for understanding the nature of a client's fluency and disfluency. Again, a substantial segment (such as 300 words or 5 minutes) may be analyzed, or separate segments may be pooled into an analysis from which average and range frequency (in numbers or percentages) of disfluency are reported. For example, suppose we have a child who spoke 274 words within the sample, of which 24 words contained one or more disfluencies. Here is how it looks:

$$DFI = \frac{24 \text{ disfluent words}}{274 \text{ words spoken (disfluent + fluent)}} = .0876 = .09 \text{ (rounded)} \times 100 = 9\%.$$

This means that in this sample, the child demonstrated an overall disfluency of 9%. This DFI can be compared to others of similar length (in terms of number of words or duration of talk time). From the comparison, average and ranges can be computed. As noted, there is greater variation in this measure compared to one of predetermined length (e.g., 100 words, 300 words, etc.).

Summarizing studies comparing children who stutter with those who do not, Zebrowski (1995) indicated the former to be at least twice as disfluent, with average frequencies of disfluency consistently above 10% of the total number of words or syllables spoken. Similarly, Guitar (2006) estimated that preschool children who are normally disfluent demonstrate fewer than 10 disfluencies of all types in every 100 words spoken. He noted that interjections and revisions are more common than part-word repetitions, and part-word repetitions usually have only one or two units of repetition per instance of disfluency. Conture (1997, 2001) advocated the use of three within-word disfluencies per 100 words as a criterion for distinguishing normal disfluency from stuttering. Conture justified this criterion by stating that individuals who produce 10 disfluencies of all types per 100 words are likely producing three or more within-word disfluencies among these 10. Furthermore, he noted that within-word disfluencies are the type that listeners are most likely to consider as stuttering and are the type of disfluencies that people who stutter produce more often than people who do not.

Recall the longitudinal work of Yairi and colleagues (Yairi, 1997, 2004; Yairi & Ambrose, 1992a, 1992b, 1999, 2005; Yairi, Ambrose, & Niermann, 1993). This literature indicated that early stuttering is often associated with very high frequencies of speech disfluency (greater than 10% of all syllables or words spoken), followed by a sharp reduction in the frequency over the next 3 to 6 months, continuing to 12 or 14 months from the time the problem was first noticed. These studies reported that most of the children who recovered naturally did so within the first 3 years of onset. Recovery rate dropped sharply after 3 years of onset, but some did recover between 3 and 5 years; none recovered naturally after 5 years of onset. See Chapter 2 for specific rates of natural recovery from 1 to 5 years post-onset in 1-year increments. A primary distinguishing characteristic of children who did not recover without treatment was a greater amount of stuttering-like disfluencies (part-word repetitions, single-syllable word repetitions, and disrhythmic phonation) after 6 months post-onset and other disfluencies (particularly interjections) during the third year post-onset. These observations emphasize the importance of detecting disfluency early, conducting the evaluation promptly thereafter, and analyzing speech samples collected at 3- to 6-month intervals after initial contact, all aimed at monitoring the speech fluency of children close to the onset of stuttering or of those suspected to be at risk. Yairi (1997) described clinicians' decisions to initiate or delay treatment as a "double-edged ethical dilemma" (p. 73). He recommended that all young children who are beginning to stutter receive a thorough communication evaluation and subsequent reevaluations combined with parent education about childhood stuttering. He also recommended that those children who have stuttered for more than 14 to 18 months without exhibiting substantial improvement receive a priority for direct fluency intervention.

Type of Speech Disfluency

Another important characteristic to assess is the type of disfluency produced in addition to the proportion of each type. This type of analysis, also referred to as the *disfluency type index* (DTI), indicates what the child is doing that interferes with the forward flow of speech and how what the child is doing changes over time. The DTI is computed by using the same sample or samples analyzed earlier for frequency of disfluency. To analyze the individual types of speech disfluency, we divide the number of disfluencies of each individual type (such as part-word repetitions, whole-word repetitions, and prolongations, among others) by the total number of stuttered words. Again, I am electing to use the word as the unit of measure, which I find adequate for most applied clinical purposes. However, clinicians need to be aware that the syllable can be and is used as the unit of measure if an individual clinician so desires. Using the word as the unit of measure, the DTI is computed as follows:

$$DTI = \frac{\text{number of disfluencies of each individual type}}{\text{total number of disfluent words}} \times 100.$$

From the example discussed earlier, let's say that of the 36 disfluent words, 18 contained part-word (i.e., sound or syllable) repetitions, 9 contained sound prolongations, and the remaining 9 contained whole-word repetitions. The number of each individual type (18 part-word repetitions, 9 sound prolongations, 9 whole-word repetitions) is divided by the total number of disfluent words, as follows:

$$\% \text{ Part-word repetitions} = \frac{18 \text{ part-word repetitions}}{36 \text{ total disfluent words}} = .5 \times 100 = 50\%.$$

$$\% \text{ Sound prolongations} = \frac{9 \text{ sound prolongations}}{36 \text{ total disfluent words}} = .25 \times 100 = 25\%.$$

$$\% \text{ Whole-word repetitions} = \frac{9 \text{ whole-word repetitions}}{36 \text{ total disfluent words}} = .25 \times 100 = 25\%.$$

This means that the sample of 36 disfluent words contains 50% part-word (i.e., sound/syllable) repetitions, 25% sound prolongations, and 25% whole-word repetitions. Again, to check your mathematical accuracy, you can do two things. Add up the frequencies for each individual type (in this case, 18 + 9 + 9); this should equal the total number of disfluent words (36). Also, add up the computed percentages for each type of disfluency (50% + 25% + 25%) and that sum should be 100%.

This more narrow form of analysis is particularly important because the frequency of speech disfluency is often so variable both within and between children (W. Johnson & Associates, 1959, and Yairi, 1981, found that at least one child in their respective studies who did not stutter had at least 25 disfluencies per 100 words). Furthermore, an analysis of the types of disfluency and fluency is an important diagnostic characteristic for distinguishing between normal disfluency and beginning stuttering. As noted earlier, while there is a great deal of overlap between children who stutter and those who do not in the types of disfluencies they produce, one significant difference is that those who stutter produce more within-word speech disfluencies (sound or syllable or part-word repetitions, sound prolongations, and disfluencies that disrupt the transition between sounds within a word) (Conture, 1997, 2001; Zebrowski, 1994, 1995). Guitar (2006) noted the following about normal disfluency:

> Revisions are common in normal children and may continue to account for a major portion of their disfluencies as they grow older. Interjections are also common, but usually decline after 3 years of age. Repetitions may also be a frequent type of disfluency around 2 to 3 years of age, especially single-syllable word repetitions having fewer than two extra units. Repetitions are also more likely to involve longer segments (e.g., phrases) as a child grows older. (p. 143)

Schwartz and Conture (1988) introduced the *sound prolongation index* (SPI), which is a measure of one type of disfluency (audible or silent prolongation). Zebrowski (1994) summarized the clinical literature indicating that children with SPIs (or DTIs for prolongations) of 25% or more (i.e., 25% of the child's total disfluencies are sound prolongations) are likely to require direct treatment for their stuttering.

Molecular Description of Disfluency

Another important measure of disfluency, in addition to the frequency and type, is a more molecular characterization for individual instances of stuttering. This includes, but is not limited to, duration (real time) and frequency (total number, mean, and range). This molecular description is particularly important for measurement of an individual's variation of speech fluency before, during, and after treatment. For example, it was useful for me to be able to document that over a period of 6 months before treatment, Robert, a 4-year-old child, had part-word (sound or syllable) repetitions consisting of between 1 and 9 units of repetition lasting 1 to 19 seconds in duration. Within 4 months of an indirect form of treatment consisting of play intervention and parent counseling, his part-word repetitions reduced to between 1 and 3 units of repetition lasting no longer than 3 seconds. This brief description does not explicitly account for the significant decrease in overall severity measured in elimination of facial and body tension. Reporting the number and duration of repeated and prolonged units provides valuable clinical information for an individual child. A reminder here for clinicians is to account, in the most molecular form possible, for the type and degree of fluency and disfluency. The computations provided earlier for frequency and type only get the processes of analysis and description started. To reflect the nature of the speech itself, we need to document other factors that can be used to describe a child's speech fluency and disfluency over time.

More specifically, tracking changes in a young child's speech fluency can be used to document progression or regression of the disorder. Zebrowski (1995) noted that "increased duration of sound/syllable repetitions (i.e., either overall or with respect to individual repeated units), a slowed rate of repetition, or both, may serve as a valid indication of the progression of stuttering in children" (p. 85). Narrowly describing a child's disfluency is invaluable for monitoring changes in the child's speech fluency and for contributing to the pool of observations (in addition to those discussed earlier and later) that are considered in making statements of diagnosis. Starkweather (1993) developed this concept and recommended that clinicians measure the duration of all disfluent speech behavior and the total speech time, and calculate the percentage of disfluency speech time. He argued that so much information is added when the duration of stuttering behaviors is measured and compared to the total speech time, which can be used to reliably measure an individual's level of fluency and the effectiveness of treatment.

The duration of disfluencies can be used to monitor changes in a child's speech fluency and to measure progression of the disorder of stuttering. It would seem likely, therefore, that differences in the duration of disfluencies (particularly within-word disfluencies) can be used to distinguish children who stutter from those who do not. Zebrowski (1995) cautioned, however, that, "empirical support for this notion has been inconsistent" (p. 83). In fact, recent studies contraindicate the predictive validity of using duration of within-word disfluencies to compare across children (Yairi & Ambrose, 2005). Zebrowski (1994) summarized that little difference was found in the duration of part-word repetitions or prolongations between young children who stutter and those who do not. She also stated that little relationship exists between stuttering duration and a child's age, length of time the child has stuttered, or overall frequency of speech disfluency. These findings, however, do not minimize the significant value of figuring the duration, frequency, and other more molecular measures of individual disfluency for monitoring changes in an individual child's speech fluency over time.

Rate of Speech

Another measure that I have found useful in monitoring an individual's speech fluency and related progress is rate of speech. As the child becomes more fluent or demonstrates fewer disfluencies, rate of speech tends to increase. The clinician can compute the rate of overall speech (both fluent and disfluent words), fluent speech only, or disfluent speech only. The differences found can be attributed to the impact of the disfluency, which should lessen throughout treatment. Rate of speech is calculated by dividing the number of words or syllables spoken (total, fluent, or disfluent) by the talk time in minutes. Again, I am assuming that the word is an adequate unit of measure for most clinical applications.

$$\text{Rate of speech} = \frac{\text{number of words spoken}}{\text{talk time (in minutes)}}.$$

When dividing, clinicians need to remember that the talk time (child's talk time only) must be in minutes in order for the result to be an average number of words spoken per minute. For example, if a child spoke the 300 words sampled earlier in 2 minutes and 15 seconds, the clinician must divide as follows:

$$\frac{300 \text{ words spoken}}{2.25 \text{ minutes}} = 133 \text{ words per minute}.$$

Remember that 15 seconds is one quarter of a minute (.25 minutes); 30 seconds is one half of a minute (.5 minutes). If the clinician has trouble converting the talk time into minutes, she can divide by the total number of seconds and then multiply by 60 in order to convert seconds to minutes, as follows:

$$\frac{300 \text{ words spoken}}{135 \text{ seconds}} = 2.22 \times 60 = 133 \text{ words per minute}.$$

Indeed, it was instructive for me to be able to report Robert's overall rate of speech increasing from 42 to 129 fluent and disfluent words per minute. Combined with the descriptions reviewed to this point, his increasing rate of speech supported the interpretation that his fluency had significantly improved. Individual methods for figuring rate of speech are in occasional disagreement across the published literature. Note that Williams et al. (1978) recommended the following for figuring rate of fluent speech:

> In counting words in speech samples, count only those words that would have been spoken had the speaker performed no disfluencies. That is, for example, "Uh, when I wuh-wuh-wuh-was 10 years old, I went—I went—I went to New York" is regarded for word-counting purposes as consisting of "When I was 10 years old, I went to New York," a total of 11 words. Count only once each word repeated singly or in a phrase. For example, count "We-we-we went home" as three words rather than five. Do not count sounds or words such as "well," "uh-uh-uh," and the like, which are not integral parts of the meaningful context. In any instance of revision, count only the words in the final form. For example, count "I started to—I went to town and bought some bread" as 8 rather than 11 words, disregarding the false start "I started to." (pp. 260–261)

Clinicians will find that even after reading a variety of standard procedures and selecting one to follow, the process is puzzling at times, and individual interpretations and decisions will need to be made. It would be nice if disfluencies were discrete entities. In other words, it would be easier if a word contained only a single instance of disfluency and if the boundaries of words were always clearly marked. In reality, of course, this generally does not happen. The message, therefore, is to be internally consistent (follow the same procedures each time) and account for what you have done and how you have done it. Then your clinical procedures will be both accountable and repeatable.

For purposes of comparison, it is helpful to know what rate of speech is considered to be average or "normal" for children who do not stutter. I have found three studies to be particularly useful for this purpose:

■ E. M. Kelly and Conture (1992) found that for boys aged 3 years 2 months to 4 years 10 months (mean, or average, age was 4 years 0 months), the average rate of speech was

153.6 words per minute (standard deviation, 18.3 words per minute), also computed as 177.6 syllables per minute (standard deviation, 18.4 syllables per minute). Kelly and Conture did not report data for girls.

⟘ Ryan (1992) found that for children aged 2 years 10 months to 5 years 9 months (mean age 4 years 5 months), boys' average rate of speech was 128.9 words per minute (standard deviation, 15.6 words per minute), or 164.1 syllables per minute (standard deviation, 20.5 syllables per minute). Girls' average rate of speech was 140.2 words per minute (standard deviation, 10.4 words per minute), or 176.3 syllables per minute (standard deviation, 20.6 syllables per minute).

⟘ Pindzola, Jenkins, and Lokken (1989) found that for children (boys and girls combined) who were 3 years old (3 years 0 months to 3 years 9 months), the average rate of speech was 140.3 syllables per minute (standard deviation, 14.2 syllables per minute; range, 116–163); for those 4 years old (4 years 0 months to 4 years 9 months), the average rate of speech was 152.7 syllables per minute (standard deviation, 17.9 syllables per minute; range, 117–183); and for those 5 years old (5 years 0 months to 5 years 9 months), the average rate of speech was 152.2 syllables per minute (standard deviation, 21.8 syllables per minute; range 109–183). Across 3-, 4-, and 5-year-old children, Pindzola et al. (1989) found that the average rate of speech was 148.4 syllables per minute (standard deviation, 18.0 syllables per minute; range 109–183). Their study did not report data for words per minute.

Secondary Characteristics

We also must quantify and qualify other speech and nonspeech factors (associated or secondary characteristics) that both impact and reflect speech fluency. The list of potential secondary characteristics is endless. They may include such nonspeech factors as facial tension, head turning, eye movement, grimacing, or body movement. Speech-related associated factors include audible inhalations or exhalations immediately before or after stuttering; rising pitch, indicating laryngeal tension; and visible oral and neck tension. Preschool children who do not stutter do not show such symptoms. However, such behaviors frequently develop early or within weeks or months of stuttering onset (Yairi & Ambrose, 2005). Typically, secondary behaviors may reflect or create the child's deepening awareness of stuttering, coping mechanisms during or after stuttering, or attempts to prevent stuttering. Associated speech and nonspeech behaviors are diagnostically significant for distinguishing between stuttering and nonstuttered behavior. Guitar (2006) noted that while children normally display "tense pauses," such behavior does not appear to be a reaction to the experience of disfluency. He advised, however, that if a child does show what appear to be normal disfluencies (such as single-word repetitions) yet consistently displays reactions such as pauses or interjections of *uh* immediately before or during the disfluencies, he should be evaluated carefully.

Severity Rating and Impact Assessment

Many school systems, clinics, and other facilities require an estimation of relative severity of stuttering. This can be interpreted by the clinician from the assessment components discussed earlier. However, the clinician must remember to keep in mind not only speech behaviors but also related attitudes, thoughts, and feelings. Recall the discussion in Chapter 5 about the woman who presented no perceptible disfluency but continued to interiorize negativity about herself as a disfluent and ineffective communicator. Many useful instruments and protocols are available as well. Haynes and Pindzola (2008) highlighted 12 instruments for assessing overt features of stuttering (p. 213) and 15 instruments for assessing covert features of stuttering (p. 218). They also emphasized the importance of information that is gained from the parents of young children who stutter.

One instrument commonly used for measuring severity of stuttering is the *Stuttering Severity Instrument–Fourth Edition* (SSI-4; Riley, 2009). It can be used with both children (i.e., preschool and school-age children) and adults, has provisions for those who can and cannot read, and measures frequency, duration, and physical concomitants of stuttering. From speech samples of between 150 and 500 syllables, the number of syllables stuttered and number of total syllables spoken are computed during reading and/or conversation. Frequency is expressed as a percentage of syllables stuttered (%SS; i.e., by dividing the number of syllables stuttered by the total number of syllables spoken and then multiplying by 100) and converted into a frequency score from 2 to 18. Duration of the three longest stuttering events is timed to $^1/_{10}$ of a second and then averaged; that average duration is converted into a duration score from 2 to 18. Four types of physical concomitants (distracting nonspeech sounds, facial grimaces, head movements, and movements of the extremities) are rated on a scale of degree of distractibility from 0 to 5 and then tallied to form a physical concomitant score from 0 to 20. The resulting total score, calculated by combining the frequency, duration, and physical concomitants scores, can range from 0 to 56. Total scores then are interpreted by using one of three normative tables (for preschool children, school-age children, or adults) that contain percentile ranks and severity equivalents (i.e., *very mild, mild, moderate, severe,* and *very severe*). Another normative table contains means and standard deviations for the three parameters (i.e., frequency, duration, and physical concomitants) and total score at each age level. Additionally, the SSI-4 recommends collection and analysis of speech samples from outside of the clinic and on the telephone, has a computerized scoring system for stuttering frequency and duration, includes a speech naturalness rating on the Examiner Record Form, and incorporates a scale for measuring self-reports by the person whose stuttering is being evaluated.

A relatively new instrument, unique for its evaluation of the experience of stuttering by and from the perspective of the person who stutters, is the *Overall Assessment of the Speaker's Experience of Stuttering* (OASES; Yaruss & Quesal, 2006, 2008). The OASES is consistent with the revised framework of the World Health Organization (2001), which addresses not only the diagnosis (i.e., the disorder) but also its impact on the individual. This framework is sensitive to both that which is observable and that which resides internally. The OASES consists of 100 items, each scored from 1 to 5, in four different sections: General Information contains 20 items related to the speaker's perceived fluency and speech naturalness, knowledge about stuttering and stuttering therapy, and overall perceptions about stuttering in general; Reactions contains 30 items exploring the speaker's affective, behavioral, and cognitive experiences; Communication in Daily Situations contains 25 items about the degree of difficulty (i.e., not the fluency) the speaker experiences when communicating in general situations, at work, in social situations, and at home; and Quality of Life contains 25 items about the degree to which stuttering interferes with the speaker's satisfaction regarding his ability to communicate, relationships, ability to participate in life, and overall sense of well-being. For each item, higher scores reflect a greater degree of negative impact related to stuttering. An impact score for each of the four sections is computed by adding the number of points in the respondent's answers, determining the number of questions completed and multiplying by 5 (i.e., at least half of the questions within each section must be completed; each item is based on a 5-point scale), and dividing the number of points in the respondent's scores by the number of possible points. Each value is then multiplied by 100. Similarly, a total impact score is computed on the basis of information gleaned from each of the four sections. Individual section scores and the total impact score, each ranging between 20 and 100, are then compared to a table in order to yield the appropriate degree of impact (*mild, mild to moderate, moderate, moderate to severe, severe*). The OASES is a relatively broad-based assessment of the speaker's experience of stuttering that also can be used for treatment planning and treatment outcomes research.

Adaptation and Consistency

As noted in Chapter 2, *adaptation* is the tendency for overall stuttering to decrease with repeated oral reading or speaking of the same material. *Consistency* is the tendency for stuttering to occur on the same sounds or words during repeated reading or speaking of the same material (Nicolosi et al., 2004). As a group, people who stutter have both effects, although some have neither. Zebrowski (1994) noted that children who demonstrate either or both effects may be performing similarly to other children whose behavior has been diagnosed as stuttering. Those who demonstrate neither effect may be unlike others who stutter as a group, be at risk for stuttering, or be normally disfluent. Because of this within-group variation and because both people who do stutter and those who do not (when considered as two different groups) show adaptation and consistency effects, Williams (1978) advised against routinely collecting adaptation and consistency scores in speech fluency assessments. Williams also cautioned against drawing conclusions about causal relationships between adaptation and consistency effects and fear of or anxiety about stuttering. Because of the possible usefulness of measuring these two types of effects for differential diagnosis of fluency disorders, however, I will outline them briefly.

Adaptation and consistency can be measured by having the child repeat a short passage or series of sentences five times (readers can read the material orally). Adaptation is calculated by subtracting the number of disfluencies in the fifth recitation from the number of disfluencies in the first, and then dividing this difference by the number of disfluencies in the first. Multiplying this quotient (i.e., the result of division) by 100 creates a percentage. Adaptation measurements of 50% or higher indicate the adaptation effect to be present. Scores greater than 50% indicate greater adaptation; scores lower than 50% indicate that the individual has not significantly reduced the frequency of disfluencies over five recitations (Williams et al., 1978; Zebrowski, 1994).

Consistency is measured by comparing the disfluencies produced in the first three recitations only. Three indices are computed: comparison of Recitations 1 and 2, 1 and 3, and 2 and 3. The indices for each comparison are computed by dividing the proportion of disfluent words in one recitation that also are produced in the second recitation by the number of disfluent words in the second reading. For example, computing the consistency index that compares Recitation 1 and 2, we would determine the percentage of disfluent words in Recitation 1 that also occurred in Recitation 2, then divide that percentage by the number of disfluent words in Recitation 2. The consistency effect is present if the individual exhibits an index of 1.0 or higher. Indices higher than 1.0 reflect greater consistency. Indices less than 1.0 reflect that the individual did not reveal consistency in the location of disfluencies within the recitation (Williams et al., 1978; Zebrowski, 1994).

More recently, Bloodstein and Bernstein Ratner (2008) noted on the basis of a review of the literature that the adaptation effect is seen on all types of disfluency, decreases with an increase in the time interval between successive readings, is temporary, demonstrates little transfer to readings of different material, is found in the stuttering of children and adults, and may be useful for predicting treatment outcome. However, not all people who stutter demonstrate adaptation (i.e., some do not demonstrate an adaptation effect and some show increased stuttering upon repeated oral readings). Further, less severe stuttering is associated with a greater tendency to adapt. Far fewer empirical investigations have addressed the consistency effect. Nevertheless, language-related factors seem to be significant in predicting the location of stuttering. Guitar (2006) indicated that most adults and school-age children tend to stutter more frequently on consonants, on sounds in word-initial positions, in contextual speech (i.e., more than in isolated words), on certain grammatical structures emphasizing content (nouns, verbs, adjectives, and adverbs) compared to those emphasizing function (articles, prepositions, pronouns, and conjunctions), on longer words, on words at the beginning of a sentence, and on stressed syllables. In contrast, preschool children tend to stutter more frequently on pronouns and conjunctions than on nouns, verbs, adjectives, and adverbs. Also, the stuttering of preschool children is more often reported to take the form of repetitions of parts of words and single-syllable words in sentence-initial positions than as repetitions, prolongations, or blocks of sounds in word-initial positions. Yet Yairi and Ambrose (2005) reported on preschool children whose stuttering began abruptly and with advanced symptoms such as sound prolongations and blocks, the persistence of which is thought to predict the persistence of stuttering. Guitar (2006) interpreted the language-based patterns predicting the consistency of stuttering among preschool children to mean that "in its incipient stage, stuttering is located at the beginning of syntactic units (sentences, clauses, and phrases), as if the task of linguistic planning and preparation was a key ingredient in the recipe for disfluency" (p. 24). Reporting similar language-based findings and in light of the consistency effect being observed among people who do not stutter, Bloodstein and Bernstein Ratner noted, "The outstanding difference in the loci of disfluency, however, is not between stutterers and nonstutterers. It is between children of preschool age and older children, whether stutterers or not" (p. 320).

Other Factors

Finally, there are other factors for the clinician to consider when analyzing the speech of preschool children (and that of people of all ages). We noted when reviewing protocols that we must consider variables such as the tempo, regularity, rate, relative tension, smoothness of transitions, and physical concomitants, in addition to feelings, thoughts, and attitudes (including avoidances, fears, and feelings of loss of control). There is just so much that can be predicted or described in a chapter such as this. Occasionally I find student clinicians who become flustered when they observe a characteristic that does not fit neatly into any of the categories noted to this point or when the complexity of an individual's speech seems to defy the methods of assessment discussed. I remember a time when one of my student clinicians and I observed a youngster who demonstrated a pattern of final-sound or syllable repetition ("Like-ike this. This-is is what I mean-ean."). The student clinician looked at me absolutely dumbfounded and sternly concluded, "This can't happen!" However, as she learned that day, anything can happen, albeit less frequently (Camarata, 1989; Defloor, Van Borsel, & Curfs, 2000; Humphrey & Van Borsel, 2001; Lebrun & Van Borsel, 1990; McAllister & Kingston, 2005; Mowrer, 1987; Stansfield, 1995; Van Borsel et al., 1996, 1998). In time and with the lessons learned from ample experience, the clinical situations that "can't happen" (those that cannot be predicted and those that we never have encountered previously) become the most challenging and instructive and, ultimately, the most inviting and rewarding.

Diagnosis

A necessary distinction needs to be made between assessment/evaluation and diagnosis (Haynes & Pindzola, 2008). The term *diagnosis* comes from the Greek word *diagignoskein*, meaning "to discern" or "to distinguish." *Dia-* means "to split apart," and *gignoskein* means "to perceive" or "to know." Therefore, diagnosis means to identify and distinguish by examination the nature of a problem from among many possibilities. If a disorder of speech fluency is present, the clinician must determine what type of disorder is operating from among the many possibilities. For example, it is possible that the child is stuttering, is at risk for stuttering, or is demonstrating normal speech disfluency. If the child is stuttering or at risk for stuttering, then the clinician also must determine if treatment is warranted and recommended and, if so, what should be the nature and focus of that treatment.

Distinguishing between various possibilities requires familiarity with the person, including how he responds, what he thinks, what he knows. The process of arriving at a diagnosis such as stuttering takes thorough assessment and evaluation, including all of the procedures discussed to this point. Furthermore, the diagnosis is not ironclad; the results of formal and informal assessment that contribute to a statement of diagnosis are, of necessity, somewhat tentative. While we use the best of our professional abilities to make necessary observations and interpretations, we must remain open to the lessons of those things that "can't happen," as well as those aspects of human behavior that only reveal themselves later. Therefore, diagnoses must be robust yet resilient and responsive to new information.

By implication, diagnoses and the foundation of information on which they stand must be both reliable and valid. *Validity* reflects the truth, or how closely an assessment actually measures what it is intended to measure. *Reliability* means that an event is reproducible. Valid assessment procedures and the diagnoses they yield will prove to be reliable. The reverse is not necessarily the case, however. Procedures that are reliable are not necessarily valid. For example, at one time it was believed by many that the Earth was the center of the universe. This was a reliable belief. However, Copernicus later proved that such a view did not reflect the truth (was not valid). In fact, he showed that the Earth rotates on its axis and, with the other planets in the solar system, revolves around the sun (the principle of heliocentric planetary motion). Just because people agree does not mean that they are right (Shapiro, 1987). As noted in Chapter 2, these concepts are essential to how we approach evidence-based practice.

Clinicians must follow their clinical wisdom based on professional training and experience. Too often, when results of standardized instruments challenge informed professional judgment of knowledgeable clinicians, I see the clinician defer to test results. Clinicians sometimes assume that external sources of information, by virtue of having been published, have greater insight than that gleaned from their own professional preparation and the most valid diagnostic instruments available—their trained eyes and ears. There will always be a place for professional judgment that occasionally defies training and logic. This part of being a professional is what is uniquely human and may be where the head and the heart meet. We need to be respectful of professional knowledge and experience and that which is sensitive, good, and empathic, and holds a positive belief in the human potential for learning and change. More will be said about this in Chapters 11 and 12, which address clinician competencies, professional preparation, and lifelong learning. Suffice it now to say that very little "can't happen." Remain open and positive, and let's have confidence in our clients, their families, and ourselves.

Prognosis and Recommendations

In addition to determining a diagnosis, clinicians are responsible for making a statement of prognosis. A prognosis is a prediction of the outcome of a proposed course of treatment for a given client, including how effective treatment will be, how far he can be expected to progress, and how long it will take. Haynes and Pindzola (2008) noted that such predictions have immediate and long-range facets, the purposes of which are to economize therapeutic efforts (focusing on those clients who hold greatest promise for improvement) and to provide families with needed direction. A more positive prognosis with preschool children, *based on retrospective and cross-sectional investigations*, requires that the intervention take place before the child develops fear and avoidance reactions (before the child internalizes that something is going wrong or that he is losing control over his speech mechanism) and that the parents and others within the child's communication system actively support and participate in the treatment. Haynes and Pindzola (2008) noted several other factors and related questions that the clinician must consider when estimating the child's prognosis for improvement:

- How long has the child been stuttering? Children who are younger, specifically those whose stuttering is of more recent onset and who have experienced relatively little exposure to adverse environmental reactions, typically have a more favorable treatment prognosis.

- What is the nature of environmental reactions to which the child has been exposed? Children who experience a more positive environmental reaction tend to have a better prognosis. Those who experience penalty and internalize the negative reaction (such as being slapped, insulted, or humiliated) have a less favorable prognosis.

- Is the child aware of speaking difficulty? Reduced awareness and a positive outlook toward communication are associated with a more favorable prognosis. Increased frustration leading to internalization of concern results in a less favorable prognosis.

- What type of disfluency is the child demonstrating? Fewer and less involved overt and covert symptoms are associated with a more positive prognosis. When danger signs are frequent and complex (such as exhibiting cessation of phonation, stoppage of airflow, dysrhythmia, tension, fear, or frustration—see Table 8.1 and Figures 8.2 and 8.3), the prognosis tends to be less favorable.

- How willing and able are the parents to become actively involved? Effective intervention requires active participation of all members within the family system; family participation is associated with a more favorable prognosis.

- What is the child's overall level of cognitive or intellectual potential? Those with reduced cognitive or intellectual potential tend to have a less favorable prognosis.

- Are there any neurogenic or psychogenic factors relating to the onset of stuttering? The presence of either factor tends to relate to a less favorable prognosis.

As noted in Chapter 2, Yairi (2004) and Yairi and Ambrose (2005) summarized other factors, *based on longitudinal investigations*, that help to distinguish children whose stuttering will be transient from children whose stuttering will be persistent. Those factors were categorized as primary, secondary, or other.

Primary Factors

- What is the family's history of stuttering? When a child has close family relatives whose stuttering persists, the child's stuttering will be more likely to persist. When a child has close family relatives whose stuttering recovered, the child's stuttering will be more likely to recover.

- What is the child's gender and history of stuttering? Boys are at greater risk for both incidence and persistence of stuttering than girls; girls recover after a shorter history of stuttering than boys. A 1-year history of stuttering without improvement indicates a greater risk for a girl's stuttering to be persistent than for a boy's.

- At what age did the child's stuttering begin? Persistence tends to be associated with later age of onset (i.e., children whose stuttering persists begin to stutter 3.5 months later than children whose stuttering recovers). Children whose stuttering onset is later tend to be at greater risk for persistence; children whose stuttering onset is earlier tend to be at less risk for persistence.

- What is the relative stability of the child's stuttering-like disfluencies? A reduction in number of stuttering-like disfluencies (i.e., part-word repetitions, single-syllable word repetitions, and disrhythmic phonation) within the first year of onset is a positive prognostic indicator for natural recovery; a more stable or increasing number of stuttering-like disfluencies during the first year of onset is a prognostic indicator for persistence.

⟶ What is the duration of the stuttering history? Natural recovery tends to occur within the first 3 years of onset. Stuttering that persists beyond the first year is viewed as a higher risk for persistence, particularly for girls.

⟶ What is the length (i.e., from molecular analysis) of the individual disfluencies? While severity of stuttering in its earliest stage is not viewed as a predictor of persistence or recovery (challenging traditional claims that longer blocks and prolongations indicate persistence), continuing disfluencies, particularly with more than three units of repetition, indicate greater risk for persistence. Increases in the duration of silent intervals between repeated units or repetitions that are slower in tempo indicate greater likelihood of recovery.

⟶ What is the duration and pattern of sound prolongations and blocks? Except during the first few months of stuttering, sound prolongations and blocks tend to predict persistence of stuttering. Reduction in the percentage of sound prolongations in the total disfluency (even if the child still stutters) tends to predict recovery; increase in the percentage of sound prolongations tends to predict persistence.

Secondary Factors

⟶ What is the severity of the child's stuttering and how long has it continued since onset? As noted, stuttering severity near the time of onset is not viewed as a predictor of persistence or recovery (children whose stuttering recovered demonstrated stuttering as severe or more severe than children whose stuttering persisted). Severe stuttering that continues for more than the first few months after onset indicates a greater risk of persistence.

⟶ What head and neck movements are associated with the child's stuttering, and how long have they continued? As with the initial severity of stuttering, the number and degree of head and neck movements near the time of stuttering onset do not distinguish between persistence and recovery. Within the first 12 months of onset, however, reduction in head and neck movements is predictive of recovery; failure to show reduction in head and neck movements is predictive of persistence. More generally, a substantial decrease in the number and severity of secondary characteristics within the first 12 months of onset is predictive of recovery; failure to show reduction in number and severity of secondary characteristics is predictive of persistence.

⟶ What are the phonological skills of the child who is stuttering? Lower phonological skills during the first year of stuttering tend to predict persistence (i.e., stuttering may emerge in children who have poor phonological skills). That predictability tends to disappear during the second year of stuttering. Yairi and Ambrose (2005) cautioned that phonological skill alone is insufficient to predict stuttering outcome and may be more predictive in combination with other factors (see Byrd, Wolk, & Davis, 2007; Nippold, 2002).

⟶ What are the expressive language skills of the child who is stuttering? Language skills alone cannot be used to distinguish between children whose stuttering will recover and those whose stuttering will persist. Yairi and Ambrose (2005) indicated, "Contrary to previous thinking, very young children who stutter tend to demonstrate expressive language skills at or above the average range" (p. 353). They suggested that stuttering may emerge in conjunction with language skills that are beyond developmental expectations, that persistence ("only in a few cases," p. 353) may be predicted by atypical patterns of language development, and that delayed language, in addition to other developmental asynchronies, may inform if not contribute to the nature of early stuttering (see also N. E. Hall, Wagovich, & Bernstein Ratner, 2007).

Other Factors

⟶ Are there any concomitant disorders? Concomitant disorders (e.g., physical, emotional, learning, speech–language, behavioral, cognitive, psychological, attentional, medical) tend to contribute to persistence of stuttering or may interfere with the recovery process.

⬚ Does the child demonstrate awareness of or emotional reaction to the stuttering experience? Yairi and Ambrose (2005) reported that there is no evidence that the child's awareness of stuttering or emotional reaction to it shortly after onset is a predictor of persistence. They indicated, however, that emotional reactions of the child or parents could have secondary effects and interfere with recovery. Such reactions should be addressed and serve as a factor in recommending intervention.

All of the information leading to the diagnosis and prognosis is integrated to form recommendations, which are discussed with the family in the post-assessment parent interview.

Post-Assessment Parent Interview

Both the initial and final parent interviews are intended to be conversational and "give and take" in nature. Nevertheless, I have found that the initial conference typically is more heavily one of collecting information from the parents, while the latter is directed toward providing information to the parents. First, we remind the parents of the purposes for the post-assessment meeting: to summarize the results of the assessment, provide recommendations, and discuss any questions that remain. In doing so, I am certain to restate and address the objectives and purposes expressed by the parents in response to my earliest questions ("Why did you meet with us today?" "What do you hope to accomplish as a result of our meeting?"). Parents frequently show both surprise and pleasure that I remembered what they said and that their objectives and purposes were and are important to me. I invite the parents to interrupt me at any time with questions for clarification or expansion.

In presenting the assessment results, I deliberately begin by providing a summary of the positive aspects of communication that were demonstrated by the child and between the child and the parents. Doing so serves at least two distinct functions. First, being sincerely positive up front establishes, if not reinforces, a positive context within which to approach the communication problem being experienced by the child and the family. Too often, professionals get right to business and describe the characteristics of the child's observed stuttering. I am not suggesting that I hold the parents in suspense, but I do feel it is critical to create by example a positive context within which to proceed with the family. The effect of our model is strong. Families tend to adopt the attitude they perceive from us. Families who seek our help often are vulnerable, if not desperate, and therefore are impressionable. I have observed that when clinicians present "gloom and doom," the family becomes negative and pessimistic. If the family is presented an accurate and realistic picture using positive terminology, particularly for serious conditions, they tend to be more positive, optimistic, and motivated to accept and participate actively within the recommendations.

There is a second reason to provide a summary of the positive aspects of communication that were demonstrated by the child and between the child and parents. After I observe the parent–child interaction, I am often aware of characteristics I wish to target for change. To prevent being misinterpreted as criticizing the parents or preaching to them about how to parent, I present a summary of what I have observed that they are doing in conversation that, in my opinion, is conducive to supportive language-based interaction and fluency facilitation. Within this positive context, parents are far more receptive to my constructive suggestions for change (incidentally, I am more comfortable in providing them as well). Some may say that I am consuming valuable clinical time, "sugarcoating the truth," or even worse, "beating around the bush." I disagree. I believe that all of us are inclined to do more of what we feel we are doing right, are more receptive to recommendations for constructive change within a positive context, and are more motivated to participate actively within a shared support system. This message conveys to the family members that the clinician shares their concern and is willing to participate in achieving a solution. It conveys that the burden is shared and that the family is not alone. It enables the family to feel empowered to approach, negotiate, and participate within the intervention planning and treatment processes.

Then, we summarize in understandable terms the nature of the child's fluency and disfluency (i.e., stuttering, if evident) and estimate the relative degree of communicative involvement. I have found it helpful for parents if we first review briefly the characteristics of normal speech fluency and disfluency and provide them adequate examples to hear. Guitar (2006) nicely summarized these characteristics:

> All of the following characteristics must be met for a child to be considered normally disfluent. The child has fewer than 10 disfluencies per 100 words; the disfluencies consist mostly of multisyllable word and phrase repetitions, revisions, and interjections. When disfluencies are repetitions, they will have two or fewer repeated units per repetition that are slow and regular in tempo. The ratio of stuttering-like disfluencies to total disfluencies will be less than 50%. All disfluencies will be relatively relaxed, and the child will seem to be hardly aware of them and certainly will not be upset when he is aware. (p. 239)

Even with guidelines as clearly stated as these, clinicians often find it difficult to distinguish between normal disfluency and borderline stuttering. On the surface, any deviation from the description above may be considered evidence of borderline stuttering. Nevertheless, it is challenging indeed to distinguish between a deviation that is attributable to borderline stuttering and that related to variation within each child. It is essential, therefore, for parents to understand the nature of normal disfluency, stuttering and its most common patterns of development, and suggestions for environmental intervention aimed at facilitating the development of the child's speech fluency. Furthermore, based on what is known about the symptom intermittency and variation in the earliest stages of stuttering (Van Riper, 1982; Yairi, 1997, 2004; Yairi & Ambrose, 2005), this meeting with the parents will be the first of several contacts to monitor the child's speech development. I explain to the parents that it is not uncommon for them to experience emotional swings in relation to their child's speech fluency. Just as they might feel, "My gosh, this really is a problem" (when their child's disfluency becomes noticeable and of concern), it might disappear. Likewise, just as they might feel, "Thank goodness, this terrible problem is gone" (when the noticeable disfluency has vanished), it might reappear. I encourage parents to listen to other young children engaged in talking to help them hear the range of variation in normal disfluency. The same advice is useful for clinicians.

Once we discuss with parents the nature of normal disfluency, we discuss the nature and development of the child's disfluency using visual representations (Table 8.1, Figures 8.2 and 8.3) and examples for them to hear. We invite and address their questions. One of the most common questions is, "What causes stuttering?" With this question, parents are often implicitly asking, "Did I cause it?" or expressing a silent request: "Tell me I didn't do it. Tell me that even though my child is having trouble talking that still I am a good parent." I take (or create) an opportunity to address, and absolve if possible, the parents' feelings of guilt for real and imagined past sins. I explain that stuttering is often the consequence of an unspecified chain of events, some of which are out of anyone's control. It is thus unlikely that the parents or anyone else specifically caused the stuttering to occur. I explain in brief the nature of child development, communication development, and specifically speech fluency development. In simple terms, we discuss the notion of predisposing factors that are not within anyone's control, precipitating factors that may be within our control, and perpetuating factors that indeed are within our control. I discuss the concepts of constitutional factors and both developmental and environmental demands that may exceed some children's capacity to remain fluent under certain circumstances. I try to emphasize that we have no control over events that are past, but that there is much we can do together to facilitate the ongoing development of the child's speech fluency and other aspects of communication. We must provide suggestions in such a way that parents feel that the future is within their grasp. Presenting a picture of a child's problem can be disabling unless strategies for improvement in which the parents and families can participate are presented and demonstrated. A discussion of these follows.

A critical part of this meeting with the parents is to present concrete suggestions for parent and family involvement to facilitate the development of the child's speech fluency. I believe these suggestions are essential, not only for parents whose children appear to be demonstrating borderline or more noticeable stuttering but for those demonstrating normal disfluency as well. Some may ask why I offer concrete suggestions for parents whose children are demonstrating normal disfluency. My response is based on the premise that such knowledge in the hands of parents can only heighten their child's communication development. While specifically aimed at facilitation of speech fluency, the suggestions are conducive to appropriate models of interpersonal communication. Furthermore, we cannot be absolutely sure that the child's speech fluency in the assessment session was representative of that outside (notwithstanding our attempts to sample the child's fluency over time from the preassessment video or audio recording and parent interview, which are compared to results collected in the assessment session). In other words, an ounce of prevention is worth a pound of cure.

In a sense, as speech–language pathologists, we are the parents' teacher. While presenting suggestions, remember that good teachers do at least three things. They tell (discuss), they show (demonstrate), and then they coach, critique, and supervise (direct). Too often we tell the parents what we expect of them, without showing them what we mean or observing them do what we intend to ensure that they understand. Therefore, I always recommend the three Ds (discuss, demonstrate, and direct). Following presentation and discussion of the suggestions, I model as many as possible with the child (who is not otherwise present during this conference), and then coach the parents as they apply the suggestions they have just heard and observed. After discussion, demonstration, and direction, I recommend several alternative readings and DVDs that are available from the Stuttering Foundation of America (see the Appendix for contact information). These help parents better understand communication development and its disorders, including stuttering, and what they can do to help their child. The readings and DVDs review and expand the suggestions already presented to them. Often the parents' concerns interfere somewhat with how much they can process and remember. The materials reinforce what they have learned, seen, and applied during the assessment session. The readings I recommend include *If Your Child Stutters: A Guide for Parents* (Ainsworth & Fraser, 2008) and *Stuttering and Your Child: Questions and Answers* (Conture & Fraser, 2007). A very useful DVD is *Stuttering and Your Child: Help for Parents* (Guitar & Guitar, 2008). Another reading, this one from the National Stuttering Association (see the Appendix), is *Young Children Who Stutter (Ages 2–6): Information and Support for Parents (Five Steps to Help You Help Your Child)* (Yaruss & Reardon-Reeves, 2006). Occasionally, I recommend a story I wrote ("Just the Way You Are"; Shapiro, 2004e; see Figure 8.4) that addresses what I wish adults had told me when I was a young child who stutters. Although written for young children, the story is useful to facilitate conversation and reactions with parents of children who stutter.

At the conclusion of the meeting with the parents, we talk about the treatment process as appropriate to the individual child and schedule a follow-up meeting. I tell them to expect a summary report within 1 week. About 2 weeks after our meeting, I make

Just the Way You Are
By David Shapiro

Hi. My name is David Shapiro and my favorite baseball team is the New York Yankees. I like them a lot because I used to live in New York and my grandpa took me to see the Yankees. I'll tell you more about my grandpa later. What's your favorite baseball team?

I am happy to share a few thoughts with you and I hope you will share your thoughts with me; that way we can become new friends. I want to tell you a few things I wish adults had told me when I was younger; those things might have helped me when I stuttered so badly. I still stutter, but only sometimes.

There is nothing we cannot accomplish together*. Living with and learning to control stuttering can be very challenging; you know that. I wish adults had told me that we would learn to control my stuttering together. Sometimes, adults felt sorry for me. Sometimes they spoke for me. A few clinicians even gave up on me; they didn't think I could control my stuttering. They were wrong. Sometimes adults can be wrong. I have learned that even the heaviest load (and stuttering can be a heavy load) seems lighter when it is shared. The load is best managed when working with clinicians and parents or guardians who understand stuttering and who are willing to work together. In the western part of the USA, there are big, very tall trees called Sequoias. Because the trees are so tall, people think their roots are very deep. Actually, they are not. The trees stand strong and tall because they grow near each other and their roots overlap and grow together. Separately, the trees would fall; together they are strong. People facing big challenges such as stuttering are like that too; together we are stronger. We can accomplish anything together. Do you have people who help you with your challenges?

Everybody needs one good friend*. I wish adults had told me that one good friend can make the whole world seem like a better place. I bet they didn't tell me because they figured I already knew. I kind of did, but I didn't realize why I was so happy when I was around my friends. I was lucky. I had three best friends. Billy was my friend in school. He never laughed at me when I stuttered and he always picked me to play on his baseball team. My grandpa was my friend too. He took long walks with me and we listened to the stream together. Once when I stuttered really badly, he told me, "I love you just the way you are." My very best friend was Buddy, a big dog with black, white, and brown hair all over his body and a wet nose. I was with Buddy more than anyone else. Nearly every day, we explored the woods and lakes near my house together. Sometimes when my stuttering was really bad and people said things that hurt my feelings, I found a sunny place in the woods to fall asleep. It always made me feel happy to wake up to find Buddy by my side and sunshine in my face. Isn't it funny that a dog can be a very best friend? All of my best friends passed away during my 17th year. That was a sad time for me. But today, I feel happy when I think of Billy, my grandpa, and Buddy. And I am really happy because I have three more best friends—my wife, Kay, my daughter, Sarah, and my son, Aaron. Do you have a best friend?

People who stutter can accomplish great things*. I wish adults had told me that I could accomplish anything I set my mind to, even though I stutter. In fact, now I know that

Figure 8.4. "Just the Way You Are." *Note.* From "Just the Way You Are," by D. A. Shapiro, 2004e, 7th International Stuttering Awareness Day Online Conference: International Year of the Child Who Stutters (J. Kuster, Conference Chair, Minnesota State University, Mankato), available at http://www.mnsu.edu/comdis/isad7/papers/bridgebuilders7/shapiro7.html. Reprinted with permission.

everybody has something to improve. Some people have trouble reading; some have trouble writing; some have trouble talking. Some are not good at sports; some have to learn how to be a friend; some forget their manners. But even though we stutter, we have many interests and talents. Stuttering doesn't interfere with playing baseball, running the 50-meter race, collecting coins and stamps, riding a bike, or being or having a friend. In fact, people who stutter have become president of the USA (George Washington, Theodore Roosevelt), prime minister (Winston Churchill), a prophet (Moses), an actor (James Earl Jones), and even a Yankees pitcher (Tommy John). All people have talents and face challenges; stuttering is just one of those challenges we face together. Knowing that others face the challenge of stuttering and have achieved great things makes me feel I can too. What are your talents? What do you want to become?

Figure 8.4.   *(continued)*

a point of phoning the parents to ask if they have any questions about the evaluation experience, the summary report, or the readings or DVD. I also discuss with them how well the suggestions are being applied and any observable changes in the child's communication behavior. Beyond the information part of this phone call, I am conveying by my actions that I care about the family as individuals and as a communication system. The family also sees that they are not alone and that help and understanding are readily available. The door is always open. By our behavior, we model open, supportive, and positive dialogue directed at facilitating the fluency of the individual child and the interpersonal interaction among the family members.

Treatment

In this section, we turn our attention to considerations of treatment, focusing first on parent intervention and then on direct intervention with the preschool child.

Parent Intervention

The parent intervention process addresses three major foci. The first two are the parents' thoughts (i.e., knowledge) and feelings (i.e., emotionally based reactions) about stuttering, their child who stutters, and themselves as parents. The third focus is the parents' behaviors when they interact with their child when he is stuttering and when he is not. The overall objective is to engage the parents in an educational experience so they understand what they already are doing that contributes to the development of their child's speech fluency and other aspects of communication, as well as what needs to be changed. We noted earlier that parents need to be informed and to feel and experience some sense of control. There are few things more worrisome to parents than when their child has a problem that they do not understand and about which they feel helpless. The clinician must respond both to the child's and the family's communication and emotional needs. It has been my experience that the parents' behaviors are more readily changed than either their thoughts or feelings. However, the behaviors they demonstrate often reflect their thoughts and feelings. Furthermore, heightening their awareness of their own behaviors and providing opportunities for behavior change often impact their current thoughts and feelings about stuttering, their child who stutters, and themselves as parents. For these reasons and for instructional purposes in this chapter, the parents' behaviors, thoughts, and feelings will be addressed separately. In reality, however, these three foci often are addressed simultaneously.

Behaviors

A number of behavioral recommendations that deliberately overlap with one another and with the domains of thoughts and feelings will be discussed first.

React to and interact with the child without drawing unnecessary attention to the disfluency. By not drawing attention to the disfluency and by preventing the child from reacting with frustration to the speaking experience, the disfluency will be indirectly controlled, will lessen, and optimally will disappear. Parents know that children often mirror their emotions and facial expressions. As hard as it may seem for the concerned parent, the message here is to respond positively to the content of the child's speech (i.e., what he says) without evidencing any concern or negative reaction to his relative fluency (i.e., how he conveys his message). This does not mean that parents need to withdraw emotionally from their child or that they would no longer feel concerned about their child's fluency. Rather, it is important for them to convey a positive attitude toward their child's communicative efforts. This in itself may help their child's fluency.

Be good listeners. I first highlight the parents' behaviors that are supportive of the child's developing communication skills, and thereby those that I wish to target for continuation. For example, we may highlight verbal and nonverbal ways that the parents have offered their support to the child, their appropriately even rate of speech, or their turn-taking skills with the child, among others. If the parents are reacting inappropriately to the child and his stuttering (e.g., interrupting the child, filling in the word before the child fully utters it, telling the child, "Don't stutter. Think about what you say first"), I discuss the counterproductive influence that such behaviors can have on the child's speech fluency. However, by identifying their behaviors that are facilitative as well as inhibiting to speech fluency, I suggest with specific examples that they replace the latter with more of the former. Clinicians need to be aware that parents need our support to confront their feelings of guilt for having made, albeit unintentionally, a parental error. We make the point that children are not fragile. In fact, in most cases children are more resilient than parents. Nevertheless, it is never too late to correct mistakes and to do even more of the things they naturally are doing right. Helping the parents know the difference indeed is within the clinician's domain.

Simplify, soften, and slow the daily speech model to which the child is exposed. Often this is a difficult concept for parents to grasp. First, slowing one's own speech model, while still sounding natural, is difficult to do. This is an example of where the three *D*s (discuss, demonstrate, direct) are critical. Parents need to know how to provide the child a slow (i.e., evenly paced with reduced rate), gentle speech model, just as clinicians need to know how to provide this model for parents. It takes not only slightly prolonging vowels but also softening articulatory contacts on consonants in addition to maintaining normal inflection, juncture, and prosody. Remember, the point is not to draw attention to the speech. Just prolonging vowels often results in a drone that more resembles robotic speech than human speech. To say the least, an inappropriate model such as this calls attention to itself.

Second, parents often feel frustrated when they believe they are expected to alter their speech all of the time, lest they hurt their child's speech fluency. Let them know you understand that there are times when speech cannot be slow, even, and gentle (e.g., when the school bus has arrived and will leave if the child doesn't move in a hurry, when the child will be harmed if he doesn't stop his behavior now, when Mom or Dad must leave for work now in order not to be late, and other instances). Because there are times when speech cannot be altered or controlled, it is helpful for the parents to set aside on a daily basis a special, uninterrupted time for talking with the child. This means that phones will go unanswered, text messages will not be received or sent, and faxes will be ignored; just quality, uninterrupted time. When events prohibit even, gentler talking, both the parent and the child deal better with the momentary urgency by looking forward to talking together later without interruption. Often I am asked, "How long should this time be?" I respond that both the quantity and the quality of time should be considered, and that the time should be as long as possible. I recommend no less than 30 to 60 minutes. It becomes instructive to see how much or little of parents' time is available to their children (as a parent, I recognize this challenge). Another frequent question is, "If we set time aside for one child, do we need to do it for all the others?" I believe it doesn't hurt. The point, however, is that the parent should be available without distraction whenever and for as long as possible. "Should we read to the child?" That is a fine activity, as long as the model of speech is appropriately slow, even, and gentle. At least as important is the dialogue about the book that should follow the reading itself, during which each takes turns speaking and the child feels he has the parent's full attention. It is important for the parent to dialogue with and listen to the child about whatever is currently on the child's mind. I have found that once there is a mechanism in place for focused, even, and gentle dialogue, most parents find ways to continue this style of interaction throughout many other daily activities in which the two may participate (such as cooking, cleaning up the dishes, making household repairs, or working on the car).

Be aware of the potentially negative effects of other forms of stimulus bombardment (visual, auditory, emotional) to the extent possible within the communicative environment. Another aspect that is sometimes difficult for parents to grasp is the degree to which the child's communication environment might be overloaded. In many homes, modern technology has provided us with cell phones, beepers, e-mail, fax machines, and so forth, which have only magnified the potential for distraction. Multisensory bombardment continues to be provided by more traditional forms of entertainment (e.g., televisions, radios, iPods, and DVD and MP3 players) and time-savers (dish and clothes washers, dryers, and microwave ovens). Some may think that I am bashing technology. I am not. I am saying that we as parents (and clinicians) need to be aware of the degree to which stimulus overload may interfere with communication and place extra demands on the child.

The presence of such stimuli can also inhibit meaningful interaction among family members. I am reminded of two relevant events. I saw a Bart Simpson cartoon with a family sitting around the television with a caption stating "Family Bonding." The irony is humorous but also of concern, particularly for children who are developing speech fluency and other aspects of communication. I was reminded of this cartoon when, during a recent camping trip, I noticed a number of other tent campers sitting under the canopy of stars, yet watching television with their children.

Give the child as much fluent talking experience as possible. We want to prevent the disfluent speech from gaining a foothold within the child's experience. Therefore, we try to manipulate the child's communicative opportunities to increase both the absolute and relative frequency of fluency experiences. This can be done in a number of ways. First, when the child is fluent, let him speak. As a speech–language pathologist, I know that children learn language and establish patterns of fluent speech by both using and hearing language. Nevertheless, being a parent of children who once were preschool age,

I know what it is like when a child seems to speak during every waking moment, apparently without taking a breath. Truly appreciating how silence can be golden, I reminded myself of how important it was for my child to both hear and use meaningful and fluent speech and language within a supportive, inviting, and reflective environment. This advice rarely presents a problem to parents. When a child is fluent, the parent has no problem knowing what to do—let the child speak. When the child is disfluent, however, many parents do not know what to do in order to help their child.

There is much parents can do to help their preschool child when he experiences noticeable disfluency. Again, the aim is to encourage the experience of speech fluency and to prevent the child from becoming unnecessarily aware of or disturbed about his disfluency. When the child is noticeably disfluent, the parents should try to take their speaking turn a little sooner than they ordinarily do. I am often asked by parents with some alarm, "Do you mean, interrupt my child?" This is another concept that is difficult to grasp. I explain that while few people realize it, we all tend to interrupt each other during conversation. When I am talking with parents, I point out to them how we tend to take our turns just before our conversational partner is finished with his or her turn. This often comes as a surprise; most people assume that we wait until our partner is finished before we begin to speak. I encourage the parents to become familiar with the conversational patterns between them and their children. Once they realize that they naturally interrupt each other, they are more receptive to the idea of interrupting a little sooner. Doing so takes the speaking burden off the child momentarily, thus enabling him to hear the slower, more even, gentler speech model from the parents. This relief, combined with an appropriate speech model, is often successful in enabling the child to regain a fluent speech pattern. Sometimes it takes several attempts to achieve the desired result.

Another common question is, "What do I do if the child continues to be disfluent after I take my turn sooner and model speech fluency?" The next two suggestions are even harder to grasp. We noted earlier that our communicative world is filled with distractions. This is one case for which I recommend a deliberate distraction. For example, the parent may "need" to remove the food from the oven, respond to the microwave beep, or move the clothes from the washer to the dryer. In this case, the distraction is brief, and the conversation continues after having been interrupted briefly. In the interim, the parent models slow, gentle, natural-sounding speech. "What if this doesn't work and the child continues to be disfluent?" Then I recommend that the parent move from distraction to a change of topic or activity. The benefit for the child (keeping the focus on fluency) outweighs the cost (interrupting the conversation). However, I stress the importance of returning to the original topic of conversation after the distraction or the shift in topic or activity. In that way, the child is reassured of the parents' interest and attention. The purpose here is to enable the child to focus on something other than talking so that he can regain his fluent speech, after which the parent re-expresses interest and the conversation continues. These patterns—distractions, topic or activity shifts—occur naturally. Thus, we gain control over a naturally occurring event and use it to the advantage of the child.

Prevent the child from becoming unnecessarily aware of or frustrated over his stuttering. Several of the recommendations already mentioned aim to prevent the child from becoming increasingly frustrated over his stuttering. The importance of responding honestly with support and compassion to the child, however, must be emphasized as well. If a child mentions his speech or disfluency, the parents (and clinicians) should not hesitate to verbalize their understanding that we all get stuck at times and to explain briefly and show (by modeling) that speaking a bit more slowly, evenly, and gently (yet naturally) helps. Parents and preschool teachers should reflect on the child's feelings while relating to the content of what the child is saying. For example, if the child runs in from the playground and is out of breath and disfluent, the listener may model more appropriate speech by saying, "Boy, I can see how excited you are. I want to hear all that you have to tell me."

Reduce the pace of activities and overall tension as much as possible. Evenly paced (with slightly reduced rate), relaxed activities are important. A slow, gentle, and natural-sounding speech model should be the rule. Again, this is a difficult concept to grasp. Many of us do not realize how tied we are to our racing internal clocks until we attempt to reduce the overall pace of our speech and general level of activity. I noted earlier that role playing helps. Through puppetry, the adult and the child might impersonate a turtle who moves and talks evenly and gently, compared to a rabbit who moves and talks fast and hard. I emphasize the importance of directing praise toward the child for what he is doing correctly (while demonstrating even and gentle speech). When the child's speech behavior is in need of correction, I prefer to create an opportunity within play for the adult to take on the child's disfluent pattern so that she (the adult) can deliberately correct herself or provide an opportunity for the child to correct the adult's speech. The child then receives praise for correcting the adult's speech, initially by evaluating the error (such as, "Too fast. You did that wrong"), then by directing the correction ("Slow down"), and eventually by demonstrating or modeling the correct form ("You have to say it lllike thhhis"). In this way, the child continually receives support for what he does right (slower, evenly paced, gentle speech; correcting the adult, and so forth) while the adult bears the weight of having been corrected, thus conveying to the child indirectly the error behavior, which is corrected into the target form. I believe this is an important message for working with children, particularly preschool children. We need to create opportunities for children to receive praise for, and thereby to become aware of, all that they are doing right. Children (and the rest of us) naturally become motivated to do more of what they believe they do well. Within play, we create such opportunities for children to succeed and for them to differentiate between the target behavior (slower, evenly paced, and gentle speech for which they receive praise) and the error (fast and hard speech for which the parent or clinician receives correction).

Other activities that emphasize slower, evenly paced, and gentle speech include "Simon Says." The parent and child can alternate between being the leader (Simon) and the follower, giving and receiving orders for various activities, including speaking slowly and gently or fast and hard. To help parents establish more evenly paced, gentle, and natural-sounding speech, it may be helpful to watch and discuss the speech model presented on *Mister Rogers' Neighborhood*, a morning program still on many public television stations (Bianco, 2003). Also, it is helpful for parents (and clinicians) to study their own speech patterns and those of people around them. Parents gain an appreciation for the variety in speaking styles, some of which encourage, while others discourage, speech fluency. Frequently I have observed in developmental day-care and other preschool settings the teacher heightening the children's body awareness through group singing of "Head, Shoulders, Knees and Toes." The pace of this familiar song increases until the children are neurophysiologically unable to coordinate the fine speech–motor movements required of the song and the gross-motor movements of touching corresponding body parts. At this point, some children fall to the ground sharing laughter with the teacher. I remember being concerned about a 3-year-old child who was beginning to stutter and who was participating in such activities. The activity was beyond the limits of this child's coordination and, I found, was exacerbating the child's disfluency. After I talked with Caroline, the day-care teacher, she replaced the activity with one that was more facilitative of children's motor and speech coordination. Caroline's speaking style was relatively fast, and on subsequent visits with the child, I used Caroline's speech as a contraexample. When I deliberately spoke too fast, the child corrected with, "You're talking like Caroline now. Slow down!"

Identify and reduce or eliminate all fluency disrupters. During the assessment, the parents were asked to describe a typical day in the life of their family in order to identify potential fluency disrupters. An extension of this activity is to talk with the parents about where their child feels comfortable to speak and free of interruption, compared to where he perceives pressure to talk because of impending interruption. This might be an activity that could begin with the clinician, be completed by the parent at home, and then be discussed with the clinician. In many families, mealtime presents potential fluency disruption for children. In these settings, individual family members gather and enthusiastically share what is on their mind (what they anticipate for the day or what has happened during the day). Typically, different people talk at once and interrupt one another. This is particularly challenging for a child who is at risk or is beginning to stutter because of the impact that time pressure and perceived impending interruption have on speech fluency. This fluency disrupter can be prevented by establishing a pattern of turn-taking whereby each person waits for the one who is speaking to finish and then takes a speaking turn without interruption (give a turn; take a turn). Without drawing attention to the concern of fluency disruption, turn-taking (with no interruptions) can be addressed as a politeness rule ("It's not polite to interrupt. Taking turns is more polite and shows better manners").

Another common fluency disrupter is *demand speech* (in which the child must respond to direct questions) or *display speech* (in which the child is directed to talk for an audience). For example, well-meaning parents might direct the child in front of relatives to tell about his new bicycle, say what he wants for Christmas, or tell a recent joke or riddle. This puts a tremendous and unnecessary burden upon the child, whose coordination for speech fluency is not yet mature. An alternative would be for the parent to relate part of the event, to which the child might independently volunteer more information. If the parents find the child in a situation calling for demand speech, they might help the child by modeling slower, evenly paced, gentle speech and by expanding what the child has already said, again enabling him to participate voluntarily rather than on demand. Another potential fluency disrupter occurs when young children become interested in talking on the phone. The excitement of talking to Grandma and the ambiguity of how she so neatly fits into the phone combines into a frequently unmanageable fluency challenge for the child. Alternative strategies might include sitting with the child who is talking on the phone and coaching him (while modeling evenly paced, gentle speech) about what he might tell his grandmother, thus providing alternative topics for sharing. This tends to reduce the demand placed on the child, enabling him to use more resources for coordination of speech and language fluency. I know in some households with multiple siblings, a ringing phone sets off a mad dash by the children. All rush to be the first to answer the phone. If the child who is beginning to stutter proves victorious, speech fluency is potentially challenged by competing for and maintaining hold of the phone. Again, turn-taking helps. In such situations, children may answer the phone in a predetermined sequence. The parent can also model the phone greeting for the child using even, gentle speech ("Hello. Who is this, please?") before picking up the phone and handing it to him. These simple politeness procedures significantly reduce the demand placed upon the child's capacities to remain fluent.

Another common fluency disrupter is filling young children's schedules too full. Many youngsters are rushed from swimming class, to soccer, to dance, to Leonard's birthday party at McDonald's. Indeed, many children become "chips off the old block." Parents are responsible for filling or overfilling their own schedules. Children, on the other hand, must be guided in making responsible choices. When all of their time is consumed in demanding, albeit creative, activities, little energy remains to meet the demand of speech fluency and other aspects of communication development. A preschool child with whom I worked in play interaction to facilitate speech fluency comes to mind. One day I observed her literally airborne, holding the hand of a babysitter who was pulling her out of the preschool setting to rush to her ballet class on the other side of town. Working with the well-intentioned parents, I explained the importance of maintaining a moderate and manageable demand on the child's time, energy, and resources, particularly when a child is at risk for fluency failure. This led into an interesting and candid disclosure from the parents about how complex and overly scheduled they were, and how these factors were causing marital discord. They meant to provide for the child, not burden her. Working with the family, while focusing on the child's communication development and the family's system of communication, resulted in significant insights by and about the parents. Independently, they sought family counseling to study, understand, and alter their lifestyle and communication between themselves as spouses. The parents reported the counseling to be productive. The play intervention with the child, which involved her parents, led to a reduction of disfluency, subsequent monitoring, and eventual dismissal.

There are many potential fluency disrupters. The parents and clinician working together identify them and subsequently reduce, and eventually eliminate, their influence. In addition to the factors already discussed, others include but are not limited to the following: inappropriate speech and language models or expectations, rapid speech rates, calling attention to stuttering, punishment for stuttering, time pressure, demand or display speech, interruption, competition, guessing what the child is about to say, speaking immediately after the child stops talking, listener loss, excitement, conflict about discipline, emotional upset, and hectic or unpredictable schedules (Gregory, 2003, 2007; Guitar, 2006; Logan & Yaruss, 1999; Van Riper, 1973; Yaruss et al., 2006). The list of potential sources of interference with the child's fluency is endless. Because every family is different, the clinician must help the parents identify both the facilitators and the inhibitors of speech fluency. Accomplishing this is a sensitive task because of the parents' thoughts and feelings.

Thoughts and Feelings

If ever a clinician experiences the essence of a therapeutic relationship, it is when she addresses with parents their thoughts and feelings about a child who is beginning to stutter. As noted previously, there are probably few experiences more frightening to parents than when their child experiences something that feels out of their control or beyond their protective umbrella. Stuttering is one such case in point, which provides the clinician with an opportunity to have a genuine and positive impact on the thoughts, feelings, and behaviors of the parents and others within the family system. The clinician, however, must be able to shift perspective in order to see through the eyes of the parents, without judgment, so as to enter and begin to understand their world as they experience it. Discussing the challenge of understanding and impacting parents' thoughts and feelings, E. J. Webster (1977) noted that each person exists in a unique and very private world made up of forces that constantly impinge from both inside and outside. Webster stated, "The outer forces help to create and shape one's inner world, while internal forces help to create and shape one's perception of the outer world" (p. 3). Indeed, clinicians must understand the parents' and family's inner and outer worlds. It may appear that one's outer world is more readily understandable because it appears to be more directly observable. However, one's world can be understood only from an appreciation of the inner world and the dynamic interaction between real and perceived internal and external forces. This concept is related to personal constructs and family systems. The clinician must work with the parents and other family members to understand their unique interpretation of their world (and specifically, the experience of the child's disfluency), their assumptions, and the patterns of communication among the family members. Only when the parents and the clinician become aware of these factors can any belief or behavior be targeted for change.

We discussed earlier how behaviors and thoughts are related. In other words, what one does often reflects what one thinks or assumes, and one's thoughts are confirmed—or challenged—by observed behaviors. By discussing with parents their observed behaviors, the clinician has an opportunity to gain insights about the parents' thoughts and their current knowledge base about stuttering. I have come to believe that at worst, most parents are doing their level best. Fortunately, with very few exceptions, parents are trying their best to provide for their children while accommodating life's demands. Most parents who innocently advised their child, "Don't stutter" or "Slow down and think about what you're saying," did not realize why this is counterproductive. Usually when we talk with parents about the nature and etiology of stuttering, they are eager to adjust their current behavior to help their child. In other words, most of the parents' inappropriate behaviors were based on inaccurate or incomplete information. One of our missions, therefore, is to be a source of information and support for parents.

Sometimes, however, when parents reflect on their well-intentioned errors and begin to adjust their behavior in order to facilitate the child's speech fluency, feelings of guilt (emotional regret for having done something wrong) and anxiety (nervousness and tension) surface. These feelings typically make it difficult for parents to confront their child's stuttering. I discussed earlier the importance of first identifying all of the parents' behaviors that are supportive of and conducive to the child's communication development. Only then, within this positive context, do we discuss possible revisions. Starkweather et al. (1990) noted that they use a similar procedure:

> We begin to alleviate guilt by showing the parents all the correct things they have done to cope with the disorder. All parents have some reactions that are less negative. If they show concern in any positive way or just provide a loving atmosphere, we compliment them on it in order to let them know that their instincts are accurate and have already led them to help the child learn to speak more fluently. If parents are speaking in a reasonably slow rate or taking turns well, we let them know that these things have been helpful. We then go on to suggest other things they might do, some of which they have probably already thought of. This kind of approach is likely to elicit a strong sense of cooperation from the parents in addition to reducing guilt. (pp. 69–70)

Parents' willingness and ability (readiness) to confront stuttering in their child varies. Some are more accepting and are ready to study and understand the situation and adjust necessary behaviors. Others are loath to confront stuttering, perhaps seeing it as their own failure, thus avoiding or denying it. Emphasizing what is positive yet realistic, we share with the parents that between 75% and 85% of all preschool children who ever stutter (and 65% to over 80% of preschool children who have just begun to stutter) recover spontaneously (without treatment), and these figures improve with treatment (Yairi & Ambrose, 2005). We also emphasize that early intervention achieves much success in preventing stuttering. In fact, one of the best prognostic indicators is the amount of time that has elapsed between the onset of the disfluent behaviors and the beginning of intervention. The longer the duration between the identification of disfluency and the beginning of intervention, the longer it generally takes to remediate the stuttering. Other prognostic indicators related to a longer duration of treatment for the child who is beginning to stutter are negative reactions of the parent toward the parent's own or the child's stuttering and anything that might make it difficult for the parents to carry out the suggestions provided in treatment (including environmental stress, financial hardship, social problems, an uninvolved parent, and marital discord) (Guitar, 2006; Starkweather et al., 1990). These and other special considerations are addressed in Chapter 5. Starkweather et al. added that the consequences of not doing anything are potentially serious enough to warrant a program of intervention, even if it is one of monitoring. Such instruction of and intervention with parents, being undertaken as soon as possible, have been supported by others as well (Yairi, 2004; Yairi & Ambrose, 1999, 2005; Yaruss et al., 2006; Zebrowski, 1995).

During this period, we invite and address the parents' questions and involve them actively in implementing the recommendations after discussing, demonstrating, and directing. These procedures tend to reduce feelings of guilt and anxiety by showing the parents that they have a partner, a comrade, who will work with them to help their child. We identify, explore, and confront as necessary thoughts, feelings, and behaviors that might have a negative impact on the child's speech fluency. We remain positive, emphasizing all of the parents' behaviors that are appropriate and monitoring and praising successes. We suggest modifications to the parents' behavior in a supportive environment. Starkweather et al. (1990) advised as follows:

> When parents have been reacting badly to stuttering, we do not try to underestimate the negative impact those reactions have on the child, but if the parents see these reactions as behaviors they were unaware of, reactions motivated by their love for the child, and accompanied by other helpful behaviors, it is unlikely that they will feel guilty about them. (p. 70)

Identifying and understanding the parents' feelings of guilt and anxiety are essential, as is modification of such feelings. The parents' guilt and anxiety potentially can consume energy that might otherwise be directed toward implementing suggestions for fluency modification. Also, the child's attitudes toward communication and beginning stuttering are influenced by those of the parent. As the child perceives the parents' verbal and nonverbal tension when the child is disfluent, the child will be inclined to try harder not to be disfluent, thus struggling and forcing as he tries harder, all the while internalizing feelings of guilt for having created unpleasantness for the parents. The parents can be helped to understand their feelings and thoughts about stuttering and their child who is beginning to stutter. With the care of a knowledgeable clinician, both the parents' concerns and the child's symptoms can normalize as all work toward the child's fluent future. The methods for adjusting behaviors, thoughts, and feelings will be discussed further in the clinical portrait at the end of this chapter.

Direct Intervention

The intervention methods discussed so far for a preschool child who is beginning to stutter have been relatively indirect. That is, the clinician works with the parents to manage the communication environment at home and elsewhere in order to achieve a reduction in the child's disfluency and a return to normal fluency. I find it helpful to conceptualize intervention for preschool children as falling along a continuum from indirect to direct. *Indirect intervention approaches* do not explicitly or overtly attempt to modify the child's speech fluency. Rather, they focus on the child and the child's communication environment. Such approaches often involve information sharing and counseling with the parents, interacting with the child in a variety of play-oriented activities in which speech is not the obvious focus, and modeling by the clinician and parents of fluent or more "easy" speech for the child. *Direct intervention approaches*, on the other hand, are characterized by explicit or overt attempts to teach the child how to change his speech or related behaviors, and may or may not be conducted within a context of play (Conture,

2001; Guitar, 2006; Onslow & Packman, 1999; Onslow et al., 2003; Van Riper, 1973; Zebrowski, 1997).

The methods discussed in this section are of increasing relative directness with respect to the child. They are intended for a child who is beginning to stutter (a child whose amount of disfluency is increasing in frequency, forms are becoming more complex, and behaviors are reflecting increased awareness or establishment of frustration). Guitar (2006) described children who are beginning to stutter as follows:

> Children with beginning stuttering are usually between 3 and 6 years of age, but some children may be 7 or 8 years old. They have probably been stuttering for at least several months, and now their parents may well be concerned that it is not a transient problem that will disappear on its own. . . . These children's most common core stuttering behaviors are part-word repetitions that are produced rapidly, usually with irregular rhythm. Some prolongations may also be present. Both the repetitions and prolongations may contain excessive tension, which can be heard as abrupt endings to the repetitions and increases in vocal pitch in repetitions and prolongations. Blocks may be present but will probably not be the predominant core behavior. Secondary behaviors are typically escape devices, such as eye blinks, head nods, and increases in pitch. A few avoidance maneuvers, such as starting sentences with extra sounds like "uh," may be observed. Children with beginning stuttering usually feel frustrated with their difficulty in talking but have not yet developed a fear of stuttering or learned to be ashamed of their speech. In rare cases, if the frequency of stuttering becomes extremely high, these children may put their hands to their mouth to push the words out or may momentarily avoid talking. (p. 322)

Within the context of play intervention, the clinician interacts with the child directly with and without the parents present (who participate actively when present). The suggestions reviewed earlier for parent intervention are continued. The direct treatment through play is an addition to parent intervention, not a replacement. The treatment process is becoming more aggressive, yet still relatively indirect, as will be seen when we review treatment for the school-age child.

Goals
The treatment goals for the preschool child in direct treatment are spontaneous (i.e., normal-sounding) fluency and maintenance of a positive attitude toward communication and oneself as a communicator.

Objectives
The objectives for the child in directed play intervention are to establish and transfer fluent speech, to develop resistance to the potential effects of fluency disrupters, to express feelings about communication and oneself as a communicator as appropriate, and to maintain the fluency inducing effects of treatment.

Rationale
Play and fun represent and create the language of childhood. Intervention with preschool children who are beginning to stutter must be done with laughter. Children want to do more of what they perceive to be fun and what they're good at. It is necessary—but not sufficient—for the clinician to sincerely enjoy working with the preschool child. When the clinician knows and understands what she is doing, feels positive about the child's and the family's potential, and is and has fun, children like the clinician and will work through play with her. Children must like and trust you. Play and fun create trust. Children are mirrors of the clinician's trust, confidence, friendship, and love. All

the clinical materials in the world cannot replace a clinician's enjoyment of children and a natural ability to talk and play with them. I particularly enjoy working with children about whom I am warned to expect behavior problems. These children challenge our professional (clinical and particularly interpersonal) skills. Although I have had my fair share of healthy challenges, I have yet to find a child who is not manageable. I remain convinced that the behavior of a disruptive child reflects as much the behavior of the responsible adult as it does that of the child. I often remind myself that when we point a finger at a child or anyone else, we have three pointing at ourselves. The procedures that follow are based on the four objectives listed above. The procedures are more direct than those presented for parent counseling, yet less direct than those presented for intervention with school-age children. While a composite is painted here of the preschool child, it is possible that the child's developing symptoms and awareness defy his age. When the symptoms (behaviors, thoughts, and feelings) are more advanced, the procedures outlined in Chapter 9 for even more direct intervention with the school-age child would be more appropriate, regardless of the child's age.

Procedures

Treatment procedures, with a brief discussion for each, are presented here.

Establish and transfer fluent speech. A first step in establishing fluent speech through play is modeling within a fun context what the child should sound like. How do I do it? We talk. That's all. We talk and I listen to and learn about the child's world. Remember, everybody has a story to tell, including young children (Shapiro, 2000, 2002a, 2002b, 2002c, 2004a, 2004b, 2004c, 2004d, 2004e, 2004f, 2004g, 2007a, 2007b, 2008). Let them tell it. Too often, clinicians' use of clinical materials hinders, rather than helps, a child's willingness to talk. Clinicians feel they must be in control, so we talk and we question. It is hard to have a real conversation when we interrogate the child, or when we repeat everything the child said for audio or video recording, or when we write down everything the child said on our legal tablet and clipboard. Just talk, listen, and have fun. In fact, the more listening we do, the more we can follow the child's lead. Children see that here they have a big person who does not need to control. In their eyes I can see them thinking, "This is mighty different." Children love to talk. Clinicians may want to review the stages of play discussed earlier in this chapter (see Figure 8.1). Somehow, most adults know how to talk with children when they meet within a social context. They say, "Hey big guy! Those are mighty nifty boots you have on. Mind if I slip them on my feet?" Or they say, "By jingo, you've got the coolest red hair I've ever seen. Do you think I could get mine that red if I used a big red crayon?" But because talking within a professional context is distinguished as "treatment," naturalness and fun, which epitomize the privilege of talking with children, go to the wind. We say things like, "I am Mrs. Smith. I am a speech–language pathologist. Do you know what that is? What is your name?" Or we say, "I am your new speech teacher. Do you know why you are here?" Let's role reverse. If we clinicians were the children listening to the latter, rather stilted, lifeless questions, would we be motivated to talk? If truth be told, I think we'd try to catch some sleep. I think I would hide under the table or throw spitballs because that seems like more fun. What about you?

So what do I do? I play and I have fun. I like puppets a lot. They tend to take the pressure off the child, even though the child is talking for the puppet. We sing songs. If the child is particularly disfluent, we may sing or speak (e.g., nursery rhymes and jingles, among others) in chorus. Throughout the activities, I model slow (i.e., evenly paced), gentle, natural-sounding speech. Starkweather et al. (1990) described this modeled speech as "naturally cadenced slow-normal speech rate with appropriate melodic contour" (p. 71). We draw and we paint. We play "Simon Says" and "Hide and Seek" right in the treatment room. If the child is disfluent, I insert both similar and more gentle disfluencies of the child's form into my speech, sometimes offering a neutral comment about my speech as I go about my play ("Oops. That was a tough one."). With children, the effect of our model is potent. They see that we and our fun are unaffected, with or without disfluency, and they follow suit. I remember a 6-year-old girl who put a large ring (from a ring toss game) on my head and said, "You're the King of Laughter." No award or accolade could mean as much to me as what she said. I believe she saw me as fun, able to communicate with her, and inviting of her story. And her fluency returned to normal in the process.

An interesting ethical dilemma has arisen on several occasions. Typically, in each scheduled meeting, I work with the preschool child first without his parents, and then I bring them into the session. When the parents are not with me, I encourage them to observe what we are doing from the observation room. I believe that the child's advantage is served when parents are kept maximally involved and informed. Literally and figuratively, I want to open the door to the parent and family. On several occasions during play interaction, however, a child shared a feeling or an event with me that would not have been shared if the observers had been present. For example, about a father who was clinically depressed and under medical and psychiatric care, the 4-year-old child said, "I don't like my daddy. He scares me. He's mean to me." Another reported, "My mommy is bad. She went to jail." In both of these cases, the parents were observing and expressed alarm at what the children had said. The children's disclosures had a positive outcome, however, resulting in additional productive dialogue between the clinician and the parents and families.

I realize the parents in these cases are the legal guardians and that they, their children, and their family are protected by confidentiality. But what about confidentiality within a family, or a child's right to express a feeling without disclosure to the parent? In some cases where the feelings or events being expressed have an impact beyond the child's communication or the family as a communication unit, I have made referrals to family counselors, social workers, and social service agencies. But when what is said has an impact within our professional domain, we neither can prevent nor predict what the child will say or when he will say it. So, until children have their own right to confidentiality, discretion and compassion must direct our standing commitment to understanding and helping communicators within families.

For the purpose of transferring fluency to the home and other outside settings, the suggestions provided in parent intervention are continued throughout treatment. Other transfer suggestions are derived from the directed play treatment experience as appropriate for each child. For example, a clinician who is providing specific feedback (such as praise) for the child's fluent speech ("I like that you just used slow, gentle speech") might have the parent continue this at home (using the three Ds—discussion, demonstration, and direction). The child's observed disfluency might serve to remind the clinician and parent to continue to praise the fluent speech when observed and to offer correction only indirectly in the form of modeling and expansion. The transfer activities should be emphasized from the very beginning of treatment, hence the importance of involving the parents and family in all aspects of the treatment experience. The individual transfer activities are limited only by one's imagination and creativity, as long as the recommendations presented for parent intervention are followed.

Indeed, from this clinical perspective, it is critical not to single out a child in a group to slow down. Nevertheless, providing models of slow (evenly paced) speech is essential, as are occasional supportive explanations. Consider the following example. A father on a picnic outing by a creek with his 3-year-old son continuously modeled slow, gentle speech, particularly when his son demonstrated noticeable disfluency. Other suggestions implemented by the father, including taking his turn sooner and engaging in gentle distractions, did not prove successful in relieving the child's disfluency. At one point, the father said to the child, "See that yellow leaf on the creek. See how it moves like this (demonstrating a slow, gentle, flowing hand movement from left to right). Let's see if we can talk like the leaf, like this (repeating the hand movement, continuing to model a fluent speech pattern)." The boy said, "Lllike thhhis (gently prolonging initial consonants)?" The father reinforced with, "That's right, just like this." This explanation represents an increase in the father's level of directness in dealing with the child's disfluency symptoms, yet still within an atmosphere of unconditional acceptance and support without any overt or negative judgment. The picnic continued, now in fluent dialogue. About a year later, when driving in the car, the father realized that both his rate of speech and that of his son were too fast. As the son's speech was becoming increasingly disfluent, the father commented, "Hold on. We both need to slow down a little" (i.e., as the father modeled slower, natural-sounding speech). The son commented, "You mean like the creek?" Having long forgotten the experience from a year ago, the father asked, "What do you mean?" The boy responded with, "You know, Daddy, like this" (i.e., moving his hand in the slow, gently flowing, wavelike pattern from left to right, while speaking in a more fluent and gentle, easily flowing manner). "That's right," the dad acknowledged with a laugh. "I had forgotten about that. That's a good thing to remember. Thanks for reminding me." The dad continued while following the child's example for slow, gentle, fluent speech. Children learn and teach by our example.

Another experience comes to mind. In directed play treatment, a 3-year-old child was provided feedback for using appropriate speech fluency ("I like the way you said that. You used slow, gentle speech"). The clinician directed the child to listen to her (i.e., the clinician's) speech and help her slow down when it got too fast. "Sometimes I forget," said the clinician, "and I need a little help from my friends." When the child's speech increased in rate or demonstrated patterns of noticeable disfluency, the clinician assumed a rapid rate with some noticeable disfluencies, thus inviting the child's correction. The purpose here was to provide the child ongoing support for what he (the child) was doing right, and for the clinician to wear the weight of correction when necessary (i.e., when the child's speech rate or disfluency increased), thus conveying the correction to the child indirectly. Again, the rationale is for speaking to continue to be a fun, positive experience. The parents were included in this experience during directed play and carried it over to the home setting. They reported that on several instances when they forgot to focus on fluency, failing to provide models of slow, gentle speech, the child reminded them, "You're talking too fast," or "Slow down!" Note that the child had never been directed to "slow down," but had internalized the correction and generalized it to the speech behavior of others. Again, children learn and teach by our example.

Here's another example. We have emphasized the importance of slower (i.e., evenly paced), relaxed activities to regulate speech fluency. What happens when the activities run out and when bedlam strikes? This happened to one family recently while they were taking a road trip of 10 hours. There were two children in the family, one of whom was a 4-year-old boy who demonstrated beginning stuttering. His speech fluency remained under control within slow, relaxed activities. When the activities ran out, as did fluency control, the mother suggested, "Let's sing songs. How about 'Itsy Bitsy Spider?'" At that, she began to sing, thus regulating a slower, gentle pace. The children joined in chorus, followed by their own selections. Slowing down the overall pace through song reestablished a comfortable speech model for all. This activity led to others (such as "I Spy" and guessing games) within which slow, gentle speech was used. Remember that such suggestions for transfer are in addition to the recommendations given earlier for parent intervention. In essence, every waking moment holds the potential for speech fluency facilitation and transfer.

Develop resistance to the potential effects of fluency disrupters. Once fluent speech is established and is being transferred to the home and other outside settings, we increasingly work to develop resistance to fluency disrupters (Van Riper, 1973). The test of any treatment is how well its effects are maintained when the conditions that formerly resulted in stuttering are systematically reintroduced. Other tests include transfer (already discussed) and maintenance of fluency, in addition to the feeling of fluency control. I find it best to conceptualize fluency challenge as falling along a number of continua. Fluency challenge is least present when the recommendations given for parent intervention are followed continuously and greatest when they are not followed at all. We might consider the recommendations separately and reintroduce fluency challenge for each.

One example already mentioned involved rate of speech. To establish fluency, we seek to model slower (i.e., more evenly paced), gentle, natural-sounding speech as much as is reasonably possible, in addition to that within special uninterrupted family time already discussed. We noted that along the way, when the child's rate or disfluency increases, we model the contraexample (fast, hard speech), inviting the child's correction in order for him to reestablish more appropriate speech patterns. Once speech fluency is established and is being transferred and maintained, we may deliberately demonstrate contraexamples, or barbs (Conture, 2001), more frequently. These barbs enable the child to gain experience withstanding potential fluency interrupters, thus minimizing their impact. Similarly, we may reintroduce interruptions and deliberately violate other conversational turn-taking conventions (by abruptly shifting topics or appearing distracted when the child is talking).

A major goal here and throughout, however, is to ensure the child's success. No positive aim is served by the child's failure. The clinician's responsibility is to ensure that the child is and remains successful. We already reviewed the motivating impact of success. If the child fails to succeed, then the learning step taken with the child between where you are (modeling slow, gentle speech always) and where you want to go (deleting the clinician's model of slow, gentle speech) is too great. You may delete your model for a minute during every 5- or 10-minute interval, systematically increasing both the frequency and duration of the periods with no deliberate model. Eventually, the child will maintain slow, gentle, natural-sounding speech in the context of no deliberate model, interruption, listener loss, increasing audience size, demand and display speech, and other challenging contexts. Sometimes it is helpful to remind the child in advance to remember to use slow, easy speech even when the clinician "forgets." That way, the child will not be confused about why the clinician's manner of speaking has changed, and he will expect increasing and deliberate challenge. The challenge of remembering to use slow, easy speech can and should become another fun game between the child and clinician and parents.

Encourage expressions of feeling about communication and oneself as a communicator, as appropriate. One of the hallmarks of the preschool child who stutters or those who are demonstrating beginning stuttering is the absence of deep emotional involvement. Part of the child's emotional neutrality reflects the absence of a long and potentially painful history of fluency failure. Another part reflects the positive, accepting, nurturing response the child receives—when he is fluent as well as when he is disfluent—from his parents and all others who function within the child's communication system. Whether the child is emotionally neutral toward his speech or better yet, overtly positive about the communication experience, is critical and a significant distinguishing characteristic of the preschool child. Our job as clinicians, and that of other communicators within the child's environment, is to make sure that the child's attitude toward communication and himself as a communicator remains positive. We do this by being open, accepting, and nurturing toward the child about his speech and all other areas of potential; by being receptive and responsive to the child's affective expressions; and by creating opportunities for the child to express feelings and to be supported for having done so.

To understand the significance of such a positive, nurturing communication context, I recommend to clinicians and parents that they record a video sample of their interactions with the child. Reviewing the video for both verbal and nonverbal factors invariably proves enlightening. We might take particular notice of the comments directed to the child. Are the comments emphasizing what the child is doing correctly and what you sincerely believe he can do ("You can do it. I know you can. Fantastic! What you just said was great slow, easy speech. You are always such a good artist.")? Or are they focusing on what the child is doing wrong, is not doing, should or should not be doing, and can't do ("Stop that now. If you do that one more time . . . Sit in your chair. Put that down. No, that's not right. I already told you how to do that.")? One of the few things that makes my uvula steam (and I don't get upset often) is when I observe clinicians verbally reward children with, "Good boy!" or "Good girl!" when a child has done something correctly, but then fail to offer a verbal reward when the child has shown his best effort but did not succeed. This concerns me for several reasons. First, this communicates to the child that he is a good person when he succeeds and implies that he is bad when he does not. Whatever happened to receiving honest recognition for doing your best, whether you win or lose? Furthermore, I recommend showing unconditional positive regard for the person (e.g., "That a boy! Way to go."), consistent recognition for the sincere effort ("That was a dynamite try. Hang in there. I'm so glad you are doing your best work."), and more discriminating feedback for the relative accuracy of the response ("Oops. That was a tough one. Why don't we try it with our slow, easy speech, like this," offering explanation, demonstration, and then supportive coaching). A scenario that invites constant correction and behavioral management might present a level of difficulty that is too challenging and might not be appropriately structured for the strengths, needs, and interests of the individual child. If the child continues to have difficulty, consider a lower level on the hierarchy or continuum of task difficulty.

How inviting are we to the child's expressions of affect? Do we create opportunities for the child to offer expressions of feeling or preferences and then support him for having done so? When we give the child a choice, do we honor his selection? As noted earlier, asking a child, "Do you want to come with me?" or "Do you want to look at these pictures with me?" invites a choice of two implied alternatives, yes and no. When the child says, "No!" and we coerce the child into coming or looking, we have not honored the child's selection. Furthermore, we convey to the child that his expression of preferences will not be taken seriously anyway. Recall the earlier discussion about how to phrase questions differently so that the child's alternatives are supportive of the treatment objectives. When a child sincerely confesses, "I don't want to do that," do we listen and respond, having considered the child's perspective, or are we locked into our own perspective (Moses & Shapiro, 1996; Shapiro & Moses, 1989, 2005)? While preschool children surely have feelings, generally they are not advanced in their expression of how or what they feel. When they offer behavioral outbursts or emotional tantrums, do we assume that they are intentionally disruptive or that they have received poor parenting? One little disfluent boy told me, "Everybody is always mad at me. Everybody blames me." Indeed these were significant expressions, as the parents were inadvertently triangulating the boy into an unstable marital relationship, vacillating between obsessive concern over his fluency and excessive criticism of most other behaviors. The concept of triangulation was reviewed in Chapter 5. Yes, it is true that not all disruptive or emotional expressions are symbolic and that some behaviors are downright and brilliantly manipulative. But we have to listen and be able to hear the child's message, which often is overlaid and rather indistinct from his feelings. To do this, clinicians must understand their own feelings, strengths, and needs, both personally and professionally, so as to shift perspective and to assume the point of view of the internal world of the child. These and other clinician competencies will be discussed in Chapter 11.

Maintain the fluency inducing effects of treatment. Once the child is speaking fluently both inside and outside the clinical setting with a variety of speakers, with and without potential fluency disrupters—all the while accepting of himself as a communicator—we begin to reduce the time spent in directed play treatment. If sessions are weekly, they may move to every 2 weeks, then once per month. Assuming that the achievements are maintained, we schedule abbreviated reevaluations every 2 or 3 months for the first year in addition to maintaining phone contact and receiving audio recordings monthly during the interim. During the reevaluations, we sample and analyze the child's speech and interview the parents. Reevaluations decrease in frequency over the following year. Should the child regress or should the parents wish to discuss the child's or the family's communication needs, they are welcomed back at any time.

▦ Clinical Portrait: Amy Stiles

Selected Background Information

Amy* was 3 years 10 months old when she was referred by her parents for a speech–language evaluation because of her "stuttering." Both Mr. and Mrs. Stiles attended the scheduled evaluation, reporting that "sometimes when Amy speaks, she will stutter. She gets real upset." Amy's disfluencies were first noticed by the parents about a year prior to the evaluation, when she told a little boy, "I-I-I am Amy," reportedly eliciting laughter from the boy. Regarding Amy's speech fluency, the parents reported fluctuation with long periods of remission and apparent awareness leading to frustration by the child, evidenced by her stopping mid-sentence and stamping her feet. Amy had had no previous speech–language intervention. Amy's birth, developmental, and medical history was without complication. She had no siblings and her family history for communication problems was negative. Because of financial hardship, Amy's family lived with her maternal grandmother. Mr. Stiles was employed as a manual laborer in a factory. Mrs. Stiles was not employed outside of the home.

Abbreviated Speech–Language Analysis

An analysis of Amy's conversational speech revealed an average rate of 140 fluent words per minute or 152 words per minute including both fluent and disfluent words. These rates represent a low-average rate of speech. Most of Amy's speech was characterized by relatively effortless, gentle articulatory transitions of even rate with normal-sounding suprasegmental features (such as pitch, juncture, and loudness). Disfluencies across the conversations were characterized by whole-word (*what-what*) and part-word (*the-they*) repetitions and occasional sound prolongations (*lllot*), which did not interrupt motor sequence, intended message, or communication effort. Based on samples of 100 words in length, Amy's overall disfluency averaged 9%. Part-word repetitions accounted for 54% of the total disfluencies and were characterized by no more than 3 units of repetition per instance. Whole-word repetitions comprised 36% of the disfluencies and again revealed no more than 3 units of repetition per instance. Prolongations, 10%, were gentle and fleeting, not exceeding

---

*All clinical portrait names have been changed to protect confidentiality.

1.5 seconds in duration. The only secondary characteristic observed was occasional inconsistent tense eye blinking during the prolongations. No disfluencies were observed during song or choral recitation of nursery rhymes. More frequent disfluencies were noted on repetition of longer, more complex words (such as *celebrate* and *incubator*). Before attempting to repeat *incubator*, Amy said, "My mouth is getting tired." Symptoms suggesting the beginning of communication interference included the high proportion of within-word disfluencies, a slight increase in disfluency in conversations with unfamiliar people and with increased linguistic demand, infrequent eye tension, and her comment about "getting tired." All other aspects of assessment (both informal and standardized) revealed age-appropriate speech (articulation and phonology) and language (semantics, syntax and morphology, and pragmatics) development. All parameters of voice and hearing were within normal limits.

Recommendations

Because all other aspects of Amy's speech, language, motor, cognitive, and social development were within normal limits, Amy's disfluency was considered to be of "borderline" concern. I elected parent intervention as a form of prevention with ongoing monitoring to ensure stability in Amy's speech fluency development. Suggestions for parent intervention were reviewed with the parents at the time of the evaluation, followed by the clinician's demonstration of the techniques and then coaching the parents in using the techniques with Amy. The parents were given supportive reading material, told that the summary report would follow within 7 to 10 days, at which time they should call me, and scheduled for reevaluation in 6 weeks. In addition, a supportive letter was sent immediately following the evaluation (Figure 8.5).

Follow-Up

Subsequent analyses of Amy's speech and parental reports for 6 months indicated that parent intervention was effective in stabilizing and reducing Amy's speech disfluency. However, the parents elected to have Amy participate in a children's presentation at their Kingdom Hall, the house of worship of the Jehovah's Witness faith, which proved to have a significant and deleterious effect on Amy's speech. This experience was discussed in advance, described as demand and display speech, and therefore discouraged. The presentation involved a number of preschool children individually going to a microphone and talking about a poster depicting a religious theme. Fortunately, the parents audio-recorded the program, from which Amy's presentation was analyzed, as summarized in the following paragraphs.

Amy spoke 62 words, of which 36 contained one or more types of disfluency, over a 90-second duration. Her overall rate of speech in this context was 41 words per minute (compared to 152 words per minute in the assessment setting), revealing an overall disfluency of 58% (figured by dividing the total words spoken by the number of stuttered words), compared to 9% in the assessment setting. Rate of speech was irregular, revealing instances of both even transitions and silent and audibly tense pauses of up to 6 seconds in duration.

Forms of disfluency included part-word repetition (e.g., *A-A-A-Adam*; 66%), which contained up to three instances of uneven and audibly forced repetition; whole-word repetition (*snake-snake-snake*; 20%) of up to 3 units of repetition; and sound prolongations (*EEEEEve*; 6%) that contained audible voiced and unvoiced struggle and vocal fry without pitch rise. Additionally, unlike that demonstrated in the assessment context, Amy's speech contained broken words (*Ca–silent pause–in*, *A–silent pause–bel*), combined repetition with tense prolongations (*f . . . f . . . for*), interjection of prolonged syllables (*uuum*) and phrases (*yyyou know*) unevenly spaced of up to 3 units of repeated interjection, and word (*picture, um, poster*) and phrase (*that's it, that's what it is about*) revision.

These selected data in this context indicated a significant decrease in Amy's fluency; increase in the observed types, complexity, and frequency of disfluency; and serious interference in her effectiveness as a communicator. In response to only her presentation, the audience applauded in empathic relief.

Treatment Snapshot

Because of the significant reduction in Amy's speech fluency subsequent to the presentation at the Kingdom Hall, she was enrolled in direct fluency treatment for the ensuing year, which utilized play both as a context and a medium for exchange. Following the suggestions described earlier in this

May 28, 2010

James and Susan Stiles
21 East Main Street
Sylva, NC 28779

Dear Mr. and Mrs. Stiles:

It was my pleasure to meet with you and your daughter, Amy, on Tuesday, May 25. Indeed, you are a beautiful and supportive family.

My assessment of Amy's speech is that she is in an early stage of the development of stuttering. Having seen evidence of her frequent repetitions during the evaluation, I feel that it is a critical period in that so much can be done now in order to prevent the disfluencies from becoming chronic.

This type of disfluency generally is most effectively treated by the parent, with advice from a speech–language pathologist. For this reason, I do not recommend scheduled direct treatment at this time. As we discussed at our meeting, I feel that the following suggestions will assist you to increase the likelihood that Amy's speech continues to develop without serious increase in the amount or type of disfluency.

I feel that you are doing an excellent job in managing the disfluency that is observed and in being "good listeners." I recommend that you continue the same approach with the following additions. First, try to provide Amy with models of slow (i.e., evenly paced), gently produced, and natural-sounding speech. As we discussed, this sounds easier than it is and will take practice on your part. Second, whenever possible, reduce any pressures on her to speak quickly or fight against interruption. If members of your family and friends can refrain from interrupting her, that should be helpful. Third, if Amy has a sudden occurrence of disfluency either when excited or in a hurry, maintain your even, gentle, natural-sounding speech model and try to get her interested in something else besides talking, so that she does not have much experience with serious disfluency. Then later, when she is less excited, you might ask her about what she was telling you. Fourth, try to keep her from becoming unnecessarily aware of or frustrated about the disfluency. If she mentions it to you, however, don't hesitate to tell her that you know we all get stuck on words at times. Suggest by showing her that trying to say them slowly or easily may help.

I hope these suggestions prove helpful and that you have had an opportunity to begin looking at the Stuttering Foundation of America resources that I loaned you. The books *If Your Child Stutters: A Guide for Parents* and *Stuttering and Your Child: Questions and Answers*, as well as the DVD *Stuttering and Your Child: Help for Parents*, should reinforce and expand upon our conversation and my recommendations. I look forward to speaking with you soon regarding these suggestions and future considerations.

If you have any questions, do not hesitate to give me a call or email me at the Western Carolina University Speech and Hearing Center. You will find my contact information at the top of this letter. Again, thank you for meeting with us and for sharing your commitment to Amy's communication development.

Sincerely,

David A. Shapiro, PhD, CCC–SLP
Speech–Language Pathologist
Faculty Supervisor

Figure 8.5.   Follow-up letter to the parents of a 3-year-old child who is beginning to stutter.

chapter, the parents both observed the first half of each session and participated directly in the latter half (the mother consistently, the father inconsistently because of schedule conflicts with work). Puppetry was used as one of many different modes to differentiate between "slow, easy" and "fast, hard" speech. Amy was provided frequent verbal rewards for remembering her slow, easy speech. Correction of the clinician's puppet was used initially to remind Amy indirectly to use a more fluent pattern, and eventually to challenge Amy's fluency control. She was told by the clinician's puppet, for example, "Sometimes when I get excited to talk with my friends, I forget to use slow, easy speech. Will you help me remember?" Then, the clinician deliberately inserted noticeable disfluencies ("What is going to ha-ha-ha-happen?"), to which Amy's response systematically increased over time in steps or levels of challenge. The same error will be used for illustration here, but in reality, both the errors presented by the clinician and the response expectation of the child vary:

⚏ Initially Amy offered, "Slow down!"

⚏ Then, she was asked, "What do you mean?" To this Amy explained, "Bird, you have to put a little stretch in that."

⚏ Still later, Amy was asked, "Would you show me how to do it?" Hearing the clinician's error, Amy was observed at one point to subvocalize the correct form of the clinician's error (the clinician said "ha-ha-ha-happen," to which Amy subvocalized, or mouthed without sound, "hhhappen"). She then offered in slow, gentle speech, "Hhhappen."

⚏ The clinician challenged, "Do you mean 'ha-ha-ha-happen?'" To this, Amy both critiqued the clinician's error ("No, that's not right") and offered the corrected form ("What is going to hhhappen?").

⚏ Then the clinician offered, "Do you mean, 'What is going to hhhappen?'" To this, Amy offered, "Yes, that's it." Then the clinician rewarded and reauditorized the correct form, "Oh, thank you. What is going to hhhappen. So, what is going to hhhappen?"

These few steps indicate how, within the context of play intervention using puppetry, the response expectation for the child moved from identification of the error, to analysis of the error (what aspect was wrong), explanation of how to correct the error, internalization of the corrected form, demonstration of the correct form, correction (response analysis) of the contraexample, reinforcement (response analysis) for the corrected form, and coaching the clinician for the correct form. Just as I have discussed the importance of telling (discussing), demonstrating (showing), and then directing (coaching and critiquing) when teaching a child or parent a new behavior, here the child is "teaching" the clinician within an opportunity created by the clinician. After completion of this sequence, the clinician created opportunities to model and expand the topic of discussion while using the correct form of the word that the child "taught" the clinician how to say correctly. A sequence such as this shows how the response expectation of the child can be increased systematically within the context of play.

Follow-Up and Epilogue

Directed play intervention worked effectively in helping Amy both regain control of her speech fluency and remain positive about communication and herself as a communicator. Furthermore, regular conferences with the parents, combined with their active participation in all aspects of the treatment process, enabled them to understand and contribute meaningfully to the treatment process. After I had worked with the family for 1½ years (6 months in parent intervention only; then 1 year in direct treatment), Mr. Stiles received a transfer to Atlanta, Georgia, a distance of 150 miles. For a short time, the family commuted from Atlanta in a most unreliable vehicle. Then, Mrs. Stiles, Amy, and her newborn sister came to live with Amy's maternal grandmother just so the family could receive fluency treatment. I remained concerned about the family being apart (between Cullowhee, North Carolina, and Atlanta). When they moved to Atlanta, I investigated treatment options there, although none were possible for the family because of the financial expense involved. We maintained phone contact nearly monthly for the next year, during which time the family continued to send audio recordings of Amy's speech. After 2½ years, we lost contact for about 18 months. Then one day, a tall girl whom I barely recognized knocked on my door. Amy had grown so in stature and maturity that, for the moment, it was hard to remember the kid I had worked with a year and a half before. I was thrilled to hear her speech fluency. We promised to exchange letters by audio record-ing, which we did for several months. She told me about Chinese cooking, Girl Scout cookie sales, and her little sister, whom she described as "a pain." Happily, Amy's rate of speech had stabilized between 170 and 180 words per minute without a trace of noticeable disfluency. The only concern was a defective /r/ production, which was receiving attention at school. Here's to good stories, happy endings, and committed families.

Guiding Principles

The clinical portrait of Amy Stiles illustrates intrafamily (personal constructs, family systems), ex-trafamily (interdisciplinary teaming and multicultural awareness), and psychotherapeutic (fluency shaping and stuttering modification) considerations. Each of these will be reviewed in turn.

Intrafamily Considerations

Fortunately, all members of the Stiles family maintained, in their thoughts, feelings, and behaviors toward and about Amy, the assumption that she is communicatively able and will communicate more fluently. This personal construct shaped the way the parents approached and participated in the treatment experience and the way Amy continued to view herself as a communicator. Also for-tunately, throughout her experiences, which potentially contributed to increased demands placed upon her (such as presenting at Kingdom Hall; moving to, from, and back to Atlanta; the birth of her sister; financial hardship; and going to school, among others) and with the ongoing and posi-tive support of her parents, Amy did not need to reconsider or revise the way she thought about herself. Although occasionally challenged, Amy continued to predict her future as she had always known her past, one of love, nurturing, and encouragement. Similarly, the Stiles family continued to function as a family unit. Every event that affected one of its members affected, in some way, all the other members. This was seen not only in Amy's fluency, but in all other family matters. When times seemed at their darkest (e.g., during miscarriages, loss of employment, and the seemingly endless repair of the family truck), the family pulled together the most and pooled resources. Both the family's view of Amy as a communicator and the networking of communication within the family were always considered in the planning and evaluation of treatment.

Extrafamily Considerations

For different reasons (distance traveled, family preference), there was relatively little involvement of an interdisciplinary team. I contacted other professionals only when treatment was considered in the Atlanta region. However, the records provided by the family were complete, ensuring my understanding of Amy's and the family's history. The family's involvement in the Kingdom Hall and other activities of the Jehovah's Witness faith provided a significant focus in their life and a source of emotional, social, and spiritual support, particularly during challenging times. I respected their faith and learned by their example. As the clinician, I needed to be sensitive to and understand their faith in the design of treatment. And, although I tried to discourage Amy's parents from having her engage in the presentation at the Kingdom Hall, I had to respect their view toward their faith and their connection to others within the congregation when they decided not to follow the advice that was provided.

Psychotherapeutic Considerations

Fluency shaping and stuttering modification treatments are least distinct for preschool children who are beginning to stutter. Parent counseling and direct treatment reflected an appreciation of both sets of assumptions. For example, providing more opportunity to talk when Amy was fluent and less when she was disfluent, structuring communication environments, establishing fluency and increasing challenge in small steps, and building resistance to potential fluency disruption all have roots in fluency shaping. Remaining positive about and toward the child as a communicator, not showing parental upset or frustration when disfluency occurred, creating opportunities for expression of feelings and supporting those expressions, engaging the child in making choices about the treatment experience, and constructing treatment within a play context originate from stuttering modification. However, these distinctions overlap. They become clearer as the stuttering enters the child's view of himself as a person and as a communicator within a social context. Such clarity will be discussed when we address school-age children who stutter, in the next chapter.

Chapter Summary

This chapter reviewed a variety of strategies for assessing and treating preschool children. Two major points were emphasized. First, distinguishing normal disfluency, at-risk disfluency, and incipient stuttering requires analysis of the child's behaviors, thoughts, and feelings, and ultimately a professional judgment on the part of the clinician. Second, intervention with preschool children and their families requires an understanding of the communication environment, full support and involvement of all members within the communication system, and identification and elimination of potential precipitating and perpetuating factors.

We noted that preschool children are in a period of intense development, are insightful, vary in their apprehension of the clinical setting, engage in play and fun, and have a story to tell. Preassessment procedures for preschool children include completing a case history form, obtaining and reviewing an audio or video recording of the child interacting with his family or other members of the household, and making a preliminary phone call to address the family's initial questions and to help prepare the child for the diagnostic evaluation. Assessment procedures include a parent interview, a parent–child interaction, a client–clinician interaction, and trial management. The parent interview is a conversational sharing of information between the clinician and parents. The parent–child interaction is observed by the clinician, who gains a better understanding of how the child and parents interact with and react to each other. The client–clinician interactions are designed to enable the clinician to directly observe the child's fluency and disfluency and the extent to which both are modifiable. These include speech–language sampling and structured activities with and without communication pressure. Trial management gives the clinician an opportunity to use different treatment activities to determine their relative effectiveness with a particular child.

Post-assessment procedures for preschool children include a thorough analysis of speech and language skills, leading to statements of diagnosis, prognosis, and recommendations, all of which are summarized in a post-assessment parent conference. Speech analysis addresses the frequency, types, molecular description, rate, secondary characteristics, severity, impact, and adaptation and consistency of the child's disfluency. A diagnosis is an integration of all information available to determine if the child is stuttering, at risk for stuttering, or demonstrating normal speech fluency. If the child is stuttering or at risk for stuttering, then the clinician must determine if treatment is warranted and recommended, and if so, the nature and focus of treatment. Before making treatment recommendations, the clinician makes a statement of prognosis, which is a prediction of the outcome of a proposed course of treatment. That prediction is based upon relevant factors from retrospective, cross-sectional, and longitudinal investigations. Treatment recommendations may take a variety of forms and are discussed with the parents and other family members.

Treatment for preschool children always includes family intervention and may include direct intervention. The goal of parent intervention is the prevention of stuttering by engaging the parents in an educational experience that allows them to understand what they are already doing that contributes to the development of their child's speech fluency, as well as what needs to be changed. Behavioral recommendations include

(a) reacting to and interacting with the child without drawing unnecessary attention to the disfluency, (b) being good listeners, (c) adjusting (by simplifying, softening, and slowing) the daily speech model to which the child is exposed, (d) maximizing the child's experience with fluency and minimizing that with disfluency, (e) preventing the child from becoming unnecessarily aware of or frustrated over his stuttering, (f) reducing the pace of activities and overall tension, and (g) identifying and reducing or eliminating fluency disrupters. Other suggestions were discussed for helping parents understand and adjust, if necessary, their thoughts and feelings about their child and his stuttering. For cases in which stuttering is indicated more clearly and direct intervention is warranted, the treatment goal for preschool children is achievement of spontaneous fluency and maintenance of a positive attitude toward communication and oneself as a communicator. Four objectives were addressed, including establishing and transferring fluent speech, developing resistance to the potential effects of fluency disrupters, encouraging expressions of feeling as appropriate about communication and oneself as a communicator, and maintaining the fluency inducing effects of treatment. Specific suggestions were presented for achieving each objective. The chapter ended with a clinical portrait of Amy Stiles, a girl who was 3 years 10 months old, with whom the assessment and treatment considerations were applied and discussed.

Chapter Eight Study Questions

1. Normally developing children create opportunities to use and develop language by interacting verbally with adults. How might stuttering in young children affect their development in speech and language and other areas?

2. We noted that there is a fine line between normal disfluency and incipient stuttering. Furthermore, distinguishing normal disfluency, at-risk disfluency, and incipient stuttering requires analysis of the child's behaviors, thoughts, and feelings, in addition to professional judgment. How would you as a clinician make these distinctions and what behaviors, thoughts, and feelings must be considered? What aspects of making these distinctions are concrete, and what is the role of professional judgment?

3. We also noted that intervention with preschool children and their families requires an understanding of the communication environment, full support and involvement of all members within the communication system, and identification and elimination of potential precipitating and perpetuating factors. As the clinician, how would you see to it that all of these requirements are met? What challenges would you foresee? How would you overcome these challenges?

4. We reviewed several precepts of preschool children. How does an awareness of the nature of preschool children impact the assessment and treatment processes? In what ways might such awareness facilitate assessment and treatment? In what ways might such awareness hinder assessment and treatment? How would you ensure the former and prevent the latter?

5. Preassessment, assessment, and post-assessment procedures provide much valuable information that is analyzed by the clinician. What components of this information do you feel are most important? How do you feel each element contributes to the important decisions being made by the clinician?

6. One post-assessment responsibility is speech analysis, which determines the frequency, types, molecular description, rate, secondary characteristics, severity, impact, and adaptation and consistency of the child's disfluency. How would this information

enable you to diagnose if a child is stuttering, at risk for stuttering, or demonstrating normal speech fluency?

7. Another post-assessment responsibility is making a statement of prognosis, which is a prediction of the outcome of a proposed course of treatment. Making such a prediction uniquely reflects the application of a clinician's knowledge and skills. Which of the prognostic indicators reviewed (i.e., from retrospective, cross-sectional, and longitudinal investigations) do you think are most useful and why? What literature supports your impressions? What literature refutes your impressions? How would you use the prognostic indictors to each child's communication advantage without creating artificial or unnecessary limitations?

8. What treatment recommendations do you have for preschool children who are stuttering, at risk for stuttering, or demonstrating normal speech fluency?

9. Results of recent longitudinal investigations of untreated stuttering patterns in preschool children (Yairi, 2004; Yairi & Ambrose, 1992a, 1992b, 1999, 2005) indicate that severe disfluency tends to demonstrate sharp reduction over 3 to 6 months after onset (boys' stuttering tended to persist longer than that of girls), continuing to 12 to 14 months from the time the problem was first noticed. A child who has just begun to stutter has between 65% and 80% chance of natural recovery between 3 and 5 years post-onset (i.e., 20% to 35% chance of persistence). What impact do these findings have on the assessment and treatment processes?

10. Chapters 5, 6, and 7 reviewed intrafamily, extrafamily, and psychotherapeutic intervention considerations, respectively. What impact do these factors have on the assessment and treatment of preschool children and on interactions with members of the family system?

Chapter Nine

School-Age Children Who Stutter

Assessment and Treatment

I watch as my child struggles with his words so much like I have done time and time again. He doesn't have a clue what to do. But he gets through it. Listeners are compassionate. He is very young. He has not missed anything for lack of speech. His awareness is growing. So I wonder how long will it be till others are not compassionate, till they move on to the next person cause they didn't know he was trying to talk, till they figure he just doesn't know what to say, till he's not cute enough for folks to go out of their way to meet him half way.

He needs to learn now what to do. He needs to learn to bring his techniques, however simple, into all of his speech, not just to impress his speech therapist. He needs one or two ways that work, to empower him to face his world with confidence.

I want it now for him. Not after embarrassment rips his confidence away. Not after he throws his dreams away. Not after he gives up dreaming. Not after he thinks he can't talk. Not after his hopes and dreams quit sprouting. Cause that might turn his words inside, words which can't come out. Not after he gives up.

I want it now. While he believes he can talk. While he believes others will listen. While he knows good things can happen. While he's still the master of his world.

I want someone to help him, someone who knows what to do.

(Letter from the mother of a 7-year-old boy who stutters. Subsequent to this letter, both the boy and his mother enrolled in fluency intervention.)

In the present chapter, we will consider school-age children who stutter. Following a structure similar to that used in the previous chapter, we will look first at general precepts, then assessment and treatment procedures and related considerations (working with children who stutter and have concomitant disorders, and working with parents and teachers), and conclude with a descriptive clinical portrait of a school-age child who stutters. In doing so, we will emphasize the following points:

⊞ School-age children who stutter must understand the nature of their own speech fluency and be in control of it before effecting reduction in disfluency.

⊞ Clinicians must manage not only the behavioral characteristics of speech fluency, but also what each child thinks and feels about communication and himself as a communicator.

⊞ Effective intervention requires an understanding of the child's communication environment and active participation of the child, his family, and others in all aspects of treatment planning, implementation, evaluation, and follow-up.

General Precepts About School-Age Children Who Stutter

The following observations can be made about school-age children who stutter. Again, such observations tend to be from a bird's-eye perspective, one that emphasizes group trends. Conture (2001) aptly noted, "People who stutter don't enter your clinical doors in a group; they walk in as individuals" (p. 89). In other words, an individual school-age child or other person who stutters may or may not show similarities to group trends. We noted in Chapter 8 that similarities between an individual and group trends (such as demonstrating adaptation and consistency effects) may indicate just that—similarity, or predictability of behaviors (see Seery, 2005). If an individual's behavior is not similar to group trends, that individual may be a person who stutters but in some respects may be unlike others who stutter, be at-risk for stuttering, or be demonstrating normal disfluency. Distinguishing among these alternative diagnoses is the clinician's responsibility. Conture (2001) noted, "Individual behavior varies around the group's central tendency (e.g., mean), and it is not at all unlikely that one particular individual who stutters may show very little consistency (or minimal adaptation), but still be a person who stutters and needs your services" (p. 89). The same could be said about any other individual characteristic when considered in isolation and compared to that of a group composite. With this caution in mind, we look now at general patterns of school-age children and of those who stutter (Conture & Guitar, 1993; Guitar, 2006; Haynes & Pindzola, 2008; Manning, 2010; W. P. Murphy, Yaruss, & Quesal, 2007a, 2007b; Shapiro, 2002a, 2004a, 2004d, 2004f, 2005):

⊞ School-age children who stutter no longer are beginning to stutter. Typically, their gentle repetitions and prolongation have progressed into struggling with, avoiding, and disguising disfluency and combating frustration and fear (Haynes & Pindzola, 2008). Guitar (2006) characterized the child with intermediate stuttering as follows:

The child with intermediate stuttering is usually an elementary or junior high school student between 6 and 13 years of age who has been stuttering for several years. . . . The typical intermediate stutterer exhibits tense part-word and monosyllabic whole-word repetitions, as well as tense prolongations; however, blocks with tension and struggle are the most evident sign of stuttering. This child may use escape devices, such as body movements or brief verbalizations (e.g., "uh"), to break free of stutters. He may also use various avoidance strategies such as starters, word substitutions, circumlocutions, and evasion of difficult speaking situations. He experiences more frustration and embarrassment than beginning stutterers do and has distinct anticipation of stuttering on specific sounds, words, and many speaking situations. His major fear is the moment of stuttering itself, and he has a definite concept of himself as a stutterer. (p. 350)

- A longer time since onset of stuttering has elapsed for school-age children than for pre-school children. While some children begin to stutter in school, most who enter the first grade have stuttered for at least a year. The additional habit strength of the stuttering acquired from cumulative experience of increasing duration presents a less favorable prognosis and, therefore, unique treatment concerns (Conture & Guitar, 1993).

- School-age children are developing increasing independence from their parents and are spending more time with children and adults other than their primary care providers, siblings, or relatives. However, they continue to be dependent upon parents for guidance, physical care, transportation, and primary needs (Conture & Guitar, 1993).

- School-age children, while becoming increasingly independent from parents, are becoming increasingly dependent on their peers for their social, emotional, and academic development. The child is introduced to and begins to participate in peer pressure, criticism, and social conformity (Conture & Guitar, 1993).

- While becoming less willing to accept advice, direction, and guidance from adults, particularly their parents, school-age children are increasingly influenced by school personnel, one of whom is the speech–language pathologist. Whereas many preschool children are referred for communication assessment or treatment by their parents, school-age children are most often referred by school personnel (Conture & Guitar, 1993). Many children tend to associate the speech–language pathologist with other school personnel who, in some cases, may be penalizing or disturbing listeners. Furthermore, children may associate speech–language pathologists with authority figures (because the child often has no choice about entering treatment), thereby potentially undermining a trusting relationship (Haynes & Pindzola, 2008).

- Generally, school-age children are reluctant or unable to verbalize internal feelings and lack the insight to analyze a problem objectively in order to establish alternative solutions (Haynes & Pindzola, 2008).

Preassessment Procedures

The assessment procedures for the school-age child are similar to those for the preschool child (see Chapter 8). Before the assessment procedures begin, the parent (i.e., primary care provider) completes a case history form in order to provide the clinician with an understanding of the child's developmental and medical history; family structure; communication strengths and limitations; and onset, development, and current perspectives regarding the communication problem. The parent is asked to make an audio or video recording of the child engaged in family interaction so that the clinician can sample the child's speech in that setting and begin to understand the communication dynamics within the family. Again, the clinician makes a preliminary phone call to help prepare the child for the evaluation, to address the parents' questions, and to convey the clinician's support and commitment.

The other people with whom the child spends much of his day need to be involved in preassessment as well. Children who stutter are often identified from communication screening in the schools or are referred by the classroom teacher. If the teacher has not already conveyed preliminary observations, he or she should be invited to do so and to provide an audio or video recording of the child talking in the classroom setting. This gives the clinician another opportunity to see how the child's speech fluency varies by setting and is influenced by other communicative demands. Typically the clinician to whom the child is referred is employed by the school system, so she has an ideal opportunity to observe the child within the classroom before the assessment procedures commence. This provides the clinician with a preliminary impression of the child's communication and social skills.

Assessment Procedures

General Considerations

Most assessments of school-age children who stutter are conducted by the clinician employed in the schools. The assessment procedures as discussed here reflect that assumption. Unlike other clinical settings, where different interviews and observations are conducted at the same scheduled appointment, assessments conducted in the schools often require several different appointments. The appointments generally include a parent interview, teacher interview, and child interview, in addition to observing the child interacting in as many different settings as possible (the recordings provided by the parent and teacher prove invaluable here). The proceedings should be recorded for review and analysis. As noted in Chapter 8, video recording is preferred, but audio recording still provides valuable information.

Parent Interview

Based on information received from the case history form, initial video or audio recordings, the preliminary phone call, and other interactions, the clinician outlines in advance for herself questions and other topics to pursue for clarification or expansion. Because interviews are typically scheduled when school is open, thus conflicting with work and other parent responsibilities, it is common for only one parent to attend the conference. In some cases, clinicians schedule appointments after school hours to accommodate the parents. After a social greeting, the clinician invites the parents to share what they hope to achieve from this meeting. Although school personnel usually initiate the referral, parents often respond with an expression of concern (e.g., "I want to know what we can do to help Billy when he stutters. I want to make sure we are doing the right thing"). The parents' response to my initial question conveys the parents' view regarding their child's and their own needs and objectives. I then share my overall purpose for such a meeting in order to orient the parents, being sure to relate directly to the parents' statement of objective. I explain that I am interested in learning more about the child's communication, past and present, and how the family members communicate with one another to help the child and understand his communication environment outside of school.

Once the parents elaborate the nature of their concern, I ask them to discuss to the best of their memory the onset and development of the problem that they just described. Many of the questions asked of parents of school-age children are the same as those for preschool children, discussed in Chapter 8. Additional questions address how the child's communication skills affect his school experience, including friendships, academic performance, and other factors. As noted in Chapter 8, the parents' description of a typical day in their household helps the clinician understand the family structure and communication dynamics and identify sources of possible communication pressure and inadvertent penalty. Williams (1978) suggested developing a profile from the parents of school-age children who stutter:

> Generally you will want to obtain the parents' views and attitudes about the stuttering problem now and the effect that they perceive it has had on their child. . . . Examples of questions that may be asked include: Why do you believe that he continues to stutter? How serious a problem is it to you or to him? How do you handle it and how do you think it should be handled by other people? In what ways do you feel it has affected your child? What kind of child is he now? In what ways do you think he would be different if he had not stuttered? How does he get along with boys and girls his own age while in school or playing? To what degree has his stuttering influenced his relationship with children or with adults (teacher, grandmother, others)? How has it limited what he has

achieved socially or educationally? How much help does he need in meeting new situations or new problems? What special allowances do you think he should receive because of his stuttering? How independent is he in comparison with other children? How has he reacted to his stuttering? How has he reacted to your help and concern about it? Questions such as these provide a picture, albeit somewhat cloudy, of the ways in which the parents have reacted to their child as a "stutterer"; and it often provides an overview of the way in which he may be reacting to himself. (pp. 68–69)

Teacher Interview

The child spends a substantial portion of each day with his teachers, who observe and interact with him regularly. Teachers know their children—all of them. In our excitement to help a child who stutters, we clinicians must be sensitive to the demands placed upon teachers to meet all of the regular and special needs of all of their children. Teachers provide a valuable and ready source of information as long as we remain interested in and supportive of helping teachers achieve their instructional mission as well. More will be said later in this chapter about how to work with teachers as partners in the intervention process.

Just as we want to learn how the child is functioning in the classroom setting, the teacher wants to understand stuttering and what can be done about it. Again, I recommend inviting the teacher to express what she would like to achieve from the meeting so that her needs are heard, met, and thereby treated as important. Just as we build relationships with children who stutter and their families, so we need to nurture relationships with our professional colleagues, including teachers. Many of the questions presented to parents can also be presented to teachers, thereby guiding the discussion with them as well. Other questions might address the child as a communicator in class and the teacher's feelings about and reactions to the child (Guitar, 2006):

- ⊞ What is the child's communication like in class?
- ⊞ How does he seem to feel about his stuttering and himself as a communicator?
- ⊞ How does his stuttering impact his classroom participation, academic performance, and overall progress?
- ⊞ How does the child interact with other children?
- ⊞ Is the child experiencing any teasing? If so, to what extent does this occur and how does he handle it?
- ⊞ How does the teacher feel about the child's stuttering, and how does it affect the classroom?
- ⊞ Does the teacher feel comfortable meeting the instructional mission while accommodating the child's individual communication needs?

Child Interview

After the necessary permission forms are signed, the clinician schedules through the teacher a relatively convenient time to meet with the child. When possible, I recommend that the child be given at least two alternative times from which to select his preference. We need to show by word and deed that he is important to us. Just as we appreciate being given alternatives from which we might accommodate our busy schedules, so does the child (as well as the parent and teacher). The child is busy and has preferences too. Too often, children are pulled without consideration from their favorite activities (e.g., playground, art, gym, music), those that contribute significantly to building the child's positive self-concept and feeling of accomplishment (see Figure 9.1). Sometimes schedule conflicts are unavoidable. However, the child's schedule, needs, and preferences should be considered.

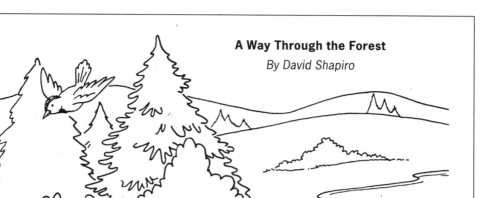

A Way Through the Forest
By David Shapiro

Once there was a boy who was 9 years old. He was not unlike many other children. He usually was happy and lived with his parents, sister, and brother in a house surrounded by a forest that had lots of streams and even a few lakes.

The boy had many friends to play with. His best friend, though, was Buddy, a funny looking dog that had long black, white, and brown hair all over his body and always a wet nose. Buddy and the boy were friends for a long time, in fact, ever since Buddy was a pup and the boy was 3 weeks old. As they grew together, they took many long walks in the woods, and they even fell asleep together in the sun by the stream. Everyone knew when they saw the boy that Buddy was not far away.

One place you would not see Buddy was in school. The boy had many other friends in school, though. He especially enjoyed playing with Billy on the playground and in gym, art, and music. These were the boy's favorite times in school because he felt that he was good at what he did. He could kick the ball higher and farther than most other children; he could run very fast; and he could climb the ropes almost without using his feet. Music was fun too because the boy liked to sing.

But the boy often did not like going to school because it was hard for him to talk in class. The boy stuttered, and he knew it.

Even when he knew the answer to a question, he would not talk because he was sure the children would laugh when he tried to speak.

One time, even the teacher laughed. When the boy tried to take his turn reading out loud, he simply could not say the words. He knew the words, but the sounds just wouldn't come out. Sometimes, trying so hard, the boy sounded like a little grizzly bear.

When the teacher said, "You do know how to read, don't you?" or "You do have a name, don't you?" (when the boy could not say his name), the children laughed. Only Billy never laughed. Billy was the boy's friend.

The boy acted like a good sport, but inside he cried. It hurt to be teased so much. He was a smart boy too. He always got good grades—usually 90 to 95 in all of the subjects, but a 65 in oral reading. That hurt too.

One thing the boy especially did not like was being pulled from the playground, gym, art, or music to go to speech class. These were activities in which the boy felt normal—almost like the other children.

Over the years, the boy worked with many different speech therapists. They usually were nice. There was one that the boy did not like because she always told

(*continues*)

Figure 9.1.   "A Way Through the Forest: One Boy's Story with a Happy Ending." *Note.* From "A Way Through the Forest: One Boy's Story with a Happy Ending," by D. A. Shapiro, March 1995, *The Staff*, pp. 2, 7. Copyright 1995 by J. B. Westbrook/Aaron's Associates. Reprinted with permission.

the boy to read. The boy knew he couldn't read out loud. Why didn't the speech therapist know that? He surely wished he could be playing with Billy or with Buddy. One time, it was so hard for the boy to keep trying to read to the speech therapist that he started to cry and ran out of the room. That was the last time he went to that speech therapist.

One day when the teacher talked to the boy's parents about how hard it was for the boy to talk in class and how unhappy it made the boy feel, the boy's parents decided to take him to a different speech therapist after school. The boy thought that might be a good idea—he didn't like to stutter one bit. "Wouldn't it be wonderful," he thought, "to be able to talk to anybody, just like talking to Buddy?" He never stuttered when he talked to Buddy.

Anyway, the new speech therapist was a man. He didn't tell the boy to read. In fact, he didn't tell the boy to do anything. He asked the boy what he wanted to do. "This is surely different," the boy thought. The boy said that he'd like to walk by a stream, just like he does with Buddy. So that is what they did. Sometimes they talked, and sometimes they didn't. The boy felt that he found another friend. In a funny way, it was like being with the boy's grandpa. The boy and his grandpa often took long walks. That made the boy feel special. Sometimes they talked, and a lot of times they just listened to the stream and walked. That was what the boy was doing with his new speech therapist.

Time passed, as did Buddy, Billy, the boy's grandpa, and the new speech therapist. Although it has been over a quarter of a century since the boy's last walk with the speech therapist, this boy remembers it well. If they could walk together again and "if words could make wishes come true," these would be the boy's words of thanks, and among the thoughts he would dream possible for other children who stutter.

Thank you for listening rather than talking.

Thank you for asking me to share my thoughts and desires, rather than demanding that I read out loud, or fit into a program that didn't fit me.

Thank you for being so interested in my feelings and for reminding me of all the things that you thought I could do so well, rather than reminding me of what I already knew I could not do.

Thank you for helping me to speak more gently by guiding me in what to *do*, rather than by directing me in what *not* to do.

Thank you for talking to me in words that I understood, rather than sounding professional.

Thank you for your patience, understanding, and support, rather than showing me frustration when I did my best, but couldn't succeed.

Thank you for being so enthusiastic and for knowing that at worst, I always did my best.

Thank you for helping my teachers understand stuttering and know how best to deal with it in class.

Thank you for reminding my parents of all of the many things that they did right.

Thank you for caring. With your help, they were all positive that the boy could find his way through the forest.

They were right.

The boy reminds other children, parents, and speech–language pathologists that things that are most meaningful and difficult to achieve often take a long time to accomplish, and those that are seemingly impossible might take a bit longer.

Remain positive. Admit honestly to when and what you don't know. Know when to seek help. Recognize feelings for what they are and are not. Continue to believe in yourselves and the healthy process of constructive change. You're in good company. Good luck.

Figure 9.1. (continued)

When meeting with the child, the clinician must convey her sincere interest in the child as a multifaceted person, not just as one who stutters (Guitar, 1997). How can we learn about the child as a person without first addressing his interests, talents, hobbies, family relationships, and friendships? Likewise, the clinician must present herself as an interesting person too, one who is inviting yet reflective, and positive and nurturing by nature. Intervention with people who stutter is about building relationships. How can we hope to convey our sincere interest in the child as a person, when seemingly within the same breath as having just introduced ourselves, we are asking the child to describe his problem? It does not take long to establish a foundation, but the time spent is irreplaceable. No dwelling will stand for long without a foundation. Building a foundation and working with a child who stutters is a form of counseling. "Simply stated, counseling involves talking *with* another person" (Williams, 2003, p. 54). Talking *with* does not mean talking *at, below, around,* or *above*. It means helping a child to see more clearly what he is good at and the nature of all of his fluency. From this positive and informed framework, the child can explore what he is doing that results in speech fluency and what he is doing that results in speech disfluency. We help the child make this distinction and guide the child in how to do more of what he is already doing that results in speech fluency. Focusing first on the speech fluency defuses the child's defenses, which more often than not have risen to the surface and are consuming the child's energies to control or deny their existence. The child comes to feel in control and successful in being able to do more of what seemed so elusive. This experience is a gateway to the child's emotions, which often are expressed in laughter or, less frequently, tears.

This section addresses how to provide school-age children such an experience by providing them guidance in what to *do*, rather than in what *not* to do. Providing guidance in what to do (what I am recommending) helps the child become focused on fluency. The child comes to see that his talking, like other behavior, is controllable. My experience has been that by providing the child guidance in how to do more of what he is already doing that facilitates fluency heightens his awareness of what he is doing right, helps him feel in control of his fluency, and brings a positive outlook and peak motivation to the experience. Within this framework, much of the disfluent speech literally drops away. The residual disfluency is addressed directly, however, within the positive framework already established.

The reader may sense my concern that much of the intervention for people who stutter (children and adults) focuses on eliminating the disfluency (directing a person in what *not* to do), rather than in facilitating the fluency (discussing, demonstrating, and directing/coaching in what to *do*). This may seem to some as just a semantic quibble. It is not. To me, this distinction is at the very heart of successful intervention and working with people who stutter. It seems that many clinicians, albeit sincere and well meaning, tend to focus on what the client should not do because that (i.e., what the client is doing wrong, or what is not facilitative to fluency) is so readily apparent. What seems puzzling to clinicians is the importance of knowing what the client is doing right (i.e., facilitative of fluency) and therefore what the client needs to do more often to increase the fluency— which effectively eliminates the disfluency. In other words, what the client should not do is clearer than what the client should do. This discussion neither ignores that fluency and disfluency are multidimensional, complex variables, nor is intended to criticize clinicians. Significantly, however, the majority of clinicians holding master's degrees have expressed a lack of confidence in treating people who stutter and a need for direction in planning and implementing such treatment (Bloodstein & Bernstein Ratner, 2008; Cooper & Cooper, 1985; Healey & Scott, 1995; Mallard, Gardner, & Downey, 1988; Manning, 2004, 2010; St. Louis & Durrenberger, 1993; Williams, 1971; Yaruss, 1999a; Yaruss & Quesal, 2002; Yaruss, Quesal, & Murphy, 2002; Yaruss, Quesal, & Reeves et al., 2002). This general attitude is not surprising given the changes by ASHA in 1993 that eliminated certification requirements for specific academic and clinical experience in the area of fluency disorders (see ASHA, 2009a, 2009b; Manning, 2010; Starkweather & Givens-Ackerman, 1997; Tellis, Bressler, & Emerick, 2008; Yaruss, 1999a; Yaruss & Quesal, 2002), combined with a discouraging influence from instructors who have been heard to say, "Don't spend your time working with people who stutter; work with people you can help" (Manning, 2004, p. 60). Manning (2010) noted, "The research leaves little doubt that some professional clinicians actively avoid assisting individuals who stutter" (p. 6; see also Tellis et al., 2008; Yaruss, 1999a; Yaruss & Quesal, 2002). (The implications of ASHA's certification requirements and training standards will be discussed in Chapter 12.)

Meeting with the child serves several functions. We already discussed the importance of establishing a foundation as mutually interested and interesting people. The clinician conveys her understanding and acceptance of the child independent of the child's speech fluency. The clinician is interested in observing the child's speech directly to determine the degree to which it is affected by structure, linguistic complexity, and communicative pressure; the degree to which it is modifiable; and the relative developmental level of the child's behaviors, feelings, and attitudes. The speech sample collected will be used for analysis and comparison to others collected from different speaking contexts. For the sake of organization, the initial interaction between the child and the clinician will be discussed in terms of speech–language sampling and structured activities with and without communication pressure.

Speech–Language Sample Without Communicative Pressure

While inquiring about the child as a person and relating to his experiences, the clinician collects a speech–language sample of no less than 300 words (Conture, 1997, 2001), or approximately 5 minutes of the child's talking (approximately 10–15 minutes of real time). As noted in Chapter 8, the purpose is to develop a corpus from which to assess the child's communication skills, including speech fluency. Once the clinician and the child have established a foundation as people with lives and interests, they may talk about their respective roles within the school. The clinician might ask the child about his friends, favorite subjects, and classroom activities. Deliberately steering the conversation toward the communication experience, the clinician asks the child how he feels about his communication skills. If an anchor is needed, the clinician may ask the child to evaluate himself on a scale from 1 to 10 for different interests and talents already discussed (such as basketball, spelling, art, and others) and then for talking skills. This invites a frank, open, accepting conversation about the child's beliefs regarding what he feels he does relatively well versus poorly; his assessment of himself as a communicator; what he feels helps him to talk better; and related thoughts and feelings. For similar purposes, the clinician might ask the child what he would want a new friend to know about him before they met. Often the child mentions his family structure, interests, and hobbies. Whether or not the child mentions his stuttering can be a significant reflection of the extent to which the child defines himself on the basis of speech fluency and can serve as a window into the child's developing self-perception.

Williams (1971) indicated that school-age children vary widely in the consistency of their stuttering and the degree to which their feelings and attitudes have been affected by the stuttering experience. And, while adults often talk about stuttering or not stuttering with children who stutter, they rarely talk about talking, how we talk, and different ways of talking. The child will come to see that both fluency and disfluency represent different ways of talking and the consequence doing things differently. Such a realization invites the child to make choices and helps him to understand that ways of talking are potentially controllable. Among the purposes of the initial meeting are to collect the child's current ideas and assessments and to begin to present the child with alternatives to consider. The child begins to talk about talking and to think about his own thoughts about his speech and himself as a communicator. The clinician guides the discussion while assessing the child's behaviors, feelings, and attitudes.

Within the process as described, many different topics are addressed. The child's level of awareness guides the directness and the content of my questions. The child may be asked why he feels he is meeting with the clinician and what he hopes to get out of the meeting. The child's response will begin to indicate his level of awareness or concern. If the child responds with, "I don't know," the clinician may do some gentle probing ("What do you think? What did your teacher or parents tell you about why we were meeting?"). If the child responds with, "I don't talk well," or "'Cause I stutter," these responses need to be probed further ("What do you mean?"). In any case, the clinician should be careful not to manipulate what the child says (i.e., not put words into the child's mouth), all the while encouraging free expression without penalty or judgment. Guitar (2006) noted that children may respond reluctantly to invitations to express feelings because adults have inadvertently rejected or negated their feelings by such comments as, "You don't need to feel that way" or "Why do you let it bother you?" Expression of feeling requires a trusting relationship that may take several meetings to establish. Indeed, the clinician should not confront the child immediately with alternative interpretations; rather, she should nurture the child's expression while actively listening and clarifying as appropriate to help both better understand the child's thoughts. Depending on the child's level of awareness, he may be asked when his stuttering was first noticed, how it has developed and changed over time, why he believes he talks this way, what he does to make talking easier, how others (such as family, teachers, friends, and others) react to his stuttering, where and with whom talking is relatively harder and easier, and how he feels about the way he talks and about himself when he talks that way.

Others recommend different strategies to gain similar knowledge about and from children within the context of conversational exchange. Williams (1978) suggested that the clinician needs to understand the child's view of the talking world and his place in it. She needs to learn the child's views regarding his verbal interactions at home and at school, specifically his perception of different people's reactions and how he feels about the experience of stuttering. Williams (1978, pp. 69–70) recommended a series of questions, summarized here as follows:

- "Whom do you like to talk to?" The clinician might ask, "Whom do (and don't) you like to talk to at (home, school, and other settings)?" "Who likes (doesn't like) to talk to you at (home, school, and other settings)?" Each reply might be expanded by asking, "Why do you think this is so?"

- "Who talks the most?" These questions include, "Who talks the most (the least) at (home, school)?" "Whom do you talk to the most (the least) at (home, school)?" "Whom does your (father, mother, brother, teacher) talk to the most (the least)?" "Why?"

- "Who interrupts?" "Who interrupts the most (the least) at (home, school)?" "Who interrupts (father, mother, brother) the most (the least)?" "Whom do you interrupt the most (the least) at (home, school)?" "Why?"

- "Who are good talkers?" "Who is the best (poorest) talker at (home, school)?" "Why?" If the child has mentioned himself directly, the clinician might follow up with where the child puts himself on the scale from best to poorest talker at (home, school).

- "When do you want to talk well?" "Are there times when you want to talk extra well?" "Where?" "Why?" "Are there times when you don't care particularly how you talk?" "Where?" Why?"

- "When do you want to talk more than you do?" These questions include, "When would you like to talk more than you do at (home, school)?" "When do you want to talk less than you do?" "Why?" "Do you think other children feel this way too?"

"Who listens?" The clinician might ask, "Who pays the most (least) attention to you when you talk at (home, school)?" "What do you like listeners to do when you talk to them (for example, look down, look at you, smile, interrupt, talk for you)?" "Who does what you like (don't like) at (home, school)?" "Why do you think they do it?"

Questions such as these are intended to facilitate the conversational exchange, not to inhibit or overly structure it. Depending on the child's unique experience (stuttering behaviors, feelings, attitudes, willingness to share, and other factors), the conversation may go in a number of different directions. As already noted, the sample is intended to foster a supportive, trusting relationship and will be used for subsequent communication analysis.

Structured Activities Without Communicative Pressure

After collecting a rich conversational sample, I engage the school-age child in a number of more structured activities that yield elicited responses for subsequent analysis. Again, we are comparing the child's communication skills, including speech fluency across speaking contexts, for assessment and differential diagnosis (to determine if a disorder of fluency is present, and if so, what type). Unlike the procedures for the preschool child, reviewed in Chapter 8, those for the school-age child include a sample of reading if the child is a reader. In kindergarten or first grade, as children are first learning to read, observed disfluency may represent more language disfluency than speech disfluency. In other words, the assessment of speech fluency within reading may be confounded by the reading difficulty as well as the demand placed on the child to remain fluent.

Ferreting out the speech disfluency that is independent of the influence of reading presents a challenge for clinicians. The same challenge is encountered when the clinician is assessing older school-age children (or adults) who have a reading disability. In such cases, the clinician compares the speech fluency within and between reading samples, as well as between reading and conversation and other more structured tasks. With these cautions in mind, I have found it useful with older school-age children to sample their speech during reading as many as three different passages. One should be easy, or below the child's reading ability; one at his reading level; and one deliberately above his level. When selecting a fairly challenging passage, I use one of the phonetically balanced passages not only to sample speech fluency but also to screen for articulation errors or phonological processes; that is, I choose reading selections that contain all of the speech sounds in the English language (e.g., "Arthur, the Young Rat," which contains 180 words; found in Williams et al., 1978, p. 276).

Other structured activities are similar to those reviewed in the previous chapter:

- Telling about a current event, holiday, or possession
- Explaining a process or procedure, such as a familiar game or activity
- Responding to questions requiring answers of differing length and complexity
- Repeating words and sentences of varied length and complexity
- Commenting on pictures (by naming objects, making short phrases in response to "What's going on in the picture?," and telling stories)
- Other activities, reviewed previously (e.g., automatic speech, echoic speech, speaking alone, monologue, talking with puppet, command speech, talking with gestures, talking with phonemic difficulty, talking on the telephone)

Speech–Language Sample and Structured Activities with Communicative Pressure

Once the speech–language sample and structured activities without communicative pressure are completed, different talking activities are entertained with communicative pressure. The purpose of having the child engage in talking with communicative pressure is to assess the relative impact of perceived communicative pressure (of time pressure, linguistic ambiguity, and violation of conversational rules, among others) on the child's speech fluency. Some activities already completed that may have involved some communicative pressure are reading a difficult passage, repeating long and complex words, and responding to questions about speaking experiences at home or at school that might be emotionally loaded for a particular child. Other activities with more distinct and deliberate communicative pressure might include playing games in which time pressure is a part of the competition (e.g., games in which each player must be the first to verbally identify something, games in which a finite time, of say 30 seconds, is allowed to complete a verbal description). Other pressured activities might involve rushed behavior (the clinician increases her own rate of speech, hand, and overall body movements and extraneous gestures, and speed of requesting answers; or directs the child to "hurry up"), interruptions (taking a conversational turn before the child has completed his, or asking a question and then asking another before the child finishes the answer to the first), loss of attention (doing something else when the child is relating an event), or requesting the child to say something else (e.g., "I didn't get that. What did you say?").

Other challenges are offered by abruptly shifting topics (e.g., introducing a topic prematurely that is unrelated to the one being discussed by the child), overstepping boundaries of the child's linguistic competence (using vocabulary that is too complex or addressing topics that are conceptual and out of the child's experiential domain), introducing linguistic ambiguity (contradicting things said by the child or clinician), or introducing verbal absurdity (saying things that border on foolishness, such as addressing the child by the wrong name, talking about a pictured girl as "he," or telling the child a joke where the punch line makes no sense). Similarly, the child may be asked to tell a joke, an experience during which linguistic demand is high. All the while, the clinician must be sensitive to the child's feelings and inform him, when appropriate, as to why she is engaging in speaking activity with deliberate communicative pressure. The clinician might say, "What I just said might have seemed a little odd. What we are doing helps us to see the impact of pressure or rush on your present degree of fluency." Incidentally, engaging in such pressure is particularly important when the child presents no observable sign of speech disfluency. Such pressure increases the demand placed upon the child's ability to remain fluent, thus eliciting disfluency when it is not otherwise observed.

Trial Management

The assessment activities discussed to this point enable the clinician to evaluate the school-age child's speech fluency, related attitudes and feelings, and other aspects of communication, in order to arrive at a diagnosis. Furthermore, the data collected provide a baseline of the child's communication behavior from which progress in treatment can be monitored. From the information collected, the clinician decides whether more formal evaluation of articulation or phonology and language is necessary. If the child demonstrates symptoms of disfluency (during the speaking activities or during elicitation) or behaviors suggestive of negative attitudes, thoughts, or feelings associated with communication, then the clinician engages the child in a variety of trial management techniques based on principles of fluency shaping and stuttering modification. The management techniques become increasingly differentiated for school-age children (compared to those for preschool children) because the stuttering behaviors and related feelings and attitudes are likely to be more developed. These techniques that are used during the assessment session (or phase, if over more than one session) help the clinician determine the child's responsiveness to different treatment strategies, thus contributing to the design of specific recommendations.

Fluency Shaping

Fluency shaping techniques include engaging the child in singing a short song and reciting a riddle or poem in chorus with the clinician. As noted earlier, these activities are essential for differential diagnosis. One would expect a child who stutters to demonstrate consistent fluency during singing (except perhaps when initiating a new passage or bar following a pause) and choral speaking or choral reading. If the child does not, the clinician must entertain the possibility that another fluency disorder is operating. Other fluency shaping techniques include establishing fluency (using slightly prolonged vowels, soft articulatory contacts on consonants, and natural suprasegmental features) through modeling, choral speaking, using mechanical devices (such as a delayed auditory feedback machine, metronome, or others referred to previously), or other externally driven methods. For children demonstrating more involved symptoms of disfluency, the clinician may first establish a fluent syllable and systematically shape it into increasingly longer and more complex units, such as monosyllabic words, polysyllabic words, phrases, and, eventually, sentences. This can be done first by imitation, moving to delayed imitation, and elicitation through picture cards, and ultimately moving to more spontaneous forms. The clinician provides verbal praise and other forms of positive reinforcement as a consequence of and contingent on a fluent utterance.

Stuttering Modification

One of the major objectives of stuttering modification is to learn that there are different ways to stutter. One can stutter hard or soft, long or short, loud or quiet, tense or relaxed, or frustrated or calm, among others. We want the child to experiment with us and thereby to realize that talking is something that we do; it doesn't just happen. Both fluency and disfluency are the consequences of something that we do differently with our speech apparatus. There are many ways to help the child achieve this discovery. In trial management, we use several different procedures and gain an impression of the child's relative responsiveness to the methodology. These and other methods will be used at a later time in scheduled treatment, should it be recommended. For example, we may use any of the following methods, among others:

⚇ Model slow, relaxed, prolonged speech with soft articulatory contacts (Clinician: "Wwhy donn't wwe llook at thhat picture nnext?").

⚇ Model easier versions of the child's stuttering in a modeling and expansion format (Child: "That that that i-i-i-i-s muh-muh-muh-muh-my buh-buh-buh-boo-k." Clinician: "I ssee thhat bbook iis yyours. Hhow abbout iif wwe take a llook aat iit?").

⚇ Demonstrate easy and eventually hard disfluencies in the clinician's speech. First offer descriptive, emotionally neutral self-comments (Clinician: "Gosh, that was a little hard") and later invite the child's comments and assessment (Clinician: "What did you think about that one?" Child: "That was wild. Was that a real one?").

⚇ Identify instances when the child uses gentle speech onset with light articulatory contact, then describe what he did ("You really used slow, gentle speech when you said the *b* in bboy. You barely touched your lips together and that was great"), and offer positive visual and verbal feedback for successful or otherwise sincere efforts (the clinician will have a positive facial expression and say something like "Yes!" in a bold voice). This procedure is intended to do two things: to heighten the child's awareness of the fluent speech that he already possesses (both how much and what types), and to model for the child how to identify his fluency, describe what he did, and offer positive feedback (three steps that at first the clinician does for the child, and eventually the child will do for himself).

⚇ Provide the child with one or two behaviors on which to focus, providing activities that he can do. For example, the clinician may model slow (evenly paced) and gentle speech, pointing out that the two behavioral foci are slow and gentle. These two will enable the child to focus his energies, thus maximizing positive change in his speech. More will be said about this in the section titled "Treatment."

⊡   Explore and support the child for expressions of feeling related to stuttering or himself as a communicator. Given the school-age child's experience with disfluency and degree of emotional involvement, discussion about feelings and attitudes tends to be more direct than that with the preschool child, but less direct than that with the adult.

⊡   Engage the child in a discussion of where and with whom he would expect his speech to be more fluent and less fluent and related feelings. This type of hierarchy can be started in the assessment session, continued in the interim before treatment, and discussed and completed in the initial treatment sessions. This activity can be conducted with significant others as well, including teachers and parents, among others. Essentially, this activity is one of several that facilitates transfer from the beginning and helps individualize treatment.

Post-Assessment Procedures

Once the clinician has collected a speech–language sample, engaged the child in more structured activities—first without and then with communication pressure—and collected her preliminary impressions, it is time to analyze the results more thoroughly. She needs to do the following:

⊡   Represent both quantitatively (using frequency counts, means, ranges, or other summary statistics) and qualitatively (narrowly describing) the nature of the speech fluency and disfluency across speaking contexts and time. This includes behaviors, feelings, thoughts, and attitudes. The reader may want to review the descriptive protocols discussed in Chapter 8.

⊡   Represent the other characteristics of communication (language fluency in terms of syntactic and morphologic, semantic, pragmatic, and phonologic and articulation competence).

From the information collected so far, the clinician conducts an analysis from which she makes statements of diagnosis, prognosis, and specific intervention recommendations, in addition to referral to other professionals as appropriate. These results are conveyed to the significant parties during individual or group meetings (involving parents, teachers, or other professionals on the Pupil Planning Teams; see B. J. Moore & Montgomery, 2008) and summarized within a report.

Speech Analysis

Analyses of the speech samples collected from preschool children, discussed earlier, are conducted on the conversational and structured speech from school-age children. These will be reviewed briefly here (see Chapter 8). The analyses, assuming the word to be the unit of measure, include frequency of speech disfluency, type of speech disfluency, molecular description of disfluency, and rate of speech, in addition to several other measures. These will be discussed in turn.

Frequency of Speech Disfluency
Frequency of speech disfluency refers to the amount of disfluency, without consideration of the individual types or relative severity, that is contained within the child's speech. Reported as a percentage, the *disfluency frequency index* (DFI) is computed by dividing the total number of disfluent words by the total number of words spoken (both disfluent and fluent), and then multiplying the resulting decimal by 100 to achieve the percentage. The frequency of speech disfluency is typically reported as a percentage of 100 words spoken, averaged over samples of 300 or 400 words.

Type of Speech Disfluency

Type of speech disfluency refers to the individual proportions for each type of disfluency. It is computed by dividing the number of disfluencies of each individual type by the total number of disfluent words, and then multiplying by 100.

Molecular Description of Disfluency

The molecular description of disfluency includes the duration and frequency (reported in terms of total, mean, and range) of the most prominent or otherwise significant forms of disfluency (particularly within-word disfluencies).

Rate of Speech

Rate of speech refers to the number of words spoken per minute. The more a person stutters, the more his rate of speech is reduced. As treatment decreases the degree and amount of disfluency, rate should steadily increase and approximate normal standards. Rate is computed by dividing the number of words the child has spoken by the child's talk time in minutes. As noted in Chapter 8, it is helpful for purposes of comparison to know what rate of speech is considered average or "normal" for children who do not stutter. Such information was provided by Sturm and Seery (2007) and Guitar (2006).

Sturm and Seery (2007) reported the speech rate in both words and syllables per minute for 36 children, aged 7 years (range = 7.0 to 7.11; mean age 7.3), 9 years (range = 9.0 to 9.7; mean age 9.4), and 11 years (range = 11.0 to 11.7; mean age 11.4), in conversation (unstructured language samples from open-ended questions) and narratives (monologues from a verbal prompt without visual stimuli, from a verbal prompt with visual stimuli, and from story retelling without visual stimuli). Each age group contained 12 children, 6 boys and 6 girls. Sturm and Seery's (2007) findings revealed the following:

⚏ In *words per minute*, the average (i.e., mean) speech rate in conversation for 7-year-old children was 117.7 (SD = 18 words per minute; range = 91.1–152.3); for 9-year-old children it was 133.5 (SD = 15.9 words per minute; range = 103.2–154.9); and for 11-year-old children it was 133.8 (SD = 14.4 words per minute; range = 112.3–160.7). In words per minute, the average speech rate in narratives for 7-year-old children was 124.6 (SD = 18.5 words per minute; range = 86.7–153.5); for 9-year-old children it was 136.9 (SD = 12.5 words per minute; range = 110.9–155.5); and for 11-year-old children it was 142.8 (SD = 16.6 words per minute; range = 113.3–177.6). Combined across age groups, the average speech rate in words per minute for conversation was 128.3 (SD = 17.4 words per minute; range = 91.1–160.7) and for narratives was 134.8 (SD = 17.4 words per minute; range = 86.7–177.6).

⚏ In *syllables per minute*, the average speech rate in conversation for 7-year-old children was 144.3 (SD = 22.9 syllables per minute; range = 108.7–194.9); for 9-year-old children it was 163.4 (SD = 20.1 syllables per minute; range = 122.8–190.0); and for 11-year-old children it was 162.1 (SD = 17.5 syllables per minute; range = 131.8–192.8). In syllables per minute, the average speech rate in narratives for 7-year-old children was 145.0 (SD = 21.1 syllables per minute; range = 100.0–174.5); for 9-year-old children it was 162.0 (SD = 15.0 syllables per minute; range = 133.8–177.8); and for 11-year-old children it was 172.2 (SD = 21.3 syllables per minute; range = 137.5–216.0). Combined across age groups, the average speech rate in syllables per minute for conversation was 156.6 (SD = 21.6 syllables per minute; range = 108.7–194.9) and for narratives it was 159.7 (SD = 22.0 syllables per minute; range = 100.0–216.0).

Guitar (2006) reported the speech rate in syllables per minute for school-age children in Vermont as follows: Children who were 6, 8, 10, and 12 years old demonstrated the following ranges in *syllables spoken per minute*: age 6 years, 140–175; age 8 years,

150–180; age 10 years, 165–215; and age 12 years, 165–220. Neither additional statistical data nor data for rate of speech in words per minute were available.

Secondary Characteristics

The secondary or associated characteristics, both speech-related (such as audible inhalations or exhalations, pitch rises, oral and neck tension) and non-speech-related (such as facial, head, eye movement or tension), are quantified and qualified. These may reflect the child's developing awareness of stuttering, coping mechanisms during stuttering, or attempts to prevent stuttering.

Severity Rating and Impact Assessment

The severity rating and impact assessment measures the child's relative degree of stuttering involvement, considering a variety of speech and nonspeech factors. As discussed in Chapter 8, use of the *Stuttering Severity Instrument–Fourth Edition* (SSI-4; Riley, 2009), the *Overall Assessment of the Speaker's Experience of Stuttering* (OASES; Yaruss & Quesal, 2006, 2008), or other instruments (including diagnostic, severity, and predictive scales for assessing overt features of stuttering and perception/attitude scales and situation/avoidance checklists for assessing covert features of stuttering; Haynes & Pindzola, 2008) helps to objectify assessment of relative severity and impact of a speaker's stuttering over time and across speakers. These data prove helpful for planning, monitoring, and adjusting treatment and for conducting treatment outcomes research. However, the information provided by such instruments is typically confirmatory, if not redundant, with the other quantitative and qualitative information collected.

Adaptation and Consistency

Adaptation and *consistency* refer to the degree to which an individual's disfluency resembles that of people who stutter (as a group). Specifically, with repeated recitation of the same material, adaptation is the tendency for overall stuttering to decrease; consistency is the tendency for stuttering to occur on the same sounds or words.

Feelings and Attitudes

The assessment of feelings and attitudes is pivotal to a clinician's understanding of a client's stuttering experience. It is an assessment of the degree to which a speaker is experiencing covert involvement related to the experience of stuttering and the relative impact of the stuttering on his view of himself as a person and as a communicator, as a member of society, and as a citizen of the world. Haynes and Pindzola (2008) reviewed 15 available protocols. These forms indeed are useful, as indicated previously. Nevertheless, I remain convinced that the most sensitive measure of a child's or any other client's feelings and attitudes related to communication is the clinician's judgment, based on objective observation, active listening, and an open heart and mind, all of which maximize the keenest of clinical tools—namely, a clinician's eyes and ears. Some years ago (Shapiro, 2000), I redefined ASHA's CCC (i.e., the Certificate of Clinical Competence) for clinical training in stuttering to represent Commitment, Compassion, and Competence, which relate directly to assessment of feelings and attitudes. More will be said about the necessary competencies of a clinician, the client–clinician relationship, and the making of a clinician in Chapters 11 and 12.

Other Factors

"Other Factors" is an open category that invites assessment of tempo, regularity, relative tension, smoothness of transitions, and physical concomitants, in addition to any other overt or covert features not yet reported. These might include interpersonal dynamics within the family and other communication systems, co-occurring challenges (e.g., learning, literacy, attention deficit, auditory processing, neurophysiological, and behavioral disorders; see also Blood, Blood, Kreiger, O'Conner, & Qualls, 2009), positive and negative reactions to the communication experience, and any evidence of social intimidation or bullying (W. P. Murphy et al., 2007a, 2007b).

Diagnosis

From the assessment and evaluation of all information available, the clinician makes a statement of diagnosis regarding the child's communication skills. This is where she determines the nature of the child's speech fluency and disfluency, stating whether he demonstrates stuttering, is at risk for stuttering, or demonstrates normal disfluency (in addition to interpreting the child's competence in language, articulation and phonology, and voice). If the child's disfluency is observed and of concern, the clinician distinguishes between stuttering and other disorders of fluency. In any case, the clinician must establish if treatment is warranted and recommended, and if so, what should be the nature and focus of the intervention. As already noted, the experience of arriving at a diagnosis is dynamic and continues to respond to new information as it becomes available.

Prognosis and Recommendations

The child's prognosis for improvement in the area of speech fluency is derived from a variety of sources. These include the assessment and evaluation results, the child's response to trial management, the clinician's professional experience with other school-age children who stutter, and relevant clinical literature. The following factors are associated with a more positive prognosis (Haynes & Pindzola, 2008):

- ⊞ *No previous unsuccessful treatment.* An absence of treatment seems more conducive to success than a history of treatment failure.
- ⊞ *A cooperative family system.* In effective family systems, family members, particularly parents, are willing to participate in a program of family counseling and to assume an active role in the treatment process.
- ⊞ *Cooperative interdisciplinary team members, including teachers and allied professionals.* The more the team members work together and communicate, the more potent the treatment effect.
- ⊞ *More severe stuttering pattern.* Although it may appear counterintuitive, school-age children with more severe stuttering tend to have a better prognosis; those with milder stuttering tend to show little improvement. As noted earlier, children with more severe stuttering have more to gain from treatment and thus may be more highly motivated.
- ⊞ *More positive self-concept of the child.* The more the child views himself as an effective, or potentially effective, communicator and the more actively engaged he is in all aspects of the treatment process, the more positive the treatment outcome.
- ⊞ *No other significant problems.* Other problems that may hinder progress include reading difficulty, learning disability, and academic difficulty, independent of stuttering.
- ⊞ *Other available resources.* Other resources include skill in athletics, music, scouting, biking, and so forth. When a child defines himself on the basis of varied interest and resources, the relative significance of stuttering to his self-concept tends to be reduced, thus leading to a more positive treatment outcome.
- ⊞ *Regular and relatively intensive treatment.* Some clinical literature (G. Andrews et al., 1983; Haynes & Pindzola, 2008) indicates a greater amount of treatment (three or four contacts per week) to be predictive of a more positive treatment outcome. As I will discuss in the treatment section, I have found that frequent contacts with a clinician tend to build communication dependence of the client on the clinician, rather than communication

independence. I have found that the more regular the treatment (i.e., weekly) and the more emphasis there is on transfer activities from the very beginning of treatment (such as engagement of the child and others in treatment that occurs between scheduled sessions), the more positive the treatment outcome and the more the child develops communication independence.

The information leading to the diagnosis is combined with prognostic indicators. These factors are integrated with intrafamily, extrafamily, and psychotherapeutic intervention considerations, all of which play a major role in designing treatment recommendations. Intrafamily considerations focus on the way the child views himself as a communicator who is successful or potentially successful (personal construct) and the extent to which members of the family system communicate openly, support each other, and sincerely participate within the clinical process (family systems). Extrafamily considerations address the degree to which the members of the interdisciplinary team communicate openly and contribute to the integrated fluency intervention program (interdisciplinary teaming), and multicultural factors that might impact planning for, conducting, and interpreting the treatment experience (multicultural awareness). Psychotherapeutic considerations relate to the degree of involvement of both overt and covert factors and seek to establish objectives that are appropriate to each individual (fluency shaping, stuttering modification). Together, this information yields informed treatment recommendations.

Post-Assessment Interview with the Parents, Teacher, and Other Participants

In clinical settings, post-assessment conferences are held immediately after the evaluation. In school settings, however, these conferences are generally scheduled by subsequent individual appointments and group meetings of the Pupil Planning Teams. In any case, the purposes are the same: to summarize the results of assessment, provide recommendations, and discuss any questions that remain (B. J. Moore & Montgomery, 2008). It always is helpful to address the needs and concerns raised by the parents and teachers, and to begin by expressing positive observations about the child's communication skills and about the adults' interactions with the child. This positive tone sets the style of interaction for all involved. Be negative, and the intervention experience will be problem focused and one of repairing the child's and the family's communication deficits. Be positive, realistic, and optimistic about designing strategies, achieving communication improvement, and working toward realizing fluency potential, and the intervention process will become solution and strategy focused, where all work together and support one another.

In the post-assessment conference, I summarize in understandable terms the characteristics of the child's fluency and disfluency. Some of the information that is reviewed for the parents of preschool children regarding the development of speech fluency and the nature of developmental stuttering is reviewed for parents and teachers. Again, protocols that help visualize the development of disfluency (see Table 8.1, Figure 8.2, and Figure 8.3) prove helpful during our conversations. I try to address their questions about causality by summarizing what we know about predisposing factors and the importance of identifying and controlling for precipitating and perpetuating factors. I offer recommendations, remembering the importance of not just telling, but discussing, demonstrating, and directing/coaching. Various resources that review and expand on the points made within the conference are recommended to parents and teachers. These resources include the booklets mentioned in Chapter 8, as well as "A Way Through the Forest: One Boy's Story with a Happy Ending" (Shapiro, 1995; Figure 9.1). Many booklets are available from the Stuttering Foundation of America (in English as well as other languages): *If Your Child Stutters: A Guide for Parents*; *Notes to the Teacher: The Child Who Stutters at School*; *Stuttering and Your Child: Help for Parents*; *Stuttering and Your Child: Questions and Answers*; *If You Think Your Child Is Stuttering: New Tips for Parents*; *7 Tips for Parents*; *8 Tips for Teachers*; *Trouble at Recess*; and *Sometimes I Just Stutter*. The Stuttering Foundation of America also has these DVDs: *Stuttering and Your Child: Help for Parents*; *Stuttering: For Kids by Kids*; *The School-Age Child Who Stutters*; *Stuttering: Straight Talk for Teachers*; and *Therapy in Action: The School-Age Child Who Stutters*. Many other excellent materials are available from the National Stuttering Association.

Treatment

Thus far in the present chapter, we have characterized school-age children and reviewed a variety of assessment procedures. Now we take a look at an integration of treatment procedures addressing the behaviors, thoughts, and feelings of school-age children who stutter.

Goals

The treatment goals for the school-age child who stutters are spontaneous or controlled fluency and establishment or maintenance of a positive attitude toward communication and oneself as a communicator.

Objectives

The objectives for a school-age child who stutters are to increase and transfer fluent speech, to develop resistance to potential fluency disrupters, to establish or maintain positive feelings about communication and oneself as a communicator, and to maintain the fluency inducing effects of treatment on communication-related behaviors, thoughts, and feelings.

Rationale

On the surface, the goals and objectives for the school-age child who stutters sound similar to those for preschool children. While the goals of spontaneous fluency and a positive attitude about the communication experience and oneself as a communicator are common to both groups, the treatment procedures differ based upon the changing needs of the child and intrafamily, extrafamily, and psychotherapeutic considerations.

The Changing Needs of the Child

Typically, school-age children who stutter no longer are beginning to stutter. A longer time has elapsed since the onset of stuttering for school-age children than for preschool children. Increased personal independence from parents is paired with greater dependence on peers and others within the social and educational context. School-age children become aware of and attend to how they are perceived by others. This social consciousness takes the form of peer pressure, criticism, and social conformity. School-age children who stutter have an additional factor that operates in how others perceive them and how they perceive themselves. Their developing independence and concomitant need for control over their lives is met with an increasing challenge. Stuttering is experienced as a loss of control, the antithesis of the social perception that children who stutter are attempting to manage. This internal conflict experienced by the school-age child who stutters forces an adjustment in how he perceives himself and what he predicts about himself. This conflict is often experienced as disequilibrium, frustration, feelings of helplessness, and despair. For these reasons, the clinician's skill in talking with children about talking and related feelings is of utmost importance. The clinician is uniquely suited to help reduce the child's burden through understanding and sharing, and to help him find a way through the forest.

Intrafamily Considerations

The school years are critical in the development of a child's personal construct, or what he thinks and expects about himself as a person and a communicator within a social context. Not surprisingly, the school years are also critical in the development of the child's stuttering. It is unusual for a school-age child to be unaware that he stutters. During these years, the overt speech behaviors are frequently seen to increase in complexity and consistency. The component feelings and attitudes are in transition as well. The clinician must come to understand both the *overt* (directly observable aspects of the child's speech fluency and disfluency) and the *covert* (internalized feelings and attitudes about communication and oneself as a communicator) features of communication. The clinician's challenge is heightened if not masked by the child's reluctance or inability to verbalize internal feelings, particularly to an adult in authority. In other words, the clinician must determine the child's unique personal construct, which is evolving, thus appearing imprecise and often ephemeral. My own observations and experiences have indicated that a major distinction between providers of effective and ineffective treatment is the extent to which a clinician shifts to and works from within the child's framework and personal perspective (i.e., the child's personal construct) (Shapiro & Moses, 1989, 2005). This means that the clinician must internalize the child's reality, yielding shared understanding, insight, and acceptance.

The school-age child's family is critically important to the success of treatment. The more the family members are aware of, participate in, and provide support for the treatment experience, the more the child internalizes and habituates the fluency facilitating controls and maintains a positive attitude about himself as a communicator. In a clinical or university-based speech and hearing center, direct meetings with one or more parents tend to be more frequent than those conducted in the school setting. In the clinic setting, I structure each treatment session in order to work individually with the child alone and then with the family members present. In the school setting, however, such regular and direct involvement of the parents proves more difficult. For this reason, the clinician must find ways to keep the family aware of, involved in, and communicating about the treatment experience. This means scheduling meetings with parents as frequently as possible, adjusting the time of treatment to accommodate the parents, phone calling, exchanging letters and audio or video recordings, and so on. Family members continue to be essential to successful treatment, although access to them may prove more difficult in school settings. While designing methods to include them in the treatment process, the clinician must remain sensitive to the child's need for increasing independence. Thus, the child must understand why the family's involvement is so important, and the parties must negotiate methods about which all are comfortable.

Extrafamily Considerations

The interdisciplinary team is a key part of the assessment and treatment of school-age children who stutter or who are at risk for stuttering. The core members of the interdisciplinary team are the clinician, the parents, and the child's classroom teachers. Together, these parties see that the communication needs of the child are met and the objectives of treatment are carried out in the classroom setting. More will be said later about working with classroom teachers. School-based clinicians have the luxury of easy access to other allied educational (learning disability and other special education specialists, psychometrists, psychologists, principals, counselors, psychotherapists, and others) or medical (physicians, nurses, physical and occupational therapists, and others) professionals as needed. The child's educational and multicultural experiences influence the content of the treatment experience and become part of the work addressed in the clinical and classroom settings.

Psychotherapeutic Considerations

With the school-age child, whose stuttering and associated thoughts and feelings are evolving, the distinction between stuttering modification and fluency shaping becomes increasingly apparent. Many clinicians are uncertain about whether to slant the design of treatment more toward fluency shaping or toward stuttering modification. As noted in Chapter 7, the decision to design treatment more in one direction than the other has relatively little to do with the severity of the child's stuttering behavior. Rather, a program oriented more toward stuttering modification is indicated when the child avoids or otherwise attempts to conceal his stuttering, demonstrates upset or embarrassment because of the stuttering, feels negative about communicating or himself as a communicator, experiences intentional or inadvertent punishment in any setting because he stutters, and demonstrates a positive response to stuttering-modification techniques during trial management. A program oriented more toward fluency shaping is indicated when the child stutters openly without trying to hide or conceal it, does not avoid speaking, exhibits a neutral or mildly negative attitude about communicating and himself as a communicator, and demonstrates a positive response to fluency shaping techniques for trial management. As can be seen, behaviors often coexist with feelings, attitudes, and thoughts. Children who demonstrate more severe stuttering behaviors often show avoidances and negativity as well. This is not always the case, however. Therefore, it is the openness with which the child stutters and the involvement of his feelings and attitudes that help guide the design and relative structure of treatment. In fact, because many of the child's attitudes are evolving, neither course is clear-cut, arguing for an approach that combines fluency shaping and stuttering modification. We also noted earlier that when fluency shaping and stuttering modification are compared, fluency shaping tends to be more efficient in changing speech behaviors, while stuttering modification is more effective in reducing fears and changing attitudes as well as strengthening generalization.

Because school-age children vary remarkably, intervention planning must be individualized. Guitar and Peters (2008) noted that the child who is 6 or 7 years old, for treatment purposes, often is more like the preschool child in terms of borderline or incipient stuttering. On the other hand, the child of 12 or 13 years may be more like the adolescent or adult who stutters. As I noted in Chapter 8, I have worked with children as young as 3 years old whose stuttering behaviors, thoughts, and feelings were severely involved, and adults whose stuttering behaviors, thoughts, and feelings represented only a minor nuisance, if that. While children who stutter may have some experiences in common, their differences remind us that each must be considered individually in all aspects of intervention.

Procedures

An integration of procedures for school-age children will be discussed with respect to each objective. Although the objectives are presented in a logical order for instructional purposes, in reality they are multidimensional and overlapping. The major objectives are the increase and transfer of fluent speech, development of resistance to potential fluency disrupters, establishment or maintenance of positive feelings about communication and oneself as a communicator, and maintenance of the fluency inducing aspects of treatment.

Increase and Transfer Fluent Speech

The first major objective with school-age children who stutter is to help them increase the amount of fluent speech and to transfer the fluency facilitating techniques learned to extraclinical settings. To do so, different but related procedures addressing the child's thoughts, feelings, and behaviors are utilized, as follows:

Construct a "safe house" within which fluency blossoms, children (and clinicians) grow, and magic happens. A clinician's treatment room must be a safe house, a retreat, a place where "a kid can be a kid" and where communication and communicators feel nurtured and secure. The clinician's role in facilitating and maintaining the child's speech fluency and positive perception of himself is absolutely critical. In an environment where the child feels unconditional positive regard and understanding, he will express himself freely—fluently or disfluently—and he should not feel even a hint of penalty. Thankfully, in most cases the clinician establishes an environment in which the child feels at home. Unfortunately, however, there are cases where the clinician is the only person the child encounters who presents a nurturing experience in which the child believes that somebody believes in him. We reviewed in Chapter 5 that some families have circumstances that overshadow the child's need for support and tangible expressions of encouragement and love. The potential influence of school personnel, particularly the speech–language pathologist, whose interactions with children are within individual or small-group meetings, is profound.

How is a safe house established? I believe the strategy varies with each clinician and with each child. Through our actions and by what we say, we demonstrate that the child is important to us as a person. We focus on all of his abilities, and only within that positive context do we provide him proactive strategies with which to increase his capacity to remain fluent. The child is shown that he is fluent most of the time and that he possesses the ability to be fluent even more often. We create opportunities for the child to succeed; we design treatment so as to prevent failure; and we guide the child to fluency accomplishments that he could not have imagined possible. We believe in the child and we help him grow. Recall how important our sincere belief in the child is as a predictor of his fluency success (Daly, 1988). This belief and this sincerity must come from within the clinician. We encourage the child's success, and we help the child see beyond predictable setbacks to future success. Increasing fluency does not occur in a straight line; it is more of a jagged profile. The child advances and then plateaus, if not regresses, until subsequent advances. We help the child understand the treatment process and his role and progress within it. We believe in the child. We accept his questions. We understand his self-doubts. We are there as an advocate, a coach, a cheerleader, a scorekeeper—a friend.

Reflecting on the importance of feeling "safe" with a clinician, Dell (2008), a speech–language pathologist, recalled his experiences as a school-age child who stutters:

Although my stuttering was not cured during my school years, the school clinicians did accomplish several very important things. They provided a place where I could come and talk, where no one would laugh at me or scorn me, where I felt free to communicate even if I did stutter. What a great feeling that was! My dog was the only other living creature with whom I felt that way. Here was a place where I could learn something about my stuttering, that mysterious thing that no one else ever mentioned. I needed a safe place where I could touch it and confront it. All of these benefited me a great deal as a young boy. . . . But most valuable of all was the gift of caring. They cared! I was made to feel some worth as a human being despite my stuttering. Because of this experience, stuttering did not destroy my self-concept the way it does in many young people. The caring and warmth I received from my school clinician helped me stay together as a person. (pp. 9–10)

There is another essential purpose in creating a safe house. A safe house and its influence endure. Throughout the process of clinical intervention, the child learns and utilizes a number of strategies (affectively, behaviorally, and cognitively) to maximize his success and freedom as a communicator. These strategies become directly associated with the safe house (i.e., the clinician's commitment, compassion, and competence, in addition to the nurturing, supportive nature of the clinical context). In other words, the communication strategies become inseparable from the safe house itself. As the child leaves the safe house, the communication strategies go with him. Consider this example. Both of my children, who now are young adults, have shared with me that their mother and I reside in their head. What does this mean? When they encounter a challenging situation in their own independent life away from home, they reflect, "What would Dad suggest? What would Mom recommend that I do?" I have never for a moment taken this blessing for granted. The clinical parallel should be obvious. The influence of the safe house continues after the child leaves the treatment setting. When experiencing communication challenge, the child might reflect, "What would my clinician suggest? What would she recommend that I do?" In this way, the clinician comes to reside in the child's head, advising, guiding, and supporting in her own absence. This too is a privilege that I have treasured as a speech–language pathologist for nearly four decades.

Invite treatment objectives from the child. Within the safe, supportive environment, invite the child to talk about and share his objectives, what he wants and hopes to achieve as a result of treatment. There are several valuable purposes in doing this. First, we want to learn the child's perspective and, in so doing, learn about his level of awareness with respect to his stuttering. Children's responses to what they hope to achieve range from general ("To talk better") to specific ("To be able to say my *B*s and *G*s without getting tight in my mouth"). In either case, appropriate follow-up inquiries may direct the child to elaborate what he said and why he does what he just described. This helps the clinician understand the information with which the child is operating. Another reason for asking the child for his objectives is to convey that the child's input is important to the clinical process. From the beginning, the child needs to see that his participation will be taken seriously and will be encouraged. I remember a 10-year-old boy who stuttered. When asked what he hoped to achieve or what he wanted to improve, he responded with, "You're supposed to tell me. I'm just a kid." When I explained that inviting him to share his wants and needs is a first step in helping him understand the treatment process, which combines our ideas and skills, he responded with a smile, "Cool. Nobody ever asked me that." Recall from the story in Figure 9.1 the boy's surprise when the clinician asked him what he wanted to do in treatment. Another boy recalled how much he appreciated his fourth-grade teacher asking him privately how he felt he would like to have his stuttering handled in class. The message to the child is that his active participation and input are essential to the treatment process.

One early activity serves multiple purposes. Designing hierarchies that contain speaking situations listed in increasing order of perceived or anticipated difficulty helps individualize the treatment experience, facilitates transfer of fluency to outside settings, and helps the child discuss objectives and related feelings and attitudes. The child is asked to think about those situations in which he would expect his speech to be fluent. Common situations include speaking alone, to a pet, with family, or with close friends.

Then he is asked to consider those in which he would predict his speech to be disfluent, those that he anticipates with a measure of dread. These often include speaking to groups of increasing audience size, unfamiliar people, persons of the opposite sex, and so on. Such hierarchies may be detailed further to include lists of speaking situations or contexts (home, classroom, stores), conversation partners (mother, father, siblings, friends, teachers, or principal), and conversation content (conversing with parents about the family pet may be easier than explaining why the child broke the garage window after having been told four times not to play near the garage door). Generally, these assignments are begun with the clinician and expanded by the child and family outside of the treatment session. The expansion then is discussed between the clinician and child. The hierarchies represent a working plan, a best guess of anticipated difficulty, and as such guide the order with which extraclinical situations are targeted for fluency facilitating control. However, the hierarchies are neither static nor permanent. They need to be discussed regularly for possible revision. It is quite possible that tasks the child thought would be easy were in fact harder than expected; those anticipated with dread might have been accomplished with relative ease. The purpose of establishing hierarchies is to increase the level of speaking challenge in minimal steps to ensure the child's successful use of fluency facilitating controls in extraclinical settings. In addition, the hierarchies individualize the treatment experience and emphasize the importance of the child's active participation from the outset of treatment.

Create opportunities for the child to experience fluency success. The beginning of treatment builds upon what was established during the assessment and evaluation and trial management. Typically I begin treatment with a short fluency shaping exercise, such as choral speaking or choral reading. Once the child is comfortable following my speech model during choral speech, I vary the volume of my speech. By reducing my volume, I allow the child to attend more to his speech and feel more in control. Eventually, I reduce my volume further to approximate lipped speech and ultimately cease modeling, but then return to modeling before the child experiences disfluency. This takes practice for the clinician. When done correctly, the clinician's and child's speech is synchronized and balanced, thus preventing the child's disfluency. I do this to establish a foundation whereby the child can feel, without reservation, "you know what, I *can* be fluent." This is the first of many attempts to create opportunities for the child to amass a foundation of successful speaking experiences. I want to begin to immerse the child in successful speaking. As noted, a child's personal construct is a prediction of his future based on his past. If he experiences regular fluency failure, then he will predict or anticipate that he will stutter. Likewise, by beginning to create a foundation of fluency success, the child will begin to anticipate the same in his future ("I can do it. I know I can. I was fluent yesterday and this morning. Maybe I can be fluent again this afternoon in reading class."). You might call this *I Can* therapy. Treatment brings children from feeling unable ("I can't") and helpless and powerless ("Why is this happening to me?") to feeling able ("I think I can. I can. I know I can.") and powerful and in control ("When I stutter, I am doing something other than what I should be doing. When I use my controls, I know I can blast those stutters. I am in control."). This means that by creating opportunities for the child to experience fluency success, we help him replace the self-doubts and negativity he has acquired from fluency failure with confidence derived from a realistically positive attitude toward himself as a potentially more fluent and independent communicator. Throughout the treatment experience, we increase the fluency challenge in minimal steps to ensure success. If the child does not succeed, then the actual challenge between where we are and the intended next step is greater than we realized.

In addition to collecting data regularly on relative fluency (specific data related to the objectives, such as self-corrections, gentle onsets, soft contacts, and slow/even rate),

I collect data on the verbal comments the child makes about himself. It is interesting to note how feelings are reflected in what children say about themselves and how what they say changes over the course of successful treatment. Such changes are seen in tandem with improvements in speech fluency. Changes in speech behaviors and comments reflecting feelings and attitudes all are observable and reportable. When the frequency (or percentage) of positive and negative self-comments is plotted over time, increases in speech fluency often coincide with significant increases in the positive statements about one's ability and control over fluency; decreases in speech disfluency often coincide with decreases in negative statements about one's ability and control over fluency. I record these data, among others, over time as a valuable measure of treatment efficacy and as a visual representation with which to discuss the child's progress and by which to help maintain his motivation.

Heighten the child's awareness of his speech fluency. Make the child's speech fluency (and only then, disfluency) the object of study. After creating opportunities for the child to experience fluency success, the clinician and child focus on and analyze together the behaviors, feelings, and thoughts that characterize what both described as "speech fluency." Initially, the clinician excitedly identifies when the child demonstrated fluent speech ("That's it! You just used your slow, easy speech!"), models what he did ("You said, 'Wwhere ddid yyou ggo?'"), and describes (using an appropriately evenly paced, gentle speech model) what was done and encourages continuation ("Tthat wwas grreat. You were really gentle on 'Wwhere.' Llet's see if yyou ccan kkeep thhat up. I knnow you can"). The clinician and child discuss the placement of the articulators and proprioceptive feedback (literally, how they felt; e.g., "The lips were nicely rounded on the *w* without any pushing"). Affective feelings are discussed as well ("It felt easy and gentle. It wasn't hard to say because I remembered to be slow and gentle").

Once the clinician and child are comfortable with this arrangement, in which the clinician identifies, models, describes, and elicits from the child subsequent feedback and feelings, the clinician gradually shifts responsibility to the child. To do this, the clinician might identify when the child used particularly slow, gentle speech by saying, "That's it! You just did it again!" followed by a leading question, "What did you do?" The child describes what he did ("I remembered to use slow, easy speech"), after which the dialogue further describes (a) which sounds in which words were affected, (b) proprioceptive feedback, and (c) affective reactions. Ultimately, the child becomes increasingly responsible by identifying instances of speech fluency, describing what he did while continuing to use an appropriate speech model, and offering a description of proprioceptive feedback and affective reactions, to all of which the clinician offers praise, appropriate speech models, and support ("You're really becoming aware of your slow, gentle speech. That's great. It surely sounded slow and gentle to me when you said the *g* in *girl*. Keep it up!").

Such activities heighten the child's awareness of his more fluent speech and convey that he already possesses within his speech much of what he needs to do even more often. The child gains a feeling of control. This approach helps the child become increasingly aware of all that he is doing right. Also, it is naturally reinforcing, in that children (and adults) gravitate to wanting to do more of what we feel we can do well. This is not a minor point. I have observed many treatment sessions in which the clinician focuses on the child's disfluency, directing him not to tense, not to look away, or not to talk so fast. In the next section, I will propose how to establish fluency facilitating control. Suffice it here to say that heightening the child's awareness of when and where he is fluent, what he does to be fluent, proprioceptive feedback, and affective reactions goes a long way toward achieving a more fluent future. I do deal directly with the residual disfluency; however, a positive approach such as this is more motivating and generates internalized feelings of success and control, especially when compared to a traditional treatment, which initially focuses on disfluency, what one is doing wrong, and relearning how to talk.

We have stressed the importance of treatment that occurs between the scheduled meetings of the clinician and client. One of the predictors of treatment outcome is time in treatment (G. Andrews et al., 1983; Haynes & Pindzola, 2008). One critical dimension of treatment that facilitates speech fluency and builds communication independence is designing outside assignments with the child that will be done regularly between treatment sessions. At first the clinician offers more initiative in designing assignments for the child. Over time, the child participates increasingly in designing the specific activities. As always, the assignments must be presented in such a way that the child is clear about what is to be done and why. The task must be specific (including what will be done, when, how often or how many times, how will it be documented, and other details) and must be one that will ensure success for the child. As stated earlier, no constructive purpose is served by the child failing to succeed.

To ensure success, we use the three Ds (discuss, demonstrate, direct). Generally I do not ask the child to do a task outside of the treatment room unless he has already mastered it with me within the treatment setting. An ideal early assignment, which actually might be initiated in the assessment or evaluation meeting, is to identify one word that was spoken fluently (i.e., with evenness, gentleness, and naturalness) and to describe telegraphically characteristics of the experience, including the setting, listener, and related feelings. At first, the child might make note of one word per day. At each weekly treatment session, after a brief social update, the child will review his activities and progress between sessions. At this point, he should have a record of no fewer than seven words that were spoken fluently, of which he might review three or at most four. The significance is that while the child is focusing on what was said and how it was said, he describes, internalizes, and thereby demonstrates the nature and process of fluent speech production, the very purpose of this stage in treatment and the follow-through assignment.

After some experience and success with an assignment such as this, the child increases the performance expectation to noting one word that was spoken fluently in the morning and one that was spoken fluently in the afternoon. Then, performance expectations increase further to noting one word that was spoken fluently in the morning, another in the afternoon, and another in the evening. Some may increase the frequency or duration of the intervals during which the child focuses on fluency. In order to increase the frequency with which school-age children and adults focus on fluency, I work toward having them associate their fluent speech (or other related treatment assignment) with a frequently occurring activity. For some people, eating or snacking occurs frequently, often around other people; therefore, fluency becomes associated with anything edible. The association is unique to each person who stutters. However, the purpose is to internalize and habituate the process of speech fluency and to heighten the child's awareness of his fluent speech and related thoughts and feelings. The importance of this expanding and positive experience in building a fluent future and adjusting one's self-concept cannot be overstated.

Over 50 years ago, Williams (1957) expressed similar concern regarding the negative or problem focus of traditional treatment on stuttering and trying not to stutter:

> The therapy procedures which appear to be most widely employed use the "stuttering" as the point of reference. The subject is asked to study his stuttering, to change his stuttering, and to control his stuttering. . . . The speaker is trained, in a sense, to keep his eyes on the stuttering and to work to reduce and minimize it. (pp. 394–395)

Williams (1957) recommended that people who stutter be directed to focus on the nature of speech fluency and how to do more of it:

From the point of view of the present discussion, it is suggested that the speaker be asked to take his eyes off the stuttering and to look instead toward the total process of talking. There are obvious advantages in looking in the direction in which one is attempting to go instead of continually glancing backward in an effort to work away from something one calls his "stuttering." The degree to which one does more things that most speakers do will be the degree that he does more things that most speakers do! This, it seems, can be considered a more meaningful use of the term "improvement." Certainly it is more meaningful than striving for "improvement in stuttering." The goal, then, is not to reduce or to stop something called "stuttering." It is to change the way the speaker talks, so that he does more and more things that most people do when they talk. (p. 395)

Williams (1957) argued that one who stutters develops a "point of view" about stuttering that affects and permeates his behavior as a communicator. A person who stutters tends to believe that stuttering is an independent entity, whether residing inside or outside of the speaker, that must be controlled, lest it will control the speaker. In other words, a person who stutters comes to be fearful that stuttering will happen "to him," failing to see that stuttering, in part, is a behavioral process created by the speaker. Behaviors are purposeful actions that are observable and modifiable. Williams advised that people who stutter should become more observant of "normal" speakers and more aware of normal speech production, including both fluency and disfluency. This same advice might well be offered to clinicians and others. From this heightened awareness, the person becomes more conscious of what he is doing as he talks. Treatment procedures, therefore, should not focus on stopping or controlling an entity called stuttering; rather, "the changes should be in the positive direction of doing more things that normal speakers do" (p. 397).

Develop or improve use of fluency facilitating techniques during instances of stuttering. Fluency facilitating control is proactively built upon the foundation described to this point. Such a foundation is characterized by a safe, supportive environment in which the child and clinician actively work and interact together, objectives are designed and planned with the child, the child is immersed in speaking experiences that highlight fluency success, and the child has become aware of the nature of his speech fluency and that of other speakers. By this time, the child understands that both fluent speech and disfluent speech are consequences of what he is doing, albeit differently. From a clear understanding of the behaviors that result in fluent speech, the child is guided in how to do these behaviors more frequently and consistently. Concrete examples and analogies are provided to help the child internalize the motor sequence and proprioceptive feedback that facilitate speech fluency. For example, the clinician and child vary the form of disfluency, as discussed in Chapter 7 and earlier in the present chapter. The child again sees the connection between his behaviors (what he does) and the characteristics of his speech. This helps the child feel in control by breaking old stereotyped habits. The child can stutter more fluently, with less abnormality. By heightening the child's awareness of what he does when he speaks, he can elect to change what he does (the essence of personal construct theory).

Once stuttering is significantly and voluntarily varied (in degree of tension, loudness, frequency, speech rate, and types), we talk about how there are two ingredients that are necessary and sufficient to eliminate the stuttering behaviors. Granted, stuttering is more than a behavior (with respect to feelings, attitudes, and thoughts). If one speaks sufficiently slowly (i.e., reduced or minus rate) and gently (i.e., reduced or minus tension), one cannot stutter. In other words, Slow + Gentle = No Stuttering. If one stutters, either one is attempting to speak too fast (i.e., + rate) for the requirements of the motor coordination or there is tension (i.e., + tension) somewhere within the speech apparatus. An increase in rate often triggers a compensatory reaction of increased tension. Likewise, an increase in tension often triggers a compensatory reaction of increased speaking rate.

While I do not make this observation the cornerstone of treatment, as do a number of behavioral programs, I do believe that it provides two appropriate foci for the school-age child who stutters. That is, we look to identify a few targets for the child, behaviors that he can do, that will have a pervasive and positive effect on his speech fluency. With appropriate models as described, working to speak sufficiently slowly and gently (with the suprasegmental features of speech naturalness) often gives the child such constructive targets. Focusing on what the child can and will *do* is in contrast to targeting behaviors that the child will *not* do (e.g., do not look down, do not interject, do not repeat, do not break words, do not tense the lips). We discuss, demonstrate, and direct/coach the characteristics of slow (i.e., evenly paced) and gentle speech. The child puts these characteristics into his own words and we design a system to evaluate such features on a regular basis.

Another illustration, represented in Figure 9.2, can help the child visualize and internalize the component concepts. I used to ask the child to visualize a milk bottle (the type with the foil seal, the original "pog"). However, since milk delivery to most homes is long bygone, I ask children to visualize a full 1-gallon cider jug fresh off the shelf, or an old water-cooler bottle. What happens when we attempt to flip it over, upside down, and pour into a glass too quickly? The child explains that the liquid doesn't come out too well. It comes out in blurps and blobs, a whole bunch at one time, nothing at

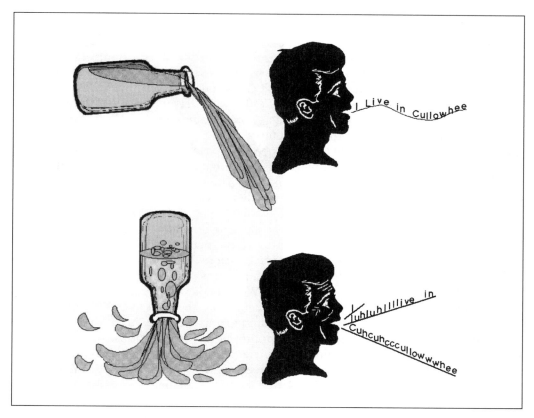

Figure 9.2.   A simple befuddling truth in vessels and speech.

another, with lots of air getting stuck inside. We compare that visual image to taking the bottle and slowly and confidently tipping it over, ever so gently. What happens then? The child explains that it all comes out slowly, steadily, consistently, evenly, effortlessly. The comparison to the speech process becomes obvious. Excessive rate and tension interfere with the forward flow of speech. In contrast, slow, gentle, and evenly and regularly produced movement facilitates natural-sounding, continuous, and forward-moving speech. After creating the visual analogy described here to represent the process of speech fluency, I was surprised, to say the least, to discover that a similar analogy was articulated by Rosalind in William Shakespeare's *As You Like It* (written circa 1599, published in First Folio in 1623):

> I have a doublet and hose in my disposition? One inch of delay more is a South-sea of discovery; I prithee, tell me who it is quickly, and speak apace. I would thou couldst stammer, that thou mightest pour this conceal'd man out of thy mouth, as wine comes out of a narrow-mouth'd bottle,—either too much at once, or none at all. I prithee, take the cork out of thy mouth, that I may drink thy tidings. (Shakespeare, 1623/2007, p. 625)

The procedures and activities described to this point help the child become more aware of what he does when he speaks fluently. I believe this awareness is essential in order to heighten the frequency of speech fluency, thus decreasing the frequency of disfluency. By increasing the frequency first, we pave the way for directly addressing the residual disfluency within a much more successful and positive context. I find this approach to be far more efficient than targeting elimination of each disfluency.

We noted earlier the importance of increasing the child's awareness in order to facilitate change. It is interesting to discover how many people who stutter are not aware of what they do when they stutter. They know when a stutter has occurred, but describe the experience only in the most global terms. As the child's awareness increases, it is not uncommon to see dramatic, albeit temporary, increases or decreases in fluency. These anticipated changes must be discussed with the child (and adult, as will be seen) in order to prepare him for their occurrence. Otherwise, left unprepared, the child will view an immediate increase in fluency as a "cure," leading to unrealistic expectations regarding his fluency and the process of intervention. Similarly, immediate decreases in fluency lead the child to believe that his speech has been damaged by treatment. Both interpretations are equally unfortunate. The fact is that the dramatic change reflects the child's heightened awareness; no more, no less. The child needs to realize that quick fixes are misleading; meaningful change usually takes hard work.

Why do dramatic changes occur at this point? I explain to the child that it is kind of like being told about a big, blue elephant standing on all fours with his ears flopping and his big blue trunk curled in front of himself, and being told *not* to think about or visualize it. Go ahead. As you read these words, try *not* to think about the elephant. When we become aware of and visualize our speech patterns, it is hard not to think about it. Thinking about speech affects how we speak. When I talk with student clinicians in class about interjections as a type of speech disfluency and they ask questions and interact in class, they become aware of how many interjections naturally occur in their speech. Typically, when they try to suppress the occurrence of interjections, the opposite effect occurs, and interjections significantly increase in frequency. So, the child needs to anticipate that an increased awareness of speech patterns, fluency, and disfluency is a necessary first step in effecting change. However, the immediate but temporary changes often observed must be discussed and understood.

There is another outcome of heightening the child's awareness of his speaking behavior. While initially aware only globally of his disfluency, the child may come to see that many of his blocks (i.e., fixed or oscillatory postures) are inappropriate articulatory postures with respect to the intended targets. For example, if one were to block on the initial sound in the word *boy*, you would expect a bilabial posture. However, if the child were to lock into an open mouth posture, this is inappropriate for the intended bilabial target. Similarly, if a child blocks on the initial sounds in words beginning with certain vowels (*eye*, *e*lephant, *a*pple, and so forth), you would expect an open mouth posture. However, if the child were to demonstrate a locked bilabial posture (with lips tense and together), this posture is inappropriate for the intended target. Occasionally, I have developed rules with children who demonstrate such patterns of inappropriate targets. When children's disfluency takes the form of a fixed posture, they are to do the following. First, they are to ask themselves, "Am I in the right posture? Are my speech helpers (articulators) where they should be?" If the answer is "yes," then they are to soften the contacts of the articulators. If "no," then they are to release the posture, move to the appropriate posture, and gently initiate the first sound in the series with soft contacts. This may sound simple on the surface, but it is challenging for the child and profound in its impact. So often, children exert tremendous effort to get through an inappropriate posture before they can focus on softening the appropriate contacts in the target sounds. I say to the children, "If you're going to get stuck, get stuck in the right position!" I would prefer that the child use his resources to establish soft contacts on appropriate targets rather than potentially exhaust such resources on an inappropriate target.

Typically in conversation, we work to establish more fluent speech with slightly reduced and more regular rate, softened articulatory contacts, gentle onsets, and continual, gentle airflow. This process adds slight prolongation to potentially difficult sounds. As noted before, establishing slow, gentle, normal-sounding speech takes practice for both the clinician and client. Each vowel and consonant will be stretched and softened. Common errors include stretching only vowels (it is harder to stretch and soften consonants) and pausing between words. Some worry about the increase in the number of prolongations, or the slight distortion that occurs on stops and affricates as a result of slowing and softening. I am not concerned about this. I find that establishing such a pattern of speaking in conversation greatly eliminates much of the existing disfluency. What remains of the disfluency (i.e., prolongations, stop and affricate distortion) gladly will be addressed directly.

Another common outcome of slow (evenly paced), gentle speech is an overall increase in rate of conversational speech. This may seem counterintuitive to some. In other words, how can slower, more gentle rate result in a faster rate overall? Typically, disfluent speech is irregular in rate and rhythm. While our ear may perceive the speech of a person who stutters to be too fast, computing rate of speech often reveals that his speaking rate is below average (between 150–180 words per minute). Slowing the speech transitions, softening articulatory contacts, and using natural-sounding suprasegmental features results in speech that is more evenly and regularly produced, thus resulting in greater overall speech output per unit of time (i.e., rate of speech). I remind children of the popular fable about the tortoise and the hare. In it, the slow, careful tortoise overcomes great odds and the fast, sly, and cunning hare to achieve unprecedented victory. The moral, therefore, is that slow and gentle wins the race.

As noted, most of the intervention is done within a conversational context. When we have established slow, gentle speech patterns, Van Riper's techniques (1973) prove useful:

⛯ *Cancellation*: Complete the word in which a block has occurred, and then say the word again, this time with a slower and more gentle production in place of the block; the form of a block is thus modified *after* it has occurred.

⛯ *Pull-out*: Change the form of the disfluency *while* the disfluency is ongoing.

⚏ *Preparatory set*: Change the form of the disfluency *before* the word in which it would be contained is spoken (change the form during the anticipatory stage).

These forms of modification were discussed in detail in Chapter 7 (see Figure 7.1). Guitar and Peters (2008) indicated that pull-outs and preparatory sets are preferred over cancellations because children tend to find it easier to replace a new form of stuttering for an old form by following the clinician's model. I agree that the clinician's models are essential. We noted that the clinician regularly inserts disfluency into her own speech and models different ways of varying the disfluency. Also, the clinician models ways to vary the child's disfluency by internalizing his forms and demonstrating alterations, followed by discussion that includes the child's assessment. Nevertheless, I have found that cancellations provide the child with a simpler, more concrete task ensuring success, particularly when the disfluency is more involved or advanced. When cancellations are used, I find that children are relatively rapid (when compared to adolescents and adults) in their transition to using pull-outs and then to preparatory sets. Every step of treatment is supported by regular activities between the scheduled meetings.

In establishing fluency facilitating techniques, treatment is often a combination of different therapy forms. Treatment frequently combines modified forms of *airflow therapy* (maintaining a continuous, gentle, and natural-sounding airflow), *relaxation* (systematic reduction in specific and general sites of tension), and *cognitive restructuring and visualization* (developing visual imagery to facilitate cognitive imaging of slow, gentle speech patterns), among others. For example, you will recall from Chapter 8 the description with appropriate hand movements of a slow moving creek given to a preschool child. This child altered his speech pattern to approximate the gentle flow of the creek, and subsequently recalled the analogy to alter the speech pattern of his conversational partner. With the school-age child, I combine such cognitive imaging with a modified relaxation technique. For example, I might direct the child to close his eyes with me and visualize a calm, relaxing image of the child's choosing. We discuss the image, clarifying the similarities and differences within our mind's eye, all the while using slow, gentle, natural-sounding speech. To use the creek example for illustration, we describe the leaf that is floating down the stream in our imagination. We discuss the slow and gentle movement of the leaf and the support given to it by the water. Initially, the clinician initiates discussion and clarification. To a lesser degree than with the adult, the child comes to initiate occasional turns discussing the leaf and the movement of the water, while using appropriately slow and gentle speech. Ultimately, the child will internalize such cognitive imaging and modified relaxation techniques and use them as needed to reestablish his fluency control. As always, the child is supported and receives praise for his active participation in the treatment process.

Transfer fluency facilitating techniques to extraclinical settings. All of the procedures discussed to this point for increasing the frequency and nature of the child's fluent speech also emphasize transferring fluency facilitating skills to outside settings. These purposes are accomplished by emphasizing the child's active role in all aspects of treatment, tailoring activities to the individual child, focusing on the child's successes, and incorporating activities and experiences that the child can internalize and thereby carry with him wherever he goes (the essence of transfer). For example, establishing a safe house deliberately nurtures and helps a child feel secure while learning and implementing a variety of communication strategies. These strategies become inseparable from the safe house itself. As the child leaves the nurturing, clinical setting, the communication strategies travel with him over time and place. The success of this objective is measured within clinical (with the clinician present) and extraclinical (without the clinician present) settings in terms of maintenance and transfer of communication strategies that are conducive to fluency freedom (e.g., use of fluency facilitating controls, expression of positive thoughts and feelings about oneself as a person and as a communicator, utilization of constructive reactions to and coping mechanisms for the experience of relapse, willingness to approach novel communication situations despite internal fear or reluctance, among others). Inviting objectives from the child emphasizes the importance of the child's participation in treatment and helps tailor the process to the individual. Similarly, creating opportunities for fluency success and heightening the child's awareness of his speech fluency enable the child to be proactive and successful, ingredients that foster heightened motivation and create natural transfer. The fluency facilitating techniques are derived logically from an understanding of the process of communication and one's role as a communicator; they both help the child internalize the motor sequence and proprioceptive feedback and address the child's related feelings, thoughts, and attitudes. Particularly important are the activities designed with the child that are completed regularly outside of the treatment setting. We discussed treatment activities that become extraclinical assignments, including designing communication hierarchies and describing with increasing frequency the characteristics of fluent words spoken. Similarly, following discussion, demonstration, and directing/coaching, other aspects of treatment are continued outside, including use of fluency facilitating controls. All the assignments to be completed outside are specific in terms of where, when, how often, and how they will be documented (typically in a small clinical notebook or electronically on a cellular phone or personal digital assistant, PDA), criteria for success, and so on.

Another significant aspect of treatment that emphasizes transfer of fluency facilitating control is the conversational context within which most of the treatment is conducted. With few exceptions, the fluency facilitating techniques are addressed within the context of conversation, rather than beginning at the sound level, moving to monosyllabic words, polysyllabic words, phrases, and sentences. There are times when individual words are analyzed for relative fluency and disfluency components. However, most of the clinical exchange is conducted within conversation, a medium that is both portable and transferable to any extraclinical setting. The use of slow, evenly paced speech transitions with gentle onset and natural-sounding suprasegmental features within conversation, combined with the regular assignments for extraclinical practice (home, school, other conversational contexts and speaking partners), facilitates the child's reliable fluency facilitating control. No less important, transfer is strengthened by (a) pointing out what the client already is doing that facilitates speech fluency, (b) encouraging an increase of the speech fluency already demonstrated, (c) focusing on what the client should *do* rather than focusing on what *not* to do, (d) building social and situational hierarchies, (e) monitoring regularly by the clinician and client, (f) engaging in regular assignments and monitoring by the child outside of the treatment setting, (g) designing specific objectives and assignments to ensure success, and (h) modeling consistently to encourage self-monitoring. Other activities that encourage transfer include bringing friends into treatment, discussing speech with friends in treatment and in the classroom, implementing specific assignments in class, and self-monitoring in class and at home. One major factor emphasizing transfer is the child's active involvement in and ownership of the treatment process from the very beginning.

Develop Resistance to Potential Fluency Disrupters

While strengthening fluency facilitating controls, the child also needs to develop resistance to old fluency disrupters. Several of the procedures already discussed promote the child's resistance to fluency disruption. Others of a behavioral nature will be discussed here; those with a primarily affective focus will be discussed in the next section. Dell (2008) emphasized the importance of heightening the child's awareness of his speech fluency and developing resistance to fluency disrupters:

We need to find ways of showing the child how fluent he is most of the time. Too many of these children think only about their stuttering. The only words they remember are those they stutter upon. We want them to shift their attention to their abundant fluency. We need to increase the amount of the child's fluency while at the same time helping him build up a tolerance for and a defense against those fluency disruptors that face him everyday. If we can design our therapy to accomplish these goals, we will not need to worry much about the child's occasional mild disfluencies. (p. 40)

Engage the child in activities with gradually increasing degrees of competition. We have emphasized the importance of conducting treatment within a conversational context. The earliest activities have little, if any, perceptible degree of competition. They are simply discussions about various topics of interest to the child. Eventually, activities with increasing degrees of competition are used. These might include games in which participants are playing against each other (such as board or card games), those in which each participant needs to be the first to respond in order to advance, or those in which deliberate time pressure increases the demand on the child's capacity to remain fluent while increasing rate of speech (e.g., increasing the number of fluent sentences spoken during a 1-minute interval timed with a sand-filled egg timer). Individual clinicians and children will determine the activities based upon their preferences.

Reintroduce direct fluency challenge. Much of the treatment experience to this point has focused on eliminating environmental stimuli that create excessive demand upon the child's capacity to remain fluent. To develop the child's resistance to fluency disruption and to increase the strength of his fluency facilitating controls, these stimuli need to be reintroduced gradually, ensuring that the child's fluency does not break down. In other words, we deliberately challenge the child's fluency control by deliberately talking too fast, interrupting him, asking a question and then asking another before the child has finished responding, or making abrupt topic shifts, among other disruptions. However, we provide fluency challenge only to the point at which the child remains successful. If the child's fluency begins to fail, we back off, discuss the experience with the child, and try to design with the child smaller steps that will ensure fluency success. Dell (2008) stated the importance of reintroducing direct fluency challenge this way:

> You can also begin to put the child under more stress now that he is talking easier, but we never put more stress on him than he can handle successfully. If we start increasing the communicative stress and he begins to have some bad stuttering, then we stop and talk about it and see if we can't solve some of his difficulty. If, after returning to the stressful communication, he is still not able to handle it, we drop the task for the moment and return to this activity at a later date. This rarely happens in our experience. After a number of these retrials, he should be desensitized enough to handle the stressful situation. (pp. 82–83)

Address the situations on the top rung of the child's communication hierarchies. The communication hierarchies are designed with the child to help individualize the treatment process, to engage the child actively in that process, and to organize the extra-clinical speaking activities and assignments. The clinician and child regularly reassess the hierarchies and adjust them as appropriate. At this point, the child should be conversing in situations and contexts, with partners, about topics, and under the circumstances described in the hierarchies that represent the most difficult level of challenge for the child. This might involve calling a child on the phone, talking to a sizable group of children with the teacher and principal present, or talking with one's parents about misdeeds that were forewarned. Whatever the experiences are, the child should feel good about his accomplishments and about his increasing ability to resist fluency disruption.

Prepare for relapse: Relapse happens! One way to prepare for relapse, the partial or total regression to pretreatment speech patterns, is to talk with the child about the likelihood of its occurrence. The worst thing for a child to experience is surprise, which results in feelings of defenselessness and helplessness. While the likelihood of relapse with children who successfully complete formal treatment is far lower than that for adults (Guitar, 2006; Manning, 2010; Starkweather et al., 1990), children still need to be prepared. Discussing this possibility with the child, the clinician reminds the child of his progress in treatment and uses appropriate visual analogies to help the child understand. For example, when talking with the child about relapse, I refer to the tool box that we might keep in our car. We don't expect to use these tools often. In fact, we may never need them. Nevertheless, it gives us confidence to know where they are and how to use them should the need ever arise. Similarly, the child may never relapse. Yet he needs to feel confident and be reminded that he has the necessary tools, the fluency facilitating techniques, if he needs them. The clinician and child may role-play a scenario of relapse to help the child prepare for its occurrence. Similarly, parents, teachers, and others also should be informed of its likelihood, so no one is surprised. Treating relapse as a probability, rather than as a remote possibility, will enable the child to respond constructively with minimal interference. Manning (2010) recommended a "buddy system" to help prevent relapse and otherwise support the child from the potential ill effects of relapse. He suggested that when entering a new and challenging speaking situation outside of the treatment setting, "the presence of someone who understands the dynamics of the situation can have a powerful supporting effect. If the clinician or parent is not there, the presence of a speech buddy may be extremely beneficial" (p. 476).

Establish or Maintain Positive Feelings About Communication and Oneself as a Communicator

The child's positive attitude about communication and himself as a communicator is critical for increasing and maintaining speech fluency. In a reciprocal arrangement, one's attitude affects one's speech fluency; one's speech fluency affects one's attitude.

Empower the child with constructive strategies for dealing with teasing: Begone, my bully! It is not uncommon for children with exceptionalities, particularly stuttering, to encounter teasing, ridicule, or bullying. In a comprehensive stuttering program for school-age children who stutter, Langevin, Kully, and Ross-Harold (2007) identified the fine line between fun teasing that is a part of every healthy relationship (i.e., no intent of hurt, both participants are having fun with mutual respect) and hurtful teasing, or bullying (e.g., name calling and mimicking—teasing that is intended to embarrass, hurt, taunt, or reduce). Bullying can be relatively direct (verbal or physical behaviors) or indirect (relational bullying, e.g., harming friendships, exclusion, spreading rumors, coercion, getting someone else to do the bullying). Without being prepared with affective, behavioral, and cognitive coping devices for the potential ill effects of hurtful teasing, children may experience frustration and humiliation (Langevin, Bortnick, Hammer, & Wiebe, 1998; Ramig & Dodge, 2010; Yaruss, Murphy, Quesal, & Reardon, 2004). Over time, such frustration and humiliation may negatively impact their self-concept (i.e., personal construct) and their motivation to continue to monitor their speech fluency (DiLollo & Manning, 2007; Manning, 2010). Bullying has been associated with long-term negative academic, psychosocial, emotional, and physical consequences, including low self-esteem, anxiety, loneliness, insecurity, depression, psychosomatic symptoms, mistrust of others, school failure, and truancy (Langevin et al., 2007; W. P. Murphy et al., 2007b). As Blood and Blood (2004) noted, children who stutter are too often predictable targets for bullying because they may be unable to respond verbally to such taunts, which may actually increase their stuttering. Enabling children who stutter to understand bullies and bullying and empowering children who stutter with constructive coping strategies and appropriate reactions have become priorities among all who support the development of school-age children.

Ramig and Bennett (1995) recommended a number of strategies for clinicians to help children who stutter counter the potential negativity associated with being teased and bullied. These strategies include the following:

1. Empower children to alter their reactions to teasing. This is done by helping children understand why others tease, why children react, and how to stop reacting.

2. Brainstorm ways children can react to teasing (e.g., ignoring the teaser or saying such things as, "Yes, I stutter" or "Would you like to know more about stuttering?").

3. Talk about possible consequences of each response to teasing.

4. Role-play teasing and selected responses. This helps children understand and communicate their feelings and alter their response pattern.

Ramig and Bennett recommended the following analogy to help children confront teasing:

> Teasing is like playing basketball. The child who teases throws the ball into your court. You have two options: tease back and throw the ball into the teaser's court or respond assertively and keep possession of the ball. When you react with a hurtful comment, you throw the ball back into the "teaser's" court. He or she now has possession of the ball and can continue to tease you. If, however, you stop reacting and keep the ball by responding in ways that take care of yourself, you take control of the situation. If you do this often enough, you take the "thrill of teasing" away from the "teaser" and "steal the ball." (p. 143)

Similarly, Langevin et al. (2007) addressed a variety of strategies to enable children who stutter to counter the effects of teasing. Such strategies include appearing nonchalant (i.e., staying calm communicates that the bully is not being taken seriously), increasing self-reliance and problem-solving skills (ignoring the bullies, telling the bullies to stop), and seeking social support (talking to someone you can trust, asking friends for help). Because being able to manage confrontation is central to the prevention of victimization, Langevin et al. provided children with three specific strategies. First, the "I Can Speak Up—Five Finger Strategy" directs the child to tell the bully to stop by saying the person's name, telling how you feel ("I don't like it when you . . .," rather than disclosing a true emotion to a bully who is unlikely to be empathic), describing the behavior that you want stopped, being respectful, and telling what you want. Second, "Rules for Working It Out" address problem solving by identifying the problem, attacking the problem—not the person—treating a person's feelings with respect, and taking responsibility for your actions. "Fouls," however tempting, that must be recognized and prevented include blaming, name-calling, threats, sneering, making excuses, getting even, and not taking responsibility. Third, strategies for conflict resolution include taking turns, compromising, using humor, and getting help.

Manning (2010) emphasized the importance of role-playing teasing and alternative responses, thus providing the child opportunities for becoming desensitized to potential taunts and insulting comments, expressing anger and frustration, and adopting more comfortable response alternatives. Furthermore, Manning discussed humor as a significant clinical device. With respect to the experience of teasing and bullying, Manning indicated that humor may help defuse or redirect the potentially hurtful comments by acknowledging the obvious and directing the comments of others back to them. For example, Manning (2001) noted that the child may say, "Yes, as a matter of fact I do stutter. But what you said was stupid and mean." He noted that in addition, depending on the circumstances and possibly the size of the children involved, the child may want to add, "And tomorrow I might no longer stutter but you may still be stupid and mean" (p. 357). Alternatively, in response to other children imitating a child's moment of stuttering, Manning (2010) suggested that the child may say something like, "Look, if you're going to stutter you ought to learn how to do it correctly. Prolong the first sound like this and add a little more tension. If you get really good at it and you're brave enough, see if you can do it with me at school tomorrow" (p. 463).

Addressing treatment for school-age children who stutter, W. P. Murphy et al. (2007b) offered a comprehensive approach to reduce bullying through role playing and self-disclosure. Specifically, Murphy et al. (2007b) presented strategies to learn about bullying (i.e., teaching children who stutter and others about bullying, the reasons children are bullied, and techniques to reduce bullying), to role-play (helping children who stutter develop appropriate responses that minimize bullying), and to educate classmates about stuttering (reducing the likelihood of bullying by making classroom presentations about stuttering and bullying that include self-disclosure). Part of a more comprehensive approach for modifying speech fluency and minimizing negative affective and cognitive reactions, the strategies focused on desensitization (i.e., reducing sensitivity to stuttering) and cognitive restructuring (learning different ways of thinking about and reacting to stuttering). Murphy et al. (2007b) presented the case of "Noah," a 9-year-old. First, Noah learned about bullying by making distinctions between comments and questions that are genuinely inquisitive (without hurtful intent) and those that are mal-intended (with hurtful intent). He also learned that the bully's behavior reflects the bully, not the child who stutters; that bullies are not born bullies (their actions reflect the way they were treated); that bullies feel weak and small inside but, when they bother others, they feel big and strong for a short time; that being bullied can rob people of their personal power and make them feel helpless, inferior, ashamed, afraid, and angry; that no one deserves to be bullied; and that children who are bullied are not alone. Second, Noah engaged in role playing via the creation of a movie with his clinician. The movie gave Noah the opportunity to develop personal guidelines in the form of "not" statements:

1. If possible, do not cry. Bullies feel encouraged when they feel power over someone.
2. Do not fight back physically.
3. Do not make threats you cannot carry through.
4. Do not ignore bullies completely. Bullies want a reaction and will just try harder if they are ignored.

Making the movie also provided Noah with the chance to brainstorm bullies' taunts, exploring both effective and ineffective reactions to such taunts, and to receive feedback and positive support from family and friends who were present for the "movie premier." The experiences of brainstorming, choosing appropriate reactions, and role playing enabled Noah to become desensitized to his stuttering ("deawfulizing" stuttering) and to become more confident in his ability to respond to bullying. Noah also learned that he could decrease the likelihood of ongoing bullying by responding in an appropriately assertive fashion, which gave him a feeling of control and power in bullying situations.

Finally, Noah prepared and delivered a classroom presentation about stuttering in order to minimize the likelihood of ongoing bullying. The primary purpose of this presentation, however, was for Noah to discover that he has the power to educate listeners and thereby to reduce unwanted comments. He indicated that he wanted those present to learn that stuttering was not his fault, that it did not help when other people made comments about his speech, and that he could not always remember to use his "speech tools." Noah also shared with his classmates other information about stuttering, including how many classmates have been to speech therapy (showing that speech therapy is common) and the fact that many famous people stutter. Noah discussed facts and myths about stuttering (demonstrating that what people think they know about stuttering often may not be true). In addition, Noah shared how it feels to stutter and described several speech management tools, explaining why they don't always work. He summarized recent research about the causes of stuttering, emphasizing that stuttering is not a person's fault or the result of insufficient effort and that stuttering is not easy to fix. Further, Noah shared how it feels to be bullied as well as some strategies for effectively responding to bullying. Finally, he invited his classmates to engage in discussion about stuttering.

Sometimes the most appropriate reaction to teasing and bullying is also the most creative and imaginative. I remember a brilliant technique used by an 8-year-old child in school some years ago. He responded to teasing by telling his taunters something of this sort: "You may call me names but, in fact, I'm the lucky one. I get to go to Ms. Baxley's speech room. She's got alligators in there. I bet you didn't know that. She lets us feed them and play with them anytime we want. Too bad you can't go." When the bullies asked how they could get to see the alligators, the boy responded with, "Only kids who stutter get to play with them. Too bad you can't." For the remainder of the year, the children who had been teasing no longer did, hoping that their good behavior would warrant reconsideration, thus enabling them to see the alligators. The clinician helped the boy turn a situation that was to be avoided (stuttering, going to the speech room) into an enviable opportunity (leaving class to play with alligators and other interesting creatures).

Even with the best preparation to withstand the ill effects of teasing and ridicule, the experience nevertheless hurts. Clinicians are reminded of the importance of providing unconditional acceptance and support to their clients who stutter and of maintaining a safe house in which the child can seek refuge at any time. As discussed previously, that refuge exists both when the clinician is present and even in the clinician's absence. The clinician is uniquely suited to help the child retain a positive self-image and to work within the family system and the interdisciplinary team to provide opportunities for the child to receive support and reminders of all that he does so well. The clinician becomes inseparable from the safe house itself. The safe house and its influence endure. An excellent resource about bullying and stuttering to initiate dialogue among children who stutter, parents, speech–language pathologists, administrators, and others is *Bullying and Teasing: Helping Children Who Stutter* (Yaruss et al., 2004), available from the National Stuttering Association (see the Appendix for contact information).

Banish negative thinking. An important aspect that must be confronted in order to establish or maintain positive feelings about communication or oneself as a communicator is negative thinking. Negative thinking inhibits fluency facilitating control among children who stutter and increases the likelihood of relapse. Manning (2010) noted the following:

> Changes in the attitudinal and cognitive aspects of the problem, often in the form of negative self-talk, may take the lead in the progression of relapse. . . . When elements of avoidance and fear begin to multiply and increasingly influence the speaker's decision making, overt stuttering will not be far behind. (p. 577)

Indeed, treatment helps the child maintain positive thinking by focusing on, understanding, and increasing the child's fluent speech; by creating opportunities for the child to succeed; by involving the child in all aspects of the treatment process; and by attending to and supporting the child's related feelings and attitudes. The child moves from feeling unable ("I can't. I'm never going to be able to talk right") to able ("I just used a gentle stretch again. I think I can do this. I know I can") and from feeling out of control ("Why is this happening to me?") to being in control ("I just self-corrected. I know I can catch those blocks before they catch me"). Strategies for maintaining positive thinking are related to those for withstanding the ill effects of teasing and bullying. Daly (1988) addressed the importance of positive self-talk in combating negative thinking and learned helplessness and in producing self-assurance and fluency success.

Ramig and Bennett (1995) recommended that clinicians help children recognize their thought patterns and help them assume responsibility for how they react to teasing, thus helping them recognize that how they think affects what they do. For younger children, Ramig and Bennett recommended that the clinician help them identify "put-downs" (hurts from the outside) and negative thinking (hurts from the inside), and replace "stinkin' thinkin" (thoughts that hurt) with "friendly thinkin" (thoughts that help). To establish a change in the thought process with older children, Ramig and Bennett recommended designing three columns—what the child says to himself ("I can't talk right"), trigger thoughts ("I should be able to talk right"), and thoughts without the negative spin ("I am doing the best I can today").

DiLollo and Manning (2007) reviewed a constructivist approach to counseling children who stutter. This approach is directly related to personal construct theory (Fransella, 1972; G. A. Kelly, 1955a, 1955b; see Chapter 5). In this approach, children who stutter are provided opportunities to reflect upon and change, or reconstruct as appropriate, the personal narrative (i.e., internalized description) they are creating of themselves. For younger children who stutter, whose personal narratives or constructs are "loose and permeable—relatively easily influenced by experience" (p. 119), DiLollo and Manning indicated the following:

> The majority of attention (therapeutic and parental/social) needs to be on the child's *fluent* speech productions rather than his or her disfluent productions. Such an approach can facilitate the development of a meaningful speaker role for the child that is primarily based on experiences and consequences of fluent speech. As the child experiences fluent speech, this experience can be made "meaningful" by being brought to the child's attention and commented on by parents and other caregivers in the child's environment. In addition, from a narrative perspective, therapy and attention focused on the child's stuttering may contribute to the development for the child of a story of "a stutterer," whereas overt, gently repeated focus on the child's fluent speech productions can contribute to the development of a story more closely aligned to that of a fluent speaker. (p. 120)

Older children who stutter tend to have a more firmly developed personal construct about themselves as communicators, typically that of a "stutterer," on the basis of relatively protracted personal experience with and about stuttering. For these children, DiLillo and Manning (2007) noted that intervention needs to focus more on changing or reconstructing their personal constructs, rather than merely establishing a meaningful fluent speaker role. DiLillo and Manning suggested experimenting with communication behaviors, helping the child to see that positive behaviors do not reside outside himself (e.g., "It wasn't me; it was just the techniques," or "I was just lucky this time") but inside (e.g., "I knew I could use that control rather than let the block run wild"). They further suggested encouraging the child to tell his story ("Children who stutter come to therapy with a story to tell. . . . It is important that the clinician accept the child's story and take it seriously" (p. 121) and helping the child elaborate alternative stories through creative play. They noted that the context of play enables children (and adults) to express emotions, thoughts, and insights that might not have been available at a more conscious level. Some children find it easier to express themselves through dramatic, creative, or otherwise playful expressions than through words. DiLillo and Manning recommended four types of play, including *embodiment play* (exploring the world through the senses, utilizing items such as play dough, slime, clay, and other tactile materials that can be manipulated), *progressive play* (discovering and exploring the world outside of oneself through the use of toys, dolls, and other objects), *role play* (playing oneself in a familiar situation and then switching to take on the role of another person), and other forms of *creative play* (e.g., engaging in artistic forms of expression such as drawing, painting, sculpting, making masks or collages, writing poetry or stories).

One experience reflecting the therapeutic value of artistic expression immediately comes to mind. For years, I have thoroughly enjoyed a professional association and personal friendship with colleagues at an international and interdisciplinary clinical facility, Občanské sdružení LOGO, in Brno, Czech Republic. There, under one roof, professionals across the health and human sciences (speech–language pathology, audiology, psychology, nursing, otolaryngology, psychiatry, neurology, internal medicine, and physiotherapy, among others) collaborate in the assessment and treatment of clients across the life span. Of particular significance, this center utilizes a variety of interventions, including creative play, art, ceramics, dance, drama, music, and even hydrotherapy (bubble baths) and therapeutic massage. Recently, I was asked to consult about one particularly challenging case. She was a 13-year-old girl whose stuttering was one of the most severe presentations I have ever observed. To most observers, this young girl appeared to be spasmodic if not epileptic, consumed in tense facial and body contortions, and nearly aphonic except for occasional, nearly inaudible, vocal fry. After meeting her in a group treatment session and upon her request, I met with her and her grandmother later that evening. Using cooking utensils in the kitchen, I explained and demonstrated how slow, even, gentle pouring from a vessel renders a nearly effortless, continuous stream (see Figure 9.2). We likened this experience to that of speech. Following the fluency facilitating procedures discussed earlier (e.g., using and fading choral reading and speaking, focusing on and increasing fluent speech, creating opportunities to succeed, illustrating through visual and concrete imagery, desensitizing systematically, supporting expressions of feeling and emotions), this girl successfully engaged in fluent speech and self-correction within reading and conversation, in both English and Slovak, before the end of the evening. My role became that of a coach, encouraging her to continue what she discovered she could do, based upon what she was told and what she heard and, significantly, what she experienced for and by herself. The following morning, she and I were happy to explain and demonstrate for her family and her clinicians what she had accomplished.

Indeed I was pleased, but not surprised, that she succeeded to such an extent and demonstrated such promise for continued success. This is what we do and what, with few exceptions, I have come to expect. What did surprise me, however, was the drawing she presented to me the following morning at breakfast (see Figure 9.3). Immediately, I was moved by the color and detail it contained, though I didn't know how to interpret its meaning. The girl's speech–language pathologist, who is also trained in art therapy and far more familiar with the girl's background, explained the drawing to me. The bottom of the drawing represents the past, the middle represents the present, and the top represents the future. In the original, the bottom is a distinct fuchsia, which, according to the girl's speech–language pathologist, is the color of fear. Notice that the past is filled with fear. The ambulances indicate medical treatment, but not necessarily relief. The figures seem to be climbing up out of the black hole, toward the light. They might represent the girl, or possibly her words. The present is where fuchsia and sky-blue meet, the transition between fear and hope. The present represents this girl's hope for the world, for her own world, and for all others who also are striving desperately to find a new way. The present approaches hope, born from fluency success, communication freedom, and nurturing from a collaborative team. Note that the location of the girl's dedication to me is in a white cloud surrounded by blue sky, the epicenter of hope. The future is green, filled with happiness. The expression of thanks is at the top of happiness, clearly within the green field. Yet, the girl is driving the car with headlights on in the middle of daylight, upside down, with a chain attached to the world. While between hope and happiness,

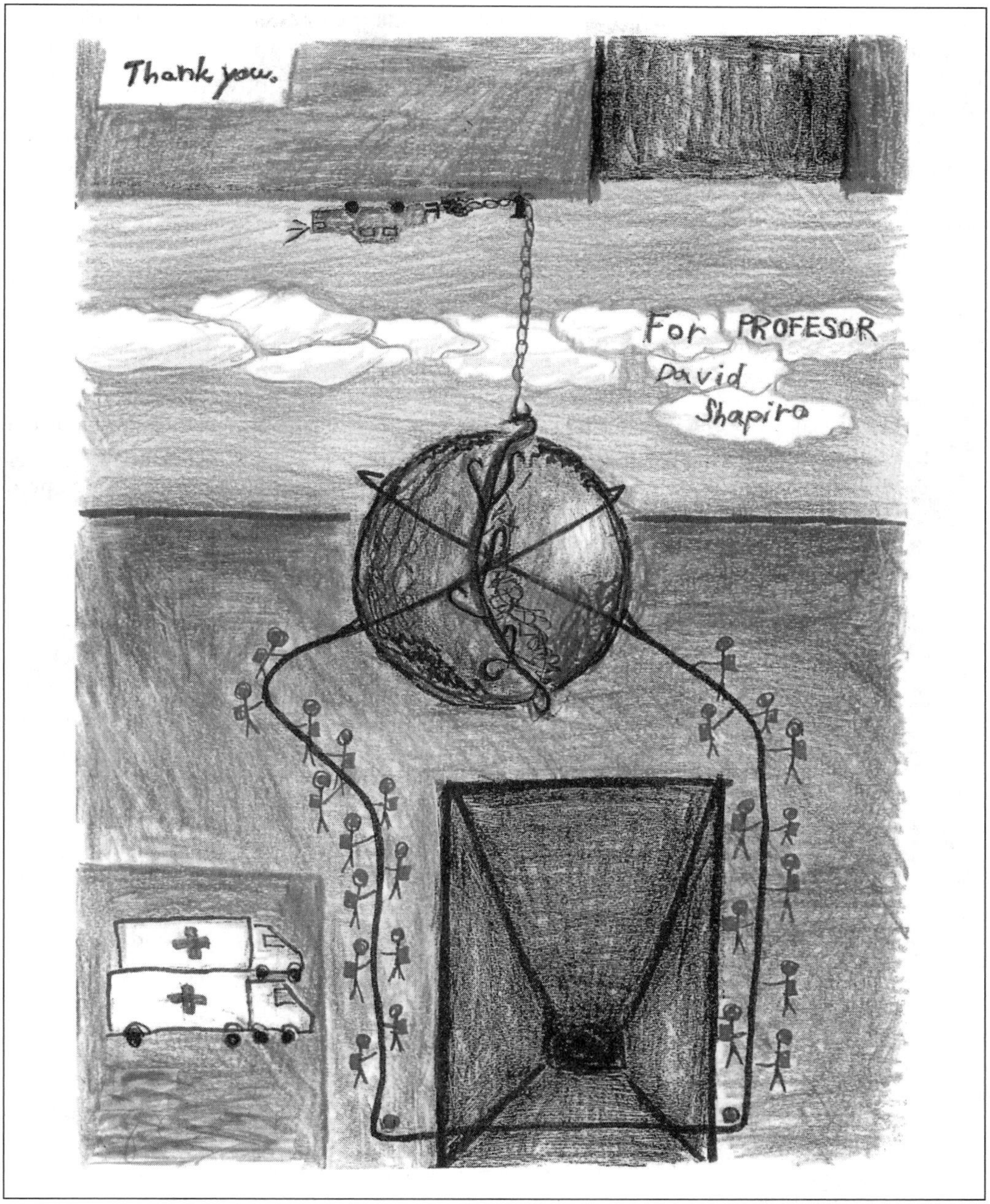

Figure 9.3. Drawing made by a 13-year-old girl after experiencing fluency success. The bottom of the drawing (fuchsia, in the original) represents the girl's past (fear), the middle (transition from fuchsia to blue sky, in the original) represents her present (transition from fear to hope), and the top (blue sky, white clouds, and green grass, in the original) represents her future (hope leading to happiness).

the girl is managing the weight of the world while she is finding her own way. Should she falter or go in reverse ever so briefly, again she will find herself in another black hole, this time alone. The black hole is bordered by hope and happiness, although it is only one misstep away. This is a girl recalling fear, experiencing hope, and striving toward happiness, acknowledging that oblivion always is near. This is a girl whose maturity of insight far exceeds her years. Her drawing reminds me of two words I learned while working in Japan. The words are *ishindenshin* and *haragei*. They mean "communication without or beyond words, heart-to-heart communication yielding tacit or unverbalized understanding," and "understanding that transcends words" (Shapiro & Moses, 2005). This is the value of artistic expression and other forms of affective and cognitive representation. This is why we are speech–language pathologists, enlightened witnesses (a concept that will be discussed in Chapter 11), and advocates for all that is good and right: communication freedom.

The drawing shown in Figure 9.3 reminds us of the emotional richness and intensity of people's reactions to their stuttering. Addressing this most important area, W. P. Murphy et al. (2007a) presented 10 treatment activities that can maintain or increase the child's positive reactions about communication and himself as a communicator:

1. *Learn about stuttering.* Acquire basic facts about stuttering to eliminate misunderstandings and stereotypes. The purpose is to understand that speech is manageable in both positive and proactive ways.

2. *Learn about other people who stutter.* Realize that you are not alone and that stuttering need not hold you back.

3. *Correspond with a stuttering "pen pal."* Participate in a program called "Stutter Buddies," sponsored by the National Stuttering Association (see the Appendix for contact information). Develop friendships with others who stutter.

4. *Engage in group interactions with other people who stutter.* Supplement individual treatment with group treatment. Feel nurtured and safe to stutter openly.

5. *Explore the moment of stuttering.* "Freeze" during a moment of stuttering (see Guitar, 2006). Heighten proprioception and understanding of stuttering.

6. *Engage in pseudostuttering.* Create stutters that are longer, louder, harder, and "sillier" than those produced by the clinician. Gain control of the structure and function of the stuttering.

7. *Create concrete representations of stuttering.* Represent stuttering blocks and fluency controls in dynamic forms, such as water balloons or modeling clay. Explore and reduce negative emotions associated with stuttering. Learn that blocks are controllable.

8. *Explore negative reactions.* Draw pictures of how stuttering makes you feel and how you would like to feel. Learn about stuttering; desensitize to stuttering; explain and understand feelings and reactions to stuttering.

9. *Engage in purposeful self-disclosure.* Acknowledge stuttering to familiar conversational partners (e.g., teacher, best friend) and eventually to less familiar conversational partners (e.g., store clerk, restaurant server). Practice fluency management controls in real-world settings. Reduce the stigma of stuttering. Discover that people often are curious about stuttering and receptive to information about the disorder.

10. *Engage in positive self-talk.* Identify negative self-talk (e.g., "People think I am stupid when I stutter") and revise it into a more positive framework (e.g., "I know I am not stupid. . . . Stuttering is just something I do when I talk," p. 131). Learn that all people have good, helpful voices inside as well as mean, hurtful ones (e.g., "When your voice talks about stuttering and is mean to you, talk back!" p. 131). Reinforce positive changes in thoughts, feelings, and behaviors.

It is indisputable that positive thinking is essential for effective communication and fluency freedom. It is also indisputable that creative and diverse strategies to maintain or increase positive thinking are vital. As noted, I have found that creating opportunities for children to experience fluency success powerfully alters their thought process in a positive direction, cementing their personal construct as effective communicators. In other words, nothing succeeds like success itself. Therefore, my best advice for clinicians working with children who stutter is to design treatment as described, while at the same time helping them cope in constructive ways with teasing and bullying, maintain positive thoughts about communication and themselves as communicators, and express their feelings within a supportive and nurturing context.

Talk with the child in positive ways. How we talk with children powerfully influences what they think about themselves. While developing independence from parents, school-age children are becoming increasingly dependent on others outside of the home for social and emotional development. What this means is that children are having experiences with an expanding variety of people, thereby confirming or challenging the impressions they have developed about themselves on the basis of interactions with family. In other words, children are vulnerable. Children's impressions about themselves and their own personal constructs are in evolution. The Golden Rule is taught and learned most powerfully during the school-age years. How we talk with children, particularly children who stutter, is critically important to helping children establish or maintain positive feelings about communication and themselves as communicators.

You might say that children, like the rest of us, are sensitive to both the *medium* (how we talk with them) and the *message* (what is conveyed or received). From a communicative standpoint, the medium and the message (Finkelstein, 1968; McLuhan, 1964; McLuhan & Fiore, 1967; Merrill & Lowenstein, 1971) are inseparable yet dynamically interrelated. The best intentioned verbal expression of support (i.e., the message) will only be as effective as the way in which it is expressed (i.e., the medium) and the degree to which the child honestly believes and relates to what is being shared. To heighten the likelihood that the message intended translates into the message received, the clinician can help the child understand directly why he is being given expressions of support. This is done by maintaining the child's active participation within the treatment process, helping the child to be keenly aware of what he is doing well, and ensuring that the message is compatible with the child's personal construct. The child must own his success. This means that he must begin to internalize the positive support received. In other words, if the child has had nurturing experiences and has internalized such a positive impression of himself, expressions of support from the clinician will "fit" or will be compatible with what the child thinks about and thereby expects for himself. Conversely, if the child has developed negative impressions about himself (e.g., I am so bad at this. I always fail. I just know I am going to fail again), all of the positive expressions of support will fall short unless the child is given deliberate opportunities to succeed, to be responsible for and keenly aware of his success, and to hear ongoing expressions of sincere and justifiable support from a nurturing clinician.

In other words, the clinician must be aware of, as well as sensitive and responsive to, the child's developing personal construct. A building is only as sturdy as the foundation upon which it stands. We cannot begin the construction process (i.e., building the fluency) without first taking stock of the foundation—the child's beliefs, thoughts, and attitudes about himself within a social context—some of which was built before we arrived. How do we assess and influence the degree to which the child's thoughts about himself are positive, while at the same time working to increase the child's fluency? Specifically, this is influenced by how we talk with children and what we say, and the opportunities we provide for children to experience successful control of their speech and to believe in themselves.

There are many wonderful illustrations of how to talk with children in positive ways (Dell, 1993, 2008; Guitar, 2006; Manning, 2010; Van Riper, 1973). In my mind, Dean Williams was the master of how to talk with children about talking. In his many publications and workshops, Williams (2003, 2004, 2006) demonstrated how to discuss *with* (not talk *to* or *at*) children their beliefs about what they believe is wrong, what they believe helps them talk better, and what their feelings are about talking. Once this is determined, children need information about what talking involves and what they can do to talk the way they want to talk. Williams explained,

> The talking that is done is structured around an active process of directing observations as the children are experiencing the ways they are talking and then helping the children evaluate and re-evaluate their interpretations of those observations. The goal is to help children explore the reality of what they are doing and to introduce and demonstrate the alternatives they have for change. (2003, p. 54)

In other words, the clinician helps the child understand his own thoughts, beliefs, and feelings, and become empowered to effect change. Understanding what the child believes is wrong and what he can do to talk better assists the clinician in knowing what information to provide and how to provide it. Furthermore, whatever explanation the child offers, whether vague ("I don't know") or specific ("Words get hooked in my throat on little fish hooks"), the child's beliefs deserve consideration because they influence what he is doing to overcome the stuttering as he perceives it. Williams noted,

> Regardless of the reasons given by a child, they deserve and require respectful discussion with the child; not from a perspective of implying that the idea is silly or wrong or unimportant, but from the standpoint of listening, of questioning, of thinking aloud with the child what it means—of sharing with the child his dilemma. No conclusions need be drawn at the time. If the child seems to be confused or frightened by his uncertainties, the clinician can reflect these or similar feelings by stating something like, "It's confusing isn't it?" Or, "It's kind of scary to not have any idea what's wrong isn't it? You're trying to talk and all of a sudden things just go whambo!" (2003, pp. 55–56)

Williams explained that children's beliefs create strong motivation for the way they behave. The child who believes that his words are caught on fish hooks will push harder to release the words from the hooks. Williams warned that changes in the way a child behaves should not be attempted without considering the motivations and beliefs that prompt the behavior. Otherwise, even if changes are accomplished, they are likely to be unstable unless corresponding changes occur in the child's motivation and beliefs. In other words, the clinician must be aware of the child's developing personal construct in order for the clinician's expressions of positive support to have a lasting impact.

In much of Williams' work, the clinician is advised to help children understand their beliefs about talking, stuttering, and themselves as communicators, and to understand that what they are doing is plausible given their beliefs. Thus, the clinician needs to help the child understand that both stuttering and more fluent talking are the consequence of things that the child is doing differently. Once the child understands this difference, he has a choice, a conscious decision. Williams stated,

> This results in his learning that he has a choice. He is free to act in accordance with his choice. This is the goal of obtaining congruence between what a person intends and the way he behaves. . . . The child should possess the basic orientation that talking smoothly involves an active doing process to be learned—with the acceptance of the mistakes that accompany any learning. (2003, p. 64)

The school-age child who stutters "may get tangled up at times when he talks," but if he does, "he can change what he is doing and talk the ways he wants to talk" (Williams, 2006, p. 35). By means of the opportunities described—helping the child understand his own thoughts, feelings, and attitudes; talking and providing feedback in candid, supportive, nurturing ways; and enabling the child to experience fluency success and control over his communication—the child discovers that stuttering is, in part, the consequence of a decision he is making. There are alternatives. He has choices. This discovery is a remarkably empowering experience for the child.

Maintain the Fluency Inducing Effects of Treatment

Of the different aspects of treatment, maintenance has proven to be the most challenging (Craig, 1998; Craig & Andrews, 1985; Craig & Hancock, 1995; Gregory, 2003; Guitar, 2006; Langevin & Kully, 2003; Manning, 2010; Van Riper, 1973). Possible explanations are many. As noted earlier, school-age children with a more severe stuttering pattern tend to have a more positive prognosis for treatment outcome. It seems that from a cost and benefit perspective, those who stand to benefit the most are more willing to invest greater energy and other resources in the treatment experience. Similarly, as children develop increasing degrees of fluency control, their stuttering problem becomes less handicapping, thus moving from being a central issue in their life (one of foreground) to a more peripheral issue (one of background). Consequently, the continuing effort and vigilance that are required for long-term maintenance may come to be perceived as less important or less worth the effort (Cooper, 1977; Manning, 2004, 2010; Perkins, 2006). Manning (2010) stated, "To the extent that treatment results in stuttering that no longer presents a major problem to the speaker, the person may choose to devote his finite time and energies to other issues and concerns" (p. 581). Manning also expressed concern that clinicians who emphasize production of fluency behavior to the exclusion of related thoughts and feelings might inadvertently promote concealment of stuttering, thus enabling such reduction in self-monitoring, if not overall relapse (Crichton-Smith, 2002; Yaruss, Quesal, & Murphy, 2002; Yaruss, Quesal, Reeves, et al., 2002). The loss of motivation in the terminal stages of treatment is a reality of consequence. Just as transfer of speech fluency must be addressed from the outset of treatment, safeguards for maintenance of fluency after the completion of treatment must be addressed directly and early. Specific suggestions follow.

Help the child become his own clinician. Maintenance of speech fluency originates at the beginning of formal treatment, not at the end, and continues throughout the treatment process. One way to facilitate both transfer and maintenance of speech fluency is to involve the client in all aspects of decision making in treatment and to deliberately shift responsibility for intervention from the clinician to the client. Initially, the clinician invites the client's ideas but is relatively assertive in establishing objectives, designing procedures and assignments, providing feedback, and monitoring speech production and progress. Over time, the client needs to assume increasing degrees of responsibility for these and other related activities. I discuss with my clients, including school-age children, that our shared objective is to reach the point where we put me (the clinician) out of a job. We want the child to become his own clinician; he monitors and regulates his own speech behavior, no longer needing the clinician to serve in this capacity. Especially for novice clinicians, it is easy to inadvertently establish a dependence of the client on the clinician. In Chapter 11, we will discuss clinicians' needs and the importance of clinicians being self-aware in order to address the needs of their clients. All clinical activities, from the very beginning, are intended to heighten the client's ownership of the treatment process and its outcome. Frequently, when I prepare student clinicians for working with people who stutter, they are inclined to assume the posture of the "great provider," intending to apply their knowledge by telling clients what they (the clients) need to achieve, by when, and by what means. Rarely do clinicians consider the importance of inviting clients to participate in these critical decisions. No one is more knowledgeable about the individual client's communication experience and related thoughts and feelings than the client himself. Sometimes the best way we can provide for our clients is to invite or elicit from them their own experiences, perspectives, and insights. That way, the client is a responsible participant from the very beginning and the process is one of shared responsibility.

I use a similar process when teaching student clinicians in their requisite courses. They, like our clients, unfortunately have become accustomed to a reactive or relatively passive role in the learning process. On the first day of the orientation preceding each academic course and clinical practicum I teach, and before I provide a copy of the syllabus, I invite the students to share with me in writing what they hope to achieve as a result of taking the course, how they would like to achieve it, and what their related questions might be. Predictably, I am greeted with dumbfounded expressions and quizzical confessions: "Nobody ever asked us that before," or "I never thought about that before." Just as we hope to sow the seeds of lifelong learning and ongoing professional development (maintenance of professional skills, addressed in Chapter 12) early in a student clinician's professional career, so we invite and expect our clients to participate actively and with increasing independence in the intervention program to facilitate their ownership of the process and internalization of self-monitoring and self-regulating skills, thus maintaining speech fluency. The more likely these skills are to be internalized and habituated, the more likely they will continue after the completion of formal treatment.

Decrease the frequency of scheduled treatment. Once the affective, behavioral, and cognitive objectives for treatment have been met (and the client is using fluency facilitating skills independently and assuming responsibility for his communication), the frequency of scheduled direct treatment is decreased. The client thereby becomes increasingly responsible for managing his communication, monitoring progress, and maintaining consistent levels of speech fluency. Essentially, this is a weaning process, one in which the client increasingly becomes his own clinician. Meetings with the clinician become maintenance checks wherein the clinician takes the role of an active listener as the client summarizes, evaluates, and projects. I must underscore the importance of the client internalizing the self-evaluating and self-monitoring skills, while assuming increasing levels of treatment responsibility and communication independence. The young driver of a standard-shift vehicle is very conscious at first of which gear he is in and all of the individual elements of a larger motor process. Ultimately, the process becomes internalized, habituated, and thereby synchronized. The driver evaluates, monitors, and adjusts as needed. While the parallel to maintaining speech fluency may be somewhat distant, the ultimate objectives are similar. The person who stutters becomes increasingly responsible for coordinating and adjusting the synchronized process of speech fluency and maintaining these skills for the long haul.

Maintain regular maintenance checks of decreasing frequency for at least 2 years posttreatment. As the frequency of scheduled treatment decreases, the importance of regular maintenance checks increases. As noted, the client becomes responsible for reporting, evaluating, monitoring, and adjusting. Initially, the maintenance may be once monthly, moving to once bimonthly, then 4 months, 6 months, 1 year, then 2 years. As noted earlier, the risk of relapse is typically greater for adults than for children and for those whose pretreatment level of fluency is less severe. Nevertheless, some type of follow-up is necessary for most clients. The process of change must be viewed as long term, so that clients have the option of returning for treatment in some form for as long as they need it. It is essential that follow-up visits not be viewed by clinician or client as an indication of failure. Rather, follow-up should be anticipated as a predictable and acceptable part of the process of change over time. While most clients do not require a return to intensive treatment, generally individual follow-up, group treatment sessions, or self-help group meetings enable clients to continue making progress and to recommit to their own communication and fluency freedom and the responsibilities that are a central part of enjoying those freedoms over time and across settings.

Build in regular, child-initiated benchmarking. A related activity that I have found useful with both children and adults for maintaining speech fluency is benchmarking. This means reassessing where one is and where one wants to be, and addressing any discrepancy. A few examples will help illustrate the usefulness of benchmarking.

A child who can do 5 sit-ups is working toward being able to do 10. He has increased from one by adding one additional sit-up per week to the daily exercise routine. By continuing to add one per week, the child should achieve his goal in 5 weeks. The child benchmarks by reassessing his progress on a weekly basis with respect to a long-term goal, making adjustments as necessary. Many of us know the increasing challenge of keeping off the extra pounds. We step on the scale every day. Seeing that we are 170 pounds and that we wish to be 165, we establish a goal of dropping 1 pound per week for the next 5 weeks. We monitor every day, but we benchmark (by stepping on the scale and reassessing current weight, projected weight, and effectiveness of current strategy) every Saturday morning.

Maintaining speech fluency is not much different. Begun at the early stages of treatment and continued throughout, we have our client benchmark with respect to each individual objective. Once we get to the stage where maintenance of fluency receives primary focus, the client benchmarks the present level of fluency-related behaviors, thoughts, and feelings with respect to pre- and posttreatment levels and previous long-term projections. With decreasing, albeit regular, frequency (weekly, monthly, bimonthly, and so on), the client reassesses his present level of functioning and determines if it is consistent with earlier projections. If it is, the client internalizes the reward for maintaining communication progress. If it is not, the client interprets the discrepancy with respect to relevant circumstances and designs a realistic, specific strategy for change. For example, if the regularity of self-monitoring speech fluency has slipped, the school-age child may commit himself to disciplined, focused self-monitoring during group reading and show-and-tell activities at school. If he experiences thoughts of inability or helplessness, he may revisit the strategies used previously in treatment to document and focus on successes and reestablish ways of positive thinking. As noted, these are the times when follow-up visits with the clinician in a supportive and nurturing environment are very useful. Likewise, ongoing support and involvement from parents, teachers, and others within the child's communication system help maintain the long-term benefits of treatment.

Deliberately revisit the past. Sometimes wishing not to relive the past helps motivate one to maintain speech fluency. As we work toward maintenance of speech fluency, I speak with the child about viewing a recording of his pretreatment communication. I do this with two objectives in mind. First, I want to celebrate with the child his accomplishments, which are so well deserved. Second, I want to increase his motivation to maintain the level of speech fluency that has been achieved. In other words, I want the client to revisit concretely how he spoke previously so that he will reaffirm his commitment to himself to do his utmost to prevent returning to pretreatment levels. This is a hard thing for a client to do and must be approached with extreme sensitivity and support. The focus of discussion before, during, and after returning to times past is, "Look at all of the things (i.e., forms of disfluency) that you have left behind."

Even though the clinician sincerely intends a positive focus, some clients are nevertheless disturbed when they are faced with the reality of how they spoke previously. This is a delicate balancing act. We want to help clients remain focused on the positive aspects of change, while at the same time deliberately presenting the sometimes shocking reality of the past. We want to encourage maintenance of fluency change and all of the constant vigilance and work it entails; we want to reward the client for progress, but we also want him to redouble his commitment to himself never to speak like he used to. We want him to recall just how painful it was to be out of control and to experience communicative helplessness in order to heighten motivation never to experience that again. Memories of a cold winter without firewood may be poignant enough to prevent ever being without firewood again.

Reexamine the child's personal construct. We have discussed that one's personal construct is a composite of thoughts, feelings, and attitudes about communication and oneself as a communicator. Personal constructs serve as a filter through which the child views his world, interprets his role within it, and thereby comes to anticipate events that are compatible with or similar to those past. In order for affective, behavioral, and cognitive changes to be maintained after the conclusion of treatment, these changes must be integrated with one's personal construct. Many clinicians and researchers have asserted that we are far more knowledgeable about how to help people who stutter become fluent than we are about how to help them maintain that fluency (Bloodstein & Bernstein Ratner, 2008; Cooper, 1977; Craig, 1998; Manning, 2004; Van Riper, 1973). I agree. At the same time, I argue that one explanation for this ongoing state of affairs is that not enough attention is being paid to thoughts, beliefs, and feelings. Unless those who stutter feel secure with the changes and feel that the changes "fit" with who they are and are becoming, the changes will not last.

Consider the parallel with overeaters. We have a friend who, over the last 2 years, dropped and then regained over 100 pounds. While Janet was losing the weight, she received ongoing social support for visible progress. In time, social support lessened as people became accustomed to and therefore anticipated Janet's relatively slim appearance. Behaviors only last as long as they are integrated within one's personal construct, however. Janet continued to "feel" obese. She enjoyed the novelty of reduced weight and the praise she received. But throughout, she felt overweight, like an impostor who would be found out. Her new behaviors, which included altered eating patterns and reduced weight, were not integrated with how she felt and what she thought about herself as a person. Consequently, old eating patterns returned, as did the extra pounds.

The feelings and attitudes of school-age children, including those who stutter, are in evolution. Clinicians must look within the child to understand how he sees himself. Those who stutter are coming to view themselves as "stutterers." Knowing the experience of fluency failure, many children internalize this experience and come to expect the same. One of the advantages of working with children is that they literally have not lived long enough for the roots of stuttering to have taken hold impenetrably. Even when life events fertilize the growth of stuttering, the roots can grow just so quickly. This is not to minimize the significance of the stuttering experience for the individual child. How do we change the child's expectation? How do we change this course of development? The answer to these questions is this: We flood the child with successful fluency experiences. We show him that he already possesses much fluency and the skills necessary to be fluent even more often. We involve the child actively in the treatment process and the related decisions, as we do the parents, teachers, and others. We create opportunities to provide the child with so much data indicative of his success and inherent potential that he has no choice but to look at those data within the context of how he views himself. Indeed the clinician's role is to help the child interpret these data and to address the discrepancy with how he feels and what he thinks about himself.

Furthermore, the clinician must help the child know how to use the fluency. Just because the child is becoming fluent doesn't mean that he automatically knows how and when to speak in socially appropriate ways. The clinician may need to work with the child to build pragmatic fluency, knowing what to say within situational constraints. Using language follows a variety of social scripts. Taking turns is a social script. Speaking at home requires a different social script, involving a different set of situational constraints, than speaking at school. Similarly, we will see in the next chapter that adults who become fluent may need to learn the social scripts for dating, interviewing, social-izing, working, and parenting. We need to help children feel fluent and internally in con-trol of their communication (by owning their fluency and feeling comfortable with it) and then to help them use their speech in pragmatically appropriate ways that are both internally and externally rewarded (ways that facilitate transfer and maintenance).

Manning (2010) supported the concept that maintenance of speech fluency must be multidimensional and address not only behavioral features but also affective and cognitive ones:

> To the listener, relapse is likely to be first observed in the surface features of the problem in terms of the quantity and quality of the speaker's fluency. However, for the speaker, relapse begins with the return of old and ingrained responses of fear and avoidance. Thus, just as the assessment of stuttering is multidimensional, the determination of the speaker's ability to maintain change must be multidimensional as well. Concentration on a single feature such as the frequency of stuttering tends to exclude the important affective and cognitive features of the problem, features that those who stutter perceive as vital. (pp. 573–574)

To help clients solidify affective and cognitive changes that are essential to mainte-nance of speech fluency, clinicians must help the client feel comfortable with and accept his new role and possibilities as a communicator. When adjusting to the new role, the person who stutters must come to view himself as something other than an individual who stutters, all the while integrating a new and unfamiliar role as a fluent speaker and making lifestyle adjustments to accommodate those changes. Through this process of adjustment, some people who stutter report feeling less than fully comfortable with their fluency, feeling that they are deceiving others and waiting for their disfluency to return. Poignantly indicating the schism between his own fluent speech behavior and the accompanying contrastive thoughts and feelings, Jezer (1997) recalled a presentation he made as a school-age child:

> I felt very much alone. So great was my fear that I seemed to go into a trance. It was a kind of out-of-body experience: A fluent person seemed to be speaking out of my mouth. I heard the words, but they did not come from me. When I was finished, the teacher complimented me for my fluency and for my courage. I think the class may even have applauded—not in sarcasm but in appreciation for my triumph and also, I imagine, in relief. . . . But my fluency mystified me. There was no way to remember how I felt being fluent, because my fluency did not seem to come from me. I was beginning to fear flu-ency. I knew myself when I was stuttering. But I felt estranged from myself when I was fluent. Fluency meant trouble. It created expectations I know I could not meet. (p. 108)

Others have long attested to the challenges incurred by a person who stutters when integrating the less familiar role as a fluent speaker (Sheehan, 1970; Van Riper, 1973, 1974, 1982). For a person who stutters, events related to the more familiar role (stutter-ing) are more predictable than those related to the less familiar role (fluency) (Fransella, 1972, 2003). Similarly, people who stutter are inclined to make a "choice" to stutter (Dalton, 1987, 1994; Fransella & Dalton, 1990), not because they want to stutter but be-cause they have defaulted to what is familiar and consistent with their view of the world and their role as a communicator within it. The clinician is uniquely suited to enable the child to discover and experience communication alternatives so that the choice between fluency and stuttering becomes a deliberate selection from among constructive alterna-tives. In short, treatment must work toward integrating and maintaining affective and cognitive changes within the context of directly observable speech fluency behaviors.

Integrate treatment changes within the communication system. Clinicians need to help listeners adjust to the "new" speaker. Conversational partners are adjusting their expectations in response to changes with the person who stutters. As noted in Chapter 5, changes affecting one person also affect all others within that person's communication system. As the person who stutters achieves fluency and becomes inclined to speak more assertively and take more communicative risks, conversational partners must adjust to different expectations. These adjustments take time and support.

Clinicians can be particularly helpful to those within the communication system (such as family, teachers, and classmates) by providing support in the form of helping them understand the nature of the changes that are occurring and ways that they can react constructively to those changes. In most cases, the clinician helps the conversational partners continue to feel needed but in different ways. Family members who have become accustomed to speaking for a child who stutters will need direction regarding when and how to allow and encourage him to speak for himself. Teachers who have become used to altering assignments to prevent penalizing a child who stutters will need guidance in learning how to include the child and what to expect of him. Friends who have protected and "looked out" for a child who stutters will need to know how to behave differently. All well-meaning people in the child's environment can continue to feel needed within the revised "rules" or expectations. The more children who stutter receive support for their communication changes from people within their communication system, and the more such people receive support for their essential roles within the change process, the more the child's changes will be integrated and long lasting. With the support of a skilled and nurturing clinician, people within the larger communication system of the person who stutters will successfully shift their perspective and adjust their roles.

As logical as this sounds, some conversational partners resist this change. Expectations based on precedent are hard to change. Listeners report feeling that the stuttering has become viewed as part of the child's personality. Change takes time and focus, both of which might be rare commodities among those adjusting to people who stutter. Other pressures occasionally placed on children who stutter inadvertently impede change. For example, pressure is often placed on the speaker following treatment to demonstrate much-improved or even perfect fluency ("How awful—after all of this time and effort and money and he still stutters!"). Any observable stuttering may be viewed as a sign of failure by the child who stutters or his listeners. Indeed, clinicians help facilitate change by helping the participants know what to expect, how to respond, and otherwise how to contribute actively and meaningfully to the change process. The integrated and overlapping processes of treatment, transfer, and maintenance indeed are multidimensional and dynamic.

Working with School-Age Children Who Stutter and Have Concomitant Disorders

Co-Occurrence of Stuttering and Other Disorders

Frequently, clinicians are faced with the challenge of serving a child who stutters and who has other communicatively relevant impairments. Bernstein Ratner (2005b) noted that this is not surprising, "given the higher likelihood of concomitant problems which accompany any primary diagnosis of a single communicative impairment" (p. 163). For example, the risk for children who stutter to have additional speech or language impairments is greater than that for children who do not stutter. Similarly, the risk for children who experience developmental communication delay (i.e., speech and language) to have additional communicatively relevant impairments is greater than that for children without developmental delay (Arndt & Healey, 2001; Bernstein Ratner, 2005b; Blood, Ridenour, et al., 2003; Bloodstein & Bernstein Ratner, 2008; Craig & Tran, 2005a; Healey, Reid, & Donaher, 2005). Estimates of school-age children who stutter and who experience co-occurring disorders vary because of issues of methodology and definition. Nevertheless, the high degree of co-occurrence is clear. The percentage of school-age children who stutter and have at least one coexisting disorder ranges from 45% (Arndt & Healey, 2001), to 50% (Yaruss et al., 1998), to 63% (Blood, Ridenour, et al., 2003), to 68% (Blood & Seider, 1981). While Blood, Ridenour, et al. (2003) identified as many as 30 different concomitant disorders potentially associated with stuttering, articulation and phonology are typically listed as the most frequent disorders that coexist with stuttering. Of the school-age children who stutter, 12.7% also presented with articulation disorder and 33.5% also presented with phonological disorder (Blood, Ridenour, et al., 2003). These figures are particularly significant compared to estimates ranging from 2% to 6% of children with articulation or phonological disorders reported for the general population (Byrd et al., 2007). The coexistence of language disorders is not as well documented, perhaps because they may not become apparent until after the fluency has improved (Bloodstein & Bernstein Ratner, 2008; Conture, 2001; Manning, 2010). Other disorders coexisting less frequently than articulation and language include learning disabilities, reading disorders, attention-deficit/hyperactivity disorder, emotional disorders, and mental retardation.

Blood et al. (2009) investigated the interactions between stuttering, race, and coexisting disorders. Based on a survey of 1,184 speech–language pathologists regarding the type and prevalence of coexisting disorders among 2,535 children who stutter, 41 different concomitant disorders were identified, of which 18 that occurred most commonly were analyzed. Results revealed that African American children who stutter, particularly boys, have significantly higher risk for coexisting learning disabilities, literacy/reading disorders, attention disorders, and behavioral disorders than do children described as White non-Hispanic, Hispanic, or Asian. Factoring out race, boys who stutter demonstrated greater risk than girls for these four coexisting disorders, in addition to central auditory processing disorders and neurological disorders. Blood et al. proposed the existence of "a double jeopardy situation with an increased likelihood of coexisting disorders occurring in African American CWS [children who stutter]" (p. 137) and questioned whether the coexisting disorders are separate and distinct disorders or symptoms of a more central disorder. Similarly, Bernstein Ratner (2005b) proposed that coexisting disorders might be attributable to genetics (i.e., fluency disorders, specific language impairment, and articulation disorder of unknown etiology may be transmitted genetically), limited or fragile resources (e.g., a primary language problem may compromise fluency abilities in a child with fragile fluency resources), or shared predisposition (conditions that provoke stuttering in some children may also predispose them to additional communication impairments).

Because of the increased likelihood that a child who stutters has additional concomitant disorders and because of the variety of disorders that potentially can coexist among school-age children who stutter, conducting a thorough diagnostic evaluation is absolutely essential. These procedures were reviewed previously. Bernstein Ratner (2005b) underscored that evaluations of school-age children who stutter must include relevant case history information, parental concerns and reactions to the child's stuttering (which will influence family counseling), behavioral features of the stuttering (frequency and severity measures), affective and cognitive components, language assessments (expressive syntax and morphology, expressive vocabulary, receptive syntax and morphology, and receptive vocabulary), speech sound production (articulation and phonology), and conversational language sampling (thorough speech and language analysis, including pragmatics).

Effects of Concomitant Disorders

There are at least two significant issues that clinicians must confront when working with children who have or are suspected to have coexisting communication problems (Manning, 2010). First, some children who are being treated for speech–language disorders have become more disfluent or have begun to stutter as a consequence of treatment (Bernstein Ratner, 1995; Conture, 2001; Starkweather, 1997). Conture suggested that the risk of stuttering onset is increased if a child is being treated for severe articulation impairment or unusual phonological problems. Furthermore, treatment for articulation or language impairment may disrupt speech fluency if the child is placed in treatment too early (i.e., before the child is capable of producing sounds correctly with relative ease), or if the treatment experience places communicative demands upon the child for speech-sound or language comprehension or production that exceeds the child's capacity to produce fluent speech (Conture, 2001; Manning, 2000, 2010; Starkweather, 1997; Starkweather et al., 1990). Conture (2001) noted,

> We have noticed this association between positive change in language and increases in speech disfluency to be particularly apparent in children around 5 to 6 years of age. We are not sure what this means or its long-term implications for recovery from disfluency, but we are inclined to speculate that increases in the length and complexity of verbally expressed languages increase the opportunities for instances of disfluency to emerge. Thus, this is probably a natural by-product of improved but still unstable expressive language skills. (p. 157)

Second, there is a "trading" relationship among fluency, language, and phonological skill within a child. In other words, demands in a variety of domains can result in fluency breakdown (Starkweather, 1997; Starkweather et al., 1990). Bernstein Ratner (1995) noted, "Efforts to remediate areas of deficiency are likely to exacerbate patterns of fluency failure. . . . This situation places the clinician in a planning dilemma—how to improve skills in one domain without further compromising skills in another" (p. 182). Furthermore, this trading relationship between communication-related resources has implications for making clinical decisions. Bernstein Ratner (1995) suggested that clinicians must realize that demands for phonological and grammatical processing compete with resources for fluent speech production; they need to organize treatment hierarchically by proceeding from language and articulation activities that the child has mastered to those that require greater demands, and determine the child's individual capacities and response to communication demands when designing intervention for multiple impairments (i.e., concurrently, sequentially, or cyclically; these styles of intervention will be reviewed shortly). Similarly, Wolk (1998) advised that clinicians planning for children who stutter and who have phonological impairment should be aware that direct articulation therapy, which works to program articulatory sequences and targets articulatory accuracy, may exert too much pressure, thereby exacerbating the disfluency (see also Byrd et al., 2007). Wolk suggested an indirect approach to phonological errors combined with direct modification of fluency. Bernstein Ratner (2005b) underscored the challenge of generalizing within-session fluency and language goals, noting that this challenge is amplified when disorders coexist: "Transfer of fluency goals is aided by programming of fluency-challenging activities that replicate real-world interactions" (p. 175). She also stated, "In all cases, bringing real-world interaction into the therapy room, and therapy goals out to the real world, are important in maintaining and expanding use of skills" (p. 176). Throughout, we have considered how to make our treatment activities most like the communication environment in which the child genuinely communicates. By doing so, we have emphasized the importance of starting the process of generalization from the very beginning of treatment.

Challenging Intervention Issues

Working with school-age children who stutter and who have concomitant disorders involves several challenging intervention issues. Before confronting these issues, however, we first must confirm that the child of interest indeed is demonstrating stuttering and a concomitant disorder. Then we must ask some key questions: To treat or not to treat? (Manning, 2010). Which disorder—stuttering or the concomitant disorder—negatively affects communication the most? (Healey et al., 2005; Logan & LaSalle, 2003). Which model of intervention—sequential, concurrent, or cycles—should be used when stuttering and a concomitant disorder coexist? (Bernstein Ratner, 2005b; Byrd et al., 2007; Healey et al., 2005; Wolk, 1998).

To Treat or Not to Treat?

Whether to treat is the question often facing informed speech–language pathologists. Manning (2010) noted that the issues and clinical decisions that must be addressed are more complex in the presence of multiple problems. Nevertheless, the answer to the question of whether to initiate treatment for a child who is disfluent and has concomitant communication problems often is "yes." Because articulation and language problems often require long-term treatment, initiation of fluency intervention typically cannot wait until the articulation and language problems are resolved because of the significant social, emotional, and educational consequences that would result. Furthermore, waiting to begin fluency intervention is contraindicated by efficacy data suggesting the importance of early intervention. For these reasons, many clinical researchers recommend a combined intervention approach. There is an increasing body of research indicating that, when the clinician is aware of the trading relationships among components of communication, treating concomitant speech and language problems does not exacerbate the child's stuttering (Bernstein Ratner, 2005b; Guitar, 2006; Manning, 2010).

Which Disorder to Treat?

When considering which disorder to treat, Healey et al. (2005) advised clinicians to determine the relative severity of the coexisting disorders and their impact on the child's communication and social functioning. Offering several case examples, the authors stressed that efforts should be made to address the most problematic disruption in the child's speech or language. For children who stutter and who present learning disabilities or mental retardation, significant delays in speech and language development are common, and the frequently observed forms of disfluency (e.g., interjections, revisions, false starts, self-interruptions) are directly influenced by the grammatical complexity of the child's constrained language formulation. For these children, facilitating linguistic competence would contribute to improved fluency. However, for children whose stuttering interferes most with communication, treating fluency as the primary disorder would be indicated and would have an overlapping benefit on the child's use of language. Once the clinician has decided to begin intervention, she must decide which disorder (stuttering, articulation, or language) deserves more immediate attention. About children who stutter and demonstrate a delay in language, Conture (2001) stated,

> Therapy oriented to modification of language seems most appropriate if the child's speech disfluencies are of a physically easy, relatively short duration and consist mainly of part- and whole-word repetitions. Conversely, therapy should probably be more oriented to modification of stuttering if the speech disfluencies are associated with visible and audible signs of physical and psychological tension, are relatively longer in duration, and mainly of a blocking or sound prolongation (audible and inaudible) type. Of course, there is nothing that says that both problems—language difficulties and stuttering—can't be simultaneously dealt with in the same session. (p. 158)

Reflecting on children who begin to stutter after, or as a consequence of, articulation treatment, Conture (2001) noted that the primary objective is to convey that speech and communication can be fun and can be done in a physically relaxed, unhurried manner. Phonetic placement or other forms of direct remediation of speech fluency and articulation are secondary. Deciding which impairment is to receive relatively more immediate or substantive focus reflects an awareness of the trading relationship among components of communication, the impact that each exceptionality has on the effectiveness of communication and social functioning, and the impact that intervention for one exceptionality has on other exceptionalities.

Which Intervention Model to Use?

Having considered the relative impact of each exceptionality on the individual child's communication process and social functioning, the clinician needs to decide whether to approach the concomitant problems *sequentially* (treating one problem before the other; e.g., treating stuttering until near mastery or attainment of the stated objectives before initiating articulation of language treatment) or *concurrently* (treating stuttering and other speech or language targets at the same time). If the decision is to move forward with a concurrent intervention, the clinician decides on the different targets that will be addressed and how to approach them simultaneously (Bernstein Ratner, 1995, 2005b).

Sequential intervention has the advantage of being able to achieve a level of success in one area before tackling another. In other words, sequential intervention prioritizes the child's goals and organizes them linearly so that secondary goals are not addressed until primary goals have been met. Whether fluency or language/phonology is addressed first, however, sequential intervention has the clear disadvantage and ethical implications of delaying treatment in an area of exceptionality deemed as secondary, albeit warranting attention. If developmental language disorder is addressed first and requires long-term management, when would one be able to address the fluency disorder (Bernstein Ratner, 1995, 2005b)? As noted previously, delaying fluency intervention is of concern in light of the accumulating evidence in favor of early intervention. Also, given the reluctance among clinicians to treat stuttering (Manning, 2010; St. Louis & Durrenberger, 1993, Yaruss, 1999a; Yaruss & Quesal, 2002; Yaruss, Quesal, & Murphy, 2002; Yaruss, Quesal, Reeves, et al., 2002), they might delay stuttering intervention indefinitely. If the fluency disorder is addressed first, a phonological disorder is not likely to worsen. However, a speech sound production disorder can limit a child's ability to be understood by others, negatively affecting his interpersonal interactions and thereby his thoughts and feelings about himself as a communicator.

Concurrent intervention treats fluency and other communication disorders simultaneously. Bernstein Ratner (1995, 2005b) suggested that fluency training be placed within linguistic and phonological contexts that the child can manage (within the lowest level of phonological and linguistic demand). For example, when treating a primary phonological disorder, a clinician can treat the fluency disorder by modeling the correct production (both speech-sound and fluency-related factors) without direct reference to the accuracy of the child's articulation. The clinician thus avoids overt correction of the child's speech, withholding direct feedback about the child's articulation to prevent possible communicative, emotional, or neurolinguistic stress being imposed upon the child. Manning (2010) reminded clinicians that each child responds differently to feedback given his unique capacity and response to communication demands, necessitating an individualized approach. Similarly, Bernstein Ratner (1995) recommended that areas within the child's language competency serve as initial fluency targets and that such competencies, targets, and related activities be determined individually, noting,

Particularly given documented trade-offs between expressive syntax and fluency . . . , the premise that all fluency therapy for children should introduce fluency skills at carefully graded levels of linguistic demand is all the more important when both expressive language and fluency are impaired. Fluency-facilitating activities should actively avoid requiring the child to produce utterances beyond those that are comfortably within the child's expressive grammatical repertoire. (p. 182)

Concurrent approaches should thus be reserved for children whose fluency system does not appear to be stressed or weakened by the requirements of feedback monitoring (i.e., children whose fluency behavior is not disrupted by the dual tasks and related processing of feedback; Bernstein Ratner, 1995, 2005b). For these children, goals for fluency intervention can be incorporated or "blended" into other remediation activities (e.g., phonology). For example, while practicing articulation targets, children in Conture, Louko, and Edwards' (1993) pilot program were encouraged to speak slowly, adjust rhythm and rate, decrease interruptions, increase the pause time between conversational turns, and adopt an overall relaxed manner of speaking. However, such intervention may not be advised when the articulation or language intervention disrupts the fluency system. In such a case, a sequential form of treatment would be advised, where a stable level of progress in one area is achieved before the clinician addresses another.

Byrd et al. (2007, pp. 178–180) reviewed and modified six intervention principles and related procedures for treating children who stutter and who have a phonological disorder (Conture et al., 1993; Wolk, 1998). This creative, concurrent approach avoids any conscious attention to articulation precision, which can worsen the disfluency. As such, this approach is a departure from traditional phonological treatment, which directly and repeatedly modifies sounds to achieve accurate place and manner of articulation. In short, this approach indirectly modifies phonological errors while directly modifying disfluency, as summarized here:

- *Use an indirect approach to the treatment of phonological errors.* This approach does not attempt to change the child's speech-sound production directly, but rather creates a relatively relaxed, enjoyable communication environment in which the clinician models slow, physically relaxed speech production. Phonological targets are introduced through play. While no explicit expectation is placed upon the child for accurate speech-sound production, closer approximations are rewarded positively. For example, rather than informing the child that the goal is to produce the *sh* sound correctly, the clinician might tell the child, "Today we are going to have fun shooting basketballs through the hoop" (Wolk, 1998, p. 73). By playing a game of basketball, the child hears multiple models of "sh" (i.e., *shoot*) each time the clinician shoots the basketball and says "sh" to help the ball go through the hoop. This is done for auditory training. Then, each time the child hears and identifies "sh," he is allowed to shoot the basketball. Later, the clinician encourages the child to say "sh" (and eventually "shoot," and then "shoot the ball") each time he shoots the basketball, helping the ball go through the hoop. While the activity does have a phonological target, it is approached indirectly through play. Pressure for accurate articulation is removed as much as possible (e.g., no correction is made for speech production errors). Wolk noted, "The entire focus of the indirect approach to phonological treatment is placed on the activity with the constant inclusion of a phonological target; however, the target is never highlighted to the child as the primary goal" (p. 73).

- *Use a phonological process approach.* Entire classes of phonological processes may be grouped and targeted to speed phonological remediation. If the child demonstrates errors on more than one sound in a phonemic class, treatment would shift to general speech practice rather than direct correction in order to reduce communicative demand on the child. The "gradualness principle" facilitates selecting stimulus items that increase in linguistic complexity, progressing from consonant-vowel-consonant (CVC) words, to consonant-

consonant-vowel-consonant (CCVC) words, to sentences, to conversational speech. To minimize the child's attention to articulatory errors, all productions (both accurate and inaccurate) are accepted; accurate productions are verbally rewarded.

⬚ *Use direct fluency modification techniques.* Fluency is modified directly by reducing the rate of speech, thus allowing more time to plan semantic and pragmatic elements and to select, sequence, and execute the articulatory motor plan (speech-sound productions). The increased time is particularly useful with phonologically complex targets (e.g., consonant clusters, multisyllabic words), which presumably increase the demand on the phonological and motor plan. Thus, the increased time for phonological organization and execution can reduce disfluency in children who stutter and have phonological disorders. Other direct fluency intervention methods that derive similar benefits include soft/light articulatory contacts, slight vowel elongation, and prolonged speech. Using light articulatory contacts facilitates gradual transitions, moving slowly from one articulatory posture to another within and across word boundaries, thereby reducing the likelihood that the child will block on a specific sound (e.g., fixed articulatory posture or sound prolongation). Using slight vowel lengthening creates prolonged speech, which also enhances fluency.

⬚ *Use a concurrent approach combining phonology and fluency intervention.* Introduce phonological targets with fluency facilitation techniques concurrently. Model slower, physically relaxed speech while indirectly working on phonological targets. Do not draw attention to or provide direct feedback for the child's speech errors. Rather, enable the child to remain involved in the fun of the activity. Introduce conceptual contrasts for both disorders (easy/hard speech, slow/fast speech, front/back sounds) within the context of play.

⬚ *Involve parents in treatment.* Solicit parent involvement whenever possible. Ensure that parents reduce their own speaking rate to facilitate the child's processing and expression, remove time pressure by increasing pause time between conversational turns, avoid direct correction of the child's error, eliminate drill and expectations for articulation accuracy, interact daily with their child while applying these techniques for at least 10 minutes per day, and listen to and demonstrate their commitment to their child.

⬚ *Use group settings to augment individual treatment.* Group settings promote ecologically valid interaction, reduce the focus and stress on an individual child to achieve accurate phonological targets, maximize friendly competition, and create an opportunity for the child to monitor his own speech and that of others. Use of groups, however, may be curtailed for children whose speech intelligibility, severity of phonological disorder, or behavior (e.g., hyperactivity, impulsivity, extreme sensitivity, attention span) presents significant limitations.

Finally, another intervention option is a *cycles* approach, in which each disorder receives treatment for a predetermined amount of time and alternation to other goals and return to prior targets is predetermined (Bernstein Ratner, 2005b). This approach is borrowed from the cycles approach in phonology (Hodson & Paden, 1991), which demonstrates spontaneous gains during times when a specific target is temporarily dropped from the therapy schedule after initial skills have been taught (Bernstein Ratner, 2005b). In this approach, specific time intervals are used to treat each of several disorders, cycling from one to the next. A criterion basis can also be used, in which treatment in one disorder continues until a predetermined criterion level of performance is achieved, followed by treatment for a second disorder until a predetermined criterion of performance is achieved, and so on for remaining disorders (Logan & LaSalle, 2003). Healey et al. (2005) provided an example of a cycles approach with a child with Down syndrome. The first cycle could focus on using a prolonged speech pattern while producing single words or phrases, pausing between phrases, and using proper turn-taking skills. Once the criterion level is achieved at these relatively simple levels of linguistic complexity, a gradual increase in length of utterance could be implemented to include sentences or short monologues, combined with an increased speech rate and reduction of pauses between utterances. The second criterion-based cycle could use another simple expressive task (e.g., rhymes, jingles) to promote the child's learning of predictable language structures. The third and fourth cycles could focus on reviewing the previously learned fluency management skills and language skills together, introducing new strategies that fall within the child's abilities within the specified communication context. Healey et al. (2005) suggested that the parents could be included in such a cycles approach by having them provide indirect support or modeling of target behaviors outside of the clinical setting. Also, the clinician should not expect the child to integrate stuttering and articulation/language skills within the same activity until he has been successful with the skills in different activities. Because different behaviors (fluency and speech/language) are being targeted simultaneously, the nature of the feedback becomes even more important. As discussed previously, generic verbal feedback, such as "Good job," is confusing without a clear referent. In contrast, when reinforcing less effortful stuttering behavior, the clinician might say, "That was even and gentle when you said 'I want that one'" (the clinician repeats the word or phrase with an appropriate model); or when reinforcing correct sound production, the clinician might say, "That was an excellent *sh* sound when you said 'I'll *sh*ow you'" (the clinician repeats the phrase with an appropriate model with verbal emphasis on *sh*).

You have probably noticed that a number of the principles and procedures highlighted for intervention with school-age children who stutter and who have concomitant communication disorders overlap with those reviewed previously for school-age children who stutter. This is no accident. In fact, the intervention suggestions herein are intended to achieve the same objective—to enable the school-age child maximum opportunity to realize his own communication potential, to access and contribute to community resources, and to experience fluency and communication freedom. For all children who stutter, with or without concomitant disorders, treatment should be designed with an understanding of the child's unique capacities and responses to a variety of demands and challenges. This understanding should be factored into the core of treatment itself. Indeed, with commitment, compassion, and competence, clients should be "pushed to the upper ranges of their ability" with full support, acceptance, and nurturing in order to significantly impact their fluency disorder. Manning's (2010) conclusion applies to all children:

> The clinician working with young children who stutter should be able to help them to learn to easily produce difficult sounds or new grammatical structures without introducing the idea that they need be concerned or frightened or should struggle with their speech. It is possible to model a smooth and flowing manner of speech production while also giving the child a real sense of command over him- or herself. (p. 468)

Working with Parents

No one influences a child more profoundly than his parents or other primary care providers. Because of this influence and the dynamic interaction between members of a communication system, the importance of actively engaging the parents within the intervention process is indisputable. In Chapters 5 and 8, we discussed these influences and the importance of working with parents. A few additional comments here will focus on the uniqueness of working with parents of school-age children who stutter.

Access to Parents

For many years in my work at a university-based speech and hearing center, I have enjoyed the luxury of relatively easy access to the parents of my school-age clients who stutter. With few exceptions, at least one parent actively participates in a part of every scheduled treatment session and in the activities that are conducted regularly between scheduled sessions. I have never forgotten, however, from the years I worked as a school-based speech–language pathologist, that such regular access to parents is rarely possible in school settings. In the school setting, direct meetings with parents take on even greater significance for the clinician, who is challenged to develop other mechanisms to inform and engage parents within the intervention process. Others have addressed such strategies, including specially scheduled meetings that accommodate the parents' schedules, phone calls, newsletters, emails, memos, "snail mail," and "backpack mail" (Conture, 2001; Dell, 2008; Guitar, 2006; Manning, 2010). Maintaining active interaction with the parents and engaging them in the treatment process are key objectives. To these ends, the quality of the interaction with parents takes on additional meaning; indeed, quality cannot be replaced by an increase in quantity.

Families often have special circumstances (see Chapter 5) that reduce their ability to attend scheduled meetings during the hours of school operation. In addition, cultural considerations (see Chapter 6) may influence the parents' willingness to participate in the intervention process or the child's ability to follow through with assignments outside of the clinical setting. The clinician must not assume that such lack of attendance, participation, or follow-through necessarily equates with a lack of interest or concern. Parents have many priorities (such as work schedules or financial considerations) that understandably may be regarded as more important than their child's speech fluency. Other limitations may exist. In mountainous, rural, or poor urban areas, some families cannot be reached by telephone, some may be functionally illiterate, and some may not speak English. Particularly when there is only one parent at home, some families may not be able to afford services and some may not be able to transport the child to treatment. These and other circumstances may interfere with the child's or parents' participation in the intervention process.

Respecting the Primary Role of Parents

A brief but significant caution is in order. In our commitment to help school-age children transfer and maintain the effects of treatment on their speech fluency, we solicit the help of others, particularly parents, outside of the clinical setting. I am concerned, however, that at times the degree and type of involvement proposed for the parents may not reflect an awareness of and sensitivity to their unique role. The parent is not the clinician in absentia. The parent is the child's primary source of guidance, support, and nurturing. This is not to say that the parents cannot or should not be critically involved in all aspects of the treatment process. Indeed, they should. However, in considering and designing methods for the parents to contribute to the intervention process, clinicians must be mindful of the parents' more primary roles.

An example might help illustrate my concern. Most clinicians would agree that parents are often inclined to provide their child with verbal feedback about the relative correctness (i.e., fluency) of the child's speech. It is hard for parents to watch their children make errors. Typically, parents (and clinicians) remember to provide feedback when disfluency is observed. In such cases, the feedback provided is typically correction ("No, that's not quite right. Try slowing down a little. Oops! You forgot the gentle stretch. Wait a minute. Let's remember to talk like the turtle."). Without advice from the clinician, well-meaning parents inadvertently create a situation in which the child becomes reluctant to talk, knowing that he is facing certain correction. In other words, while the parents believe they are being helpful, they are inadvertently penalizing the child for talking. The child ceases to participate in family conversations, and the parent or child becomes emotionally upset.

Let's cast this a little differently. To prevent a setback, we can discuss with the parents the importance of keeping verbal interaction a fun, happy experience and of encouraging the child to develop his own communication independence. One method that encourages both of these objectives is to provide the child with positive feedback. That is, we need to continually point out to the child the many things that he is doing right. All of us are inclined to do more of what we feel we are doing well. Showing the child that he is succeeding will encourage him to be a more active conversationalist; constantly correcting him will close him down. Some parents will say, "But he is so disfluent. Listen to the way he struggles." Such disclosures remind us that we need to show (discuss, demonstrate, and then direct/coach) parents that even when the child is highly disfluent, much, if not most, of his speech is fluent. The fluency is what we want to highlight. In fact, the child's disfluency should serve as an additional reminder to the parents to compliment the child's fluency ("You said that great! That was really gentle. You remembered to use your slow, easy speech just now when you said 'ttthat.'"). Other parents will say, "Sure, I can give feedback for the fluency, but I'm not doing anything about the disfluency." This is where modeling and expansion come in.

I explain to the parents that a good way to correct the disfluencies is to show the child by example how to talk more slowly and gently. When the child is disfluent, his parents may use the word that the child spoke disfluently in a different but related sentence while using slow, gentle speech. For example, if the child says, "I cuh-cuh-cuh-can't find the duh-duh-duh-dog," the parent might respond with, "You cccan't fffind the dddog. I bbbet hhhe'll be bbback sssoon to bbbe fffed." The parent is being encouraged to compliment the child on all aspects of his speech that are slow and gentle and to model and expand the child's sentence during instances of disfluency. It is also helpful for the parents to demonstrate ongoing models of slow (evenly paced), gently produced, relaxed, natural-sounding speech for the child. In this way, fluent speech is encouraged and modeled, all within a positive framework in which the child develops or maintains his active role and independence as a communicator. Other suggestions discussed in Chapter 8 for parental intervention apply here as well (be good listeners; simplify, soften, and slow daily speech models; reduce the pace of activities and overall tension; and identify and eliminate interruptions). The reader may want to revisit Chapter 8 to review these suggestions.

Despite the best coaching from the clinician, some parents find it difficult to remember to accentuate the positive rather than dwell on the negative. I remember one mother who made this challenge absolutely clear to me. After doing my best to explain the rationale for the positive focus by the parent, she said, "Oh, I understand. But what you're saying is that I should notice when there are no cobwebs in the corners by the ceiling. I notice the cobwebs when they are there, but it is so hard to remember to notice the ceiling when the cobwebs are not there." The mom has a good point; sometimes it feels as if a clinician's job is never done. We agreed that seeing the cobwebs will remind us to take notice of the many clean corners in the house.

One additional mention is in order. As noted in Chapter 5, the Lidcombe Program identifies the parent as the primary agent of change in the intervention process. Indeed, the Lidcombe Program presents a contrast to the caution I offer here to respect the primary role of parents. As also noted in Chapter 5, the Lidcombe Program directs the clinician as well as the parents to provide correction to the child—an aspect of the treatment that concerned me before I witnessed it in action; the delivery of feedback to the child could not have been more gentle or positive by the parent or the clinician, who was training the parent. The apparent conceptual contrast and concern over the nature of parental involvement are both reduced significantly when the nature of the feedback is taken into account. Nevertheless, contrasts are good; no field or discipline has ever advanced without it. There are many treatment venues for people who stutter; this too is good. Their worth is interpreted by the extent to which they enable people who stutter to achieve fluency freedom, to experience communicative empowerment, and to feel at peace with themselves and their place in the world.

Meeting Parents' Needs

To this point, we have addressed how parents can help respond to the communication needs of their child. In most cases, the child's welfare is the parents' primary concern. We cannot overlook, however, that parents have needs of their own. Parents' needs, like those of their children, are behavioral, affective, and cognitive. We have addressed the parents' behavioral needs (what the parents can do to help their child establish, transfer, and maintain speech fluency). But meeting the parents' needs does not end there.

Many parents have intense feelings about their child's stuttering. Some feel responsible, some feel helpless, some feel resentment. Many parents are not aware of how they feel. Parents experience multiple demands upon their time and energy; thus, many feel they cannot afford the "luxury" of focusing on, understanding, or addressing their own feelings. Dell (2008) recommended that clinicians provide parents with "an opportunity to unburden themselves of some of their pent-up feelings of frustration, guilt or anxiety resulting from their child's stuttering. . . . The parents need to talk and talk freely" (p. 88). Parents so often are advised by well-meaning peers and professionals not to worry about their child's stuttering. We noted in the last chapter that "worry" is a factor in most parents' job descriptions. Telling them not to worry not only is useless advice but also reflects neither an understanding of nor a sensitivity toward the parent as a person. Dell suggested asking parents general but leading questions combined with active listening and reflective speech. Such techniques help parents see that we are interested in and relate to their story, which encourages them to talk further. For example, the clinician might say, "Tell me about Juan. What are some of his strengths and weaknesses, his likes and dislikes?" When the parent talks about the development of the child's speech, and particularly his stuttering, the clinician asks about what they think might have caused it and what they are doing to help the child when he stutters. Dell suggested the following as a lead-in for parents to express their feelings: "I'll bet you've had lots of advice from relatives and friends? It seems that everyone is an expert on the problem of stuttering, and they all feel that you are not using the right methods to cure his stuttering. People love to give advice to us about our children" (2008, p. 89).

Along with offering leading expressions and reflective listening, clinicians must be tolerant, if not nurturing, of silence. Without constructive silence, parents are often unable to unburden themselves and share their feelings, and clinicians are unable to gain insights about clients and their families.

Such interactions with parents often reveal their feelings of guilt (the painful feeling that results from doing something we think is wrong; B. Murphy, 2005) and personal responsibility. Some parents conceal their feelings by appearing calm and confident. However, when provided the opportunity, many parents express somewhat emotionally loaded feelings of accusation from society or self-condemnation for their child's stuttering. Dell (2008) emphasized the importance of alleviating the parents' feelings of guilt, even when parents have done things that are harmful to their child's fluency, because such feelings impede the parents' ability to follow the clinician's guidance and facilitate the child's fluency. Also, the parents' feelings of guilt are often communicated to and affect the child. The child may feel that he is at fault for causing the parent distress and may become even more reticent. Clinicians can alleviate such feelings of guilt by accepting and supporting the parents' expressions of feelings and insight and providing more accurate information about communication, stuttering, and strategies available for intervention. In other words, we cannot change what has already passed. However, the clinician is a source of support and a resource of information, the combination of which alleviates the parents' fears by showing them that both the burden of stuttering and the commitment to successful intervention are shared.

The clinician also must meet the parents' cognitive need, or need for knowledge. That is, parents' actions, what they typically do or say to help the child while he is stuttering, reflect what they think or know about communication and stuttering. One of the first questions parents ask is, "What causes stuttering?" An implicit request is, "Tell me I am not the cause of it. Tell me that I am OK as a parent even though my child stutters." Again, we need to determine the parents' beliefs and assumptions, offering support for all the parent might be doing that facilitates fluency. At the same time, we must provide information that reflects our collective knowledge base in these areas and offer constructive suggestions for intervention and change that will facilitate the child's fluency. These discussions, however, must be responsive not only to the child's needs but also to the parents' ability to understand the information provided and to contribute meaningfully to the intervention process. Most parents are willing and able to contribute to the intervention process and help with follow-through activities at home. We must remain mindful of the multiple and pressing demands experienced by parents.

I have been working with a boy who is being raised by his grandparents. They came to me despondent over the boy's clinical depression, resulting from his severe stuttering. As often as possible, the grandparents are included in the boy's treatment, enabling them to understand the process and to be an essential part of it. Their questions are important; their needs are real. My meetings with them deliberately focus on responding to their need for information, emotional support, and an opportunity to be heard and nurtured. Recently they left me a note that reflects the importance of responding to the cognitive and affective needs, in addition to the behavioral needs, of all participants in the treatment process:

> We love this young man so much and, when we first came to you, we had no idea how to make his life better. We tried everything we knew to do. You gave him something to live for and you took an interest in us. Words cannot express our appreciation for what you have done for our family. I hope you know that the time and effort you have taken has saved his life. We will always be thankful.

Working with Teachers and Other School Personnel

School personnel, particularly teachers, play a key role in the management of school-age children who stutter. Many of the suggestions discussed earlier for parents also apply to classroom teachers. Excellent instructional materials are available with constructive suggestions for teachers and intervention in school-based settings (e.g., Cooper & Cooper, 2003; Dell, 2000; Guitar, 2006; Manning, 2010; Ramig & Bennett, 1995; Ramig & Dodge, 2010; Reitzes, 2006; see also the Appendix, which lists useful websites that offer materials in English and other languages). Given the importance of such school-based instruction about stuttering (Ivoškuvienė & Makauskienė, 2009; Langevin, 2009; Makauskienė, 2008), a few other suggestions are provided here.

Build Rapport and Establish Colleagueship with Teachers

Most teachers know their children so well, even before the school year begins, that they proactively seek appropriate information when they anticipate working with a child who stutters. Nevertheless, before we can expect teachers to help contribute to our communication mission with children who stutter, we must first establish rapport with teachers as colleagues in education. One way to accomplish this is by initiating a meeting with the teacher. If at all possible, ask the teacher for her preferred times, or at least give several options from which the teacher might choose. Again, this shows our respect for the teacher's time-consuming responsibilities. The purpose of the meeting is to exchange information so that the clinician can work with the teacher to achieve the child's communication objectives. However, just as we must be mindful of the parents' primary role, so we must respect the teacher's instructional mission, seeking to determine how we can help her achieve that mission, particularly with children who stutter. Collegial collaboration is a two-way street.

Mutual respect and support must rule. In the initial meeting, teachers often ask about the nature of stuttering in general, and with more specific questions about the child who is now in her classroom. At the same time, clinicians should inquire about the curriculum and the teacher's objectives and related plans. The classroom (and the curriculum) provide an excellent context to facilitate transfer and maintenance of speech fluency. There is no reason why the clinician cannot apply the fluency facilitating techniques to discussions of the content being addressed in the classroom. Teachers appreciate our interest in their work and individual missions. In fact, the degree of commitment shown by some teachers to support the fluency intervention process is a direct reflection of that shown by clinicians toward the curriculum and classroom activities. Dell (2008) noted the importance of an initial meeting with the teacher. He indicated that there are too many distractions during recess or in the teachers' lounge for good communication. After the first meeting, however, interactions can be less structured and even held in passing.

Manning (2010) noted that the character of the relationship between a clinician and a teacher will depend partly on the model used for service delivery in the schools. In a *consultative model*, for example, the clinician works through the teacher and parents to help the child. In a *collaborative–consultative model*, the clinician works with the child on an individual basis and collaborates with the teacher and parents in planning activities for transfer and maintenance of fluency into the child's daily activities. In a *pull-out model*, children are taken out of the classroom and are seen individually or in small groups by the clinician. The first two models are more conducive to creating long-term change for the child, as well as fostering positive professional interaction and a sense of colleagueship between the teacher and the clinician (Gregory, 1995, 2003; B. J. Moore & Montgomery, 2008; N. W. Nelson, 2007).

Providing communication workshops is another strategy for building rapport and colleagueship between clinicians and teachers and involving school personnel in the communication intervention experience. This is relatively easy for clinicians to do, partly because of the ready availability of instructional brochures, pamphlets, and audiovisual materials (e.g., DVDs) (see the Appendix). And, I have always found teachers and administrators highly receptive to my willingness to present such a workshop. An opportune time is the weekly faculty meeting, typically held after school. This is an excellent time to build teachers' understanding of the nature and treatment of children who stutter, in addition to those with other communication exceptionalities. I have found that video clips from actual treatment easily hold teachers' attention and generate rich questions and lively discussion. Also significant is the clinician's willingness to share not only what she knows, but a glimpse of what she does. By example, this invites such sharing among all teachers and provides an excellent opportunity for clinicians to express interest in what teachers know, what they do, and how the clinician can learn from and help the teachers.

Banish Elitism—All Colleagues in Education Are Equal

Elitism means thinking that one is part of a superior or privileged group. Clinicians, particularly those who are itinerant, run the risk of inadvertently communicating a sense of elitism. Clinicians are in short supply. Clinicians hold an advanced and specialized degree. Clinicians often receive a pay supplement for serving the needs of school-age children with exceptionalities. Clinicians work with fewer children than teachers do. Itinerant clinicians are in an individual school for less time than classroom teachers, guidance counselors, and other school personnel. Clinicians generally do not do bus duty, hall duty, cafeteria duty, and other such chores. However, the beauty of working in the schools is that all educators are colleagues in the same bunker. All within the educational team seek to help children achieve their full potential. That is our mission. Nothing more; nothing less.

However, some teachers have expressed understandable resentment when itinerant clinicians assume that their time is in shorter supply and communicate that their instructional needs should take priority. How do we avoid acting or being perceived as elitist? We become an indistinguishable part of the educational team. We volunteer to do all the things that teachers do, even the mundane chores they get stuck with. I recommend that we volunteer to do bus duty and cafeteria duty, sit through faculty meetings, and chaperone school events. I remember visiting and eating with teachers in the teachers' lounge. It is amazing what you can learn from and about teachers just by listening. I even contributed to the "sunshine fund," the kitty of money that was used to recognize significant events in teachers' lives (birthdays, weddings, anniversaries, births, deaths). Even though I circulated to three schools, I enjoyed birthday cake as much as anyone else. More than that, I enjoyed being a member of the educational team. I still maintain some of the friendships that were forged during my first position in the schools more than 30 years ago.

Since that time, I have held several positions. One position in the schools was under contract with the university where I was employed. I established a speech–language–hearing program in a local school district, coordinated related services, and supervised the student clinicians from the university. The school reimbursed the university for my time (2 days per week). One day I was approached by the principal, who invited me to chaperone the annual sixth-grade trip to New York City. He explained that I was one of several teachers who were chosen by both students and teachers to go on this 3-day trip. Flattered to be an indistinguishable part of the educational team, I responded, "Sure, I'd love to." It was not long before I remembered that the university was paying me to provide assessment and treatment services to the school, not walk the streets of the Big Apple. The principal and superintendent officially made their request of my supervisor at the university. All agreed that if I were willing, the school's request of me would be supported and my time during those days would be spent on the school trip. Indeed, we all had a wonderful time in New York City.

Provide Teachers with Strategies to Facilitate Fluency in the Classroom

As noted earlier, teachers provide a pivotal role in helping children who stutter transfer and maintain the positive effects of treatment. Within an educational context in which all professional colleagues are equal, learn with and from each other, and strive to hold paramount the needs of all children, teachers and other educational personnel welcome and are receptive to our suggestions for facilitating fluency in the classroom. Teachers frequently ask questions such as the following:

"When and under what conditions should a child who stutters be expected to recite in class?"

"Should you talk with him about his speech or ignore it?"

"What should you do if the other children laugh at or tease him?"

A few suggestions for teachers follow.

Advocate for all children, particularly a child who stutters. Advocating for a child means showing understanding, being available to the child, and rewarding what he recognizes as progress in behavioral or affective change (Manning, 2004, 2010). This advocacy, like that provided by the clinician, parents, and others, can powerfully reduce the potentially handicapping influence of stuttering. Teachers need to feel sincerely positive about the child who stutters and communicate that feeling to him and others. Negative reactions toward and discomfort about a child who stutters most likely reflect a lack of experience and understanding on the part of the teacher. Clinicians can provide information and instructional materials to help teachers understand the nature and treatment of stuttering. By understanding and being a part of the intervention process, teachers are in a better position to help the child transfer and maintain the positive effects of treatment. The teacher will also more likely have and communicate a positive attitude toward the child as an effective communicator who is working toward self-improvement.

Provide the child with more opportunity to speak on days when he is fluent, less when he is more disfluent. Stuttering, particularly in the early stages of development, tends to be intermittent if not cyclic. In other words, it comes and goes with long periods of remission. In fact, there is some evidence to indicate that early stuttering is situation or context specific (Bloodstein & Bernstein Ratner, 2008; Byrd & Gillam, 2011; Van Riper, 1982). The child may be relatively fluent in most situations but may be more disfluent on the playground or in the lunchroom. As stuttering becomes more firmly established, the child demonstrates disfluency in an increasing number and variety of situations with increasing consistency (i.e., reduced intermittency). Therefore, while intermittency may be frustrating to the child, teachers, parents, and others around him, it is positive in that it indicates incipiency.

By understanding the cyclic nature of stuttering, teachers can encourage the child's participation by calling on him more and providing more opportunities for him to speak on his fluent days. As discussed in the previous chapter, providing opportunities for fluent talking experience helps the child remain positive about communication and the prospects for treatment (Dell, 2008). Conversely, the teacher may reduce the frequency of the child's participation by calling on other children first on days when he is relatively disfluent. Manning (2010) noted that as teachers understand the effect of time pressure and other stimuli on stuttering, they may be inclined occasionally to call on a child unexpectedly or early in the class, when stuttering is less likely to occur. After being called on, the child can relax somewhat and be more attentive to classroom activities. Similarly, teachers may call on a child who stutters when the anticipated response is relatively short, particularly on those days when the child's fluency is more challenged. As always, an open, positive interaction between the child and his teacher is critical for building an understanding of stuttering and enabling the child to discuss his stuttering openly.

Expect the child to participate in regular assignments, but provide flexibility and support when adjustments need to be made. Teachers frequently find themselves in a dilemma when considering how much verbal participation to expect from a child who stutters. Should a child who stutters be expected to recite a poem or book report or read aloud in front of the class, or should the child be excluded to avoid embarrassment? There is no easy or clear-cut solution. On the one hand, forcing a child who stutters to embarrass or humiliate himself seems unnecessary, if not unfair, yet granting special privileges (such as handing in a written report instead of doing an oral report, presenting to the teacher alone, or not doing the assignment) may result in teasing from the other children and a loss of confidence and self-respect. One solution would be to talk with the child privately to discuss this dilemma, thereby conveying understanding and support. The teacher might inquire about how this challenging situation has been handled in previous classes and about the child's preferences. Similarly, the child's parents, clinician, and teachers might be involved in a meeting with the child present in order to problem-solve together. Importantly, the teacher conveys her concern for the child's feelings and her commitment to understand and support the child. The discussion should be positive, based on all of the child's significant abilities. All children have strengths and limitations. No pity or sympathy should be conveyed or tolerated. The teacher and others are interested in and supportive of discovering ways to ensure the child's continued success.

The teacher might also consider a variety of other strategies, working together with the clinician. First, the clinician and the teacher might design a project for the child that involves oral reading, presenting an oral report, or recitation, thus enabling the child to use the classroom setting as an ultimate transfer context for fluency facilitating control. This experience might follow similar transfer activities conducted at home or among friends. Second, the clinician and child might design some instructional aids (e.g., an outline of topics distributed or projected to the class, charts, or tangible materials) that might direct the immediate attention away from the child, thus reducing the demand placed upon the child. Third, the clinician might talk to the child about engaging in some audience participation, again, to reduce the immediate demand. Fourth, we know that stuttering tends to reduce somewhat as audience size decreases, and to disappear during reading or speaking in chorus (in unison) with someone else. Therefore, teachers might consider having the children participate in group activity whereby each child presents to smaller groups of children. Similarly, teachers might consider having children recite or read orally in unison as appropriate, preparing the child to read in unison with groups of decreasing size and ultimately alone.

Manning (2010) acknowledged the importance of both preventing children who stutter from escaping school assignments and responsibilities and making adjustments as indicated. Rather than excluding children from class presentations or plays, he suggested that clinicians should help teachers understand that such children typically do not stutter when they play a role, speak with a dialect, or sing. Therefore, if children who stutter are reluctant to participate in a speaking part in presentations or plays, teachers might consider involving them in nonspeaking or nonverbal parts. Again, there are no simple solutions. Each strategy must reflect an understanding of the child's strengths and needs, expectations in the classroom context, and the sensitivity and creativity of the teacher. Most important, the strategy implemented should be jointly decided so that the child understands the positive support he is being provided; burdens are lessened by virtue of being shared.

Shift perspective to see through the eyes of the child who stutters. The clinician should encourage the teacher to shift perspective, looking at the world through the child's eyes. For example, teachers often ask, "Should I fill in for a child when I know the word he is trying so hard to say?" or "Should I continue to look at the child when he is struggling so miserably? I don't want him to think I am staring." When seen from the child's perspective, solutions might become more apparent. Generally, I recommend not filling in for the child, yet continuing to look at him as one would any other conversational partner. Filling in the word may seem expedient, helping the child in the short run. However, think about how the child will come to feel in the long run, knowing he failed and that the teacher had to talk for him (e.g., "I couldn't even say my own words. Ms. Brown had to say it for me"). Also, looking away might seem expedient until one considers the child's perspective (e.g., "Was it that bad? Did I look so grotesque that the teacher couldn't bear to look at me any longer?"). Teachers should be encouraged to treat children who stutter as "normally" as possible. This means continuing to function as an active listener, engaging in appropriate eye contact, and patiently waiting for the child to finish what he is saying. The clinician might also remind teachers to reward evidence of speech fluency and any indication of treatment progress, and to model and expand occasional words that the child speaks disfluently in evenly paced, gently produced, natural-sounding speech. It is important for children to feel that they have as much time as they need to express themselves and that their teacher is sincerely interested in what they have to say and confident in their ability to say it.

Provide all children, particularly those who stutter, regular support for their daily victories. When the teacher recognizes that a child is electing to participate in class despite his stuttering, she might reward the child either during or after his participation, verbally or nonverbally. With help from the clinician, the teacher will know when and how to respond when a child adjusts his tense and fragmented speech into a more gentle, forward-flowing pattern. She also will recognize when he transfers a fluency facilitating technique (such as cancellation or pull-out) from the treatment setting to the classroom. The teacher will also be pivotal in rewarding these events when they occur in other school settings, such as the playground and lunchroom. When the teacher recognizes these seemingly small events as personal victories, she will recognize and reward their occurrence, thus facilitating the intervention process and cementing the child's positive self-image.

Prevent singling out a child who stutters. In their attempt to protect a child who stutters, teachers may be inclined to speak to the class to build their understanding and acceptance of stuttering. This is not necessarily a bad idea, but it must be handled with care. Consider the following statement of a teacher to her class: "We all know that Johnny tries as hard as the rest of us. We know that he stutters, so let's show him our undivided attention and patience." Such expressions may be well meaning but may invite ridicule from other children and embarrass the child who stutters, bringing unnecessary attention to him. Alternatively, the teacher might do any of the following: First, establish classroom-wide rules against interruption. All children will have a chance to speak (to initiate or respond) without being rushed, but interruption will not be permitted. Second, demonstrate a pattern of active listening, paraphrasing or verbally confirming what each child has said so as to reward, clarify, and encourage the effort. This way, when such restatement follows the response of the child who stutters, he will not feel singled out. Furthermore, such a response is much more affirming than simply ignoring a stuttered response or reacting with silence, thus communicating that what was said by the child who stutters was unimportant. Paraphrasing and clarifying what children say is a valuable instructional tool for the classroom. Third, accept and positively reward the contributions of all children. The teacher should not look tense, uncomfortable, or alarmed when a child verbally contributes to the classroom activity. Teachers need to be aware of the forms of feedback they provide, both verbal and nonverbal. Finally, address exceptionality as a topic of instruction. Stuttering can be discussed as one of many exceptionalities. The children may talk about their interests and strengths and acknowledge the area or areas in which each is working toward self-improvement. Likewise, the child who stutters may talk about his strengths (e.g., he can run the 50-yard dash in 6.9 seconds, a school record) and interests (e.g., sports, photography, nature and wildlife) and indicate that his area of self-improvement is speech fluency. He might choose to share his speech-related objectives and how he is transferring his fluency skills to the classroom. Different school professionals may be invited to talk about exceptionality. For example, the speech–language pathologist may talk about stuttering in addition to other communication disorders; special educators may address learning exceptionalities; the nurse may address diseases, syndromes, and sensory impairments. In this day of heightened appreciation of human diversity, all efforts to build understanding, and thereby acceptance of each other, are consistent with our collective educational mission—to enable each person to become all he or she is capable of and to learn with and from each other in this collaborative, lifelong process.

▦ Clinical Portrait: Thomas Wells

Selected Background Information

Tommy* was 9 years 1 month old when he was referred by his parents and school-based speech–language pathologist for a communication evaluation because of "severe stuttering." Only Mrs. Wells accompanied Tommy to the evaluation, and she reported, "His speech gets better and then worse. Now it is so bad that he gets mad, cries, and says, 'I can't talk. I'm choking.'" Reportedly, Tommy demonstrated average to early developmental milestones and had an unremarkable birth and medical history. Tommy's disfluency first was noticed when he was 3 years old. Its onset was gradual, without any significant co-occurring events. Having been told to "ignore it" and that he would "outgrow it," Mr. and Mrs. Wells did not seek professional advice until Tommy entered kindergarten. Since that time, he was enrolled, dismissed, and subsequently re-enrolled in school-based intervention. Treatment focused on a modified fluency shaping approach in which Tommy received a token for use of slow and gentle speech. The parents reported being informed of his progress but otherwise uninvolved. Tommy was an above-average student in the fourth grade who reportedly felt "singled out" because of having to leave class to go to the school clinician and because of teasing. Tommy resided with one older brother and both parents. Family history for communication disorders was negative. Mrs. Wells was a teacher. Mr. Wells was a professor at a community college.

Abbreviated Speech–Language Analysis

Tommy's communication was analyzed on the basis of a variety of tasks, including conversation, reading, structured and unstructured play activities, imitation of words and sentences, and responses to questions. Tommy's speech rate revealed an average of 98 fluent words per minute in conversation and 79 in reading, both significantly below average. Conversational speech ranged from 6% to 16% disfluency, averaging 14 disfluent words per 100 words spoken. Types of disfluency, based on samples of 100 words spoken, included part-word repetitions (sound or syllable repetitions, 47%), whole-word repetitions (6%), audible sound prolongations (20%), inaudible sound prolongations (13%), word and phrase interjections (10%), and word and phrase revisions (4%). Tommy spoke up to 20 fluent words between disfluencies. However, rhythm and phrasing were irregular. Part-word repetitions (e.g., *luh-luh-luh-luh-like*) contained up to seven units of repetition per instance; whole-word repetition contained somewhat less (i.e., up to three units of repetition per instance). Audible and inaudible sound prolongation ranged from 2 to 17 seconds, the former containing pitch rise indicative of significant laryngeal tension, and both containing rapid eye blinking, facial tension, and irregular, horizontal movement of the head. Interjections ranged from one to six units per instance; revisions were one unit per instance. Reading proved more difficult than conversation, as did repetition of longer words and sentences and responses to questions

---

*Names have been changed to protect confidentiality.

that were longer and more complex. The only other secondary characteristic was aversion of eye contact during disfluency. No disfluency was observed during singing, choral speaking, or choral reading. All other aspects of assessment (informal and standardized) revealed age-appropriate speech (articulation and phonology) and language (semantics, syntax/morphology, pragmatics). All parameters of voice (except the instances of laryngeal tension) and hearing were within normal limits. Tommy's response to trial management combining fluency shaping and stuttering modification during the evaluation was favorable, if not dramatic. Tommy candidly discussed his feelings and frustration about stuttering and significantly reduced the relative frequency and severity of his disfluency.

Recommendations and Objectives

Based on the results of the evaluation, the positive influence of trial management, and the ready support of his family, the recommendation was that Tommy receive direct intervention for 1 hour per week. The objectives were as follows:

- ⊞ to heighten Tommy's awareness of his fluent speech
- ⊞ to increase the frequency of Tommy's fluent speech
- ⊞ to establish fluency facilitating control during instances of disfluency
- ⊞ to transfer fluency facilitating techniques to extraclinical settings and to maintain the effects of treatment
- ⊞ to heighten Tommy's understanding and thereby acceptance of himself as an effective communicator
- ⊞ to invite, encourage, and expect Tommy (and his parents) to participate actively in all aspects of the treatment process (including planning clinical and extraclinical activities, implementing activities, evaluating effectiveness of procedures, and participating in follow-up and revision, as appropriate)
- ⊞ to provide a forum for candid, supportive dialogue and shared problem solving

Treatment Snapshot

Treatment began by establishing a social, human connection between Tommy and the clinician. The clinician learned that Tommy was an avid coin collector, photographer, swimmer, and biker. To Tommy's surprise, the clinician invited Tommy to share what he hoped to accomplish as a result of the intervention process, during which the clinician listened to and took notes about Tommy's ideas and verbally rewarded Tommy for his many instances of gentle fluency. At one point, Tommy broke out into an awkward laughter. The clinician inquired, "What's so funny?" noticing that Tommy's eyes were watering with emotion. Tommy explained, "No one ever asked me what I wanted to do. I was always told what I was going to do. They think we're just dumb kids. And I thought you were going to correct my stuttering, not tell me I was doing great." This gave the clinician an opportunity to explain the nature and process of treatment. "In other words," the clinician explained, "you're going to learn first that most of your speech is fluent. And there seems to be no reason why you can't, with my help and a lot of work, learn to do more of what you already are doing when you are fluent. You will see that being fluent and disfluent aren't things that happen to you, but are results of things you *do* differently." "You mean, I *can* be fluent?" Tommy asked. "Why not? While I cannot promise, we learn to do lots of things by setting our mind to it. We learn to ride a bike. We learn to swim. We learn to use a camera. Why can't we learn to speak just as fluently as you do, even more often?" the clinician responded. Tommy continued, "You're saying that I have a choice? I can be fluent or disfluent?" The clinician said, "That's a big part of it." The clinician added, "You'll see."

The clinician explained that because most of Tommy's speech was fluent, fluency seemed like a good place to start. Indeed, because Tommy's conversational speech ranged from 84% to 94% fluent, why not first work to increase Tommy's control over his fluent speech, thereby increasing its frequency? Rather than direct him *not* to blink, *not* to repeat, *not* to interject, and so forth, this strategy provided Tommy guidance in what he *could do*, and what he *could do more often*. This presented a positive, optimistic, empowering foundation. Tommy increasingly took control over his speech by adopting foci (such as slowness and gentleness) that had a pervasive effect on his communication. Within such a positive foundation, the remaining disfluencies were then addressed directly (e.g., "Hey, wait a minute! What happened there?"). The focus was on what Tommy *could do*, rather than on what he *couldn't do*. With these procedures and others discussed in this chapter, most of the major forms of disfluency virtually disappeared.

To establish a slow, gentle speech model, the clinician engaged Tommy in a choral reading exercise during which she faded her speech volume but then increased it before Tommy became disfluent. Again, Tommy laughed with delight. Initial treatment activities were used to design speaking hierarchies and to narrowly describe the fluent experience. Assignments were designed to be completed at home on a daily basis, following the procedures used in treatment. At first Tommy focused on what it felt like to be fluent when talking to his dog (the lowest or easiest end of one hierarchy), and reported in a little speech notebook one fluent word he spoke in the morning and one in the afternoon (specifically, the word, perceptual and proprioceptive feedback, and the surrounding circumstances). These activities continued up the hierarchy of perceived difficulty and increased in frequency and performance expectation.

One activity that Tommy particularly enjoyed was role-playing an announcer for a swimming competition. A video-recorded swim meet was played with the volume turned off. Tommy sportscasted the event, demonstrating his use of fluency facilitating control and his knowledge of swimming. One day, the clinician video-recorded Tommy in the role of the sportscaster, so that the two could review and critique it, attending particularly to the speech fluency that was maintained as the rate of speech increased (toward the end of the meet).

Tommy's mother was involved in the last quarter of every 1-hour treatment session. His father attended less regularly but was involved nevertheless. At each session, Tommy explained to his mother what he had accomplished. The clinician helped Tommy keep the discussion focused on his successes and maintain a positive attitude about successes he was yet to achieve. On infrequent occasions, Tommy's brother, special friends, teacher, and school speech–language pathologist (with whom Tommy continued to receive treatment, with the clinician's support) attended the sessions. In general, discussions addressed Tommy's successes and the importance of providing praise for Tommy's fluent speech and ongoing models and expansions using slow, gentle speech. Tommy's behaviors, feelings, and thoughts were addressed directly, as were those of the other participants.

Tommy demonstrated increased fluency and successful use of fluency facilitating controls inside and outside of the clinical room. He reported feeling more in control of his speech as well as experiencing more enjoyment of the communication experience. At the top of his hierarchy, Tommy successfully used his controls when speaking to the class, to the principal, and on the phone. His teachers reported marked increase in his willingness to participate and the speech fluency with which he did so. His parents reported that the recommendations provided enabled them to feel that they could actually support his communication needs, resulting in his increased fluency at home and away with family and friends. Others reported to the parents and teachers having noticed Tommy's significant improvement.

Follow-Up and Epilogue

Treatment continued for just under 2 years. During the latter stages, frequency of direct treatment was reduced steadily, requiring increased vigilance on Tommy's part to transfer and maintain fluency. Tommy's fluency facilitating techniques were challenged deliberately by the clinician in the treatment setting, and by his parents, teachers, and the clinician in the home and school settings. Eventually, Tommy was dismissed with an explicit welcome to return anytime.

Follow-up continued for 2 years after treatment concluded, at the end of which time Tommy's rate of speech in conversation and reading had stabilized at between 150 and 160 fluent words per minute. His frequency of disfluency remained no greater than 1% (1 disfluent word per 100 words spoken). Tommy reliably adjusted his oral posture to facilitate fluency before the block occurred (preparatory sets), although occasionally he needed to perform the adjustment while the block was occurring (pull-outs). The only remaining disfluency, therefore, was gentle prolongation of a fleeting nature, lasting no longer than 1 second. These behavioral data, combined with self-reports indicating positive feelings and thoughts about himself as a person and as a communicator, revealed significant fluency progress.

Guiding Principles

Tommy Wells' clinical portrait illustrates the three fundamental types of treatment considerations: intrafamily (personal constructs, family systems), extrafamily (interdisciplinary teaming and multicultural awareness), and psychotherapeutic (fluency shaping and stuttering modification).

Intrafamily Considerations

Feelings of isolation and negativity brought on by his stuttering were beginning to influence Tommy's personal construct (as a person and as a communicator). That Tommy was conversant about such feelings, however, was a positive prognostic indicator that his feelings still were in evolution. Treatment was designed from a positive perspective, accentuating Tommy's understanding of and control over his fluent speech. This control and internalized experience of success then was applied to his disfluent speech. Tommy learned and insightfully expressed that fluency and disfluency were both consequences of his actions, a realization that provided Tommy with a deliberate and responsible choice. Tommy's family was consistently supportive, adjusting aspects of their interaction and discipline to cast Tommy and his older brother in a positive and constructive light. The parents were welcoming of support and constructive suggestions, even when these necessitated behavioral and attitudinal change on their part. They willingly shifted their assumed posture from the clinician in absentia (correcting and charting Tommy's disfluency and reminding him to do his speech homework) to Tommy's advocate at home, praising him for his frequent use of gentle speech and self-corrections; providing ongoing models of slow, gentle speech; offering correction only by example (demonstrating models and expansions of words on which Tommy was disfluent, rather than telling him what to do); and identifying and eliminating sources of interruption and time pressure. Most important, the family members were supportive of Tommy's strengths and needs and rallied to participate in and support each other through the intervention process. The parents and brother were as candid in expressing feelings of uncertainty as they were willing to receive praise and constructive suggestions.

Extrafamily Considerations

The teacher and other school personnel were key figures in helping Tommy transfer and maintain his speech fluency. Specifically, the classroom teacher, the specialty teachers (of physical education, art, and music), the school-based speech–language pathologist, and the principal, among others, understood what Tommy was trying to accomplish and were active on the treatment team, contributing meaningfully to the decisions within the intervention process. These school personnel also felt relatively comfortable in responding to Tommy and making adjustments to meet his needs. Significantly, all members communicated regularly with each other, thus feeling involved, informed, and supported in helping meet Tommy's needs, while also feeling valued for possessing unique areas of expertise and for handling multiple, and occasionally conflicting, responsibilities. The most significant multicultural consideration was Tommy's age and stage of development. All participants in the intervention process acknowledged Tommy as a person whose thoughts, feelings, and behaviors as a communicator were evolving. Other factors of diversity addressed or acknowledged during intervention were the professions held by Tommy's parents and the unique interests of Tommy and his family, which were discussed and valued during the treatment process.

Psychotherapeutic Considerations

Tommy's feelings as a person and as a communicator were becoming negatively influenced by the experience of stuttering. In order to help Tommy preserve his personal construct, treatment combined fluency shaping and stuttering modification techniques. Tommy was provided with opportunities to gain control over his fluency and to generalize these methods to instances of disfluency (fluency shaping), while participating actively in all aspects of the treatment process, discussing his thoughts and feelings about communication and himself as a communicator, and becoming increasingly responsible to function as his own clinician (stuttering modification). Significantly, the people in Tommy's communication system (including parents, teachers, and friends) all participated in planning, implementing, and evaluating the treatment process, all with Tommy's communication-related behaviors, thoughts, and feelings in mind. Tommy realized that fluency and disfluency each represented active and deliberate choices available to him. Perfection was never a goal. Rather, Tommy set out to achieve as much control over his communication skills as he could, treating his errors (disfluency, temporary communication-related setbacks) as constructive stepping stones to learning. Within this positive, constructive, and integrated communication system, Tommy achieved significant gains that have been maintained over time.

Chapter Summary

This chapter presented a variety of strategies for assessing and treating school-age children who stutter. First, each child who stutters must understand the nature of his own speech fluency and be in control of it before effecting reduction in disfluency. Second, clinicians must address what the child thinks and feels about communication and himself as a communicator. Third, effective assessment and treatment require that the clinician understand the child's communication environment and that the child, his family, and others participate actively in all aspects of treatment planning, implementation, evaluation, and follow-up.

School-age children who stutter typically have been doing so for some time. They are developing independence from their parents, while spending more time with children and adults outside of their family. School-age children are also becoming increasingly dependent on their peers and being influenced by school personnel, yet frequently are reluctant or unable to verbalize internal feelings and lack insight to analyze a problem objectively in order to establish alternative solutions. The potential influence of a speech–language pathologist on school-age children who stutter is profound.

Preassessment procedures include completing a case history form, obtaining and reviewing an audio or video recording of the child, and making a preliminary phone call to the parents, teachers, and others. Assessment procedures include a parent interview, teacher interview, child interview, and trial management. The parent and teacher interviews are conversational exchanges of information conducted to foster understanding of the child in a variety of communication settings. Because of potential schedule conflicts during the school day, these meetings are often held before or after regular working hours. The child interview is an opportunity for the clinician to convey her sincere interest in the child as a multifaceted person, not just as one who stutters. The interactions with the child enable the clinician to directly observe the child's speech fluency and disfluency and the extent to which his speech is modifiable, and to gain a better understanding of the child's thoughts, feelings, and attitudes that may relate to his stuttering. The child interview contains speech–language sampling and a variety of structured activities with and without communicative pressure. The clinician uses different forms of fluency shaping and stuttering modification treatment during trial management in order to determine their relative effectiveness with the particular child. Post-assessment procedures for school-age children include a thorough analysis of speech and language skills. This analysis leads to determination of diagnosis, prognosis, and recommendations, all of which are summarized in subsequent meetings with the child, parents, and teachers. Speech analyses for school-age children are similar to those reviewed in the previous chapter, including the frequency, types, molecular description, rate, secondary characteristics, severity and impact, and adaptation and consistency of the child's speech disfluency, in addition to assessment of the child's related thoughts, feelings, and attitudes. The diagnosis integrates all of the information available to determine the nature of the child's speech fluency and disfluency and whether or not treatment is warranted. If intervention is indicated, the clinician estimates the child's prognosis for improvement within a proposed course of treatment. Treatment recommendations vary with each child, particularly with respect to intrafamily, extrafamily, and psychotherapeutic considerations, and are discussed with all parties involved.

Treatment goals for school-age children who stutter are spontaneous or controlled fluency, as well as establishment or maintenance of a positive attitude toward communication and oneself as communicator. Specific and comprehensive treatment strategies were presented, discussed, and applied for the purpose of achieving four objectives: (a) establishing or increasing and transferring fluent speech, (b) developing resistance to potential fluency disrupters, (c) establishing or maintaining positive feelings about communication and oneself as a communicator, and (d) maintaining the fluency inducing effects of treatment on communication-related behaviors, thoughts, feelings, and attitudes. Increasing and transferring fluent speech involves constructing a "safe house," inviting treatment objectives from the child, creating opportunities for the child to experience fluency success, heightening the child's awareness of his speech fluency, developing or improving use of fluency facilitating controls during instances of stuttering, and transferring fluency facilitating controls to extraclinical settings. Developing resistance to potential fluency disrupters involves engaging the child in activities with gradually increasing degrees of competition, reintroducing direct fluency challenge, addressing the situations on the top rung of the child's communication hierarchy, and preparing for relapse (relapse happens!). Establishing or maintaining positive feelings about communication and oneself as a communicator involves empowering the child with constructive strategies for the likelihood of being teased (begone, my bully!), helping the child maintain positive thinking about communication and himself as a communicator, and talking with the child in positive ways. Finally, maintaining the fluency inducing effects of treatment requires helping the child become his own clinician, decreasing the frequency of scheduled treatment, implementing regular maintenance checks of decreasing frequency for at least 2 years post-treatment, building in regular child-initiated benchmarking, deliberately revisiting the past, reexamining the child's personal construct, and integrating treatment changes within the communication system.

Other suggestions were provided for working with children who stutter and have concomitant disorders, and for working with parents and teachers. Working with children who stutter and have concomitant communication impairments requires that clinicians understand the nature and impact of coexisting disorders and address at least three challenging intervention issues (whether to treat, which disorder to treat, and which intervention model to use). Working effectively with parents involves access to parents, respecting the primary role of parents, and meeting parents' needs. Working effectively with teachers and other school personnel requires building rapport and establishing colleagueship, banishing elitism, and providing teachers with strategies to facilitate fluency in the classroom. Such strategies include (a) advocating for all children, (b) providing the child who stutters with more opportunity to speak on days when he is fluent and less when he is disfluent, (c) expecting the child to participate in regular assignments but providing flexibility and support when adjustments need to be made, (d) shifting perspective to see through the eyes of the child who stutters, (e) providing all children regular support for their daily victories, and (f) preventing a child who stutters from being singled out.

The chapter ended with a clinical portrait of Tommy Wells, a 9-year-old boy, in order to apply and discuss the assessment and treatment suggestions in addition to intrafamily, extrafamily, and psychotherapeutic intervention considerations. Presented were selected background information, an abbreviated speech–language analysis, recommendations and objectives, a snapshot of treatment, and a follow-up and epilogue.

Chapter Nine Study Questions

1. This chapter began with a review of general precepts about school-age children who stutter. How might the factors reviewed impact the clinical process (assessment and treatment) involving the child, parents, teachers, and others?

2. We discussed preassessment, assessment, and post-assessment procedures primarily as conversational exchanges of information for a variety of purposes. What is the significance of using the medium of conversation, and how does that medium impact the process and products of assessment?

3. Assessment and treatment of school-age children who stutter are multidimensional and dynamic processes. How do the processes relate to and impact each other? In working with school-age children who stutter, what are the demarcations of assessment and treatment? In what ways might assessment continue into treatment? How is treatment begun during the period of initial assessment? What do you feel are the necessary tasks and competencies for effective assessment and treatment?

4. We have addressed the significant impact of intrafamily, extrafamily, and psychotherapeutic considerations on the intervention process. How do these factors affect assessment and treatment with school-age children who stutter? What similarities and differences are there in the influence of these factors on intervention with school-age children compared to preschool children?

5. This chapter reviewed two goals and four objectives for school-age children who stutter. For each objective, multiple clinical procedures were provided. Despite being presented in linear order for instructional purposes, the goals, objectives, and procedures, in reality, are addressed simultaneously. In what ways do the clinical procedures relate to and impact each other? In what ways do the clinical procedures for one objective impact another objective as well? Which clinical procedures do you think are the most important, and why? How will the individual client's intrafamily, extrafamily, and psychotherapeutic factors ultimately determine which clinical procedures prove to be most important?

6. Clinicians must be aware of a number of considerations when working with school-age children who stutter and have concomitant disorders. What do you believe are the critical issues to be addressed when assessing and treating such children? How will you use what is known about the trading relationship between components of communication to the child's advantage in designing intervention? How will you approach each of the three challenging intervention issues? For whom would each model of treatment (sequential, concurrent, cycles) be most appropriate? On what basis will you make such decisions?

7. Many strategies were reviewed for working effectively with parents and teachers. What are the most critical ingredients for effective clinical interaction with these people? What might parents and teachers hold to be the most important elements of effective interaction with speech–language pathologists? How will the knowledge you gained from this and previous chapters impact your interactions with parents and teachers? How will this knowledge influence the design and implementation of workshops you might present for these audiences?

8. We indicated that working effectively with parents entails gaining access to parents, respecting the primary role of parents, and meeting parents' needs. Specifically, by respecting the primary role of parents, we advised against treating the parents as if they

were the clinician in absentia. Yet, we argue for active engagement of the parents in the treatment process. In what ways might we engage parents actively while respecting their primary role? How would a parent (or clinician) know when that invisible line has been crossed? How might that line be different for different parents and families, and what factors should be considered in making such a determination?

9. The Lidcombe Program (Harrison & Onslow, 2010; Harrison et al., 2007; Onslow et al., 2003) identifies the parent as the primary agent of change for young children who stutter (primarily preschool children) and follows a "rule of thumb" (provide five times the amount of acknowledgment and praise for stutter-free speech than for acknowledgment of stuttering and direction for self-correction). The Lidcombe Program thus presents an apparent conceptual contrast to one of the premises presented here (respecting the primary role of parents). In what ways do you believe the premises and procedures presented in this book and those of the Lidcombe Program are in conflict? In what ways are they compatible? Is there a middle ground? On the basis of what you have learned, how will you determine what is the best form of intervention for the individual child on your caseload?

10. Working effectively with teachers and other school personnel entails building rapport, banishing elitism, and providing teachers with constructive strategies to facilitate fluency in the classroom. When serving school-age children who stutter, how will your work with teachers reflect your attention to each of these three priorities? For example, how will you serve a teacher's educational mission while expecting a teacher to serve your communication mission? How will you become an indistinguishable part of the educational team? Finally, how will you advise a teacher to interact with a child who stutters? What recommendations do you have to enable the teacher to best meet the communication needs of a child who stutters?

Chapter Ten

Adolescents, Adults, and Senior Adults Who Stutter

Assessment and Treatment

I have been a stutterer since I was 5 years old. I am now 61 years of age. Although I have learned to live with it, I would like very much to be cured. I have retired from the city of Asheville after 36 years of service. My children are all grown and on their own. So I feel that now I could give this problem my full time. It would be the greatest thing in the world to be able to talk fluently. Do you think it would be possible to talk with you about this problem?

(From a client's letter of initial contact. This man achieved controlled fluency after 2 years of treatment. He is able to order for his wife in restaurants, introduce himself on the golf course, and lay-read in church—the three most challenging yet appealing objectives he set for himself.)

In the present chapter, we turn our attention to adults who stutter. Specifically, we will consider what it means to be an adolescent, adult, or senior adult; how to assess the communication of an adult who stutters; and how to design and implement treatment with such individuals. We will examine how stuttering impacts the behaviors, thoughts, and feelings of adults who stutter and will conclude with a clinical portrait of one man's intervention experience. We will make the following points:

- Adults who stutter must understand, be in control of, and thereby increase their speech fluency before they can effectively reduce their disfluency.
- Clinicians must help adults who stutter manage not only the behavioral aspects of stuttering but also the more central thoughts and feelings about communication and themselves as communicators.

⌘ Effective intervention must consider and be responsive to intrafamily (personal constructs and family systems), extrafamily (interdisciplinary teaming and multicultural awareness), and psychotherapeutic (fluency shaping and stuttering modification) factors.

⌘ Change is realistic, desirable, and possible at any age across the life span.

⌘ Intervention with senior adults who stutter is a positive, inviting, and enlightening opportunity.

General Precepts About Adolescents, Adults, and Senior Adults Who Stutter

This section addresses what it means to be an adolescent, an adult, or senior adult. We will entertain commonalities first before addressing each group separately. As always, such patterns represent group trends and may or may not relate to a particular individual who stutters.

Precepts Common Across These Three Groups

⌘ Typically, adolescents, adults, and senior adults who stutter have been doing so for a number of years; stuttering usually begins before school age. G. Andrews (1984) noted, "Most children begin to stutter before they are of school age and virtually none, unless they become brain damaged, begin after puberty" (p. 11).

⌘ The stuttering behaviors, thoughts, and feelings tend to increase in complexity the longer one stutters. However, there are many adults whose stuttering symptoms are described by both the speaker and listeners as "mild." Nevertheless, Guitar (2006) characterized the "advanced stutterer" as follows:

Individuals with advanced stuttering are usually older adolescents or adults who have been stuttering for many years. Their patterns, which are well entrenched, consist of blocks, repetitions, and prolongations that are usually accompanied by tension and struggle, as well as escape and avoidance behaviors. Typically, these individuals have developed negative anticipations about speaking situations and listener reactions. Sometimes, their stuttering has been such an important factor in their lives that they have chosen occupations beneath their abilities. (p. 392)

⌘ The duration of the stuttering is thought to be more significant prognostically than the age of the person who stutters (Conture, 2001; Daly, Simon, & Burnett-Stolnack, 1995). Yairi and Ambrose (2005) found that duration of stuttering following its onset is related to persistence of stuttering among young children. This means that the older the stuttering (i.e., the longer one's history of stuttering and, presumably, the more pervasive the experience of communication-related frustration and effort), the less favorable the treatment prognosis. However, I will argue anecdotally that this is not always the case. We will discuss significant communication improvements experienced by adults and senior adults who, for the first time in many years if not the first time in their lives, are able to focus on themselves, their communication, and their own self-improvement. As a consequence, there is no externally imposed limit to their potential progress, including establishment, transfer, and maintenance. The extent to which they wish to progress (and implicitly, the extent to which they are willing to invest in the process of self-improvement) is individually defined and, indeed, an active and constructive choice.

⌘ People who stutter, particularly those who have lived the longest, have stories to tell. Stories and dialogue provide a real (not artificial) and meaningful (ecologically valid) context for human interaction that promotes through modeling the very communication skills we are trying to establish with adults who stutter (Shapiro, 2004c, 2004g, 2007a). Conversation, therefore, provides an ideal context for clinical interaction and for all participants to learn with and from each other.

Precepts About Adolescents

⟁ Adolescence is the period of transition between childhood and adulthood. This transition and others that characterize the life cycle were discussed in Chapter 5. Adolescence begins with the physical and emotional changes accompanying puberty and ends when the adolescent becomes more independent and self-sufficient, typically leaving home or starting a career. Adolescents no longer consider themselves to be children, yet may recognize that they are not quite adults (Blood, 2003; Novak, 2002b; Schwartz, 1993; Zebrowski, 2002, 2003). Conture (2001) noted that adolescents' mood swings and struggle with independence are similar to an approach–avoidance conflict (see also Sheehan, 1958, 1970, 1975). One minute adolescents want freedom and independence from parents; in the next minute they are asking for their parents' advice and support. Similarly, they seem to want the freedoms and privileges of adulthood while occasionally refusing the responsibilities that come with them. Speech–language pathologists must use their professional judgment in deciding whether to treat the adolescent who stutters more like an older child (Conture, 2001) or like an adult (Guitar, 2006; Manning, 2010).

⟁ Adolescence is a confusing period for an individual and his family. The challenges faced by the adolescent and all within the family system are, however, somewhat predictable. Willa Cather (1992/1913, p. 51) noted, "There are only two or three human stories, and they go on repeating themselves as fiercely as if they had never happened before." Nevertheless, the challenges are unique to each person and each family. The local bookstore and library have numerous titles addressing adolescence and teenage years as topics of both research and self-help (e.g., *Get Out of My Life, But First Could You Drive Me and Cheryl to the Mall?*, Wolf, 1991; *Yes, Your Teen is Crazy! Loving Your Kid Without Losing Your Mind*, Bradley, 2003). There are moments, tempered with humor, when we might conclude, "Adolescence is not a stage of life; it is a psychiatric diagnosis" (Chapman & Chapman-Santana, 1995, p. 154; cited in Manning, 2010, p. 406). As a parent of two children, one adolescent and one young adult, I remember vividly the moment when we realized and discussed just how difficult it was going to be to raise a set of parents. We laughed at the magnitude of our shared challenge; significantly, we laughed and we talked. We continue to do so.

⟁ Adolescent changes and pressures are significant and real. These include rapid physical growth, sexual maturation, conflicts between dependence and independence, development of self-confidence and interpersonal skills, the search for personal identity and ultimate meaning, group loyalty, and career choices. Additionally, adolescents confront many high-risk behaviors on a nearly daily basis, including substance abuse, suicide, unsafe sex, teen pregnancy, AIDS, eating disorders, teen violence, school underachievement, delinquency, terrorism, and global crises (Dolby & Rizvi, 2008; Haynes & Pindzola, 2008; Kindlon & Thompson, 2000; Milner, 2004; S. L. Nichols & Good, 2004; Novak, 2002b; Pollack, 1999; Skott-Myhre, 2008; Von Drehle, 2007; Way & Chu, 2004). For these and other reasons, adolescents often are overloaded with personal concerns and do not always welcome clinical intervention. Despite our best efforts to build motivation on the part of the client (specific methods to do so will be discussed later in this chapter), some clients will reject therapy. There are times when it is prudent to support a client's wish to decline therapy or to volunteer that declining therapy is an option. Personal timing is essential. I remember one adolescent who clearly stated, "I don't want to come to therapy." To his parents' chagrin, I suggested that we support his wish, demonstrating our confidence in his judgment. In doing so, however, I made it equally clear that my door was always open and that he should feel welcome to return at any time. Not surprisingly, several years later, he returned as an adult for 2 years of individual and group treatment, achieving controlled fluency that has been maintained for 2 years since. He is now completing a 4-year college degree in social work.

⟁ Adolescents often demonstrate a strong desire to be like, and liked by, others, and not to appear in any way weak or insecure. Revealing that one stutters, even if help is needed and desired, may be perceived by the adolescent as an indication of weakness. Indeed, Conture (2001) cautioned that the last thing some teenagers want is to touch, see, feel, and discuss their speech, the very thing that is bothering them most. Some adolescents have been sent for intervention without their consent; others may be growing weary of continued treatment. Some will mask their true feelings with a "No big deal" appearance or message, concealing their feelings, thoughts, and attitudes. Haynes and Pindzola (2008) recommended a straightforward approach whereby the clinician acknowledges the pressures on the individual, discusses the successes experienced by others, and addresses the academic, social, and economic penalties that result from communication impairments such as stuttering. Others stress the importance of placing the client in the role of the expert about his stuttering, emphasizing the therapeutic alliance as one of mutual dependence, following the client's lead, using humor for strengthening the therapeutic relationship, engaging in writing activities for developing responsibility and expanding insight and coping responses, developing positive self-talk, using creative imagery, adjusting motor and mental focus (as is done with athletes), and engaging in cognitive restructuring to alter core constructs about self and others (Manning, 2010; Zebrowski, 2002).

⬚ While occasionally appearing stalwart and confident to a fault, adolescents are remarkably vulnerable. Indeed, they appear to be self-focused, immune to the many stresses that befall them, always "cool" in family and social situations, committed to relationships with peers above all else, and constantly rendering judgment of adults as "jerks" who are irrelevant and "clueless." We will discuss again the importance of building meaningful rapport where the clinician and client are sincerely interested in each other as people; where the treatment room is a safe house; where the client feels free and without penalty to express himself with or without fluency; and where the clinician is herself offering sincerity, confidentiality, personal commitment, ongoing positive regard, and deliberate opportunities for systematic fluency success. Haynes and Pindzola (2008) advised clinicians to explain the assessment and treatment processes thoroughly, to encourage questions, to listen without judgment to criticisms of parents or school officials, and to discuss the results of intervention with the adolescent who stutters before talking with the parents or school personnel. Zebrowski (2002) noted, "As (adult) clinicians, we will improve our credibility with teenagers who stutter by providing them with a model of adulthood that they can envision themselves attaining and that they respect" (p. 93). That is our challenge, to present ourselves in our most honest light—flawed but accepting, knowledgeable but not all-knowing, focused but flexible. That light, as will be seen, is genuinely inviting.

⬚ Despite the "adolescent mandate" (Wolf, 1991) to let go of childhood and the simultaneous inherent conflicts in doing so, adolescents who stutter provide a remarkably rewarding opportunity for clinicians. Adolescents often demonstrate a degree of energy, enthusiasm, and passion that may be refreshing to the clinician. Working with adolescents provides an opportunity to see through the eyes of someone who is in transition, if not in evolution. It is an opportunity to learn from and with someone who confronts forces and influences about which we might be unaware, someone who has diverse interests and talents, and someone who is more knowledgeable than anyone else about his own private stuttering experience. It is an opportunity to discover and to use our own communication skills and to demonstrate the difference between *human beings* (people engaged in a timeless, placeless, and purposeful presence and focus with another person where words only augment communication and understanding) and *human doings* (people who talk before they reflect, act before they think, and set out to resolve problems they do not understand). Every load can be lightened by sharing; there is no limit to what two people with a joint focus can achieve. Our clients are our best teachers.

Precepts About Adults

⬚ Distinguishing between the end of adolescence and the beginning of adulthood is an inexact science at best. Adulthood begins when the individual becomes relatively independent and self-sufficient, typically coinciding in mainstream United States with leaving home or starting a career. We discussed in Chapters 5 and 6, however, how such separation is culturally mediated; in some cultures, emotional or geographic separation is not a hallmark of adulthood. For our discussion, adulthood will be assumed to represent the working or parenting years, the end of which signifies the beginning of senior adulthood. In other words, adulthood is assumed to begin approximately between 18 and 21 years of age and end between 55 and 65 years of age.

⌘ Adulthood is a period of multitasking. Adults manage and juggle their own personal responsibilities (e.g., establishing and maintaining a marriage or partnership, finances, a home) and professional responsibilities (e.g., career, professional relationships, continuing education), while attending to those of significant others (spouses, children, aging parents, community members). It is a time when many adults report being their busiest and when stress seems to be at its peak.

⌘ Stuttering is thought to be fully developed in adulthood (Guitar, 2006; Haynes & Pindzola, 2008; Manning, 2010). As will be reported, stuttering tends to decrease in severity and significance, combined with a reduction in rate of speech, between later and senior adulthood (Benjamin, 1988, 1997; Searl, Gabel, & Fulks, 2002; see also Cooper & Cooper, 1995; Manning & Monte, 1981; Manning & Shirkey, 1981; Rosenfield & Nudelman, 1991; Van Riper, 1991). Haynes and Pindzola (2008) presented a helpful portrait of stuttering in adulthood:

The disorder is fully developed in adult clients: Speech interruptions are more complex and characteristically compulsive; fears and apprehensions become chronic; avoidance, disguise, and negative attitudes hamper and distort the individual's relationships with others. At this stage, a speech breakdown is not simply a response, it is also a stimulus—the problem has become cyclic and self-reinforcing. Clinicians agree that the treatment of stuttering at this advanced stage is complicated—but far from impossible. (p. 227)

Precepts About Senior Adults

⌘ For the purposes of this discussion, *senior adulthood* refers to those years after one has completed his or her career, when the adult children are grown and on their own, beginning roughly between 55 and 65 years of age. In Chapter 5, we referred to this period as one of review and integration, in which we see shifting generational roles; maintaining individual and marital functioning and interests during physiological decline; exploring new family and social role options; supporting the more central role for the middle generation; making room in the system for the needs and wisdom of the older generation; preparing for and dealing with the loss of a spouse, siblings, and peers; and preparing for one's own death.

⌘ Senior adulthood is a time of aging and later development. Every person ages; however, "old" is a relative concept. For example, my children and my students think of 30 years old as ancient, whereas I view 50 as relatively young. Age, obviously, is interpreted from one's own vantage point. And what is age? Should "old" be determined by chronological age (the number of years one has lived, the metric used most commonly in gerontological research) or biological age (the relative wellness of one's body and cognitive functions) (Worrall & Hickson, 2003)? I remember attending a ceremony to honor a senior professor who was retiring after serving our profession for nearly five decades. Addressing several hundred people assembled, he said slowly, "I am older than most of you here, and younger than every one of you." Nevertheless, as we age, we gray. The "graying of America" refers to the increase in the elderly population. This population has been characterized as representing three different stages, namely the *young-old* (age 65–74), *middle-old* (75–84), and *old-old* (85 and over). While childhood (dependence, immaturity, and education) often is interpreted as the first age and adolescence and adulthood (independence, maturity, employment, and responsibility) as the second age, young-old (retirement from the workforce, personal fulfillment) is often associated with the third age and old-old (final dependence) with the fourth age (Worrall & Hickson, 2003).

⠿ In the United States, people 65 years and older constitute the fastest growing segment of the population; those 85 years and over represent the fastest growing segment of all. While people 65 years and older constituted only 4.1% of the population in 1900, this percentage grew to 12.4% in 2000 and is projected to be 20.4% by 2050. The number of people in the United States over the age of 65 was 3.1 million in 1900 and 35.1 million in 2000, and is projected to be 87 million in 2050. People 85 years and older made up 1.5% of the population in 2000 and are projected to be 4.8% in 2050. People 100 years old in the United States numbered 37,306 (by estimate) in 1990; this number climbed to 64,6587 in 2004 and is expected to be 1.1 million in 2050 (Himes, 2006; O'Neill, 2009; T. R. Palmer & Hunter, 2007; Whitbourne, 2008; Wilmoth & Longino, 2007; Worrall & Hickson, 2003). One centenarian reported, "I had to wait 110 years to become famous. I want to enjoy it as long as possible" (cited in Whitbourne, 2008, p. 1). The rapidly increasing number of senior adults has significant implications for delivery of speech–language pathology and audiology services. At present, approximately 19% of the current speech–language pathology caseload and 33% of the audiology caseload in the United States are senior adults. By 2050, those figures are projected to be 39% and 59%, respectively. Surely, speech–language pathologists and audiologists need to be prepared to address the communication changes associated with healthy aging, including speech fluency (reviewed below), hearing (decreased sensitivity to pure tone and speech discrimination in adverse listening conditions), language (decreased word retrieval and comprehension of complex messages), conversational discourse (reduced understanding of complex and lengthy utterances, reduced cohesion within and between utterances, increased number of words per clause and expressive ambiguity), speech (reduced articulatory precision, rate of speech, and respiratory support), and voice (increased pitch for males, reduced pitch for females, decreased vocal quality) (Benjamin, 1988, 1997; Lubinski & Welland, 1997; Mueller, 1997; Shadden, 1997; Worrall & Hickson, 2003; Zraick, Gregg, & Whitehouse, 2006).

⠿ People age 65 years and older represent a particularly diverse and heterogeneous group in terms of race and ethnicity. While nationally about 86% of people over age 65 are White (i.e., non-Hispanic White), the culturally and linguistically diverse population of elderly adults is growing faster than those who are White. Between 2000 and 2030, the population of senior adults who are White will increase 81%, compared to 131% for seniors who are African American and 328% for seniors who are Hispanic. By 2050, the population of senior adults who are White will have dropped to 64% of the total senior adult population in the United States. Compared to the total senior adult population in the United States, the population of seniors who are African American will increase from 8% in 2000 to 12% in 2050; the population of seniors who are Hispanic will increase from 5% in 2000 to 16% in 2050. Despite higher fertility rates among non-White populations, the population of senior adults who are White will continue to be larger in number because African Americans, Hispanics, and other minorities continue to experience higher mortality rates than Whites from illness and other causes. Such higher morbidity and mortality among African Americans reflect longitudinal disparity in education, employment, and income, all of which limit access to and use of health care (Himes, 2006; National Center for Health Statistics, 2009; Rakowski & Pearlman, 1995; Worrall & Hickson, 2003). In addition to being prepared to address the communication changes associated with healthy aging, clinicians also need to be competent regarding, and responsive to, the cultural and linguistic diversity of their clients.

⠿ The chances of surviving to senior adulthood are related to a person's gender. In the United States in 1900, the average life expectancy for White males was 46.6 years; for White females, 48.7 years; for males of other races, 32.5 years; for females of other races, 33.5 years; and for all groups combined, 47.3 years. In 2005, average life expectancy for White males was 75.7 years; for White females, 80.8 years; for males of other races, 69.5 years; for females of other races, 76.5 years; and for all groups combined, 77.8 years. By 2030, life expectancy for all groups combined should increase 3.4 years for men and 3.3 years for women (National Center for Health Statistics, 2009). Another way to look at life expectancy is to project beyond age 65 years. In 1950, after living 65 years, White males were expected to live an additional 12.8 years, White females an additional 15.1 years, African American males an additional 12.9 years, and African American females an additional 14.9 years. In 2005 after living 65 years, White males were expected to live an additional 17.2 years, White females an additional 20.0 years, African American males an additional 15.2 years, and African American females an additional 18.7 years (National Center for Health Statistics, 2009). These data indicate that elderly women outnumber elderly men. In 1900, the number of males for every 100 females in the population of people (all groups combined) over 65 years of age was 102, in 1930 was 100.4, in 1990 was 67.2, in 2000 was 70.4, and in 2008 was 72.4. The number of males for every 100 females in this population is projected to be 82.9 in 2025 and 84.3 in 2050 (Kart & Kinney, 2001; Whitbourne, 2008; Worrall & Hickson, 2003). This gender gap continues in the United States until the age of 100 years; there are 4 times as many male centenarians as there are female centenarians (Whitbourne, 2008). Further, men over 65 years of age become widowed less frequently (14%) than do women (44%). This means that most elderly men are married; most elderly women are widowed. The disparity between being married and widowed widens with age. By age 85 years of age, 34.6% of men are widowed compared to 78.3% of women (Whitbourne, 2008).

People over 65 years old are not evenly distributed across the United States. Distribution of people over 65 years of age can be interpreted both in terms of *absolute frequency* of occurrence (the number of people over 65 years old residing in a particular state) and in terms of *relative frequency* of occurrence (the number of people over 65 years old compared to the total number of people residing in a state). In terms of absolute frequency, as of 2005, slightly over half (52%) of the people over 65 years of age lived in nine states: California (3.9 million people over 65 years of age), Florida (2.8 million), New York (2.4 million), Texas (2 million), Pennsylvania (1.9 million), Ohio (1.5 million), Illinois (1.5 million), Michigan (1.2 million), and New Jersey (1.1 million) (Vierck & Hodges, 2005; Whitbourne, 2008). Although the largest number of people over the age of 65 live in California, the relative proportion of older adults in California is only 11%. The largest relative proportion of people over 65 years of age live in Florida, where estimates range from 16.8% (Whitbourne, 2008) to 20% (O'Neill, 2009). In terms of relative frequency, there are nine states in which at least 14% or more of the total population are over 65 years of age. In addition to Florida, those states are Pennsylvania (16%), West Virginia (15%), Iowa (15%), North Dakota (15%), Rhode Island (15%), Maine (14%), South Dakota (14%), and Arkansas (14%) (Vierck & Hodges, 2005; Whitbourne, 2008). The geographics of aging, or where the elderly live, is significant because speech–language pathologists in these states will be expected to respond to a greater than average demand for intervention services for the senior adult population. The information we are considering about senior adults has focused on the United States only. It is beyond the scope of this book to consider the international geographics of aging. However, it is interesting to note that world trends confirm an aging population. As of 2006, there were 483 million people worldwide over 65 years of age; that number is predicted to nearly double to 974 million by 2030. Also, the country with the largest number of older adults now and projected to 2030 is China. Italy has the highest relative proportion of people 65 years and older (Whitbourne, 2008). Life expectancy is longest in Japan (81 years) and shortest in Zambia (33 years) (Corliss & Lemonick, 2006).

There continues to be a relative paucity of clinical literature on older adults and senior adults who stutter. Nevertheless, there seems to be general agreement that a less favorable prognosis for treatment is associated with older stuttering (Bloodstein & Bernstein Ratner, 2008; Conture, 2001; Daly et al., 1995; Guitar, 2006; Manning & Shirkey, 1981; Van Riper, 1982). Older speakers, however, demonstrate an interesting paradox. People who do not stutter increase in disfluency as they reach senior adulthood, particularly in the forms of interjection of sounds and words, whole-word and phrase repetition, and revisions or incomplete phrases in the absence of any obvious tension (i.e., between-word, formulative, supramorphemic, or "normal" disfluency). Also observed, as summarized by Searl et al. (2002), are reduced rate of speech (Amerman & Parnell, 1992), increased consonant and vowel durations (Morris & Brown, 1987), and reduced maximum phonation duration (Mueller, 1982). During the same years, people who stutter tend to demonstrate a decrease in sound and syllable repetitions, sound prolongations, disrhythmic phonation, tense or silent prolongations, and pauses with cessation of airflow or voicing between small linguistic units (i.e., within-word, motoric, coordinative, or "stuttered" disfluency) (Benjamin, 1988, 1997; Manning & Monte, 1981; Manning & Shirkey, 1981; Rosenfield & Nudelman, 1991; Searl et al., 2002; Yairi & Clifton, 1972; Van Riper, 1982, 1991). The findings of reductions in disfluency among senior adults who stutter have prognostic implications for this population. Clinical wisdom holds that treatment prognosis is directly and positively related to age of stuttering (i.e., the younger the stuttering, the more favorable the prognosis; the older the stuttering, the less favorable the prognosis). If research addressing older people who stutter continues to indicate reductions in stuttering and the number of people who stutter, then we must reconsider these prognostic assumptions. As Manning and Shirkey (1981) indicated, "It may be that stutterers are at least as likely to recover from stuttering during the last few decades of life as they were during the teenage years" (p. 185). My work with senior adults who stutter indicates that factors other than age of stuttering are at least as relevant when one is estimating prognosis for improvement in fluency as a consequence of treatment. For these reasons, the nature and efficacy of treatment for older people who stutter must receive a more careful and optimistic review.

▣ Recent data emphasize the importance of considering multiple perspectives when researching or treating the "elderly." In fact, the heterogeneity of this vast population commands us to reconsider our old assumptions, typically those of a downward trajectory in function or competence and inevitable and irreversible loss (Bengtson & Schaie, 1989). Clearly, a more positive perspective is indicated by changes in human demographics related to age and social activity (i.e., increases in life expectancy, relative proportion of senior adults, retirements, and the like) and increases in public awareness of both normal and pathological changes with age. Moreover, a more positive perspective of senior adulthood must include one of vitality, wisdom, and relevance; living longer, healthier, better; getting to know one another, again and again; 84 going on 50; seeing anew; and still at work on oneself ("The Age Boom," 1997). A comment made by Sir Edmund Hillary, the first person to reach the summit of Mount Everest, captures a more modern perspective on aging: "I'm eighty-four, but I still fly around the world two or three times a year. Why not? When I'm old, I can sit at home and enjoy the garden" (Hillary, 2004, p. 192).

▣ Senior adults are not necessarily any more like each other than are children or adolescents; they are individuals. In my work with senior adults who stutter, they have proven to me, individual by individual, that change is realistic, desirable, and possible at any age across the life span, and intervention with such persons is a most positive, inviting, and enlightening opportunity.

▣ Highlighting the diversity among the population of senior adults, Haynes and Pindzola (2008) noted that some older clients may present some special problems requiring clinicians to make behavioral adjustments in treatment. They advised clinicians to be alert to fatigue, disorientation, failing eyesight, and hearing loss, and to structure, organize, and pace clinical procedures to ensure understanding. They indicated, "Following standard procedures may not be as important as providing an environment in which the person is able to perform at an optimal level" (p. 30).

▣ Clinicians should expect and invite senior clients to share their stories. Haynes and Pindzola (2008) noted that because of feelings of uselessness or disintegrating health, older clients may need to talk to a clinician as a listening audience about past accomplishments or medical concerns. Indeed, Hooper (1996) suggested that clinicians not only should expect clients and family members to tell "what grandma was like before" but also should facilitate such a process by encouraging use of photographs, pictures, stories, videos, and other memorabilia from past work or home life. Hooper also suggested that clinicians should identify and understand the client's belief systems as they relate to the condition being treated; views of power and control, specifically with respect to service delivery; and differences in professional, family, and client points of view, communication styles, and abilities. Doing so helps "to enhance a positive therapeutic alliance" (Hooper, 1996, p. 45). In the courses I teach and in my writings and clinical workshops, I emphasize the importance of encouraging people who stutter, particularly adults, to share their own story and for clinicians to learn about their clients from these stories. These stories provide a web, a network, a system of communication that connects the participants in the clinical process to each other in a shared focus that transcends time and place. They express the client's developing belief that the world of communication can improve, that good things can happen to good people, and that good things can become even better.

As with all generalizations, these snapshots of the adolescent, the adult, and the senior adult are offered only as a starting point, a set of considerations that inform the clinician but do not keep the clinician from listening carefully, individual by individual.

Preassessment Procedures

The assessment procedures for adolescents, adults, and senior adults are similar. Where significant differences exist, they will be highlighted.

Case History Form, Audio or Video Recording, and Preliminary Phone Call

Several weeks before the assessment appointment, the client completes and returns a case history form. This form provides the clinician with information about the client's developmental, medical, and educational history; family structure; communication strengths and limitations; and onset of, development of, and current perspectives about the communication problem. Because this form is somewhat generic (it requests information that would be appropriate for different individuals and for other speech and language disorders), the clinician can get a preliminary idea about whether the presenting fluency disorder is stuttering and if other communication disorders coexist. For example, typical case history forms ask the following:

- ▦ Who referred you to for this evaluation?
- ▦ What is the reason for the referral?
- ▦ Describe the problem you are experiencing with speech, language, and/or hearing.
- ▦ What do you think caused this problem?
- ▦ How does this problem make you feel?
- ▦ How has this problem changed since it was first noticed?
- ▦ How has this problem affected you (e.g., family/social interactions, education, occupation)?
- ▦ What communication situations are challenging for you?
- ▦ Have you ever sought professional advice about your communication problem? If yes, what were the locations, dates, and results of previous evaluations and/or treatment?
- ▦ Have any relatives had a communication problem? If yes, explain.
- ▦ Describe any illnesses, injuries, operations, or other health problems you have or have had.
- ▦ In what ways might these experiences contribute to your communication problem?
- ▦ Have you been hospitalized in the last year? If yes, please explain.
- ▦ List all prescription and nonprescription medications you have used over the past year.
- ▦ Have you ever had a neurological examination? If yes, indicate the date, location, and results.

Other important questions might include the following:

- 🔢 What do you hope to accomplish as a result of the communication evaluation?
- 🔢 What questions and concerns would you like to see addressed?
- 🔢 What factors (such as family, home, or work) do you feel are influencing your speech?
- 🔢 Describe your areas of strength and special interests or hobbies.
- 🔢 Please feel free to provide any other information that might be helpful in the evaluation.

The client is asked to make an audio or video recording of himself while engaged in family interaction to help the clinician assess his relative speech fluency in that speaking context and begin to understand the communication dynamics within the family or partnership. The clinician also makes a preliminary phone call to help prepare the client and his family for the evaluation, to address preliminary questions, and to convey from the outset the clinician's support and commitment. When possible, the clinician is encouraged to provide the client with at least two alternative times for the assessment appointment. These procedures establish mutual respect, joint decision making, and shared ownership from the beginning of the clinical process.

Significant others with whom the client communicates should be involved in assessment-related experiences to the extent possible and appropriate. Indeed, the longer we live, the more our lives affect and become affected by family and friends with whom we interact closely. Many adolescents are referred by their classroom teachers or parents. If teachers and parents have not already provided preliminary observations and impressions, they should be invited to do so and to provide an audio or video recording of an interaction with the client from their respective settings. Adolescents are encouraged to complete the forms and preassessment procedures themselves, but parental help is welcomed. Adults and senior adults often discuss, if not decide, with their spouses or families the prospect of pursuing fluency assessment. Helping to prepare all members of this significant therapeutic alliance and addressing their questions, therefore, is critical. Hooper (1996) reported one client as advising, "If you want to help me, help my family" (p. 43). Indeed, Hooper recommended intervention from a family, rather than individual, perspective and distinguished between "primary kin" (spouse, children, and siblings) and "secondary kin" (others who may function as family, such as friends and neighbors). Hooper noted that secondary kin "may provide as much, or more, quality of life and happiness for the older adult as the primary kin. They often provide support in tandem with other family members" (p. 44).

Preassessment Conference

Another procedure that I have found useful with prospective clients and their families, particularly with adolescents, adults, and senior adults, is a preassessment conference. Sometimes, inquiries from these individuals or their families or friends about assessment or treatment seem somewhat tentative, if not reluctant. Such reluctance results from a variety of reasons (e.g., discouragement with previous treatment, anticipated pressure from professionals to enroll in treatment, pressure or ambivalence from family or friends, misinformation, embarrassment, fear). In such cases, I invite a preliminary conference in which the clinician interacts informally with prospective clients and their families. This is not a time for structured assessment. Rather, it is a meeting of people, as people, to discuss in a positive, inviting context the questions of our prospective clients and their families and the preliminary aspects of the presenting concern.

The clinician has an opportunity to observe the communication dynamics among the family members; the family has an opportunity to learn about communication, its disorders, and the nature of intervention. I believe firmly that clients and their families make the best decisions when they are fully informed and involved. Helping the client and the family decide whether they wish to pursue a diagnostic assessment is central to the purpose of the preliminary conference. Other avenues of intervention are available and indeed may be more appropriate for some (e.g., fact-finding, reviewing literature or instructional materials for the public about stuttering, reading personal accounts of successful adults who stutter and have had positive treatment experiences). Another avenue that might be pursued before, in tandem with, or instead of intervention is self-help and mutual aid (Reeves, 2006; Yaruss, Quesal, & Reeves, 2007). It is very important to me that the client should experience no pressure. Too many clients report having previously experienced pressure by prospective clinicians in addition to receiving un-realistic promises (Jezer, 1997), only to have their hopes dashed and their readiness for productive change delayed (Floyd, Zebrowski, & Flamme, 2007; Manning, 2006). As a consequence, precious years pass until the client even envisions pursuing treatment again.

Starkweather (1993) discussed the importance of preventing clients from experiencing the placebo effect, explaining that the stuttering severity of some people is strongly attributable to the desperation they feel to find relief:

> When the stutterer believes that he has finally found, perhaps after years of unsuccessful treatment, something that is really going to help him, the desperation gives way to relief, and, since the desperation was causing all or some part of the behavior, the behavior diminishes or disappears. The emotional high that some stutterers feel as they begin a program that they believe in advance will finally resolve their problem may itself have a direct effect on muscle activity levels. (p. 163)

I support the importance of understanding and preventing a placebo effect in fluency assessment and intervention. Also, I agree that our discussion of treatment options and their potential for success needs to be "realistic" and that we must not guarantee outcomes (ASHA, 2010). However, I do not agree that we should present a "pessimistic perception of how successful therapy is going to be" (Starkweather, 1993, p. 163). Clients deserve an opportunity to learn from a clinician who is positive yet realistic within an inviting, supportive, interactive context where they feel understood and secure. In such a preassessment conference, clients directly experience the clinician's competence and interpersonal skills. I find that after a conference of this sort, the client and family are more fully prepared and, with few exceptions, elect to pursue the assessment appointment, now with confidence and heightened understanding.

I remember conducting a preliminary conference with a young man of 16 years and his parents. Having been through a variety of fluency shaping programs without elimination of noticeable stuttering, the family conveyed feelings of shared failure and related frustrations. Essentially, they were "shopping" for other approaches. They expressed frustration that previous treatment seemed to work as long as the young man was "plugged in," but once he left the treatment setting he was no more fluent than before. I took this to mean that they were displeased with the relative lack of transfer of fluency shaping techniques (delayed auditory feedback, or DAF) and his lack of communicative independence. They were intrigued to learn that some therapies address the cognitive and affective aspects of stuttering in addition to the observable behaviors, individualize the design of treatment, involve all members of the family system as active participants in the treatment process, require active participation between all treatment sessions, and emphasize the importance of increasing fluency as a means to decreasing disfluency. Also, they were intrigued when encouraged not to make a treatment decision but, rather, to leave and discuss their options as a family and to feel welcome to call if I might be of help. Indeed they called, and achieved their shared objectives over the next 18 months of scheduled treatment.

I remember another preliminary conference, this time with a man in his 60s who stuttered and his wife. He recalled a history of intermittent treatment spanning more than 50 years. Treatments included immobilizing alternate sides of his body and crawling to stimulate the contralateral cerebral hemisphere, engaging in elocution exercises, receiving psychotherapy and medication, and undergoing hypnosis. They too were intrigued with an alternative approach that maximized their participation in all aspects of the treatment process in order to facilitate communication independence. Abbreviated differential diagnostic procedures indicated that the man indeed stuttered and that he possessed the ability to speak more fluently. He discussed being denied promotions because of his stuttering, which had a negative impact on his retirement. His wife discussed all of the compensations she and their sons made to minimize the impact that his stuttering had on the family (e.g., she always ordered in restaurants for the family, she or the sons answered the phone, and the like). At this, I asked them to consider if they wanted to "open a can of worms." This was not to discourage them, but to invite them to think seriously about the positive effects that his increased fluency would bring and the impact such changes would have on them and their lifetime of adjustments. Some of the effects of stuttering would be irreversible. Specifically, the man had retired; his working years were over. I knew that once he experienced speech fluency and communication independence, he would think about how different his retirement might have been had he achieved his promotions.

This family, like so many others, pursued the assessment appointment and subsequent treatment. During the first day of treatment, as the man was participating in modified fluency shaping techniques (choral reading with the clinician, who reduced and systematically eliminated her speech model), the man exclaimed, "Tell me why! Why couldn't I do this 40 years ago? Why couldn't I do this while I was still working?" We recalled together the "can of worms" and how some tender issues surface and need to be addressed as a part of the change process. Talking candidly with the couple and their adult sons in advance helped them make a joint and informed decision about pursuing treatment, and helped prepare the family for the shared problem solving and adjustments that would be necessary at tender moments of discovery such as these. This man's treatment lasted 2 years, during which time he established communication independence (exhibiting controlled fluency with minimal noticeable stuttering) and mastered the speaking challenges he had identified as being at the top of his individualized hierarchy—ordering for himself in a restaurant, introducing himself on the golf course, and lay-reading in church.

Assessment Procedures

General Considerations

Interacting with adolescents, adults, and senior adults within a supportive, nurturing, conversational context provides an ideal opportunity to invite and dialogue about the client's story. Indeed, it often seems that those who have lived the longest have the richest tales to tell. For years, student clinicians and practicing speech–language pathologists have told me that when I am engaged in assessment or treatment with people who stutter, it looks like we are just talking. Indeed we are, with a shared focus, mission, and bond. I noted earlier that conversation creates a context for the clinician to model appropriate speech and communication skills and for the client to practice these skills within a medium of conversational dialogue that is relatively natural and therefore generalizable to the client's extraclinical communication settings. The importance of involving the client's family and significant others in the decisions and procedures related to the clinical process cannot be overstated. Doing so facilitates changes experienced by both the client and significant others, all of which are brought about by improvements in the client's fluency. Working with and within families ensures that the change process will be productive and constructive.

Assessments of many adolescents who stutter are conducted by the clinician employed in the schools. In these cases, the sequence of procedures is similar to those outlined in Chapter 9 (conferences with parents, teachers, and the adolescent; observations of the adolescent interacting in as many different settings as possible; and a critique of audio- or video-recorded interactions in extraclinical settings). Readers may wish to review these procedures in Chapter 9. Haynes and Pindzola (2008) noted that assessment of older students who stutter is even more challenging because adolescents are more likely to deny the problem, be uncooperative, and lack motivation. As discussed, adolescents present unique and formidable challenges. Nevertheless, the passages being experienced by many adolescents are real, confusing, and somewhat frightening for them. Recognizing and understanding such passages from the individual adolescent's perspective is a critical skill for clinicians (and parents), one that transforms the treatment setting into a safe house and enables the adolescent to feel understood and secure. This does not mean "swinging" with the adolescent, attempting to be "cool," or otherwise relinquishing one's professional role. It does mean, however, that clinicians must avoid preconceptions or stereotypes of adolescents and interact with each client from the perspective of an open mind. Clinicians must realize that stereotypes of adolescents are no more just than adolescents' preconceptions or stereotypes about speech–language pathologists. Many adolescents are remarkably supportive, cooperative, and motivated. Adolescents, like clients of all other ages, present opportunities to rally, use, and improve our own clinical skills.

The remainder of this discussion on assessment procedures will assume that adolescents, adults, and senior adults are being seen at a clinical facility other than that provided in schools. Adolescents are grouped with other adults for discussion purposes because the main emphasis at these ages is on the effect that stuttering has had on their lives and the ways they have learned to react to it (Hayhow et al., 2002; J. F. Klein & Hood, 2004; Klompas & Ross, 2004; Plexico et al., 2005; Stewart & Richardson, 2004). Also, with few exceptions, people of this age who stutter serve as the primary informant for assessment purposes.

Client and Family Interview

Preparation

Before the interview and based on preliminary information (including case history form, audio or video recordings, phone calls, allied medical or educational records, etc.), I prepare myself a telegraphic outline of information that I want to receive and information I want to provide. As always, I remind myself in writing to *listen* and to facilitate an opportunity for the client's story to unfold. This outline helps me to organize my thoughts and procedures, thus enabling me to focus more attention on the client and the dialogue between us. The outline, however, must never be used inflexibly. We must adapt and adjust continuously to the needs, questions, and concerns of those with whom we are interacting. The proceedings should be recorded (video is preferred) for later review and analysis. The clinician should observe the adult's speech directly and determine how it is influenced by structure, linguistic complexity, and communicative pressure; how it is modifiable; and the relative developmental level of the client's behaviors, feelings, and attitudes. The speech sample collected will be used for analysis and comparison to others collected from other speaking contexts.

Social Greeting

The interview should begin with a social greeting. I feel strongly that before we can interact effectively within a professional domain, we must recognize and respect each other as people. In the previous two chapters, we discussed the importance of establishing a foundation as mutually interested and interesting people. The clinician seeks to understand and conveys her acceptance of the adult and his family, independent of the stuttering. In the old days, establishing a personal foundation was referred to as "establishing rapport," a critical first step in the clinical process. It seems that today, with our faster pace, instantaneous technological connectivity, emphasis on evidence-based practice, and unavoidable accounting of "patient contact hours," something risks being lost. We might be inclined to get right to business, to use clinical time "efficiently." We might ask questions immediately about the problem (e.g., "So, tell me about your stuttering"), rather than connecting as people (e.g., "Did you find the clinic OK?" or "What do you think about this crazy weather?"). We have discussed the importance of intrafamily and extrafamily considerations in designing assessment and treatment. Occasionally, such "small talk" leads to discussion that helps us understand the client's assumptions about himself and his communication (personal construct), his family structure (family system), previous treatment or professional contact (interdisciplinary teaming), or unique cultural or personal perspectives (multicultural awareness). While the clinician structures the assessment context, there is no replacement for talking and communicating with the people and families we are trying to know, understand, and serve. At this point, permission forms and releases are signed, and the client is given a general orientation of the assessment process. The clinician explains that she is interested in learning more about the client as a person and as a communicator and about the network within which the client interacts. To do so, she explains, she will be asking a number of questions about the client's communication experiences and related feelings and engaging the client in a variety of speaking tasks. Each of the procedures, which will be audio- and video-recorded, will result in speech samples that will be analyzed for speech fluency and communication competence. The results of this analysis, including a diagnosis and related intervention recommendations, will be discussed in a closing interview at the end of the meeting and will be followed by a written report detailing the items discussed.

Questions and Dialogue

The assessment of adults who stutter is primarily an interview consisting of many direct and open-ended questions. Readers will recognize parallels in the interview presented here with those presented in earlier chapters. After social "icebreakers" in which we have established a conversational context, a series of questions is begun that address the client's and family's general orientation to the assessment experience, followed by those that address the past (onset and early development, causal assumptions, family history, previous treatment), present (experience with the problem educationally, socially, vocationally; variability, learned responses; feelings and attitudes of self and others), and future (outlook toward change, inherent motivation and priority) with respect to communication and the communication impairment (Guitar, 2006; Williams, 1978). It is important to remember that the questions that are asked and discussed should be in the form of a dialogue (an exchange of information, thoughts, and feelings), not an interrogation. The extent to which such an interaction is conversational reflects the clinician's skill and experience. The clinician learns about the client's background by asking, responding, commenting, and probing, all the while exercising an invisible but effective balance between conversational structure and clinical flexibility. The first general orientation questions are as follows:

▓ "What do you hope to achieve as a result of our meeting today?" A related question is, "Why have you come to meet with us today?" Responses to these initial questions provide me with an idea of what the client perceives as his own needs and objectives, to each of which I respond directly before the conclusion of the evaluation. These initial questions also invite the client's participation in the clinical process from the very beginning and communicate the clinician's interest in understanding and serving the client as a member of a communication system. We must remember also that clients are referred for many reasons. We cannot presume that we know our clients' needs before we ask about them. Even if they are referred for "stuttering," we cannot assume that they and we mean the same thing by the word *stuttering*. The clinician then shares her overall purpose and a general orientation to the assessment process, being sure to relate directly to the client's or family's statement of objective.

▓ "When you use the word *X* [*stuttering, stammering, hesitating*], what do you mean?" The questions noted earlier (regarding why the client has come and what he and his family hope to accomplish) provide an opportunity for the client to begin to explain the nature of his concern. If he has not already done so, I ask the client to discuss the nature of his concern and to elaborate on whatever words he uses to describe his concern. I generally do not use the word *stuttering* until the client does because the term is evaluative and is relatively useless without narrow qualification (description) and quantification (summary statistics).

From these questions of general orientation, we move to those that help us learn about the client's communication past:

▓ "Describe the best you can when and how your stuttering began. How has it developed or changed over time?" Once the client has articulated his concern, I ask him to describe the onset and development of the problem he has just characterized, highlighting any patterns or changes that have been noticed. The clinician should try to determine the source of the client's information. Specifically, does he recall its onset, or is he relying on reports of parents or other family members? We noted earlier that family reports, while well intentioned, often contain errors of memory and association. Patterns of late or abrupt onset may need to be investigated for the possibility of neurogenic acquired stuttering, psychogenic acquired stuttering, or other disorders of fluency (discussed in Chapter 4). Guitar (2006) noted that events associated with changes in the stuttering (such as job changes or family or personal events) might be precipitating or perpetuating factors and therefore might require more focused attention.

▓ "What do you think caused your stuttering? What did your parents or other family members believe caused your stuttering?" The discussion of causal assumptions is often easily tied to previous questions about onset and development. These causal assumptions can reveal the attitudes and beliefs that the client has held about his stuttering and about himself as a person and as a communicator. The clinician will better understand the client's personal construct once she appreciates his assumptions about his stuttering and the general orientation with which he operated growing up and from which he has attempted to cope with the problem. Responses to these questions also have implications for the client's motivation. For example, if stuttering is viewed as a divine punishment, efforts to change may be viewed as conflicting with the client's religious beliefs (see Chapter 6). Similarly, clients who assume that stuttering is inherited or caused by a psychological disorder will be relieved and thereby motivated to learn other causal interpretations and to take heart from the clinician's assertion that he possesses the ability to speak more fluently. Clinicians need to understand the client's causal assumptions and relative accuracy of information, thereby determining what can and should be changed.

▓ "Have you ever had previous treatment for stuttering? If so, for how long and what did it involve? What did you feel were the most and least helpful aspects?" Williams (1978) emphasized that the client's attitudes and beliefs about previous treatment experiences will affect directly the way he responds in future treatment. The clinician should thus determine the degree to which previous treatment left the client with discouragement and negative ideas about himself and his stuttering, which must be addressed directly for present treatment to be successful. The clinician also needs to determine what the client expects from treatment and from the respective roles of the clinician and client within the process. From an understanding of the client's past treatment experiences and related attitudes and beliefs, the clinician will be in a better position to facilitate the design and implementation of effective intervention.

⟨⟨ "Does anyone else in your family have a communication impairment? Does anyone else in your family stutter?" Guitar (2006) indicated that determining if other family members stutter may help the clinician understand the factors that influence the client's attitudes toward himself and his communication skills.

From these questions about the client's past experiences, we move to those that investigate the client's perceptions of how his stuttering has impacted his experience educationally, socially, and vocationally:

⟨⟨ "How would you describe yourself as a communicator? How do you think others would describe you as a communicator?" It is important to determine whether the client acknowledges his communication strengths and the extent to which he perceives stuttering as a central part of himself. Similarly, it is important to see how he believes he is perceived by others. Lasting change in fluency intervention must be based on a foundation of communication strengths. Therefore, one of the first steps of treatment must help the client recognize and identify with his strengths as a communicator. Such questions also help assess the degree to which stuttering might be interiorized. There are times when the client perceives his stuttering as far more intrusive than do his listeners. In such cases, clients need to appreciate their listeners' perspective in order to realize and build on their communication strengths.

⟨⟨ "How is your stuttering affecting you at the present time?" Responses to this question often provide insight into the factors that motivated the client to initiate or return for treatment. For example, one woman indicated that her stuttering is worst at work, where she felt she had been passed over for promotions because of her stuttering. By pursuing intervention, she wished to eliminate any question over her competence to ensure professional advancement. Another client, a physician in his 40s, indicated that his stuttering rendered him unable to give oral depositions in court. This man wished to pursue his fluency; otherwise he would relinquish his position as chief psychiatrist.

⟨⟨ "Where and with whom would you expect your speech to be best (where do you experience no disfluency)? Where and with whom would you expect your speech to be worst (where do you to experience significant disfluency)? What strategies do you use in each of these situations to help keep your speech as fluent as possible?" Responses to these questions have direct implications for treatment. They provide the clinician with a picture of the client's perceptions and attitudes about his speaking experience outside of the treatment setting and his current use of fluency facilitating controls versus tricks (postponements, avoidances, and word substitutions, among others). Designing communication hierarchies such as these helps tailor treatment to the needs of each individual, facilitates the process of transfer from the very beginning, and engages the client actively within the clinical process.

⟨⟨ "How have your educational, social, or vocational activities been affected by your stuttering? How would your participation in these activities have been different had you not stuttered?" Responses to these questions reflect the client's beliefs and attitudes about ways that his stuttering has interfered with or facilitated his progress in life experiences. This information can be used in treatment planning, particularly with respect to establishing hierarchies for transfer of fluency facilitating controls, and can indicate the need for appropriate referrals (interpersonal counseling, psychotherapy, and vocational counseling).

Finally, the clinician needs to assess the client's outlook on the future and the extent to which he sincerely believes that he possesses the ability to change his communication behavior:

- ⬚ "How do you see your communication skills as affecting your future (including school, career, retirement activities)?" A related question might be, "How would improvement in your communication skills change your life?" By discussing topics such as these, the client offers a glimpse of his feelings, thoughts, and attitudes toward stuttering in addition to his personal degree of motivation to change this condition. The clinician might ask, "On a scale of 1 to 10, where would improving your fluency fall as one of your life's priorities?" In order for an adult to improve his speech fluency permanently, the change must be among one of his top priorities in life and he must have the support of those within his family system. However, for an adult to be unable to project how reducing his stuttering would change his life is not necessarily an indication of lack of motivation or a negative prognostic indicator. Some people have stuttered for so long that they cannot even imagine how their communication might be improved. Many of my adult clients have confessed that they even stutter in their dreams. One aptly said, "Stuttering is all I have ever known." For some, it is as though their motivation has enabled them to approach and knock on the door of fluency, yet they have no idea what is on the other side of the door. For these adults, their dreams begin to take form as they experience fluency success and communication independence within individualized treatment.

- ⬚ "What are your feelings about enrolling in fluency intervention? What would you expect from such a prospect? What are your family's feelings about your interest in pursuing fluency intervention?" These questions seek to determine how the client's motivation might be affected by others around him and the extent to which family members might be actively involved in the treatment process. As noted earlier, the client's inability to articulate his idea of treatment structure and outcome is not necessarily a negative indicator.

- ⬚ "Thinking about yourself as a communicator, are there any other questions you have or topics you think we should address?" This kind of question invites dialogue, a conversation in which the client can ask questions that he feels are pertinent. A follow-up question such as this invites the client to participate actively and to share any additional thoughts that might have surfaced during the process of interaction.

Speech–Language Sample Without Communicative Pressure

When meeting with an adult, the clinician must demonstrate sincere interest in the adult as a multifaceted person who also is a member of a communication system. The client is not merely someone who stutters; he is someone with interests, talents, hobbies, community responsibilities, family relationships, and friendships. In short, he is someone with a life story. Before addressing aspects of the person's communication skill and experiences, the clinician has an opportunity to convey a powerful message regarding her interest in knowing, understanding, and relating to the person who has come for help. Meeting as people first creates a foundation upon which a solid clinical relationship can be built. It does not take long to establish this foundation, but the time spent building it is invaluable and irreplaceable. Relationships are built on shared interests and sincere feelings of mutual respect. Clinical relationships are no exception.

I am working with a man in his 50s who, in addition to working in a precision tool and die plant, is an expert carpenter and woodworker, maintains a farm, likes to travel, and enjoys fine food—and, he stutters. We have a lot in common. We always seem to have a home repair project ongoing at any given time; we always seem to be returning from or planning a trip; and we always have a recent tale of the best or worst meal we just experienced. I have sought his advice on numerous occasions regarding the fixes I find myself in when tackling home repairs I know I should not have attempted. We respect each other; we like each other. Why do I mention the farm? Because he enjoys a frequent laugh on my account given my lack of experience in this area. Just as Eskimos know snow, he knows cows. I feel accomplished that I can distinguish a cow from a pig. I enjoy learning from his experience, particularly in those areas about which I am unfamiliar. We talk and we laugh. We laugh at ourselves and, occasionally, at each other. His wife is a dignified and delightful woman who participates in every treatment session. She recently commented how much she appreciates that we have interests in common other than our communication focus, and indicated that this, in part, is one causal explanation for his significant communication success compared to previous treatments. Are our commonalities so deep, so significant, that we become kindred spirits or bonded to each other? Hardly; but meaningful relationships are often based on sharing life's simple joys, and occasionally life's disappointments. Does this mean that clinicians and clients must be friends in order to work effectively with one another? No again; but relationships are built on those commonalities from which people often come to care for and about each other as people. Does this mean the fluency and stuttering take a backseat? Absolutely not. Our commitment to understanding and improving communication is the primary focus and that which bonds our relationship. All of the commonalities we share only contribute to our foundation as caring, interested, and committed people, a foundation on which a meaningful and constructive clinical relationship is based.

The interview questions discussed in the previous section, in addition to the clinician's sincere interest to become familiar with the client as a person, create an ideal opportunity to collect a speech–language sample (without communication pressure) from the client. As noted in the previous chapter, the sample should be no fewer than 300 words (Conture, 1997, 2001), or 5 minutes of the client's talking (approximately 10–15 minutes of real time). This sample provides one of the bases on which to assess the client's communication skills, including speech fluency. Such conversational interactions invite candid, open, accepting exchanges about the adult's beliefs regarding what he does relatively well versus poorly, what he does to speak as fluently as he can, his self-assessment as a communicator, and his thoughts and feelings related to the experience of stuttering. While often thinking about stuttering or not stuttering, adults rarely think or talk about talking, how we talk, and different ways of talking.

The client will come to see that fluency and disfluency both represent different ways of talking and are the direct consequence of doing things differently. Coming to realize that stuttering is not something that happens to you, but something you do, implies that speech is potentially controllable; thus the adult has choices to make. When sharing his ideas and assessments and receiving alternative ideas to consider, the adult begins to think and talk about talking in different and positive ways. He begins to consider his own thoughts about his speech and himself as a communicator. Invariably, the adult begins to question ways he has viewed himself as a person, including social, educational, and vocational choices he has made. In some ways, conducting assessment and treatment with adults who stutter and their family is like opening Pandora's box. Neither the clinician nor the client knows exactly what lies inside. However, a relationship has begun in which each is committed to pursue the journey together, discovering communication-related behaviors, thoughts, feelings, and attitudes, all the while working, learning, and growing together.

Structured Activities Without Communicative Pressure

After collecting a rich conversational sample, the clinician engages the adult in a variety of relatively structured activities. These are used for subsequent analysis and comparison across speaking contexts in order to assess and differentially diagnose the individual's communication skills, including speech fluency. In other words, in addition to assessing the individual's competence in parameters of speech sound production, language, and voice, we are determining if a fluency disorder is present, and if so, what type. The following activities are among those used:

⚙ *Reading.* For readers, three different passages are typically used (below, at, and above the client's reading level). Easy passages might include the morning newspaper; moderate passages might include one or two different phonetically balanced passages, such as the Grandfather Passage and the Rainbow Passage, reproduced by Shipley and McAfee (2009, p. 188 and p. 189, respectively); difficult passages might include a page from an advanced statistics textbook or *The New England Journal of Medicine.* The phonetically balanced passages contain all of the speech-sound productions (phonemes) in the English language and thereby provide an opportunity for screening articulation and phonology as well as speech fluency. People who stutter typically become more disfluent as the level of reading difficulty increases. However, the clinician must be mindful that assessment of speech fluency may be confounded by reading competence. While the clinician interprets the influence of increasing linguistic demand on speech fluency, she must also ferret out the linguistic disfluency that reflects inadequate reading skills (e.g., those with a reading disability or bilingualism, those for whom the passage is too difficult).

⚙ *Recalling and describing events, holidays, possessions.* The client is asked to describe both simple/concrete and complex/abstract events and things. Theoretically, the former impose less demand on the individual's ability to remain fluent than the latter. For example, to elicit simple or concrete recall, the clinician might ask the client, "If I were to visit your home or work, what would I see?" In comparison, to elicit complex recall, the clinician might ask about a technical aspect of the client's work (e.g., "I understand that the plant where you work makes tool and die equipment for the production of zippers. What is the process that results in a finished zipper?").

⚙ *Word and sentence repetition.* The clinician prepares on her outline words and sentences of increasing length and complexity. When asking the client to repeat them, however, the clinician presents them in random order, thus not conveying the pattern inherent in the task (increasing length and complexity). The clinician then looks for a relationship between length/complexity and fluency. Typically, the simpler or shorter words and sentences impose less demand and therefore result in less disfluency than longer or more complex items.

⚙ *Questions and answers.* The client is directed to respond to questions requiring answers of differing length and complexity. Again, for people who stutter, shorter/simpler questions and answers are frequently associated with greater fluency than those that are longer/more complex. One explanation is that the former impose less linguistic demand than the latter. For example, answers to questions like "What is your favorite X [television show, food, sport]?" are often less disfluent than those to questions like "Which presidential candidate do you feel had a more convincing economic policy and why?" There are predictable exceptions, however. Most people who stutter report that responding to "What is your name?" is one of the most difficult fluency challenges. This question, while both simple and concrete, provides no alternatives (if your name is David, you cannot respond with Susan), thus superimposing a type of demand speech over a relatively simple linguistic construction. I believe that is why answering the phone is so difficult for so many people who stutter (there are few acceptable alternatives to "Hello," combined with internalized time pressure). Similarly, several other types of questions whose surface structure suggests less demand often result in more disfluent responses because of factors at an underlying or deep structure level that produce greater demand. For example, questions that elicit emotional, affectively awkward, politically polarized, or otherwise "off limit" responses tend to impose more demand than that predicted from the surface structure of the question alone (e.g., "What's going on in this picture?" when presented a picture of sexually suggestive or explicit content; or "How much money do you make?" "Are you voting as a Democrat or Republican?" "What do you think of the gender gap today?"). These and other factors must be considered when the clinician is identifying patterns and variability of stuttering.

⚏ *Other*. There are a number of other relatively structured activities that clinicians might use. These include commenting on pictures, naming objects, telling stories, using automatic speech, using echoic speech, speaking alone, speaking in monologue, using command speech, talking with gestures, talking with phonemic difficulty, and talking on the telephone.

Speech–Language Sample and Structured Activities with Communicative Pressure

After the clinician completes the speech–language sample and structured activities without communicative pressure, she engages the client in different activities with deliberate communicative pressure. The clinician is seeking to determine the effect of communicative pressure (e.g., time pressure, linguistic ambiguity, violation of conversational rules) on the adult's speech fluency. Some of the activities already completed contain differing degrees of communication pressure, including questions about the adult's communication past, which can evoke sensitive memories.

For example, I remember a man who was 63 years old at the time of the diagnostic assessment. Addressing questions about how his parents and family responded to him when he stuttered, the man recalled the physical abuse he incurred as a child. Describing vividly and emotionally what his father's hands looked like as they reached for him when he stuttered, the man articulated how his father either beat his head on the barn door or submerged his head into a barrel of water until he promised he would not stutter again. The man showed us the remaining scars on his forehead. I remember that while listening to this human tragedy, the two student clinicians each had a tear running down their cheek. Interestingly, as I write these words years later, my own eyes still water as I share this man's experience. Indeed, his treatment was interdisciplinary, and it included his wife, friends, a psychiatrist, and psychiatric social worker, among others.

Other activities involving deliberate, albeit less emotional, communicative pressure include rushed verbal and physical behavior (the clinician increases her rate of speech, hand and overall body movements and extraneous gestures, speed of requesting answers and responding; and directs the client to "hurry up"), interruptions (the clinician takes a conversational turn before the client has completed his, asking a question and then asking another before the client finishes answering the first), loss of attention (the clinician does something else when the client is relating an event), or requesting the client to say something else (the clinician says, "I didn't understand that. What are you trying to say?"). Other deliberate verbal challenges include abruptly shifting topics (introducing a topic prematurely that is unrelated to the one being discussed), overstepping boundaries of intellect or experience (using words about topics that are unfamiliar to the adult), introducing linguistic ambiguity (contradicting things said by the client or clinician), or verbal absurdity (treating foolish statements as if they were legitimate, e.g., addressing the client by the wrong name, making deliberate errors in topics discussed or pictures described, or telling a joke with a punch line that makes no sense and asking the client if he understood it). The clinician also may direct the client to tell a joke, deliberately creating a high linguistic demand on the client. The clinician must remain sensitive to the client's feelings and inform the client as to why she is engaging in activities that might seem odd or rude. These activities are important even when the adult client is not showing observable signs of disfluency. By increasing the demand on the adult's ability to remain fluent, the activities may elicit disfluency that otherwise is not apparent. As stated earlier, such pressure may affect the fluency of different clients in unique ways.

Trial Management

The activities described so far enable the clinician to evaluate the adult client's speech-related fluency, feelings, thoughts, and attitudes, in addition to other aspects of communication, and to arrive at a diagnosis. The data also provide a baseline of the client's communication behavior from which the effects of treatment can be measured. Furthermore, the data help the clinician determine if more formal evaluation of articulation or phonology and language is necessary. If the adult demonstrates observable disfluency or negative communication-related attitudes, thoughts, or feelings, the clinician engages in trial management techniques based on fluency shaping and stuttering modification. Trial management, a necessary part of the evaluation process, enables the clinician to help the client directly by exploring and adjusting his behaviors, thoughts, and feelings to determine the client's responsiveness to different and specific treatment strategies, and thereby to design specific treatment recommendations.

Fluency Shaping

The clinician should engage the client in a variety of fluency shaping techniques for the purposes of differential diagnosis and determining the client's relative responsiveness to such techniques. For example, I often engage the client in singing, choral speaking (such as reciting the Pledge of Allegiance, a poem, or some other familiar verbal passage), and choral reading. People who stutter should demonstrate consistent fluency during such experiences, except when initiating a new passage or bar of music following a pause. If the client does not demonstrate remarkably improved fluency, the clinician should consider the possibility that some other disorder of fluency is operating. Manning (2010) noted, "Some of the fluency-enhancing activities can provide highly dramatic results, and such instantaneous improvements in fluency tend to have the effect of making anyone who uses them an 'expert' in helping those who stutter" (p. 356). The clinician must communicate why she is using such techniques and the fact that their effect is temporary at best, to prevent the client from developing inappropriate expectations.

The activities are extremely effective, however, in enabling the client to "feel" fluent speech directly, sometimes for the first time, which often has the effect of significantly heightening the client's motivation. Other fluency shaping techniques include establishing fluency (characterized by slightly prolonged vowels, soft articulatory contacts on vowels and consonants, natural suprasegmental features) through modeling, choral speaking or reading, using electronic devices with altered auditory feedback (delayed auditory feedback, masking auditory feedback, or frequency altered feedback; see Chapter 7) or other externally driven methods, speaking loudly or in a whisper, using a dialect, or speaking to a rhythmic stimulus (such as the movement of a finger or the head, or the beat of a metronome). For a client who demonstrates more severe symptoms, the clinician may first establish a fluent syllable and systematically shape it into increasingly longer and more complex units (using a progression—monosyllabic word, polysyllabic word, phrases, sentences). First using imitation, the clinician may move to delayed imitation, elicitation through pictures, and eventually more spontaneous forms. The clinician provides praise and other forms of positive reinforcement as a consequence of a fluent utterance.

Stuttering Modification

The clinician wants the client to discover that there are many different ways to stutter (e.g., hard or soft, long or short, loud or quiet, tense or relaxed, and so on). Modeling for the client, we want him to experiment with how he talks, thereby realizing that talking does not just happen; it is something that we do. Both fluency and disfluency are consequences of something we do differently with our speech apparatus. For many adults, this will be a new perspective. Telling an adult is not as effective as enabling him to discover for himself that he can modify his own speech. If it can be modified, he must have choices. Such an awareness (that I can change and thereby control the way I talk, that I have choices, and that fluency and disfluency represent the consequence of different choices), once discovered, is remarkably empowering and motivating. While self-discovery is generally the most effective teacher, adults tend to be more disbelieving than children. Adults typically have longer histories of stuttering; fluency failure therefore has become more predictable. Many adults have been wounded by stuttering; they form inflexible impressions about themselves and the world; they doubt their abilities; they lose faith in themselves. Individualized fluency intervention seeks to work with them to create opportunities for fluency success, thus yielding an alternative set of data from which the adult must reconsider his beliefs about his communication skills, himself, and the world. A variety of stuttering modification techniques contribute to this self-discovery process (see also Chapter 9):

- Explain to the client that you will be putting his disfluencies into your own mouth. You are not mocking him; rather, by internalizing what he does, you can better understand it. This conveys a powerful message to the client regarding the clinician's commitment and willingness to share the same bunker. The clinician is communicating, "Do as I do, not just as I say." Furthermore, once internalizing what the client does, the clinician is in a better position to model ways of stuttering differently.

- Model slow, relaxed, prolonged speech. Use an even (regular, steady, consistent) rate, gentle articulatory contacts, and natural-sounding suprasegmental features with slight prolongation ("Yyou ssaid eearlier thhat yyou llike ssports. Wwhich ssport iis yyour ffavorite?").

- Demonstrate easier versions of the client's stuttering. Use a modeling and expansion format (Client: "I-I-I-I huh-huh-huh-had a huh-huh-hard t-ime ffffinding a-a-a-a puh-arking p-lace." Clinician: "II knnow. Ffinding a pparking pplace ccan bbe a rreal bbear aarround hhere.")

- Demonstrate easy and eventually hard disfluencies in the clinician's speech. Initially, the clinician will offer descriptive, emotionally neutral self-comments (such as, "Hey, that was a tough one") and later invite the client's comments and assessment (Clinician: "What did you think about that one?" Client: "That was pretty tough. You're starting to sound like me!")

- Identify instances when the client uses gentle speech onset with light articulatory contact, describe what he did, and offer positive feedback. These procedures heighten the client's awareness of how much and what type of fluent speech he already possesses, and model for the client what he will eventually do for himself (i.e., identify his fluency, describe what he did to produce fluent speech, and offer positive feedback).

- Provide for the client one or two foci for positive assertions of behavior. For example, the clinician will model slow (evenly produced) and gentle (easy, relaxed) speech (see Figure 9.2), pointing out that the two behavioral foci are "slow" and "gentle."

- Supportively explore with the adult expressions of feeling related to stuttering or himself as a communicator. As always, such interaction is conversational, informal, and safe. These interactions, particularly with adults, may be tender subjects. The clinician should feel comfortable listening actively; reflecting; asking a blend of open-ended and directed questions; commenting, inquiring, clarifying, and reassuring; and understanding and demonstrating the constructive value of silence. More will be said about essential interpersonal and intrapersonal characteristics of effective clinicians and the transformative nature of the clinician–client relationship in Chapter 11.

- Extend the discussion of where and with whom the client would expect his speech to be more and less fluent, and discuss his related feelings. Hierarchies such as these help explore the client's feelings and perceptions, tailor treatment if recommended, and facilitate transfer from the outset of the clinical process.

Post-Assessment Procedures

After engaging in conversation and more structured activities first with and then without communicative pressure and delineating preliminary impressions, the clinician needs to analyze the results more thoroughly in order to quantify (numerically account using summary statistics) and qualify (narrowly describe) the nature of fluency and disfluency within and across speaking contexts and to describe competence in other areas of communication (including language, articulation and phonology, and voice).

The clinician analyzes the data collected and makes statements of diagnosis, prognosis, and recommendation for intervention, in addition to statements of referral to other professionals, if appropriate. These results, in preliminary form, are conveyed to the client and his family in a conference at the end of the evaluation and summarized subsequently in more complete form within a written report. Frequently, the clinician and client meet again, either in person or on the phone, once the report has been received.

Speech Analysis

The analyses of conversational and structured speech samples from adults are similar to those from children. The procedures used for speech analysis are reviewed more thoroughly in Chapters 8 and 9; they are summarized here. Words are the units of measure.

Frequency of Speech Disfluency

Frequency of speech disfluency, a general measure of the amount of disfluency without consideration of the individual types or relative severity, is estimated on the basis of the *disfluency frequency index* (DFI). Reported as a percentage, the DFI is computed by dividing the total number of disfluent words by the total number of words spoken (disfluent and fluent), and then multiplying the resulting decimal by 100 to achieve the percentage. The frequency of speech disfluency is typically reported as a percentage of 100 words spoken, averaged over samples of 300 or 400 words.

Type of Speech Disfluency

The type of speech disfluency is assessed to identify the individual proportions for each type of disfluency. It is computed by dividing the number of disfluencies of each individual type by the total number of disfluent words, and then multiplying by 100.

Molecular Description of Disfluency

The molecular description of disfluency includes the duration and frequency (reported in terms of total, mean, and range) of the most prominent or otherwise significant forms of disfluency (particularly within-word disfluencies).

Rate of Speech

Rate of speech is a measure of the number of words spoken per minute. The more a person stutters, the more his rate of speech is reduced. As treatment decreases the degree and amount of disfluency, rate should steadily increase and approximate normal standards. Rate is computed by dividing the number of words the client has spoken by the client's talk time in minutes. For purposes of comparison, it is helpful to know what is considered to be an average or "normal" rate of speech for adults who do not stutter.

Those figures, expressed in *words spoken per minute*, range from approximately 116 to 164 for conversation (G. Andrews & Ingham, 1971), 114 to 173 for monologue (e.g., talking about one's job) (Williams et al., 1978), and 148 to 190 for reading (Williams et al., 1978). Duchin and Mysak (1987) provided additional detail for speech rates, also expressed in *words per minute*, for adults (males only). Average (i.e., mean) rate of speech for adults aged 21 to 30 years was 182.7 in conversation (i.e., $SD = 17.2$ words per minute), 151.4 in monologue (picture identification; $SD = 49.6$), and 219.9 in reading ($SD = 37.1$). For adults aged 45 to 54 years, average rate was 153.7 in conversation ($SD = 26.7$), 133.7 in monologue ($SD = 27.4$), and 182.1 in reading ($SD = 18.5$). For those aged

55 to 64 years, the average rate was 168.7 in conversation (*SD* = 37.6), 141.7 in monologue (*SD* = 30.7), and 190.1 in reading (*SD* = 19.2). Adults aged 65 to 74 years revealed an average rate of 155.1 in conversation (*SD* = 35.9), 131.0 in monologue (*SD* = 21.7), and 182.5 in reading (*SD* = 29.1). Finally, for adults aged 75 to 91 years, the average was 133.3 in conversation (*SD* = 14.9), 117.8 in monologue (*SD* = 16.8), and 167.9 in reading (*SD* = 19.2). Expressed in *syllables spoken per minute*, the average rate of speech ranges from approximately 162 to 230 for conversation and 210 to 265 for reading (G. Andrews & Ingham, 1971; Calvert & Silverman, 1983; Guitar, 2006).

As noted previously, rate of speech tends to decrease with age, as is characteristic of senior adults and, particularly, centenarians. Caruso, McClowry, and Max (1997) reported on the case of a 105-year-old woman whose conversational speech rate was 105 words per minute. Searl et al. (2002) analyzed the speech of seven centenarians (four males, three females) ranging in age from 100 to 103 years old (mean age, 100.6 years). Their rate of speech in conversation ranged from 101 to 135 words per minute (mean, 111.6 words per minute).

Secondary Characteristics

Secondary characteristics, both those related to speech (e.g., audible inhalations or exhalations, pitch rises, and oral and neck tension) and those not related to speech (e.g., facial, head, and eye movement or tension), are quantified and qualified. These may reflect the client's developing awareness of stuttering, coping mechanisms during stuttering, or attempts to prevent stuttering.

Severity Rating and Impact Assessment

The severity rating and impact assessment utilizes both speech and nonspeech factors to determine the client's relative degree of stuttering involvement. The *Stuttering Severity Instrument–Fourth Edition* (SSI-4; Riley, 2009), the *Overall Assessment of the Speaker's Experience of Stuttering* (OASES; Yaruss & Quesal, 2006, 2008), and other instruments (e.g., diagnostic, severity, and predictive scales for assessing overt features of stuttering and perception–attitude scales and situation-avoidance checklists for assessing covert features of stuttering; Haynes & Pindzola, 2008) help provide an objective assessment of relative severity and impact of a speaker's stuttering over time and across speakers. The information collected is used for planning, monitoring, and adjusting treatment and for conducting treatment outcomes research. However, the information provided by such instruments is typically confirmatory of, if not redundant with, the other quantitative and qualitative information collected.

Adaptation and Consistency

Adaptation is the tendency for overall stuttering to decrease with repeated recitation of the same material; *consistency* is the tendency for stuttering to occur on the same sounds or words. As a group, people who stutter have both effects, although some show neither (see Chapter 8).

Feelings and Attitudes

The assessment of feelings and attitudes—the assessment of the degree to which a speaker is experiencing covert involvement related to the experience of stuttering—is pivotal to a clinician's understanding of a client's stuttering experience. Published protocols are available (see a review of 15 such protocols by Haynes & Pindzola, 2008), but as Guitar (2006) noted, the most reliable measure of the client's feelings and attitudes is the clinician's judgment. Haynes and Pindzola, too, acknowledged that "ultimately, the most important diagnostic tool is the diagnostician" (p. 22).

Other Factors

"Other Factors" is an open category that invites assessment of tempo, regularity, relative tension, smoothness of transitions, and physical concomitants, in addition to any other overt or covert features not yet reported. For example, the clinician might determine that she needs to explore further interpersonal dynamics (e.g., within the family, social, educational, or employment settings), coexisting challenges (communication, learning, emotional, health, financial), or possible experience of social intimidation or bullying (Blood, 2003; Blood & Blood, 2004), in addition to the client's dreams, goals, and objectives.

Diagnosis

The clinician analyzes and synthesizes all available information about the adult's communication skills and makes a statement of diagnosis. In doing so, the clinician determines if the client is demonstrating a communication exceptionality, namely stuttering or any other disorder of fluency. If an exceptionality is identified, the clinician determines if treatment is warranted and recommended and, if so, the nature and foci of treatment. The clinician also determines if there is a need to make a referral to other professionals and estimates the client's prognosis for improvement in the area of speech fluency.

Prognosis and Recommendations

The clinician estimates the client's prognosis for improvement based on a variety of sources. As noted previously, prognosis is a prediction of the outcome of a proposed course of treatment. This includes how effective treatment is likely to be, how far the client is expected to progress, and how long it will take (Haynes & Pindzola, 2008). We have noted also that estimating prognosis is an inexact science at best. Daly (1988) stated, "We cannot predict which clients will make significant improvements in their fluency and which will not" (p. 34). Stressing the importance of the clinician's attitude as a prognostic factor, Daly recommended that clinicians be positive and enthusiastic with every client who stutters. Indeed, "I would rather err in the direction of optimism than pessimism" (p. 34). In the following sections, we review general predictors of successful treatment based on group trends (Craig, 1998; Florance, 1986; Haynes & Pindzola, 2008; Huinck et al., 2006; Iverach et al., 2009; Prins, 1993), followed by a discussion of chronic perseverative stuttering syndrome (Cooper, 1987a, 1990a, 1990b, 1993a, 1993b, 1993c), a potential subcategory of stuttering that presents unique challenges to clients and clinicians.

Never Say Never

Nowhere is understanding the distinction between group trends and individual performance more important than in estimating prognosis. Group trends reflect general patterns that surface from the population of people under study, without regard to individual differences. Conture (2001) noted that people who stutter enter our clinical facilities one at a time, not as a group. I want to caution clinicians to avoid ascribing greater predictive validity to the general prognostic indicators than they deserve. Too often, clinicians themselves are doubtful about a client's potential for improvement. Sometimes, this doubt (which can easily be communicated to the client) stems from clinicians' insecurity about their own professional skills (Conture, 2001; Manning, 2010; F. H. Silverman, 2004). As Daly (1988) noted, the sincerity of the clinician's attitude regarding the client's ability to effect improvement is predictive of the change achieved. This means that a positive outlook is itself part of the treatment.

Who is to say what one individual can and cannot achieve? I know that we must be realistic with our clients so that they do not form unrealistic performance expectations. I know that our Code of Ethics (ASHA, 2010) prohibits us from offering guarantees and that issues of accountability and liability are real. However, clinicians must take seriously the importance of understanding both the visible and invisible aspects of each individual client's personal construct and his potential to dream. Just as clients learn about dreams and dreaming from clinicians, so many clinicians can take a lesson from the great advances many clients make, some of which are unpredictable or come from clients who demonstrate clearly negative prognostic indicators. *Never* say never. *Never* even think never. An effective clinician will enable a client to imagine, work toward, and realize dreams, occasionally far beyond that imaginable to either participant. To say that "the sky is the limit" only conveys the limitations of our thinking and our inability to imagine the unimaginable. There should be no limits imposed on our clients who stutter. Stuttering may be viewed from one perspective as a limitation; from another as an opportunity for change, learning, and growth by the client, his family, and the clinician.

Prognostic indicators, or predictors of treatment outcome, are inexact and are particularly so with adolescents, adults, and senior adults who stutter. Guitar (2006) offered the sobering thought that "most people who stutter severely for a long time or who are not treated until after puberty make only a partial recovery. They usually learn to speak more slowly or stutter more easily and are less bothered by it. However, some people will not improve, despite our best efforts" (p. 7). It is equally if not more important to recognize that some older people who stutter severely and who have a variety of other negative prognostic indicators achieve remarkable fluency freedom, independence and control over their lives, and advances as people and communicators. The most critical and effective ingredients of the change process within stuttering intervention are yet to be determined (Franken et al., 2005; Manning, 2006). That uncertainty, while discouraging to some people, is for me—as a speech–language pathologist and as a person who stutters—a clarion call for optimism. Van Riper (1974) noted that for many years he accepted onto his caseload one client who, for him as a clinician, held a "zero prognosis" (p. 105). Reflecting on such experiences, he indicated the following:

> With a few of them a most successful result ensued; with the others either some improvement or at least no harm occurred. They taught me much. Most important of their teachings was the revelation that I had more potential for growth than I had realized—and so had they. Over and over again I have found that they knew what they really needed to solve their problems or at least to make them more bearable and that if I could only understand their needs, I had something to give. Perhaps it was not enough, but it was something. Often out of many such moments of partial understanding and inadequate therapy came surprising changes for the better. (p. 105)

We owe it to our clients to assume that each can achieve great things. There is no telling what one can achieve knowing that one person believes in us. Prognostic indicators are thus a snapshot, a picture reflecting group means, not individual potential. They are useful only if the clinician keeps this caveat in mind.

Prognostic Indicators with Adolescents, Adults, and Senior Adults

The following indicators tend to be associated with a more positive prognosis for adult clients with speech disfluency (Bloodstein & Bernstein Ratner, 2008; Craig, 1998; Daly, 1988; Florance, 1986; Haynes & Pindzola, 2008; Huinck et al., 2006; Iverach et al., 2009; Prins, 1993).

No record of unsuccessful treatment. An absence of treatment seems more conducive to treatment success than a history of therapeutic failure. However, I have worked with many adults (ages 18–70) who have had treatment on and off for most of their lives without permanent success, only to achieve their speech fluency goals later in life.

A cooperative and supportive family system. Treatment outcome seems most promising when family members are willing to participate meaningfully in family counseling and the treatment process.

Cooperative interdisciplinary team members. Similarly, the treatment effect is most potent when team members (teachers, allied educational and medical professionals, and associates) work together and communicate effectively.

More severe stuttering pattern. Those with a more severe stuttering pattern tend to demonstrate greater motivation and therefore greater likelihood of improvement. Those with a less severe stuttering pattern tend to show less improvement. Those with a more severe stuttering pattern also tend to show greater likelihood for relapse than those with a less severe stuttering pattern.

No significant concomitant problems. Problems that may hinder progress include other communication disorders; reading or learning disabilities independent of stuttering; intellectual, sensory, or motor limitations; and mental health disorders or psychopathology.

Other available resources. Those with areas of interest or expertise (in areas such as outdoor interests, reading, or music) are often more well rounded in their way of living and tend to achieve greater fluency success.

Positive pretreatment motivation and voluntary enrollment. Not surprisingly, motivation (one's internal drive) to change is associated with greater improvement. Florance (1986) found that self-referred clients were significantly more motivated and achieved greater fluency success than those who were referred by parents or other family members. Therefore, she made voluntary enrollment a prerequisite for treatment. The client is given time after the evaluation to consider the benefits of treatment and to render an independent decision. She reported that most of the adults, particularly teenagers, who chose not to enroll immediately did so later, with dramatically positive results. Similarly, Watson (1995) noted, "Given the effort and time that therapy demands, it is important that a client has made the decision to address his problem and that such a decision was not made by a spouse, employer or other individual" (p. 149). Notwithstanding the importance of positive pretreatment motivation and attitude, I have found that clients typically believe not what they are told but what they experience for themselves. This means that clients must be provided with regular opportunities to experience fluency success; creating such opportunities is the clinician's responsibility. Nothing less should be believed by the client; nothing is more motivating than success itself. Indeed, success begets success.

Significant timing and readiness for change. Clients' motivation for treatment often interacts with critical life experiences. People who have reached a point at which they feel blocked because of their stuttering (e.g., limitations in job advancement, education, employment, marriage, or family relations) and who voluntarily enroll in treatment often have a more positive prognosis. Many of the senior adults with whom I have worked acknowledged that previous decades of treatment had not been successful. But they wanted to try once more, particularly because they finally had the time to focus on their own communication needs. I have found intervention with such people to be remarkably successful. Success is always sweet, particularly when one has wished and worked for it for so long. The clinical portrait at the end of the chapter profiles one such client.

Commitment to a jointly determined treatment plan and schedule. The client must share the process of determining a comprehensive treatment plan and appropriate schedule, which must be followed with sincerity and internal motivation. Recommended plans and schedules vary with clinicians (e.g., no less than twice per week, Daly, 1988; daily treatment initially with subsequent reduction, Florance, 1986). However, I have found that the shared establishment and ownership of such factors is key in predicting prognosis.

Personality variables. Tolerance for ambiguity, positive self-reinforcement, and internal locus of control contribute to a positive prognosis. Florance (1986) described a high tolerance for ambiguity as the ability to cope with uncertainty, often associated with creative people who like to be involved in different activities. In contrast, low tolerance for ambiguity is often associated with clients who fight to maintain the status quo, prefer structure and order, and follow rules carefully. High self-reinforcers monitor and focus on increasing the positive aspects of their speech fluency; low self-reinforcers focus on the disfluent behaviors and decreasing their frequency. Those with an internal locus of control see both disfluency and fluency as the consequence of something they actively do. Those with external locus of control feel that their speech behavior is controlled by their environment (believing that they are victims of fate) and blame people and external events for their stuttering and for personal shortcomings they perceive to be associated with their stuttering.

Therefore, high pretreatment tolerance for ambiguity, positive self-reinforcement, and an internal locus of control have been associated with greater readiness for change and successful treatment outcome. Significantly, however, I have found that previous unsuccessful treatment has left many clients with negative prognostic indicators in these areas—low tolerance for ambiguity, infrequent positive self-reinforcement, and external locus of control—at the time of reassessment. These clients are lacking in motivation and doubtful regarding the likelihood of a positive treatment outcome. Yet, they have come for a reevaluation; this is positive. Effective management in which the client experiences heightened awareness of existing fluency and production of fluent speech (i.e., opportunities for fluency success) can improve early prognostic indicators (such as increased degrees of tolerance for ambiguity, positive self-reinforcement, and internalized locus of control, resulting in greater motivation). I noted previously that the positive effects of early treatment experiences are seen in client statements that reflect a shift from feeling unable ("I can't be fluent; I never could") to able ("By golly, I did it. Did you hear the gentle *g* when I said *girl*? I love it!"), and from feeling controlled externally ("Why is this happening to me?") to being in control ("I used my controls seven times yesterday, and five the day before. I know I can do this. I know I can catch those blocks before they catch me").

More recently, Manning (2010) addressed relevant if not predictive personality variables, referred to as "principles of change" for people who stutter. Such variables include demonstrating a sense of agency (autonomy, acting for oneself, and speaking on one's own behalf), moving toward rather than away from the problem, assuming responsibility for taking action, being willing and able to restructure one's own internal view of oneself as a person and as a communicator, and being inclined to recruit the support of others. As noted, much is yet to be learned about how client factors, clinician factors, and clinical process factors interact and how they relate, individually and collectively, to a positive treatment outcome.

Positive yet realistic expectations regarding the commitment required for fluency intervention. Necessary life adjustments and readiness for change accompany the process of addressing and resolving stuttering-related behaviors, feelings, and attitudes (Floyd et al., 2007; Guitar, 1976, 2006; Guitar & Bass, 1978; Prins, 1993). Perkins (1979) underscored the importance of assessing the client's attitudinal readiness for change and targeting that change. He stated, "We have serious doubts about the long-term effectiveness of any behavioral program that is not systematically concerned with evaluating and effecting improvement in the stutterer's attitude" (p. 109). Indeed, as Daly (1988) pointed out, "too many of our clients get fluent in their mouths but not in their heads. Despite success, they feel threatened and helpless when trying their new skills alone" (p. 35). Similarly, Perkins stated the following:

> So much of their lives has been built around stuttering that, suddenly freed of it, they realize the extensive role it has played for them. When fluent, they feel like unwelcome strangers to themselves. If stuttering has been used as a defense against an unrealistic self-concept, then its removal will arouse anxiety. . . . But for some it is more a matter of identity. They wish to feel like themselves, and stuttering is part of that self-image. (1979, p. 121)

Positive clinician attitudes and expectations. The clinician's attitude and expectations toward the client are both prognostic indicators and critical elements of treatment. Daly (1988) noted that "the clinician's attitudes toward stuttering and people who stutter have as much to do with the successful treatment of this disorder as the methods selected for therapy" (p. 34). In other words, the clinician must sincerely believe in the client and his potential for change, just as the client must believe in the clinician's ability to facilitate such change. Relating the efficacy literature on treatment of terminally ill cancer patients to those who stutter, Daly noted that a positive attitude toward treatment was a better predictor of treatment outcome than the severity of the disorder. Therefore, the attitude and expectations demonstrated by the clinician significantly impact those of the client, and thereby predict the outcome of treatment. Daly stated,

> Might our clients detect any insecurities or uncertainties in the clinician's attitudes or feelings about the treatment advocated? Clinical experience repeatedly demonstrates that intelligent persons will expend effort and energy in treatment only when they expect substantial results. When the clinician concentrates on negative behaviors or problems rather than positive objectives, clients are apt to get discouraged. Such incongruity between the clinician's expectations and the client's expectations may account for the high dropout rate among our stuttering clients. Roughly one-third of stuttering clients withdraw from treatment prior to completion. . . . We have expended tremendous effort studying clients who stutter. Perhaps it is time we study ourselves. (pp. 34–35)

A Prognostic Caveat—Chronic Perseverative Stuttering Syndrome

Distinguishing between three distinct types of stuttering, Cooper (1993b; see also Cooper & Cooper, 2003) indicated that out of every five people who stutter, two demonstrate developmental stuttering, two remediable stuttering, and one "chronic perseverative stuttering (CPS) syndrome," or "incurable stuttering." Reportedly, developmental stuttering is characterized by achievement of normal fluency control by 7 years of age without professional help; this type of stuttering involves no sense of loss of control during disfluency, infrequent interpretation of disfluency as problematic, and no recall of earlier difficulty with stuttering. Remedial stuttering is characterized by achievement of normal fluency after 7 years of age by means of adjustments (behavioral, affective, and cognitive) made as a result of stuttering intervention; this type of stuttering involves loss of control during episodic moments of disfluency and recall of earlier difficulty with

Table 10.1 Chronic Perseverative Stuttering Syndrome Checklist

---

- The individual's fluency disorder developed concomitantly with the development of language and speech.
- The individual's fluency disorder has persisted for 10 or more years.
- The individual's disfluencies are, or have been, accompanied by a fleeting but generalized feeling of loss of control.
- The individual has experienced periods of normal fluency accompanied by the feeling of control.
- The individual experiences a persistent fear of a catastrophic loss of fluency although, in fact, such occurrences occur rarely, if ever.
- The individual has identified one or more adjustments in speech production that generally, but not always, enhance fluency.
- Although capable of predicting the level of fluency to be experienced in most situations, the individual continues to experience unpredictable fluency failures.
- The individual has experienced fluent periods after a heightened and sustained period of psychic and physical concentration on attaining fluency, but has been unable to maintain that level of concentration or fluency.
- The individual's predominant self-perception is that of being a stutterer.
- The individual experiences periods of obsessive absorption in striving for normal fluency.

Note. From "Chronic Perseverative Stuttering Syndrome: A Harmful or Helpful Construct?" by E. B. Cooper, 1993a, *American Journal of Speech–Language Pathology*, 2(3), p. 13. Copyright 1993 by the American Speech-Language-Hearing Association. Reprinted with permission.

stuttering, but no thought of oneself as still stuttering. Finally, Cooper defined (1987a) and inventoried (1993a; see Table 10.1) chronic perseverative stuttering:

> The chronic perseverative stuttering syndrome is an adolescent and adult disorder in the fluency of speech resulting from multiple coexisting physiological, psychological, and environmental factors, distinguished by (1) recurrence after periods of remission; (2) characteristic cognitive, affective, and behavioral response patterns; and (3) susceptibility to alleviation but, given the present state of the healing arts, not to eradication. (1987a, p. 386)

Cooper and Cooper (1995, 2003) argued that speech fluency is a by-product of the feeling of fluency control. The loss of such control is a significant indicator that distinguishes remedial stuttering from chronic perseverative stuttering. In other words, the feeling of loss of control during disfluency is prominent in remedial stuttering, whereas it is present but not prominent in chronic perseverative stuttering. Cooper (1993a) argued that the feeling of fluency control, rather than demonstration of fluency itself, must be a top priority in fluency intervention, advising that attempting to achieve speech fluency before the feeling of fluency control is premature and a "fluency trap" (1993a, p. 14); such an end goal of treatment is not realistic in many cases. Acknowledging that the construct of CPS syndrome is controversial and may be interpreted as "dream-shattering" (1993a, p. 14) for some, he countered that it is a positive construct that relieves guilt and self-deprecation for those who remain "abnormally disfluent" (1993a, p. 14) despite years of treatment and self-help. Cooper (1987a) recommended that at the end of the diagnostic interview with an individual who presents with CPS syndrome indicators, the clinician should give the "bad news" first ("The bad news is that you have the chronic perseverative stuttering syndrome which means that there is no cure for your stuttering," p. 387), followed by the "good news" ("You most likely will still be disfluent, but you will . . . have the skills to alter your speech and to communicate effectively. You will have the feeling of control," p. 387).

Indeed the construct of CPS syndrome is controversial. It is undeniable that for some people who stutter, speech fluency is an unrealistic treatment objective. It is also undeniable that many people who stutter are put to unnecessary and unfortunate feelings of frustration and failure. However, when and how a CPS syndrome diagnosis can be made remains debatable. I have seen too many senior adults achieve their lifelong fluency goals after many years of unsuccessful treatment to accept that a diagnosis of CPS syndrome can be made at the end of the initial diagnostic evaluation. I am convinced that prognosis is a dynamic, rather than static, entity. This means that one's prognosis fluctuates on the basis of various factors. For example, timing and readiness (Floyd et al., 2007) are critical factors impacting prognosis. Many young adults who are establishing marital relationships, raising children, building careers, and securing financial foundations do not have the time or financial resources to focus on their own needs, including speech fluency. Once such individuals have the resources (e.g., children grown, career established or completed), they can focus on their own needs and achieve remarkable fluency progress. While I see a value in Cooper's construct, I am concerned about its potential overuse and misuse, namely by clinicians who already are reluctant to treat people who stutter (Manning, 2010; St. Louis & Durrenberger, 1993; Yaruss, 1999a; Yaruss & Quesal, 2002; Yaruss, Quesal, & Murphy, 2002; Yaruss, Quesal, & Reeves, et al., 2002). After achieving her objectives for speech fluency and communication, one "chronic perseverative stutterer" or "incurable stutterer" I worked with told her discriminating employer what she thought of him and his company, and is now extremely financially successful as a private practitioner in computer programming; another became the chief psychiatrist at a developmental evaluation center; another is enjoying his retirement, "going out fluent," as he says. All beat the odds against them and now feel in control; all demonstrate spontaneous fluency or, occasionally, controlled fluency.

Another "incurable stutterer" comes to mind—the author of this book. Many well-intentioned clinicians who worked with me ultimately threw in the towel—they became frustrated with my progress and gave up. It is as though the checklist for CPS syndrome was written to describe me and my stuttering. Without treatment success, I stuttered severely for most of my first 25 years. Thankfully, for over three subsequent decades, I have enjoyed spontaneous fluency, although occasionally I resort to controlled fluency. *Never* throw in the towel. Too many well-meaning people become obstacles, inadvertently snuffing out the light of hope of someone else's dream. Within the limits of realism, which are individually defined, I am convinced that the most difficult challenges require the most time and energy, and those that seem impossible require even more. *Never* give up. Both clinicians and clients must be and remain real. Perhaps "being real" will be empirically validated as an effective component of the clinical process and of life. Recently, I shared my thoughts with adolescents who stutter and are working to achieve fluency freedom (Shapiro, 2007a; see Figure 10.1). The forum was the 10th International Stuttering Awareness Day Online Conference (archived on the Stuttering Home Page; see Appendix for contact information). I share these thoughts with you because they seemed to resonate strongly with those at the conference, including teenagers who stutter, families, student clinicians, speech–language pathologists, and others from around the world. I also hope it enables you to reflect on what "being real" might mean for you and for all those you are striving to serve.

Recommendations

All of the information collected for the purpose of making the diagnosis and statement of prognosis is integrated with intrafamily, extrafamily, and psychotherapeutic considerations in order to form treatment recommendations. As noted previously, intrafamily considerations focus on personal constructs (the way the adult views himself as a person and as a communicator, the extent to which he sees himself as successful or potentially successful as a more fluent or effective speaker), and aspects of the family system (the extent to which members of the family unit communicate openly, support each other,

Being Real

By David Shapiro

"What is REAL?" asked the Rabbit one day, when they were lying side by side near the nursery fender, before Nana came to tidy the room. "Does it mean having things that buzz inside you and a stick-out handle?"

"Real isn't how you are made," said the Skin Horse. "It's a thing that happens to you. When a child loves you for a long, long time, not just to play with, but REALLY loves you, then you become Real."

"Does it hurt?" asked the Rabbit.

"Sometimes," said the Skin Horse, for he was always truthful. "When you are Real you don't mind being hurt."

"Does it happen all at once, like being wound up," he asked, "or bit by bit?"

"It doesn't happen all at once," said the Skin Horse. "You become. It takes a long time. That's why it doesn't happen often to people who break easily, or have sharp edges, or who have to be carefully kept. Generally, by the time you are Real, most of your hair has been loved off, and your eyes drop out and you get loose in the joints and very shabby. But these things don't matter at all, because once you are Real you can't be ugly, except to people who don't understand."

"I suppose *you* are real?" said the Rabbit. And then he wished he had not said it, for he thought the Skin Horse might be sensitive. But the Skin Horse only smiled.

"The Boy's Uncle made me Real," he said. "That was a great many years ago; but once you are Real you can't become unreal again. It lasts for always." (from *The Velveteen Rabbit*, by Margery Williams, 1922)

In order to understand what I have to say, you may need to know a little about who I am. I am a person who is blessed. I married my best friend 24 years ago. Her name is Kay. We have two remarkably wonderful children, our daughter, Sarah, who is 18 years old, and our son, Aaron, who is 15. We laugh and we are happy. Also, I am a speech–language pathologist and have been one for 30 years. I am a professor at Western Carolina University, which is right in the middle of the Great Smoky Mountains of North Carolina in the USA. North Carolina is between Washington, DC, and Florida, the home of Disney World. And I am a person who stutters.

Being Real—For Me

For me, being real is realizing that life, at its essence, is about relationships. Relationships, all relationships, take time. And being real is about loving and being loved, being giving and forgiving despite being hurt, living and learning in every moment and growing every day, seeing beauty in things when others may not, laughing until your sides hurt, remaining young and passionate despite the passage of years, dreaming and enabling those around you to realize their dreams, and bringing a smile and comfort to those in need.

Being real is about stuttering and the anguish of being unable to communicate with a single person on the planet. But it is also about having a dog, Buddy, who for 17 years did not care if I stuttered or not. It is about seeking peace in the woods and, after falling asleep, waking to find Buddy by my side and sunshine in my face.

Being real is about having a grandpa who, when walking with me hand in hand and unable to understand me because of my severe stuttering, said, "I love you just the way you are."

(continues)

Figure 10.1. "Being Real." *Note.* From "Being Real," by D. A. Shapiro, 2007a, 10th International Stuttering Awareness Day Online Conference: Stuttering Awareness—Global Community, Local Activity (J. Kuster, Conference Chair, Minnesota State University, Mankato), available at http://www.mnsu.edu/comdis/isad10/papers/messages10/shapiro10.html. Reprinted with permission.

Being real is about being Jewish and being unable to become a Bar Mitzvah, which is accomplished by leading a service on your 13th birthday, because of severe stuttering. But being real also is about going through confirmation by playing a solo on the saxophone in synagogue rather than speaking publicly, and about a Rabbi who wished me the strength to find my words and the ability to speak.

Being real is about going to a school dance and stuttering severely when trying to ask girls to dance, only to hear them say, "I'd rather not." But being real also is about Lynn and Linda Kall, two beautiful twin girls who asked me to dance, and about feeling so happy inside. It is also about Margaret's smile. Margaret was a nice girl who wore metal leg braces; nobody was asking her to dance. When I asked her to dance, she was so pleased. Her legs moved very little, but her arms and smile were all over the gym floor.

Being real is about making something of myself after speech–language pathologists stopped believing that I could overcome my stuttering, teachers told me not to go to college, and professors advised me not to pursue the profession of Communication Sciences and Disorders. And being real is about learning that sometimes grown-ups, even smart grown-ups, can be wrong. It is about stuttering through an oral final examination and receiving an "F" in the mail, about continuing to believe in yourself even when others may not, and about knowing that saying "the sky is the limit" only reflects the limitations of one's own thinking. There is no limit.

Being real is about electing to take a public speaking course when it is no longer required and earning an "A" in the third and final speech, entitled "Breaking Barriers and Controlling Stuttering." Being real is listening to people applaud.

Being real is about going to Indiana University to earn my PhD, where I met Kay, a girl with the prettiest blonde hair and eyes as blue as the clearest sky. It is about getting up the nerve to call a beautiful girl, knowing that I would not be able to say her name.

Being real is about asking your best friend to be your partner in marriage for life and hearing her say, "Yes." It is about waking up every day to your best friend, witnessing your child's first breaths of life, and looking into their eyes as they grow into adulthood and experience the world beyond.

Being real is about losing all of my hair and having a wife who explains that it has been loved off, a son who when he was younger collected hair from the barbershop floor and when asked why explained that it was for his dad, and a daughter who sees the lines of age on her father's face and around his eyes and explains that they are there because I smile a lot.

Being real is about being thankful for the privilege of working with people of all ages who stutter and their families, about sincerely believing that the work and the relationships are important, and about being as excited in one's career after 30 years as if it were the first year on the job. It is about having wonderful friends and colleagues, all of whom are committed to understanding stuttering and helping people who stutter, literally all over the world.

Being real is about counting our blessings, realizing that sunflowers grow into the horizon, hearing birds sing, and remembering what is true.

Being Real—For You
Being real is about knowing that coping with stuttering may hurt deeply and be more difficult than anyone else can understand. But it is also about realizing that stuttering is only a part of who we are and that it is our choice whether or not to define ourselves on the basis of stuttering. Each of us represents a composite of many abilities and interests, talents and challenges. If you were to meet a new friend, what would you want that friend to know about you? What are your talents? What are your interests? Who are you? Who do you want to be? Are you working to become that person?

(continues)

Figure 10.1.   *(continued)*

Being real is about realizing that life presents challenges. Indeed, stuttering can be a big challenge. Yet we must face our challenges with courage and do our best to become the best we can be. Other people who face the challenge of stuttering have been very successful. Did you know that people who stutter have become president of the USA (George Washington, Theodore Roosevelt), prime minister (Winston Churchill), a prophet (Moses), actors (James Earl Jones, the voice of Darth Vader; Nicholas Brendon, Xander in *Buffy the Vampire Slayer*), basketball stars (Bob Love and Ron Harper, Chicago Bulls), and baseball stars (Tommy John, New York Yankees)? Being real is knowing that stuttering never needs to hold us back. Only our imagination limits what we can do and become. There is no limit. Do you always do your best? What do you want to become?

Being real is about having one real friend. You may be fortunate to have family, friends, teachers, clergy, speech–language pathologists, and others who believe in you. Through life, you may become rich and famous. But if you have one friend, then you are blessed. What makes you feel fortunate? For what do you feel most thankful? Who is your best friend?

Being real is knowing that usually we are stronger together than we are alone and that there is nothing we cannot accomplish when we put our hearts and minds to it. It is knowing that when we focus on a common area of interest or shared concern, such as stuttering, all differences that could separate us tend to drop away. It is about knowing that we, anywhere all over the world, are far more similar than we are different. To whom are you most alike? From whom are you most different?

Being real is knowing that we always have choices. Being real is making the right choices. Even when we make mistakes or wish we had done things differently, we have a new assortment of choices to make. What choices have you made? Do you wish you had made different choices? How will you alter the choices you've made by making new choices?

Being real is doing what is right, even when doing what is right is unpopular. It is about always doing your best and making good decisions. It is so important to do well at whatever you choose to pursue and to do good (i.e., that which is meaningful and right as a service to oneself and to others). People who do what is right don't always receive recognition or reward. However, we know when we have done what is right and we carry a smile inside. That is the best reward of all. What have you done that is right? How did it make you feel?

Being real is giving back. Those of us who have encountered challenges such as stuttering know how hard it can be to confront and overcome our challenges. We have an obligation to give to those who have not yet been successful and to help them along their journey. When have you helped another person who is facing a challenge? Are there other people you know of who could use a helping hand?

Finally, being real is living and giving and loving and being loved and cherished just like you are. I wish for you the confidence to feel equal to and as good as any person present or past, and the humility and civility to feel better than not a single one. I wish for you to be real—for always. Good luck.

Figure 10.1. *(continued)*

and sincerely participate in the clinical process). Extrafamily considerations address interdisciplinary teaming (the degree to which members of the interdisciplinary team communicate openly and contribute to an integrated fluency intervention program) and multicultural factors (the individual differences that might impact planning for, conducting, or interpreting the treatment experience). Psychotherapeutic considerations are those factors that help individualize the treatment plan based on the relative degree of involvement of overt and covert factors, and help to establish objectives that are appropriate to each individual (i.e., fluency shaping and stuttering modification). When integrated, this pool of information yields informed treatment recommendations.

Post-Assessment Conference

The post-assessment conference, held immediately after the evaluation, is intended to summarize the results of assessment, provide recommendations, and discuss any remaining questions. It is helpful first to address the objectives, needs, and concerns expressed by the adult and his family, and to express positive observations about the adult's communication skills and the interactions among the family members. The tone in which the results are summarized and discussed establishes the style of interaction among all participants of the clinical process. Negativity generates a problem focus and one of repairing the adult's defective speech and the family's deficient communication. A more positive, albeit direct and realistic, approach yields a solution and strategy focus directed toward achieving communication improvement and realizing fluency potential where all work together and support one another.

One of my student clinicians recently asked me if being so positive might be "sugarcoating the truth." I don't believe so. Being positive yet realistic by nature provides a model for the clinical process, as noted, but it also helps the client and family be more receptive to the results being presented, the seriousness of the concern, and the recommendations for constructive change. As long as the truth is represented objectively and fairly, the clinical process can become a collaborative, positive endeavor in which all participants actively contribute, support each other, and share the outcome. The alternative, which I do not find appealing, is one in which the communication problem and clinical process are conceptualized in the light of misfortune or as gloom and doom. I guess I have always felt that everyone has unique strengths and limitations. People who seem least able have hidden strengths; those who appear to be most successful have limitations to offset their strengths. For some, the limitations may not be as visible as for those who stutter. The clinician's personal construct about the clinical process and the respective roles of the participants within it significantly influence the nature of the process that results.

In the post-assessment conference, I summarize in understandable terms and with sufficient audible and visual illustration the nature of the adult's fluency and disfluency. I address the family's questions about causality by summarizing briefly what we know about predisposing factors and the importance of identifying and controlling for precipitating and perpetuating factors. I offer recommendations, remembering the importance of not just telling, but discussing, demonstrating, and directing/coaching the adult and family implementing the recommendations. Having discussed with the family the importance of making a joint decision and commitment to return to treatment (deciding they are ready to "open a can of worms"), I determine the relative confidence and consensus of the family's decision. If they are not fully decided, I encourage them to take their time, without applying any pressure or offering undue encouragement. Many of the adults I have worked with have pursued false promises and endured high pressure in the past. Perhaps I overcompensate, but I want to ensure that a decision to pursue treatment reflects a shared and confident decision without any external pressure.

I explain this premise as well as the nature of treatment. I explain that I have no magic and that I can offer no promises. Treatment is likely the hardest work the client will ever do, requiring increasing degrees of vigilance. Treatment is a shared process that is tailored for each individual. I explain that I tend to be more directive toward the beginning of treatment and deliberately shift greater responsibility onto the client and family as the process unfolds. I make it clear, however, that if the client ever does not fully understand what we are doing or why we are doing it, he should speak up. No instructions are to be followed blindly. Many clients have followed instructions without complete information in the past, and therefore may be expected to do so again. I want all of the clients and their families to understand and participate in, and thereby own, all aspects of the treatment process. The client-related factors discussed to this point—making independent decisions to enter or reenter treatment, understanding and committing to the clinical process, demonstrating strong internal motivation, maintaining a positive yet realistic attitude regarding the treatment process and one's role within it, and contributing actively and independently to the treatment process—essentially screen or handpick clients who are likely to be successful. When possible, I prefer to stack the deck in favor of the client's potential for success. Some prospective clients may not have expected to be so involved in the process, or still may be in pursuit of the "quick fix." For others, the timing may be wrong. They may be viable candidates for intervention, but cannot commit to the time involved or degree of internalized vigilance and concentration required. For such individuals, I recommend that they consider seriously when might be a more appropriate time for them to enroll and I offer a welcome for whenever that time comes.

Various resources available from the Stuttering Foundation of America and elsewhere may be discussed with and loaned to prospective clients. The SFA has brochures (*Myths, Beliefs, Straight Talk; Using the Telephone: A Guide for Those Who Stutter; 6 Tips for Speaking with Someone Who Stutters; Myths About Stuttering; Why Speech Therapy; Did You Know: A Fact Sheet About Stuttering; Stuttering: Answers for Employers*), booklets (*Do You Stutter: A Guide for Teens; Advice to Those Who Stutter; Self-Therapy for the Stutterer*), and DVDs (*Straight Talk for Teens; If You Stutter: Advice for Adults; Alan Rabinowitz: Keynote Address*). Other resources include personal accounts (*A Stutterer's Story*, Murray, 2008; *Tangled Tongue: Living with a Stutter*, Carlisle, 1985; *Stuttering: A Life Bound Up in Words*, Jezer, 1997) and electronic websites (National Stuttering Association, Stuttering Foundation of America, and the Stuttering Home Page; see the Appendix for contact information).

Treatment

In this section, we discuss integrating treatment procedures to address the behaviors, thoughts, and feelings of adolescents, adults, and senior adults who stutter.

Goals

Treatment goals for adolescents, adults, and senior adults who stutter are spontaneous or controlled fluency and the establishment or maintenance of a positive attitude (i.e., feelings and thoughts) toward communication and oneself as a communicator.

Objectives

Objectives for adolescents, adults, and senior adults who stutter are to establish or increase and transfer fluent speech, to develop resistance to potential fluency disrupters, to establish or maintain positive feelings about communication and oneself as a communicator, and to maintain the fluency inducing effects of treatment on communication-related behaviors, thoughts, and feelings.

Rationale

The goals, objectives, and treatment approaches for adolescents, adults, and senior adults, on the surface, appear similar to those for school-age children who stutter. The significant differences, however, are revealed in *how* the procedures are implemented, reflecting differences in intrafamily, extrafamily, and psychotherapeutic considerations. Adolescence through senior adulthood is a time of transition that has been described variously as life after youth, an urge to merge, a solo flight, a predictable series of passages or adult crises, or otherwise a time of change (Sheehy, 2006). A poet's words, on the occasion of our country's Independence Day, apply also to the passages experienced between adolescence and senior adulthood. He said, "We live in a postmodern world, where everything is possible and almost nothing is certain" (Havel, 1994). The conflict between the establishment of increasing independence and self-sufficiency and the loss of control experienced by people who stutter intensifies for adolescents, adults, and senior adults. Those central and guiding considerations that both distinguish and impact the design of intervention for adolescents through senior adults will be addressed now.

Intrafamily Considerations

People who continue to stutter throughout their life span often develop an entire system of coping mechanisms to accommodate their life and communication needs. Van Riper (1982) noted, "It is difficult for those who have not possessed or been possessed by the disorder to appreciate its impact on the stutterer's self-concepts, his roles, his way of living" (p. 1). Similarly, Guitar (2006) stated, "By adulthood, his fear of stuttering and desire to avoid it can permeate his lifestyle. An adult who stutters often copes with it by limiting his or her work, friends, and fun to those people and situations that put few demands on speech" (p. 7). What this means is that the adult who stutters has often established a clearly defined personal construct (about himself as a person and communicator) and a consistent lifestyle (involving educational and employment ambition, social dynamics, family relationships, and partner selection), both of which increase the individual's resistance to change. Just as the stuttering behaviors have developed and become habituated over time, so have the thoughts, feelings, and attitudes of the person who stutters. Identifying and understanding the client's personal construct provides a major challenge to both clinicians and clients. Clients need to be able to envision how life as a communicator could be better by being fluent; they must develop the ability to imagine things that have never been.

It has been said that it is hard to imagine freedom until one has experienced it. That is why creating opportunities for clients to experience fluency success, and thereby fluency freedom, is so important. Clinicians must be able to observe objectively without judgment; to internalize another adult's reality; to consider alternative points of view (i.e., to distinguish between an event and its multiple interpretations); and to strive toward understanding, insight, and acceptance. These and other clinician competencies are discussed in Chapter 11. Such competencies and component tasks present a particular challenge to clinicians when working with clients whose life passages they have not experienced. For example, although many clinicians have not yet experienced later or senior adulthood, they must be able to learn from and relate to their clients in order to meet their clients' diverse needs. Whereas the personal constructs of younger people who stutter are in evolution, those of older people tend to be more firmly established. While personal constructs are not impenetrable, attitudes, thoughts, and feelings that have a longer history make intervention and the process of change uniquely challenging for clinicians and clients. As will be discussed, the treatment events around which older clients experience fluency success must be so salient as to create a catalyst that compels them to reconsider the way they have viewed themselves and their communicative futures.

Also potentially impacting the intervention process are the communication dynamics within the family system. A change experienced by one member of a family unit affects all other members in some way. For this reason, all family members must be considered if not involved directly in treatment. As discussed in Chapter 5, communication dynamics are affected by the diversity, characteristics, interactions, functions, and life cycle of the family. As the person who stutters and his family grow and mature, certain aspects of the interpersonal dynamics tend to become patternized or ritualized (in terms of who speaks to whom, who orders for whom in restaurants, who seeks whom for advice, who is responsible for providing discipline, and so forth). Clinicians must be aware of and sensitive to such dynamics in order to design, with the family, the treatment procedures that will be the most effective for achieving the changes desired. The family members are absolutely critical participants on the intervention team. The clinician must understand the family system and the feelings, thoughts, and needs of each member. The changing needs of the person who stutters and those of all other family members must be met simultaneously. This creates unique challenges for clinicians, yet is a key to effective intervention. The importance of forming a "therapeutic alliance" with older clients is evident in the advice offered by a client: "If you want to help me, help my family" (Hooper, 1996, p. 43).

Extrafamily Considerations

In Chapter 6, we discussed the importance of working collaboratively with members of interdisciplinary teams, as well as with an awareness of the client and his family's unique system of beliefs and traditions. We noted earlier that for adolescents who stutter and are receiving treatment in the schools, clinicians have the luxury of relatively easy access, as needed, to other allied educational, medical, and health professionals—learning disability and other special education specialists, psychometrists, psychologists, principals, counselors, psychotherapists, physicians, nurses, physical therapists, occupational therapists, nutritionists, and dietitians. While access to allied professionals may not be as easy or affordable for people being treated in clinical settings outside of the schools, such collaborative opportunities are available and should be explored as needed. The adult's educational, vocational, and multicultural experiences impact the content and process of treatment. The clinician must strive to understand and relate to all these aspects of the client within the treatment process. In addition to unique ethnic or cultural beliefs or traditions, clinicians must also understand the client's stage within, and individual interpretation of, the life cycle. These domains overlap with the client's personal construct and family system. The clinician must also understand each individual client's experience as an adolescent, adult, or senior adult, realizing that such life experiences are dynamic. In other words, each individual experiences and is affected by life differently. This means that while generalizations of any group may be tempting, clinicians must recognize and address the uniqueness of each person who stutters.

Toner and Shadden (2002) provided several valuable suggestions for working effectively with older clients while valuing their unique beliefs and abilities. Specifically, they advised clinicians against both negative bias and positive bias, temptation to control, and behaviors and manner that trivialize or otherwise devalue clients or their contributions. Negative bias may take the form of preconceived assumptions about aging, age-related disorders, and what older people should and should not be doing, feeling, or wanting. Such negative bias and stereotype must not influence or inappropriately restrict decisions about the length, nature, and prognosis of therapy. Toner and Shadden stated, "The clinician must be careful not to assume anything simply because the client or caregiver is old" (p. 70). Positive bias is no better. Overpersonalizing, while positive on the surface, may be interpreted as condescending, insulting, or otherwise offensive. For example, comments such as "Isn't she a sweet, little old lady" and "You remind me of my grandmother" assume a degree of familiarity or intimacy that might not be appropriate. Controlling the content and flow of information minimizes the importance of the client's role. A clinician's respect for the client and family can be conveyed by the way information is solicited, the types of information requested, and the manner in which information is used. Clinicians need to prepare clients and families for the clinical process (e.g., inviting them to organize background information, issues and concerns, questions, and any other information they believe the clinician should be provided), to utilize casual conversation moving from familiar topics to more critical information, and to provide open-ended opportunities for sharing issues and raising questions. Finally, comments that devalue ("I hope I'm doing as well when I'm your age"), trivialize ("I know how you feel; I forget things all the time"), or reflect stereotypes (e.g., "elderspeak," a patronizing form of baby talk characterized by exaggerated intonation patterns, higher pitch, markedly simpler vocabulary and grammar, excessive redundancy and reduced speaking rate, and use of the assumed "we," as in "Are we having a good day today?") are inconsistent with our treatment mission of building independence through improved communication. Rather, Toner and Shadden noted that genuine empathy (earnest attempts to understand the problem, genuine expressions of concern, and a sincere desire to assist the client/caregiver) within a trusting relationship (one in which the professional is viewed as a long-term partner) is more successful. Similarly, Shipley and Roseberry-McKibbin (2006) indicated that older clients respond favorably to clinicians who demonstrate spontaneity, flexibility, concentration, openness, honesty, emotional stability, trustworthiness, self-awareness, belief in people's ability to change, commitment, cultural competence, knowledge and wisdom, communication skills, and academic and clinical competence. Characteristics of effective clinicians will be elaborated in Chapter 11.

Psychotherapeutic Considerations

Just as the behaviors, thoughts, feelings, and attitudes of people who stutter typically evolve across the life span, so do the relative merits of stuttering modification and fluency shaping. As noted in Chapter 7, a stuttering modification emphasis is indicated when the client avoids or attempts to conceal his stuttering, demonstrates upset or embarrassment because of the stuttering, feels negative about communicating or himself as a communicator, experiences intentional or inadvertent punishment in any settings because he stutters, and demonstrates a positive response to stuttering modification techniques during trial management. A fluency shaping emphasis is indicated when the client stutters openly without trying to hide or conceal it, does not avoid speaking, exhibits relative emotional neutrality about himself as a communicator, and demonstrates a positive response to fluency shaping techniques during trial management. Recall that most often, fluency shaping and stuttering modification procedures are combined uniquely for each individual. Significantly, the severity of stuttering has little directly to do with the relative emphasis of treatment. The severity of stuttering behavior, however, often impacts and is impacted by the thoughts, feelings, and attitudes of the person who stutters. Therefore, stuttering severity may indirectly impact the design of treatment. As discussed in Chapter 7, when fluency shaping and stuttering modification techniques are compared, fluency shaping tends to be more efficient in changing speech behaviors, while stuttering modification tends to be more efficient in reducing fears, changing attitudes, and strengthening generalization.

Procedures

A discussion of the integration of treatment procedures with respect to each objective follows. The order in which the objectives are presented reflects a logical sequence that facilitates instruction. In reality, however, the objectives and procedures are multidimensional and overlapping. Although the procedures discussed here are similar to those discussed for school-age children, major distinctions are seen in how they are implemented; how the intrafamily, extrafamily, and psychotherapeutic considerations impact the design of treatment; and how thoughts, feelings, and attitudes are addressed.

To minimize redundancy, the procedures will be summarized herein with distinctions highlighted as they relate to adolescents, adults, and senior adults. See Chapter 9 for a fuller discussion of treatment procedures.

Increase and Transfer Fluent Speech

Adolescents, adults, and senior adults who stutter first need to increase the absolute and relative amount of fluent speech—the degree and frequency of fluency compared to itself and that of disfluency over time—and to transfer the fluency facilitating techniques that are learned in treatment to extraclinical settings. To do so, the behaviors, thoughts, and feelings are addressed directly.

Establish the treatment setting as a "safe house" where clients and clinicians learn with and from each other and, as a consequence, grow together. A safe house is a retreat, a refuge or shelter, where people feel accepted, nurtured, and secure. People of all ages, not just children, need to feel safe. How do we help our client feel safe? We express our sincere interest in him as a person, in his family, his work, his interests. We focus on his communication abilities, what he already is doing well, and only within that positive context do we provide constructive strategies to increase his ability to be and feel fluent. By learning that he is fluent most of the time, that both fluency and disfluency are consequences of what he does, and that he already possesses the ability to be fluent even more often, the client feels empowered and motivated. We help the client maintain such feelings by designing treatment activities in which he will succeed, and we celebrate with him his effort and his success. Within such an environment, dreams are born. Clients begin to consider how they have viewed communication and themselves as communicators, and reconsider the appropriateness of such constructs; ultimately, they come to believe in themselves and their communicative potential.

We noted that within a "safe" environment, clients often express themselves freely, whether they are fluent or disfluent. In fact, the degree of expression and self-disclosure occasionally takes the clinician by surprise. Two former clients, both in their 40s, come to mind. One was a successful attorney who presented the picture of poise and confidence. Seeing him handsomely dressed in the finest clothing and sporting a winning smile, my student clinicians concluded that he felt positive about himself as a person and as a communicator. When I provided him with an opportunity to receive positive feedback about his fluent speech and to consider what he wanted to achieve from the treatment experience (a procedure discussed in the next section), my student clinicians were astonished when his eyes began to water and he emotionally described his "impossible dream," a dream that he could be as confident about himself inside as he knew he projected on the outside. He discussed his success as an attorney, noting that he can act, or adopt another persona, all the while continuing to feel insecure about himself as a communicator and continuing to expect impending doom. Another client was a social worker. She ably masked her inner feelings about herself, projecting the picture of confidence and communicative assertiveness. When gently asked about her present level of fluency and her family and work, she described herself as an "impostor," always trying to be something she was not. She also described ongoing turbulence in her marriage and in her work. Both clients, through speech intervention and professional counseling services, ultimately were successful in achieving, transferring, and maintaining more positive feelings and thoughts about themselves, in addition to improved speech fluency. People of all ages flourish within a safe house, and clinicians should not be fooled by deceptive appearances. Recall earlier discussions about the "interiorized stutterer" (Douglass & Quarrington, 1952) and the importance of both understanding the client's personal construct and approaching treatment from an interdisciplinary perspective.

Invite treatment objectives from the client. I discuss with my clients what they want and hope to achieve as a result of treatment. Some clients express astonishment at having a professional invite their input. Such clients report being accustomed to being told what will be accomplished and how it will be done. I explain that of course I have ideas, but before sharing them, I must understand how the client envisions the treatment experience and what he hopes to accomplish. Some clients know specifically what they want to accomplish (e.g., "I want to be able to speak freely without having to scan my words; I want to be able to present psychiatric depositions in court"; "I want to be able to introduce myself on the golf course without waiting to be introduced"). Others are less specific. Recall the man who could not even imagine what it would be like to be more fluent "because stuttering is all I have ever known." Dialogue of this sort gives the clinician an understanding of the client's previous communication and clinical experiences and attitudes about himself as a communicator. The client also begins to understand that his active participation is critical to the process of treatment and its outcome, and that treatment is a joint, collaborative venture.

Discussing what the client hopes to achieve in treatment often leads to designing communication hierarchies, which are lists of speaking situations in order of increasing perceived difficulty. These lists help individualize the treatment experience, facilitate transfer of treatment gains to outside settings, and help the client discuss and thereby understand objectives and related thoughts, feelings, and attitudes. Such hierarchies address a variety of speaking contexts, including individual conversational partners (e.g., family, friends, superiors, strangers), audience size (few to many people), location (home, school, work, stores, restaurants), content (e.g., casual conversation about family scheduling vs. talking with a professor about a grade), and other contexts. Hierarchies, preliminary estimates of anticipated communication difficulty, are designed initially with the clinician and are expanded by client and family between scheduled treatment meetings. As a working plan, hierarchies are discussed regularly by the clinician and client and revised as necessary. Hierarchies individualize the treatment experience, reinforce the importance of the client's active participation in treatment, and facilitate generalization of treatment gains to outside settings from the beginning of treatment.

Create opportunities for the client to experience fluency success. Nothing stimulates motivation to achieve speech fluency more than fluency success itself. For this reason, I begin with a fluency shaping exercise to enable the client to experience speech fluency, thus helping the client to visualize, internalize, and personalize the goals to which he is striving. Some clients may be unable to project treatment objectives or to visualize themselves as more fluent speakers. I remember one such client in his 50s whose wife was responsible for his pursuing assessment and treatment. During the evaluation experience, he was skeptical at best about the possible benefits of treatment. I recall vividly his disbelieving glances at his wife, as if to say, "Look what you got me into now," and his disparaging comments, which conveyed the attitude, "What does this person who calls himself a professional think he has that I might be interested in?" When he was engaged in a choral reading experience, his stuttering dramatically (predictably) disappeared. The client was visibly stunned. He began to laugh, then cry, exclaiming, "What is going on? I've never been able to speak like this." I use a fluency shaping experience deliberately, both to confirm the presence of stuttering (through differential diagnosis) and to provide the client an experience, sometimes his first, to feel or own fluency directly. Clinicians must heed Manning's (2010) warning, however, not to mislead clients with such procedures, which sometimes yield dramatic results. These results are temporary at best and do not by themselves generalize. Clinicians must be mindful not to generate false hopes in clients. Specific procedures, including how the clinician establishes an appropriate model, varies and fades her volume, and returns so as to prevent the client's disfluency, among others, were reviewed in the previous chapter.

Many adolescents, adults, and senior adults who stutter expect to stutter. This is part of their personal construct. When the client and clinician form a foundation of successful speaking experiences that is as strong as that of stuttering, the client will need to reconsider his expectation of disfluency. Regular fluency failure has led the client to predict that he will stutter. Deliberately helping the client to amass successful fluency experiences, he will begin to expect speech fluency over stuttering. Therefore, we design treatment so as to create opportunities for speech fluency. The fluency shaping exercise, the development of speaking hierarchies, the focus on fluency before disfluency, and the emphasis on taking small steps are intended to contribute to such an alternative foundation. Data collected on self-comments and speech fluency often result in predictable covariance. Increases in speech fluency often coincide with significant increases in the positive statements about communication ability and control over fluency; decreases in speech disfluency coincide with decreases in negative statements about communication ability and control over fluency. These data provide a valuable record of treatment efficacy to maintain the client's motivation (Gouge & Shapiro, 1989–1990).

The main point, however, is that clinicians must design treatment activities so as to ensure the client's fluency success. The experiences must be dramatic in their effect on the client and facilitate an internalized feeling of control, from which the client will be compelled to reconsider his view of himself as a communicator and how these views have developed, and to begin to entertain adjustments to such views (his personal construct) for the future. Indeed, seeing is believing. This is particularly true for older clients, who have longer histories of stuttering and who thus require more successful fluency experiences on which to base alternatives to present personal constructs. Creating such opportunities both within and outside of the treatment setting is clearly within the domain of the speech–language pathologist.

Heighten the client's awareness of his speech fluency. Make the client's speech fluency the object of study. After creating initial opportunities for the client to experience fluency success, the client and clinician analyze and discuss the behaviors, thoughts, and feelings that characterize "speech fluency." At first, the clinician assumes greater responsibility by *identifying* when the client uses gentle speech (e.g., "Right there! You just did it!"), *modeling* what the client did (e.g., "You said, 'Shhe'"), and *describing* what the client did and encouraging its continuation (e.g., "Ffantastic! Yyou wwere rreally ggentle on 'Shhhe.' Keep it up!"). The clinician and client discuss articulator placement, proprioceptive feedback, and the client's thoughts and feelings about his speech and himself as a communicator. As discussed in Chapter 9, responsibility gradually shifts to the client, who ultimately identifies instances of speech fluency, describing what he did while demonstrating an appropriate speech model, and offering description of proprioceptive feedback and affective reactions, to all of which the clinician offers support and encouragement. Treatment activities of this nature heighten the client's awareness of his fluent speech, convey that he already is doing much of what he needs to do more often, and enable the client to gain a feeling of control by becoming aware of what he is doing right in addition to proprioceptive feedback and his affective reactions.

Jointly design extraclinical assignments. Extraclinical assignments are critical. Jointly designed between the clinician and client, these assignments must be clear and specific so as to ensure success. Typically, assignments are mastered with the clinician before they are conducted by the client outside of the treatment setting (using the three Ds: discuss, demonstrate, direct/coach). For example, to heighten awareness of his own speech fluency, the client may describe in a pocket notebook or in an electronic device one word per day spoken fluently. These assignments may increase in frequency or focus. For instance, assignments may increase the frequency or duration of the client's attention to his fluent productions. As noted previously, such fluency focus is ultimately associated with frequently occurring events (e.g., when around anything edible, when using the phone, when asking questions, when engaged in social small talk).

Another common assignment is to have clients attend to the speech of others, particularly those whom they consider to be exemplars of superior or inferior speaking effectiveness. Such assignments help the client discover that much of the speech of people who stutter is fluent; much of the speech of people who do not stutter is disfluent. Watson (1995) noted, "As a group, adults who stutter may have unrealistic expectations about their speaking capabilities as they view the speech of others as unrealistically excellent" (p. 154). Assignments evolve as treatment progresses, reflecting and supporting treatment progress. In this way, while assignments have commonalities across people who stutter, there are unique features reflecting the individual treatment of each client. Daly et al. (1995) underscored the importance of having clients keep "success journals," which help maintain motivation. Actually documenting assignments ensures completion (Daly et al., 1995).

Occasionally, clients complain that there is not enough time to do speech assignments outside of treatment. At this, I acknowledge and offer my respect for their busy schedules, restate the importance of treatment conducted between scheduled sessions, and emphasize that the assignments are to be done as much as possible during one's regular activities. Clinicians must be familiar with the client's daily routine and obligations in order to help design assignments that will not interfere with these activities. Assignments require that the client attend to speech fluency during his regular activities in ways that he otherwise would not. Regularly attending to speech fluency is absolutely critical for identifying and replacing habituated speech patterns. Too often, clinicians and clients assume that speech-related assignments are done apart from one's daily speaking interactions. On the contrary, the assignments need to be integrated with one's regular activities. The client may be the only one aware that an assignment is being implemented (his conversational partner may not be aware). He may internalize his focus, thus gaining a feeling of fluency control, recording in the speech notebook or electronic device what has been designed and agreed to when he feels appropriate. This means that the client need not report completion of his assignment in front of his unsuspecting conversational partner. Clients indicate that they want their assignments to be "their business," not drawing additional attention to themselves. I respect and support this need, as long as the client reports his progress regularly and as soon after completion of the assignment as appropriate and possible.

Develop or improve use of fluency facilitating techniques during instances of stuttering. Before working to improve fluency control, the clinician must establish a safe clinical environment, design and plan objectives with the client, immerse the client in speaking experiences that highlight fluency success, and help the client become aware of the nature of his speech fluency and that of other speakers. Once the client understands that speech fluency and disfluency are consequences what he is doing, then he can both increase the frequency and consistency of the behaviors that result in fluency (i.e., slow/even pace, gentle/soft articulatory contact, natural prosody) and vary the forms of disfluency in order to stutter with less abnormality. The knowledge of and ability to vary what he does enable the client to break the habit strength of stereotyped behaviors and to realize that he has choices. Exercising choice is the essence of the feeling of fluency control, a significant factor leading to the behaviors, thoughts, and feelings of speech fluency (Cooper, 1993c; Cooper & Cooper, 1995, 2003; Dalton, 1987, 1994; Fransella & Dalton, 1990; Williams, 2003).

We select with the client one or two behaviors that he can do that will have a pervasive and positive effect on his speech fluency. Important procedures were reviewed in the previous chapter for how to discuss, demonstrate, and direct/coach the characteristics of slower, evenly paced, and gentle speech (see Figure 9.2); discuss the importance of advising clients about dramatic, albeit temporary, increases or decreases in speech fluency during the early stages of treatment; and help clients become more aware of and in control of their articulatory postures. Intervention typically occurs within the context of conversation, resulting in more fluent speech with slightly reduced and more regular rate, softened articulatory contacts, gentle onsets, and continual, gentle airflow. Other procedures reviewed include establishing and modeling fluent speech; fluency modification techniques (e.g., cancellations, pull-outs, preparatory sets; Guitar, 1998; Van Riper, 1973; see Figure 7.1); and combining different forms of treatment, including airflow therapy, relaxation, and cognitive restructuring and visualization.

Address thoughts, feelings, and attitudes directly. One distinction in working with adolescents, adults, and senior adults compared to working with school-age children is how thoughts, feelings, and attitudes are addressed. Generally, such discussions, including positive and negative expressions of feeling, are more direct. We may ask the following: "About that slow, gentle fluency we just heard coming out of your mouth, what does it make you think or feel about yourself?" "How did you feel when you asked Amy to go out with you and she did not maintain eye contact when you stuttered?" "What do you feel when you discipline your children and you find yourself stuttering?" "What was it like ordering for your wife in a restaurant for the first time in your 35-year marriage?" Such questions and the resulting dialogue assume a maturity of expression within the affective domain, for both client and clinician.

Clients vary with respect to their comfort and willingness to interact affectively. Some are not comfortable because of lack of experience, others because of negative previous experience. For example, listeners may have minimized or negated sincere expressions of feeling by responding, "Don't sweat the small stuff" or "Don't let it bother you. Just remember, 'Sticks and stones may break my bones but names will never harm me.'" Some people, particularly older adults, are unwilling to share feelings because, in the words of a former client, "that is something grown men just don't do." Similarly, clinicians vary in their ability and willingness to engage affectively. I have had a number of student clinicians and practicing speech–language pathologists in workshops acknowledge the importance of addressing the thoughts and feelings of a client and his family but also confess to feeling discomfort and a lack of preparedness to actually engage affectively (W. P. Murphy & Quesal, 2004; Plexico et al., 2005; Reeves, 2006; Stewart & Richardson, 2004; Watson, 1995; Yaruss et al., 2007). Interacting affectively is one of the areas of a clinician's preparation and competence that will be discussed in the next chapter.

Transfer fluency facilitating techniques to extraclinical settings. All the aspects of treatment discussed to this point emphasize the transfer of speech fluency to extraclinical settings. This is accomplished by emphasizing the active role of the client and his family throughout the treatment experience, individualizing activities for each client, and helping the client gain the feeling and experience of fluency control. For example, specific strategies help construct a foundation on which the client can begin to address developing or improving his use of fluency facilitating techniques during stuttering and understanding and adjusting, as necessary, his thoughts, feelings, and attitudes about himself as a communicator. These strategies include building an environment within which the client feels safe to take risks with the ongoing and unconditional support of the clinician, inviting objectives from the client, creating opportunities for fluency success, and heightening the client's awareness of his speech fluency and that of other speakers. The fluency facilitating techniques themselves are built upon our knowledge of communication and one's role as a communicator, and they help internalize the motor sequence and proprioceptive feedback, as well as addressing the client's thoughts, feelings, and attitudes. Furthermore, extraclinical assignments deliberately extend the treatment experience beyond the treatment room; the hierarchies tailor the treatment process for each individual client; and the conversational context within which most treatment is conducted creates a medium that is portable and transferable to any extraclinical setting.

As noted in the previous chapter, other aspects that facilitate transfer of increased fluency and fluency facilitating control include (a) emphasizing what the client already is doing that is facilitative of speech fluency, (b) encouraging an increase of the speech fluency already demonstrated, (c) providing strategies for the client to *do* (rather than focusing on what *not* to do), (d) building social and situational hierarchies, (e) monitoring client progress, (f) encouraging regular assignments and monitoring by the client and family outside of treatment, (g) designing specific objectives to ensure success, (h) modeling consistently to encourage self-monitoring, (i) shifting responsibility from the clinician to the client, and (j) engaging family and friends in all treatment phases. The client's active involvement in and ownership of the treatment process, from the very beginning, also fosters transfer.

Develop Resistance to Potential Fluency Disrupters

While clients are engaged in increasing and transferring behaviors, thoughts, and feelings consistent with fluent speech, they need to develop resistance to the potential effects of fluency disrupters. Several techniques for establishing resistance to behavioral interference will be reviewed here. Those for establishing resistance to affective and cognitive interference will be addressed in the next section (see also Chapter 9).

Introduce direct fluency challenge. Behaviors cannot be considered to be established until they withstand direct, varied, and repeated challenge over time. Therefore, those stimuli that have been eliminated in order to prevent the client from stuttering need to be reintroduced gradually within the treatment setting. These stimuli vary with each client. For example, we may begin to deliberately compete with the client, talk too fast, interrupt, ask a question and then ask another before the client has finished responding to the first, shift topics abruptly, contradict ourselves or our clients, or overestimate the client's familiarity with the topic being discussed. This stage of treatment provides a challenge for the client and clinician but should be conducted with a light spirit within a context of collaboration and fun. Challenge should be varied so that the client successfully maintains his fluency, in terms of both ease and effort. While challenge needs to systematically vary and increase, no constructive purpose is achieved by enabling the client to experience persistent failure. Success begets success; success enhances motivation to achieve increasing levels of challenge. Failure begets failure; failure when sustained causes clients to recoil, solidifying old constructs of being unable and out of control. Clinicians, and ultimately clients, need to regulate the degree of challenge presented to ensure internalized feelings of control and resulting fluency success.

Revisit and advance toward the top rung of communication hierarchies. The hierarchies designed with the clients individualize the treatment process, actively engage clients in that process, and organize extraclinical speaking activities and assignments. Throughout treatment, the client and clinician have reassessed and revised the hierarchies as necessary. In other words, hierarchies were established on the basis of the client's perceptions of how, where, and with whom speech fluency would be increasingly challenged. Experience reveals errors; some contexts prove more difficult, while others prove less difficult, than expected. At this advanced stage of treatment, adolescent, adult, and senior adult clients should be conversing fluently with partners about topics and under circumstances listed in the hierarchies as representing the most difficult level of challenge. This might involve asking or responding with a question in class, asking someone out for a social engagement, making phone calls, ordering for one's family in a restaurant, introducing oneself on the golf course, or negotiating with the Social Security office about funds to be received. Whatever the specific experiences of each client are, he should feel accomplished about his increasing ability to remain fluent and to use fluency facilitating controls in the face of persistent and varied communication disruption.

Prepare for relapse: Relapse happens! Indeed, relapse is more likely among adults than among children who stutter (Bloodstein & Bernstein Ratner, 2008; Craig, 1998; Huinck et al., 2006; Guitar, 2006; Manning, 2010). Van Riper (1973) described relapse as more the rule than the exception among adults who stutter. Clients need to be prepared for this likelihood in order to deal constructively with its occurrence. The course of relapse has been described in different ways. Starkweather (1993) noted,

> With adults the typical scenario is that the controls are given up slowly, behavioral piece by behavioral piece, as the stutterer says to himself, "Oh that was just a little one, hardly anyone could notice; I won't be bothered with it." From this point on, "little ones" are not worried about. Then pretty soon, a behavior that is a little "bigger" is let go without control, and the level of uncontrolled behavior is recalibrated to a higher level of acceptance. Slowly, the old behaviors return, until suddenly the client realizes that he has begun to stutter again. . . . Occasionally, the relapse does occur suddenly, when the stutterer makes a kind of decision that he just cannot stand the burden of using controls any longer—he would rather stutter. Then there is a sudden crash. (p. 164)

Manning (2010) emphasized the role of thoughts and feelings:

> The frequency of stuttering is not the initial or only indicator of regression. . . . Changes in the attitudinal and cognitive aspects of the problem, often in the form of negative self-talk, may take the lead in the progression of relapse. . . . When elements of avoidance and fear begin to multiply and increasingly influence the speaker's decision making, overt stuttering will not be far behind. (p. 577)

Despite our best efforts at prevention, relapse may be unavoidable. Nevertheless, we must help clients and their families understand the nature of relapse and prepare them for the likelihood of its occurrence. Talking with the client about relapse is the first step in preparation. It has been said that "forewarned is forearmed." Once informed, the client can develop behavioral, affective, and cognitive strategies in advance in order to respond constructively should relapse happen and to view the experience as a developmental opportunity within the progression of fluency establishment, transfer, and maintenance. If the topic of relapse is left unaddressed, the client will be unprepared, and the emotional consequences resulting from the client's communicative defenselessness and helplessness can be deleterious to the process and progress of treatment.

I remember an experience vividly that reflects a critical moment in my growth as a communicator. It also indicates the benefits of being prepared for relapse and developing constructive strategies for dealing with its recurrence. For more than 20 years, I experienced severe stuttering behavior and feelings of incompetence as a person and as a communicator. Over the years, I achieved a level of spontaneous fluency and positive feelings and thoughts about myself, reverting to controlled fluency during rare times of extreme fatigue or stress. A university meeting some years ago was a doozy! Meeting in the chancellor's conference room, the chairperson suggested that we go around the boardroom table and introduce ourselves. "No, don't do it! Not today! We all know each other," I thought to myself. I had been up at 4:00 a.m. grading papers, and the meeting was at 4:30 p.m. The participants were all senior faculty members and high-ranking administrators within our university. In other words, I was exhausted and these were to me very important people, a sure formula for disaster! To make matters worse, the first to introduce himself established a quick, crisp, staccato pattern of introduction. It went something like, Bum-Bum, (pause) Bum! I could tell we were each allowed two (and only two) bursts of sound. Each member followed the same pattern—Alvin Jerkface, Psychology; Rita Repulsa, Criminal Justice; and so on. Great way to get up close and personal. On with the sweaty palms, the beating heart, the red face. No way out!

As it came to my turn, I was rehearsing internally, telling myself, "You can do it. Just sound as pitiful as everyone else." As I began to introduce myself, I felt my articulators tensing slightly, but not locking. I knew I could do it. I indulged in the slightest delay, the most minute deviation, before beginning to say the first sound, poised and relatively relaxed given the circumstances. Just as I was shaping the *d* in *David*, I heard—to my horror—the person who was to follow me say, "David Shapiro, Communication Disorders. Come on. Say it!" Could this really be happening? While seemingly the entire boardroom started to laugh, I reflected—for one humiliated moment—on many things timeless, placeless, nameless. As the laughter subsided, I regrouped and said, "David Shapiro, Communication Disorders." After a momentary, tensionless pause, I did my Bum-Bum, (pause) Bum. As the introductions continued, I heard very little. While I was tempted to indulge in feelings of self-pity and worthlessness (wondering, "How could I have been so stupid? How could they have ever hired me and tenured me and promoted me to full professor?"), I stopped and realized that this experience was not about me at all. It did not reflect on me in the least. Instead, it reflected on the person who interrupted me and demonstrated his professional immaturity, intolerance, and impertinence. Acknowledging his lack of professionalism only to myself, I felt so glad to be me. We all have to live with ourselves. Feeling proud despite my faults, I smiled so big inside. What is the story about the last laugh? It has to do with coping strategies and continuing to feel successful and maintaining integrity in the face of potential adversity. At least, that's how I remember it.

Blood (1995a, 1995b, 2003) developed a relapse management program for adolescents and adults who stutter in the form of a cognitive-behavioral board game. The program's name, POWER-R, is an acronym standing for *Permission, Ownership, Well-Being, Esteem of Self, Resilience,* and *Responsibility.* Each step addresses different topics and related activities including stuttering, the impact of stuttering on clients' lives, ways to cope with the challenges of stuttering, and the concept of resilience, or hardiness. According to Blood, the program provides an opportunity to teach and discuss awareness of the problem, problem-solving techniques, negotiating and owning short- and long-term goals (for speaking, feeling, and thinking), facilitators and inhibitors of carryover, self-esteem issues related to relapse (e.g., speaking assertiveness, self-talk, enhancing feelings and thoughts about stuttering and oneself), perceived control issues (e.g., control over and reactions to relapse, realistic objectives, mental and physical persistence), social support factors in maintaining fluency, and assumption of responsibility (i.e., change and functional use of motor and cognitive skills, identity change, and different types of coping).

Establish or Maintain Positive Thoughts and Feelings About Communication and Oneself as a Communicator

We have noted repeatedly that one's behaviors, thoughts, and feelings are intricately and dynamically interrelated. In other words, one's attitudes (i.e., thoughts and feelings) affect one's behavior (i.e., speech fluency); one's behavior affects one's attitudes. This is particularly true among adolescents, adults, and senior adults who stutter because they have had longer to solidify their personal construct.

Establishing or maintaining positive thoughts about communication and oneself as a communicator requires taking proactive steps to protect the evolving personal construct of a successful communicator. This includes the adolescent or adult's strategies for coping with teasing and bullying. Systematic investigations indicate that as many as 43% (23/53) of adolescents who stutter, compared to 6% (11/53) of adolescents who do not stutter, routinely experience teasing and bullying (Blood & Blood, 2004). The relationship between communicative competence and the risk for being bullied is not surprising. Significantly more adolescents who stutter (57%) reported poorer self-perceived communication competence than did adolescents who do not stutter (13%) (Blood & Blood, 2004; see also Blood, Blood, et al., 2001, 2003). As discussed previously, bullying can take many different forms (e.g., hurtful verbal comments, shunning, spreading rumors, unwanted physical contact, beatings, stealing, threats). Also, bullies tend to target those with visible differences (e.g., physical, intellectual, sensory disabilities; learning challenges; special needs) and those perceived as more reserved (e.g., cautious, quiet, withdrawn, unassertive) (Garrett, 2003; Geffner, Loring, & Young, 2001; Thompson, Arora, & Sharp, 2002). These data must be taken seriously, particularly by the strongest advocates of adolescents who stutter, namely we speech–language pathologists. Blood and Blood (2004) discussed the implications of these findings for stuttering intervention:

> If bullies tend to select targets who show poor communication skills, avoidance strategies, and unassertive behaviors, then treatment strategies and programs that work on attitudes and feelings appear to be warranted as a technique to build general communication and social skills. For some adolescents who stutter, changing motor speech behaviors may not result in accompanying attitudinal and cognitive changes. Programs that reinforce assertive skills, positive communication models, acceptance of stuttering, and ways of dealing with stuttering may actually assist in dealing with potential co-occurring issues like bullying. (p. 76)

Similarly, Cooper and Cooper (1995) noted that behaviorally focused fluency intervention programs that do not address attitudinal and cognitive features "may be the single major factor leading to the needless guilt and shame" (p. 130) experienced by people who stutter. They concluded, "From the beginning of therapy, the focus should be on the development of feelings, attitudes, and motor skills that enhance the feeling of control" (p. 130).

It seems clear that we must address cognitive and attitudinal changes (i.e., personal constructs) among adolescents and adults who stutter, in addition to and concurrent with behavioral change required to master fluency facilitating controls. To do less risks leaving clients searching for coping strategies and for solutions to the guilt, shame, and fear (B. Murphy, 2005) that too often result from the stuttering experience. *Guilt* is the painful feeling that results from doing something we think is wrong or not doing something we think we should. Guilt concerns behavior. Guilt results from avoiding activities like phone calling or speaking in class, or changing the name of your child before he is born because you know the first sound will be hard to say. *Shame* is the painful feeling we experience when we realize that part of us is defective, bad, or a failure. Shame is thus about being, not doing. Shame is the feeling that results from being told to sit down in class or hearing the phone go dead after trying your best to talk but being unable because of severe stuttering. *Fear* is the painful feeling caused by awareness or anticipation of danger (dread, fright, alarm, panic). Fear results from accepting the chancellor's invitation to present the university's commencement address, the keynote speech at the graduation ceremony, and then anticipating stuttering to an audience of over 1,000 students, their families, all my faculty colleagues, administrators, and board of governors. It went really well; more later in this chapter. Attitudinal and cognitive strategies for developing and maintaining a positive perspective about oneself as a communicator are at least as important as the behavioral strategies for maintaining the motor skills associated with speech fluency. The attitudinal and cognitive strategies presented below systematically target the behaviors, thoughts, and feelings of adolescents, adults, and senior adults who stutter, while providing opportunities to explore and develop positive communication and social skills, assertiveness, and coping mechanisms.

Treat teasing and relapse as probabilities rather than possibilities. Empower clients with constructive strategies to withstand the potential ill effects of teasing, bullying, and relapse. Clients need to be prepared with strategies to remain positive about communication and themselves as communicators in the face of teasing, bullying, or relapse. As noted, adolescents who stutter are at greater risk for teasing and bullying than adolescents who do not stutter. One might assume that the rates for bullying of older adolescents, adults, and senior adults who stutter would be lower, but anecdotal reports from clients indicate that teasing and bullying warrant attention. Further, if teasing does occur less frequently among older clients than among children, this relative infrequency might exacerbate the potential ill effects.

A former client in her later 30s comes to mind. Carrie was a computer technician who, in her second year of fluency intervention, had nearly mastered her fluency controls, accompanied by a feeling she described as "a freeing feeling" and "a feeling of power." She described the pleasure she gained from using the words she really wanted to use instead of using words that would be easier to say, and making phone calls instead of delaying or finding excuses. She explained that her fluency controls were in the background. She said that if she needed to, she could move the controls to the foreground. "Now when I get apprehension," she explained, "I just do what I have to do." However, Carrie recalled a disturbing event that had occurred a week prior to our meeting. At a formal gathering related to her work, she "got stuck" on the word *now*. The woman she was speaking with began to laugh and demonstrated an exaggeration of Carrie's block, puffing her cheeks and spitting, to the amused chagrin of others gathered. Carrie had anticipated such unlikely events from treatment exercises and remained emotionally and personally integrated, albeit somewhat embarrassed. She recalled, "I was just horrified. Shocked actually. This wasn't for a second or two. She went on mocking me, doing this thing with her face, for at least 15 seconds. This is probably the most painful experience I have had since I was a child. I did not know there were people so truly ignorant out there." Such experiences illustrate the importance of treating teasing and relapse as probabilities rather than possibilities and of empowering clients with strategies to remain positive and in control.

Negative thinking inhibits fluency facilitating control and increases the likelihood of relapse. The treatment described here helps clients maintain positive thinking. By focusing on, understanding, and increasing the client's fluent speech; by creating opportunities for the client to succeed; by involving the client and his family in all aspects of the treatment process; and by attending to and supporting the client's feelings and thoughts related to speech fluency, the client moves from feeling unable and out of control to feeling able and in control. Other strategies, however, often are necessary to combat negative thinking and learned helplessness and to achieve positive thinking, self-assurance, and fluency success.

A variety of cognitive coping strategies can be used to help clients adjust to their improved speech fluency and to react constructively to teasing and relapse. Daly (1988) noted, "Too many of our clients get fluent in their mouths but not in their heads" (p. 34). Before a person can change, he must understand and adjust how he views himself. Relaxation, mental imagery, visualization, and positive self-talk may be used as discrete elements for cognitive intervention or may be used in combination (Daly et al., 1995).

Relaxation is the refreshment of body and mind resulting from being aware of and voluntarily adjusting the relative tension perceived in specific or general body locations. This is done with or without external stimuli (auditory, visual, proprioceptive, and so on). *Mental imagery* is picturing or mentally rehearsing an event before it occurs. Just as anticipation of fluency failure can contribute to its occurrence (as in a self-fulfilling prophesy), so rehearsing, visualizing, and internalizing fluency success (specific to the task or stage in treatment) can contribute to its occurrence. During the recent Olympic Games, several athletes who were interviewed after their successful events reported having mentally imagined their entire performance before it actually occurred. I remember another remarkable event. In 2008, during the Pacific Rim Gymnastics Championships in San Jose, California, 15-year-old Samantha Shapiro (no relation to the author) began her floor routine. Because of a malfunction in the sound system, her music ceased 26 seconds into the routine. Without hesitation, as if the music were present, Samantha completed her brilliant program in front of millions of people. One of the commentators noted that Samantha was hearing the music and visualizing the entire routine in her mind. Samantha confessed, "I had to pull my focus back and do my routine." Much has been written about and by persons in athletics, science, and business who use or recommend mental imagery.

Visualization involves creating soothing pictures in one's mind that contribute to a more relaxed state, a more positive self-image, and positive behavioral adjustment. We discussed earlier visualization and relaxation exercises in which initially the clinician led the client through a description of a leaf moving gently on a flowing stream; eventually the client led the clinician through the exercise; and ultimately the client internalized the experience completely with no verbalization. *Positive self-talk*, also referred to as "affirmation training" (Daly et al., 1995), involves making statements about oneself in positive, first-person language. These statements may reflect the current situation or what the client would like to happen in the future. Daly et al. noted, "Repeating positive, success-oriented statements increases positive expectations of future improvement and strengthens the students' belief in their own abilities" (p. 166). In the example cited earlier in this chapter, as I was sitting around the boardroom anticipating introducing myself, I deliberately relaxed my articulators, mentally rehearsed what I was about to say with both fluency and confidence, and engaged in positive self-talk ("You can do it. You are fluent. Picture yourself relaxed. Now just do it slowly, gently, and natural sounding, and with confidence.").

Another personal example related to positive strategies for coping with fear and preventing relapse comes to mind. Earlier in this chapter I mentioned the fear I experienced after accepting the chancellor's invitation to present the university's commencement address. Around that time, I received some positive recognition as a teacher, clinician, and researcher in the area of stuttering; I read that I was an expert. As pleasurable as these experiences were, they also created in me an intensified pressure to perform. At that time, I had experienced 20 years of successful speaking, relying on controlled fluency when I needed. Prior to those 20 years, however, I had been consumed by stuttering, unable even to visualize fluency freedom. As my dread mounted, I reflected on my success: "You can do this. You have spoken in so many different settings over the last 20 years and have experienced reliable fluency." Memories of my earlier failures kept interfering, however: "You're going to fall flat on your face. You're going to show them some expert stuttering." Clearly, I was experiencing a conflict in constructs: "You can!" versus "You can't!" I enjoy writing and prepared the speech in 2 days. The weeks before the event were both a blessing and a curse; I had ample time to prepare and to worry. I used the time to escape into the Smoky Mountains, to a place that I find particularly peaceful, and presented the speech to the trees while visualizing the stadium where the event would be held, all of the people in attendance, and me on the stage. Thankfully, through this process and before the event, I mentally embraced the more recent data, holding the earlier data at bay, anticipating a successful speaking event. Nevertheless, I could anticipate every sound and every word that would be disfluent, if I were not able to harness my fluency controls. I was ready and looked forward to getting this new experience behind me. At the dinner before the event, the chancellor's wife, who knows about my professional and personal experience with stuttering, noticed my anxiety (perhaps because I could eat or drink nothing) and shared some very kind and supportive words. She also said that, if I needed, I should look up and I would see her in the center of the first row in the balcony. She would be wearing a black, large-rimmed hat, and she would be smiling at me.

Time seemed to pass so slowly before the event began. Eventually, after the established protocol and preliminary speeches, I was introduced and walked to the lectern. As I was about to begin, I found that I was blocking on the "g" in "Good evening." After just a moment of fear mixed with dread, I recalled and internalized where I had practiced the speech for several weeks. I visualized many presentations to the trees and the calmness of trees swaying back and forth. I must confess that I also recalled the tourists' quizzical expressions, wondering what this man was doing talking to the trees. Then, inadvertently, I looked up. As promised, there was the chancellor's wife, wearing a black, large-rimmed hat, smiling at me. I will always remember her genuine kindness and compassion. Then, I tried again. The visualization, the imagery, and the smile; that is what I needed to choose fluency control over fluency failure. The speech went very well and, before I knew it, many people wanted to be photographed with me. This event was another turning point in my life as a communicator. I would welcome such an opportunity again, knowing even better this time that, indeed, "I can." This is the confidence I want us to bring to our clients who stutter, not to be perfect or *the* best, but to do *our own* best. Being positive, patient, and persistent. To visualize, to affirm, and to imagine. This is fluency freedom.

Help clients maintain positive thinking about communication and themselves as communicators. Treatment procedures and coping strategies reviewed previously to help clients withstand the potential ill effects of teasing, bullying, and relapse also help clients maintain positive thinking about themselves as communicators. Several additional procedures can help clients remain focused on their successes and, as a result, remain positive and optimistic. For example, such techniques as reframing, confronting, encouraging, empathic listening, and using humor (Blood, 2003; Manning, 2010) may be used singly or in combination. Let's consider those who "get fluent in their mouths but not in their heads." These are the clients who, despite remarkable improvement in the fluency of their speech behavior, continue to reflect "I can't" and to view themselves as communicatively ineffective, unable, and out of control. *Reframing* means shifting perspective to consider another point of view. When the client says, "I always stutter" or "I never will be able to talk right," the clinician can help the client realize that such a global assessment is not based on fact. Indeed, the data collected by both clinician and client reflect that the client is steadily improving, although there seems to be a mismatch between what the client does and how he thinks and feels about himself. *Confrontation* is a direct form of bringing something to someone's attention for identification or confirmation. For example, when the client demonstrates speech that is slow (even, steady rate), gentle (with easy or soft onsets), and natural sounding (with varied inflection), the clinician might say, "That's it! Did you catch it? You just said the *b* in boy really gently." I noted previously that ultimately we want the client to identify, describe, and praise himself when he hears himself using speech fluency or successfully completing any other treatment procedure or assignment. *Encouragement* is another clinical technique. It helps the client build on what he has just said or done. For example, when the client begins to identify his own disfluency and says, "I just did it," the clinician might say, "That's right, you surely did. Tell me more about what you just did and how it felt." *Empathic* or *active listening* is yet another technique, although somewhat less direct, of seeking clarification or confirmation of what the client just said. It reinforces that the clinician is interested, engaged, and understands what the client is sharing, and that she is sensitive to the needs and emotions being expressed. It confirms to the client that he is operating within a safe house. The clinician might say, "So you're saying that you feel you were denied the promotion because of your stuttering," or "It sounds like you feel excited about the successes you just shared."

A final method of helping clients maintain a positive outlook on communication and themselves as communicators is the use of *therapeutic humor*. Manning (2010) discussed the clinical implications of humor by indicating its positive correlation with personality characteristics such as enthusiasm, playfulness, hopefulness, excitement, and vigorousness, and its negative correlation with fear, depression, anger, indifference, and aloofness. Humor invites a natural expression of amusement (laughter) in response to an immediate conceptual shift using contradiction, incongruity, or integration of contradictory ideas. Manning noted that humor reflects the spontaneity in timing within a therapeutic relationship that has achieved some level of intimacy, and that humor and laughter frequently occur during successful treatment sessions. Clinicians need to be able to model the ability to see humor in life, to value humor as a tonic, and to laugh at oneself. The ability to laugh at oneself and life's ironies enables a client (i.e., and the clinician) to remain positive for the long haul. Manning (2010) provided an excellent example of therapeutic humor:

> One afternoon during our group therapy session, Marcy was reporting to the others that she had finally, after many failures, willed herself to order something at a drive-through restaurant. Since we were at the early stages of treatment, the goal of this activity was simply to do the task regardless of any stuttering that might occur. In vivid detail, Marcy described her fear as she approached the enclosed microphone-speaker and her attempt to place her order. The typical semi-intellectual voice asked for her order, and she promptly responded by saying, "I would like an order of fries, coke, and a ham- ham- hambur- hambur- hamburger." The group responded with applause at her courage for taking such a risk of carrying out an action that she had rigorously avoided for many years. She thanked us all but added that the only real problem she had was when she pulled around to receive her lunch. The cashier handed her an order of fries, a coke, and five hamburgers. The laughter of Marcy along with the other members of the group suggested that she had achieved some distance from an event that had always been thought of as an absolutely dreadful experience. (p. 38)

Here is another instance of therapeutic humor. I still remember fretting with two of my colleagues years ago in a hotel room the night before our first presentations at a national conference. While each of us had a personal background of severe stuttering, we had achieved different levels of fluency success. Discussing our concern about being able to control our fluency the following day, one of us began to stutter deliberately, the next out-stuttered the first, and before long we were convulsively stuttering and laughing at ourselves. Does this mean that we are insensitive to the problem of stuttering? I don't think so. We were among friends and we felt safe. Being able to laugh at ourselves and each other enabled us to reframe our concern (to realize that our global concern was unfounded), to shift perspective (to realize that we were all well prepared and that we should derive confidence in that), and to enjoy the therapeutic catharsis resulting from contradiction and incongruity (three academics demonstrating their worst nightmare in Technicolor). Ultimately, this experience enabled us to succeed the following day, knowing that we had the necessary fluency facilitating controls, knowledge, confidence, and strength of friendship.

Talk with clients in positive ways. Help clients understand how they speak, think, and feel about themselves. Clinicians ask, "How do we assess and influence the degree to which a client's thoughts about himself are positive, while at the same time increasing the client's fluency?" Enlightenment awaits both clinicians and clients who video-record and analyze their own talking. Clinicians should listen to what they say to their clients, as well as how they say it. Does the clinician convey sincere enthusiasm about the client's potential, focus on what the client can rather than cannot do, address fluency at least as often as disfluency, use positive terminology even when offering corrections, invite the client's input for treatment-related decisions, reflect on what the client has shared, involve the client actively in the treatment process, and demonstrate both patience and persistence regarding the client's self-discoveries? Clients should listen to how they speak about themselves. Does he emphasize what he can do and has done successfully? Does he reflect an awareness that both fluency and disfluency reflect the consequences of things he is doing, albeit differently? Does he take charge, remaining active in his role within the treatment process, or does he defer passively to the clinician? The importance of the client–clinician relationship and understanding the essential nature of each participant's role within it will be discussed further in Chapters 11 and 12.

Maintain the Fluency Inducing Effects of Treatment

We noted in the previous chapter that maintenance of speech fluency after the completion of treatment, of all the treatment objectives, proves to be the most vexing. As the client improves throughout treatment, his remaining speech disfluency comes to be less handicapping. The communicative need, which has been the source of great motivation, wanes. Therefore, safeguards for maintenance of speech fluency must be addressed early, directly, and throughout treatment. Some specific suggestions follow.

Help the client become his own clinician, right from the start. Both transfer and maintenance of speech fluency originate at the beginning, rather than the end, of formal treatment. In word and deed, the client must assume increasing degrees of responsibility for monitoring and regulating his speech behavior. Both the client and clinician must understand and be committed to this basic objective and must be able to relinquish and assume different responsibilities as appropriate. The clinical process is dynamic. The feedback loop (the process by which a client receives feedback and adjusts his behaviors, thoughts, and feelings) must move from being externally controlled (by the clinician) to internally controlled (by the client). Clients must resist the temptation to become dependent upon the clinician. Clinicians must be aware of and address their own need to be needed, so as to serve, rather than exploit, their client. Maintenance of speech fluency is accomplished by discussing the roles and responsibilities of each participant and jointly establishing objectives, designing procedures and assignments, providing feedback, and monitoring speech production and progress. Initially, the clinician is more assertive. However, as the client comes to understand the process and share in its ownership, he assumes increasing responsibilities for these and other responsibilities related to clinical decision making. The more the client participates actively in treatment and both internalizes and habituates the key elements of the process, the more he will maintain the behaviors, thoughts, and feelings conducive to speech fluency.

Decrease the frequency of scheduled treatment. Once the treatment goals addressing behaviors, thoughts, and feelings related to speech fluency have been met and are being maintained, the frequency of scheduled direct treatment is decreased. This reflects the client's success and increasing responsibility for managing his communication and himself as a communicator. The scheduled meetings of decreasing frequency become maintenance checks, wherein the clinician actively listens while the client summarizes, evaluates, and projects his ability to internalize communication responsibility.

During several recent monthly meetings of this nature, one client who was 22 years old discussed how excited and proud she was to have self-monitored and adjusted her fluency during a series of oral reports and other presentations in college classes. As she reviewed and shared the notes she had collected about these experiences, she indicated, "I knew I could do it. It felt so good to be in control and I am so happy inside." A 55-year-old client recalled on the basis of his notes how he had remembered to focus on his fluency facilitating controls during visits to the barbershop, the auto-parts store, the physical therapist, and his physician. He shared that the experience at the barbershop was particularly noteworthy because he elected to speak knowing that he did not need to, and because his audience grew from only the barber initially to eight others who entered consecutively. He said, "The fluency was good and I was in control. I am so pleased about that." These experiences are no small victories. They reflect the importance of enabling the client to become his own clinician.

Maintain regular maintenance checks of decreasing frequency for at least 2 years posttreatment. As noted, the client becomes increasingly responsible for reporting, evaluating, monitoring, and adjusting his behaviors, thoughts, and feelings. Initially, the maintenance checks with the clinician can be once monthly, moving to bimonthly, and then every 4 months, 6 months, 1 year, then 2 years. Most clients do regress at some point and experience the need for follow-up. They should be prepared for this and should feel welcome and encouraged to return for as long as they need. Needing to return for some type of refresher should not be seen as failure; rather, it should be seen as a necessary and predictable component of long-term change. Individual follow-up, group treatment sessions, or self-help group meetings generally enable clients to continue making progress.

Institute regular, client-initiated benchmarking. Benchmarking means reassessing where one is and where one wants to be, and addressing any discrepancy. The client benchmarks by reassessing his progress regularly with respect to each long-term goal and makes adjustments as necessary. Once maintenance of fluency is receiving the client's primary attention, he benchmarks his present level of fluency-related behaviors, thoughts, and feelings on the basis of pre- and posttreatment levels and projections. If the client's present level of functioning is consistent with earlier projections, he internalizes the reward for maintaining progress. If not, the client interprets the discrepancy with respect to relevant circumstances and designs a realistic, specific strategy for change. Occasionally, when a client feels he has dipped with respect to expectations, a follow-up visit with the clinician in a supportive, nurturing environment proves beneficial. Similarly, ongoing support from other members within the communication system proves invaluable for maintaining the long-term benefits of treatment.

For example, I met recently with a 44-year-old client whom I dismissed from formal treatment over a year ago. She is a mother, wife, and successful professional and had been benchmarking successfully with respect to behaviors, thoughts, and feelings. However, recently she noticed an increase in her disfluency, which generated old feelings of being out of control. She described her feelings as follows: "It's like I am falling from a building not knowing how far I will fall, what's at the bottom, or whether or not someone is there to catch me." When we met, she brought a friend who is also a professional colleague. It became evident that the client was using fluency facilitating controls successfully, but was internalizing an unfounded fear that her controls would fail her. It further became evident that she was experiencing stress within her family because her husband lost his job several months prior to our meeting. She decided to increase the frequency of her benchmarking from biweekly to weekly, during which she reviewed her daily log of use of fluency controls and resulting positive feelings and thoughts about herself as a communicator. During the meeting, she discovered that she had been triangulating the financial and emotional concerns resulting from her husband's unemployment onto her speech, which she perceived as a loss of control. She decided to explore the family counseling that she and her husband had already discussed. She wrote to me later that her speech fluency gains were being maintained, as was her positive attitude about herself as a communicator. She also shared that the family counseling sessions were successful, that she and her husband were talking openly, and that his employment options appeared bright. This example illustrates the importance of fluency-related benchmarking, supportive follow-up visits with the clinician, and monitoring personal constructs and family systems.

Deliberately revisit the past. The clinician should help the client prepare to view a video recording of pretreatment communication both to celebrate the client's accomplishments and to maintain the posttreatment level of speech fluency. The clinician should discuss with the client how the video viewing will help the client focus on the forms of disfluency that he has left behind and the fluency that has resulted. When viewing the video, the client is encouraged to discuss his previous thoughts and feelings about himself as a communicator and how these have improved as a result of treatment success. It is particularly important for clinicians to be sensitive and supportive at this time. Viewing the video can be disturbing for some clients. It is hard to return to times past and see oneself struggle and contort. Even within the supportive context of "Look at all you have left behind," some clients experience such feelings as, "How could I have been so dreadful for so many years?" Clinicians are challenged to maintain a delicate balance between remaining focused on the positive aspects of change while revisiting a disturbing, albeit past, reality.

This stage in treatment, and specifically this procedure, must be handled with *extreme care.* It is not uncommon for clinicians to follow up with clients by phone after such a visit to times past to ensure the maintenance of a positive attitude. Sometimes, clients feel positive and accomplished when reviewing the video with the clinician, but find that reality strikes after they leave the security and support provided by the clinician. Some clients reflect on the video and center on the bizarre or grotesque nature of their earlier disfluency. Older clients occasionally confront feelings of how things could have been different had they accomplished fluency success earlier in their life. Some wonder about career choices, financial status, family issues, and even selection of partners. Again, intervention with adolescents, adults, and senior adults can involve opening a can of worms. Every person has his own Pandora's box. Nowhere is ongoing support and understanding of the client and his family more important than now. And at no point is an appreciation of the dynamics of the client's personal construct and the uniqueness of his family system more important than at this stage. Memories are dear and exist in the soul of a person; they can be tender and painful. Clinicians must be aware of the territory they are exploring.

Reexamine the client's personal construct. In order for affective, behavioral, and cognitive changes to be maintained after the conclusion of treatment, the changes must be integrated into the client's personal construct. Unless the client feels that the changes "fit," they will not last. We have discussed the importance of helping the client shift from feeling unable and externally controlled to feeling able and internally in control. We accomplish this by helping the client understand the nature of his fluency and that he already possesses a great deal of fluency and the skills necessary to be fluent even more often. We have deliberately designed opportunities for the client to experience fluency success, and we have involved him and his family actively in the treatment process and related decisions. From amassing a foundation of fluency success, the client was compelled, with our support, to take a closer look at how he has viewed himself as a communicator. We have helped him to know what to say and how to speak within social constraints (i.e., to develop pragmatic fluency) now that he can predict speech fluency. We have helped the client to think of himself as something other than a person who stutters and to make changes in his lifestyle throughout the treatment process that support his evolving view of himself. Despite our best efforts to enable the client to change and to feel comfortable with the changes, some report not feeling like themselves. They feel that they have deceived everyone but themselves. How we integrate such changes into the client's personal construct represents a major difference in our work with adolescents, adults, and senior adults.

Behaviors, thoughts, and feelings about which we remain unaware stubbornly endure. Older clients tend to develop more firmly held opinions about communication and themselves as communicators; yet they also tend to possess the relative emotional and cognitive maturity to be able to analyze directly, with our assistance, such opinions and constructs. These opinions form the core of an individual's personal construct, the cumulative and integrative filters through which he views his world and predicts his future. The combination of opinions and potential for insight and change can be used to the client's communication advantage by a knowledgeable clinician. I have emphasized the importance of identifying and understanding the client's personal construct, which provides a window into his affective self. In order to help clients establish and maintain positive feelings about communication and themselves as communicators, the client and clinician need to identify the client's feelings, assess the extent to which such perspectives are justified, and determine whether a reconsideration is warranted. This process must be systematic, as it addresses sensitive issues including thoughts, feelings, and behaviors—essentially, the heart of the client.

In earlier publications (Moses & Shapiro, 1996; Shapiro & Moses, 1989, 2005), a colleague and I presented a model of problem solving based on cognitive learning theory that has applications when a client encounters a novel situation that presents a clinical problem. Adjusting one's personal construct to changes experienced in communication competence is one such situation. The model contains a series of component operations that generate a variety of procedures enabling the client to identify his own perspective and ultimately to shift perspective so as to consider, if not to construct, alternative points of view. For purposes of illustration, this model will be applied briefly to a client who is adjusting his personal construct to accommodate a communicative change— improved speech fluency and communicative independence. This discussion assumes that the client understands how his thoughts, feelings, and behaviors are interrelated and represented within his personal construct.

The clinician asks the client to write or present an autobiographical account of himself as a communicator, focusing particularly on behaviors, thoughts, and feelings. Early in the treatment process, such accounts typically reveal thoughts and feelings expressing inability ("I can't be fluent. I never could talk well") and being external in locus of control ("Why does this stuttering have to happen to me?"). As the client builds fluency success over the course of treatment, his accounts of himself as a communicator should shift to thoughts and feelings of ability ("I can do this!") and internal control ("I know I can be fluent by remembering to speak slowly, gently, and naturally more often"). This positive shift in thoughts and feelings, when paired with improved behavior, should be discussed explicitly with the client so as to solidify the adjustment in how the client views himself as a communicator. Continued feelings of inability and external control despite observable evidence to the contrary are of clinical concern and must be addressed directly. To do so, it is useful to understand a series of component operations of problem solving (Shapiro & Moses, 1989) from the client's perspective:

1. *Identification*—identifying a problem from one's own perspective
2. *Disequilibrium*—feeling uncomfortable or anxious as a result of identifying a problem
3. *Reflection*—thinking about and initiating causal interpretations
4. *Exploration*—discovering and differentiating one's own from another's perspective
5. *Solidification of conflicting perspectives*—believing even more strongly in one's own perspective (disequilibrium typically intensifies during this process)
6. *Negotiation*—internal distancing and abstraction from one's own perspective
7. *Modification of perspective*—applying or constructing knowledge, thereby reducing disequilibrium
8. *Evaluation*—evaluating the efficacy of procedures and solutions in terms of the resolution of the problem
9. *Construction or modification of causal theories*—constructing (or modifying) causal theories by reflecting on and interpreting events with reference to causality

These component operations generate a variety of possible strategies for the client who is adjusting his personal construct to accommodate observed changes. These procedures will be discussed briefly and applied to the experiences of one former client. Specifically, the client's feelings about himself as a communicator were resistant to change, despite his improved speech fluency:

1. The client must come to see that a problem exists (recognizing the mismatch in thoughts and feelings compared to behaviors) and be able to describe the problem from his own perspective ("I feel like an impostor." "I don't feel fluent even though I behave fluently").
2. The client identifies and reflects upon his assumptions about the problem situation and about learning and change. The client reflects on the mismatch, causal elements, and similarities to and differences from other life events. The client may become anxious because the feeling "just doesn't make sense" and is inconsistent with the observed behavior. Interestingly, the client's increase in disequilibrium occasionally may lead to increased disfluency. This turn of events may be circular, leading the client to feel, "You see, I don't feel fluent inside because I just stuttered again," which may reduce disequilibrium temporarily. The client needs to be reminded that he is and has been fluent.
3. The client evaluates the problem situation from the perspectives of all participants involved or affected. Those affected might include the clinician, family members, friends, and coworkers, among others. The client reflected, "Everybody is telling me that I sound so good. I have improved. I know I have. Why can't I believe it? Why can't I feel as fluent as I sound?"
4. The client and clinician specify and define the desired change. Once the client is aware of his own perceptions and assumptions and those of others, the desired change is discussed. Specifically, the client wanted to integrate his improved speech behavior into his thoughts and feelings (he wanted to feel fluent and internally in control of his communication abilities, and thus to think of himself as a relatively fluent speaker).
5. The client and clinician plan a strategy for provoking change with respect to the problem situation that has been identified and evaluated. Specifically, the client agreed to do three things—to engage in visualization and cognitive imagery one time per day of himself as a fluent speaker (i.e., to mentally rehearse the behavioral synchrony and proprioceptive feedback, thoughts, and feelings of fluency, like the gymnast visualizing the perfect routine); to engage in one additional speaking interaction per day that would not otherwise occur (i.e., deliberately flooding himself with successful speaking opportunities); and to evaluate and benchmark his progress every weekend. The client and clinician agreed to meet to discuss and evaluate the strategy implemented.

6. The client and clinician implement the strategy for provoking the change that has been described. The plan was implemented as described.

7. The client and clinician evaluate the effectiveness of the strategy. The client and clinician met as described, agreeing that the data collected were indicative of a successful strategy. The client reported that the strategy enabled him to focus more on his thoughts and feelings, and that the flood of additional successful speaking experiences resulted in greater confidence as he approached unplanned and more challenging speaking encounters.

8. The client and clinician reflect on their assumptions about the problem situation, learning, and change in light of the progress achieved. This opportunity to reflect enabled the client and clinician to clarify their assumptions, agreeing that behaviors, thoughts, and feelings about which we become aware can be changed; that about which we remain unaware perpetuates. The client noted, "I really feel in control now, knowing that I can feel as fluent as I sound. I guess you can teach an old dog new tricks."

9. Finally, the client and clinician, individually or jointly, approach new problem situations with clarified assumptions and the wisdom gained from focused and shared experience.

These nine procedures originated from the component operations noted earlier and can be applied to the resolution of novel or problem situations. Systematic problem solving contributes to the client's and clinician's growth as people, communicators, and clinical colleagues (i.e., "comrades in a common struggle"), and particularly to the client's communicative skills.

Integrate treatment changes within the communication system. It is not only clients who need to adjust to the affective, behavioral, and cognitive changes resulting from increased fluency and communication independence. Conversational partners within the client's communication system (including family, friends, and coworkers) need to adjust to the "new" speaker as well. With increased communication skills, the client will participate more and will take increased communicative risks, and conversational partners must adjust their expectations. Clinicians can help conversational partners understand the nature of the changes that are occurring, how to react in ways that are supportive of such changes, and ultimately, how to continue to feel needed in different ways. Family members who have become accustomed to speaking for a family member who stutters will need direction in when and how to let him speak for himself (e.g., in restaurants, on the phone, at family gatherings). Teachers and employers who have become accustomed to altering tasks so as not to penalize the person who stutters will need guidance in how to include the client and what to expect of him. I have found that spouses need to get used to their partners talking so much more. Grandchildren are not accustomed to grandpa talking so much, or vice versa. There are new rules, and all people within the communication system must be supportive of these rules and be supported throughout the change process.

In most cases, people within the communication system are more than willing to change with the person who stutters and appreciate guidance and support along the way. Parents are happy to see their adolescent children become more independent on the phone, in social settings, and in school or work activities. Spouses or significant others are more than happy to be introduced, rather than always scanning the social situation to determine whether to introduce the person who stutters so as to prevent him embarrassment or wait to be introduced. In most cases, change is welcomed by those who care for and communicate with people who stutter. However, there are situations in which conversational partners are resistant to change, particularly when the relationship is based more on need than mutual support. In such relationships, a partner who has felt needed and important as a ready spokesperson may feel threatened by the increasing communicative independence of the person who stutters. Recall from

Chapter 1 the woman who conveyed that although she would do anything to support her husband's fluency goals, she was concerned that he would find her "less attractive" when he achieved fluency independence.

I always will remember with regret a family for whom the changes created by one member's improved fluency could not be integrated into the interpersonal dynamics. A 35-year-old man referred himself to me after a 15-year hiatus from fluency shaping treatment. Interestingly, his earlier clinical reports indicated that he was dismissed because all of his fluency goals had been met; however, his prognosis was "guarded." He and his wife had two sons. He explained that his continuing stuttering was interfering with his parenting and his work. In an individualized program that combined stuttering modification and fluency shaping, his progress was steady. I met with both of his sons during the first several months, but was unable to meet with his wife. I made several appointments at times that were intended to accommodate her work schedule, but she ultimately canceled each one. When I initiated phone contact, she seemed rushed and I always felt that my calls were at times that were inconvenient for her. I expressed to her early that everyone within a communication system affects and is affected by everyone else. I expressed to her the belief that his improvement would continue and that the changes caused by it would need to be integrated into the family system.

I never met with the man's wife. At my suggestion, he pursued family counseling; however, they were divorced within a year. Did the improvement in his speech cause the divorce? Probably not, but the changes imposed by his increasing communication independence probably contributed to and revealed the instability of the marriage. In other words, the changes created demands that exceeded the family's capacity to remain integrated as a family unit. Perhaps the communication changes constituted the proverbial "last straw." In most cases, one family member's gain contributes to the gain of all (creating a win–win situation). In this case, the one family member's gain was seen as another's loss (yielding a win–lose, or zero-sum, situation). According to my client, his wife no longer felt useful because she was not needed as his spokesperson. Had I not actively pursued involvement of his wife and the integration of the communication changes within the family system, I would have felt directly responsible for the dissolution of the family. The moral here is to be mindful of the impact of communication changes within the family system, and to do everything possible to facilitate those changes, while being sensitive to the unique roles and contributions of each family member.

Respect the primary role of the conversational partners and help support their needs. In the previous chapter, I cautioned clinicians to remember the primary role of those within the communication system who are helping the person who stutters to transfer and maintain his fluency. Too often, clinicians and clients assume these people to be "clinicians in absentia," expecting them to provide correction and other forms of feedback, as would the clinician; for example, "Wait a minute. What about your gentle speech?" or "You forgot to correct that one." Taking on the role of the clinician in this manner ultimately inhibits communication because the person who stutters becomes reluctant to talk, knowing that he is facing certain correction. In fact, emotional upset may result. Clients find themselves feeling or saying, "You're my [mother/father, girlfriend/boyfriend, wife/husband], not my clinician!" Indeed, the role of clinician in absentia may interfere with the interpersonal dynamics within the family. Inadvertently, a dependence on the clinician shifts to a dependence on the conversational partner, rather than fostering a communication independence by the person who stutters. I have had spouses express feelings that they are letting their partners down if they do not correct them. I have also found that clients will enable their partners to assume this role because it is easier than internalizing responsibility for self-corrections.

Clinicians need to talk with the clients and their families to help them understand that the client must become his own clinician. Family members should be advised to offer supportive comments for all they see that the client is doing right (e.g., "Hey, you're doing great today! You really are remembering your controls. I am so proud of you!"). Surely, they can offer correction occasionally, but they should not feel compelled to do so. We have noted before that all of us are inclined to do more of what we feel we are doing right; constant corrections close one down as a communicator and encourage conversational passivity. In fact, the client's occasional disfluency may serve to remind supportive family members to comment on the fluency when it is observed, and to model and expand slow, gentle, natural-sounding speech with even more deliberateness and frequency. Clients should be reminded that they, not their supportive partners, need to internalize the responsibility to monitor and control their speech fluency. While it is tempting and understandable for the client to want his partner to take the monitoring and correction load off his shoulders, this must not happen. Becoming his own clinician is the client's job.

A related reminder is that we must recognize and support the ongoing and dynamic needs of the conversational partners within the communication system. It would be easy to address only the communication needs of the adolescent, adult, or senior adult who stutters. The significant others have behavioral, affective, and cognitive needs as well. We have addressed the importance of clinicians helping the significant others know how best to contribute to the client's establishment, transfer, and maintenance of speech fluency. Addressing the affective and cognitive needs of significant others tends to be more challenging for clinicians. Many parents, siblings, spouses, and others have intense, albeit initially inarticulate, feelings about the client's stuttering. We noted before that some feel responsible, some feel helpless, some even feel resentment. Some are not precisely aware of what they feel. Again, asking general but leading questions, combined with active listening and reflective speech, enables the significant others to see that we care about them. Caring about significant others invites them to tell their story, enabling them to clarify and communicate their thoughts and feelings to both themselves and the clinician. Occasional constructive silences encourage them to share their feelings, forming insights about themselves, their family member who stutters, and the family system. Clinicians need to alleviate feelings of guilt by inviting, accepting, and supporting expressions of feeling and insight, yet providing information and alternative suggestions where appropriate.

Related to the significant others' affective need is a cognitive need, or need for knowledge. What people do or say to help the person who stutters generally reflects what they think or know about communication and stuttering. Again, clinicians need to determine the beliefs and assumptions of significant others, offering support, information, and alternatives. I meet regularly with the significant others, both with and without the client present, to ensure that I understand their experiences related to the change process and their unfolding needs. I might ask any of the following:

⚏ "So, how do you think things are going?"

⚏ "How do you feel about your role in the change process both inside and outside of treatment?"

⚏ "How are you all adjusting to the changes in Paul's speech fluency?"

⚏ "Are there any things that you feel we need to talk about regarding the communication environment at home?"

In other words, we need to check in occasionally with significant others to ensure that their needs are being met (one of which is their need to be needed), that they are contributing meaningfully to the treatment process and perceive themselves in this way, and that the family system is adjusting to and supportive of the changes resulting from the client's improved communication skills.

◫ Clinical Portrait: Bill Rice

Selected Background Information

Bill* was 55 years old when he was referred by his family physician for a communication assessment because of "severe disruption of speech fluency." An informal preassessment meeting was held with Bill and his wife, Frances, to address initial questions and discuss general intervention options and implications. After deciding to pursue a diagnostic evaluation, Bill and Frances attended the scheduled evaluation. Bill described his stuttering as "aggravating." Frances described Bill as a "severe stutterer" who never let his disfluency hold him back and who persisted until his listeners understood what he had to say. Bill's disfluency reportedly began early in childhood and had remained constant in degree and type as long as both Bill and Frances could recall. Bill had received no treatment over the last 30 years, but he had experienced brief periods of treatment before that time involving oral elocution (exercises requiring him to practice consonant and vowel combinations, and to squeeze his abdomen and contract his neck muscles while speaking, among others), neuropharmacology (medication by prescription), and psychiatric intervention. Reportedly, Bill was told by numerous physicians that he would in time outgrow his stuttering. While typically severely disfluent, Bill could predict fluency when talking alone or to the family dog. When asked how improvement of communication skills would affect his life, Bill indicated that he could not respond because he had always stuttered and could not imagine what it would be like not to stutter. He said, "This is all that I've ever had." Bill had no causal explanation, but acknowledged that his parents associated the onset of stuttering with a car accident in which he was involved as a child. No hospitalization or loss of consciousness was reported, however. Bill's sister reportedly demonstrated mild stuttering behavior when she was young, and his father demonstrated imprecise articulation of speech sounds. Both Bill and Frances reported that his disfluency at the time of the evaluation was representative of his regular communication skills. Bill shared that his pursuit of the evaluation and related intervention options resulted from the ongoing support and encouragement he received from his wife. Bill was a longtime factory employee; Frances was an educator in a local public school. Bill and Frances' adult son was employed and lived in their home.

Abbreviated Speech–Language Analysis

Bill's communication was analyzed on the basis of conversation, reading, and word and sentence repetition.

Conversation

Bill's conversational speech revealed an average of 41 fluent words per minute (163 in 4 minutes), significantly below the normal average of 115 to 165, reflecting the severity of Bill's disfluency. His disfluencies included the following:

- ▨ initial (e.g., *tuhtuhtuhtuhtuhto*; i.e., *t + uh* vowel = *tuh*) and medial (e.g., *remuhmuh-muhmuhmember*; i.e., *m + uh* vowel = *muh*) syllable repetitions (units rapidly repeated from 1 to 16 seconds)
- ▨ word repetition (e.g., *I-I-I-I-I would say*; 1 to 9 units repeated) and part-word repetition (e.g., *under-under-understand*; 1 to 6 units repeated)
- ▨ phrase repetitions (e.g., *It is—it is—it is—it is a rhythm*; 1 to 7 units repeated)
- ▨ syllable interjections (e.g., *uh-uh-uh socially*; 1 to 9 units interjected/repeated)
- ▨ word and phrase interjection (e.g., *Well, I a-a-a-a-a usually*, 1 to 10 units interjected/repeated; *That well-a-well-a-well-a-well-a gets people*, 1 to 6 units interjected/ repeated);

---

*Names have been changed to protect confidentiality.

occasionally, words were interjected within word boundaries (e.g., *under- well––stand*; 1 unit interjected)

▤ combinations of disfluency types noted above (up to 50 distinct units chained together for a sentence of 13 words that lasted 55 seconds, e.g., *Well socially I'd say well that it a that it uh uh uh that it a a a well that it it it it a a a it you know a a a well well a a a chose well a social that well luhluhluhluhluh well a well a well luhluhluh well luhluhluhluh . . . life. I don't know.*)

Bill's disfluency was associated with tight eye closure, pitch increases indicative of laryngeal tension and rapid vertical jaw movements during syllable repetitions, and visible facial tension. The disfluency reduced Bill's rate of speech, general communication output, and overall speech intelligibility. Within Bill's conversational speech, there were islands of fluency of up to 16 words (e.g., "That's what they say but I don't know whether that had anything to do with it"). This fluent speech was characterized as gentle with good (natural-sounding) intonation, inflection, phrasing, and juncture.

Reading
Bill read the initial part of a phonetically balanced passage (the Grandfather Passage, also used to evaluate sound production skills). His rate of speech in this context was 12 fluent words per minute (37 words/3 minutes). Forms of disfluency were consistent with those noted above. However, the severity and intensity of the forms were more pronounced. For example, syllable repetition (e.g., *guhguhguhguh . . . grandfather, nuhnuhnuhnuh . . . nearly*) was extremely rapid and lasted up to 90 seconds in duration. After a 90-second repetition of the *g + uh* vowel targeting the *g* in *grandfather*, Bill stopped without having stated the complete word and remarked, "I can't say that word" with absolute fluency. Word interjection (e.g., *a-a-a-a-a-a-a-a to know*) lasted for up to 20 seconds per instance. The reading exercise was terminated due to Bill's difficulty with this context.

Word/Sentence Repetition
Bill repeated 6 of the 10 monosyllable words (e.g., *to, you, hat*) without disfluency and 1 of the 10 multisyllabic words (e.g., *statistics*) without disfluency. All of the sentences of increasing length and complexity contained disfluency (i.e., from 1 to 3 disfluent words in sentences of up to 8 words in length). The form of disfluency was consistent with those noted above. The difference in overall fluency within this context (i.e., greater disfluency on longer, more complex words and sentences) was consistent with stuttering behavior.

Other
All other aspects of assessment revealed appropriate speech (articulation and phonology) and language (semantics, syntax, and pragmatics) consistent with regional dialectical patterns. All parameters of voice, except during instances of laryngeal tension, and hearing were within normal limits.

Trial Management
Several trial management techniques, including both fluency shaping and stuttering modification, were used during the evaluation. These techniques focused on helping Bill experience more fluent speech and gain a better understanding of the nature of his fluent, as compared to his disfluent, speech. A particular objective of the trial management was to provide Bill with an opportunity to experience speech fluency (to get a glimpse of "fluency freedom"), an experience he reported having never had previously. No disfluency was observed during song or choral speaking or choral reading. Bill was successful at discussing the nature of his fluency and disfluency and related feelings. It was emphasized that disfluency is much less likely to occur in the context of slow, gentle speech, and that both fluency and disfluency are the consequences of something we actively do. Results indicated that Bill's disfluency indeed was stuttering behavior and that a combined fluency shaping (direct manipulation of symptoms) and stuttering modification (analysis of fluency, disfluency, and related feelings) approach would prove successful in reducing his disfluency.

To indicate the improvement resulting from the trial management, another sample of Bill's conversation and reading after the trial management was transcribed and analyzed. The conversational sample revealed an average rate of 120 words per minute (120 words in 1 minute), containing a total of 6 disfluent words. Reading the Grandfather Passage in its entirety revealed a speech rate of 89 words per minute (133 words in 1.5 minutes), containing a total of 3 disfluent words. All of the disfluent words were characterized by silent articulatory fixations or syllable repetitions, however, with significantly reduced struggle and tension behavior. Bill and Frances both acknowledged that they have never observed this degree of fluency in Bill's speech. These data revealed a marked improvement as a result of trial management and suggested that Bill possessed the ability to speak with greater fluency and communication independence. Also discussed in the evaluation and trial management was the importance of making a joint family decision regarding initiating the treatment process. Bill and Frances indicated that they intended to pursue scheduled treatment. The significance of the family communication system was addressed, as all members of this unit would be directly or indirectly affected by Bill's fluency focus and projected improvement.

Recommendations, Goals, and Objectives

Recommendations
Based on the results of the evaluation, the positive influence of trial management procedures, the internal motivation demonstrated, and the ready support of his family (his wife and his son, with whom I spoke separately), I recommended that Bill receive direct fluency intervention for 1 hour per week.

Goals
The goals for Bill to accomplish by the end of scheduled direct treatment, tentatively projected for 1 to 2 years from the beginning of treatment, were as follows:

  ⊞ Bill will develop and use specific fluency facilitating controls and self-monitoring skills.

  ⊞ Bill will replace the present forms of disfluency with the fluency facilitating controls of pull-outs and preparatory sets (Van Riper, 1973). This means that he will replace an instance of stuttering while it is occurring within a word (pull-out), and eventually before it occurs (preparatory set).

  ⊞ Bill will transfer fluency facilitating controls to outside settings.

  ⊞ Bill will understand and discuss his communication-related feelings.

  ⊞ Bill will participate actively in all aspects of treatment planning, execution, follow-up, and evaluation.

These goals were considered appropriate for Bill on the bases of baseline data, status of fluency at the time the goals were designed, success in trial management during and subsequent to the diagnostic evaluation, and dialogue with Bill and his family members. Furthermore, the goals resulted from an understanding of Bill's views toward himself as a person and as a communicator within a social context and the cognitive, behavioral, and emotional dynamics that were operating within Bill's family.

Rationale and Procedural Approach to Goals
The procedural approach to achieving Bill's goals took the form of a combined stuttering modification and fluency shaping approach within a family systems context. The combined intervention approach provided an opportunity to help Bill experience more fluent speech and gain a better understanding of the nature of his fluent speech, compared to his disfluent speech. This approach also provided an opportunity for Bill to experience controlled, volitional fluency and to identify, discuss, understand, and gain control of his communication-related feelings and attitudes. It also enabled all members of Bill's family, particularly his wife, Frances, to participate actively and regularly in all aspects of the intervention process. The approach was interactive and collaborative.

The design of treatment resulted from an awareness of cognitive, behavioral, and emotional dynamics that tended to perpetuate Bill's stuttering. Of significance and related to cognitive factors, Bill indicated that he could not imagine how improvement in communication skills would affect his life because he had always stuttered and knew nothing else. Providing Bill with an opportunity to experience fluency success was essential in enabling him to begin to visualize, internalize, and personalize the goals that he helped design and was striving to accomplish. Behaviorally, Bill reported being unable to control his disfluency and being unaware that his articulatory postures during fixations were frequently inappropriate in relation to his target sound. Giving Bill an opportunity to heighten his understanding of his fluency and disfluency in addition to gaining control was essential in order to break the habit strength that had persisted for so many years. Emotionally, Bill's family, particularly his wife, shared Bill's commitment toward a brighter fluency future and expressed a willingness to do all they could in active pursuit of shared goals. However, life was so busy and chaotic that there was at best minimal time for real communicative dialogue, and what did exist was rushed and fractured. As will be seen, this maintaining or perpetuating factor was integrated into the design of goals and the objectives and procedures.

Objectives

The objectives for Bill to accomplish approximately within a 2-month period included the following:

- ▦ Bill will heighten his awareness of the nature of his fluent speech.
- ▦ Bill will discuss specifically what he does when he is fluent, and compare that to what he does when he stutters.
- ▦ Bill will compare the feelings associated with fluency and those associated with stuttering.
- ▦ Bill will reduce the severity of his stuttering by varying and experimenting with the form and degree of disfluency.
- ▦ Bill will begin to "cancel" (Van Riper, 1973) instances of disfluency. This means that he will finish uttering the word that contains an instance of stuttering. Before going on, he will return to the beginning of that word to institute a slow, gentle, natural-sounding posture to replace the instance of stuttering. In this way, Bill will begin to gain control over his speech after an instance of stuttering has occurred.
- ▦ Bill will determine with his family a regular, predictable time for uninterrupted, quality family interaction.

The objectives were determined from an awareness that they are elemental to the goals described earlier. Bill needed to gain an understanding of the nature of his fluent speech. In the speech of most people who stutter, even among those who stutter severely, fluency is more prevalent than disfluency. However, because disfluency tends to draw more attention to itself, fluent speech often is not as noticeable as stuttered speech. Bill needed to understand and be able to describe specifically what he does when he is fluent in order to be able to do it even more often. This is highly motivating and a necessary step for beginning to control his stuttered speech and ultimately replacing it with fluency facilitating controls. Also, Bill and his family needed to find time to communicate, discuss the intervention process, and share responsibility for it. For these reasons, intervention helped Bill and his family develop a communication context that was more conducive to meaningful, less frenetic, interaction. This could only happen through involvement with, and an understanding of, the family.

Rationale and Procedural Approach to Objectives

The client's home might have been a more ecologically valid setting for conversational interaction, but the university speech and hearing center was used for practical reasons. The treatment room was arranged to encourage informal dialogue and sharing of ideas. This was achieved by the clinician's supportive, professional manner of encouragement, active listening, positive facial expressions and eye contact, and unconditional positive regard.

The objectives and procedures were designed in order to afford Bill experiences that would enable him to consider alternative and expanded perceptions of himself. They allowed him to move from "I cannot succeed. I am a stutterer" to "I am able, and since I know I have achieved some fluency success, I know I can achieve more." As noted previously, tracking the client's comments about himself over time is an important part of treatment (Gouge & Shapiro, 1989–1990; Shapiro,

2004a, 2004b, 2004c, 2004d, 2004e, 2004f, 2004g, 2005, 2007b). Typically, such comments move from expressions of inability ("I can't speak fluently. I never could do that") to ability ("I just used a gentle slide. I know I can do this"), and from being out of control or externally controlled ("Why is this happening to me?") to being in control or internally controlled ("I just self-corrected. I know I can blast those blocks before they get me"). These experiences had direct cognitive implications, enabling Bill to study and revise his personal construct of himself as a communicator. Furthermore, recall that Bill initially demonstrated a lack of fluency control and inappropriate articulatory postures. The setting, objectives, and procedures provided a supportive context encouraging Bill's active participation, systematic approximations for success, and heightened auditory, visual, and proprioceptive feedback, all of which are prerequisites to fluency control. The ongoing involvement of Frances and other family members in Bill's fluency treatment provided both the opportunity for and model of meaningful conversational interaction, which was carried over into the home and other settings outside of the clinic.

Treatment Snapshot

Two days after Bill's evaluation, I received an audio-recorded letter from him containing spontaneous speech and a reading sample. Both samples revealed appropriate use of the fluency facilitating controls we had discussed in the evaluation, including reduced and more even rate, soft articulatory contacts, and slight prolongation on initial sounds in words. He explained that he had never sent an audio recording as a letter before, and wondered, "Why can I be completely free of stuttering when I am alone, yet when I am with people, stuttering shows its ugly head?" I phoned Bill immediately and pointed out to him that while he stated that he was "alone," he actually was speaking to an audience once removed (the clinician). I explained that the fluency he demonstrated in addition to his ability to integrate the suggestions discussed during the initial evaluation were indicative of his ability to speak more fluently and his motivation to improve his speech. I also reminded him of our discussions regarding the predictable yet temporary effects he might expect (such as a significant increase or decrease in fluency) as he increased his communication awareness. Bill expressed his interest to "get started in treatment" and followed up with a postcard in which he stated, "Thanks again for your time that you gave me yesterday. I am looking forward to being involved in your program and working with you in any way that I can."

In the preassessment and assessment conferences, Bill, Frances, and I talked about the dynamic nature of the family system and how all members affect and are affected by each other. We discussed treatment as an exciting multidimensional process that takes a lot of work and commitment for all involved. I encouraged Bill to consider his family members when entertaining intervention decisions and let him know that I would be doing just that. I explained that making a decision to return to treatment is a major decision for all involved, often not unlike "opening a can of worms." "In other words," I explained, "sometimes you just don't know exactly what you are getting into. Others will be expected to change along with you and typically need support to know how to change and to feel good about it. Furthermore, sometimes change triggers thoughts and feelings that you may not have known you even had." Bill's son was less directly involved in treatment meetings because of the travel distance involved and resultant schedule conflicts. However, the following was taken from one of his letters:

> I enjoyed talking with you this morning and especially appreciate your generosity of time, knowledge, and personal experiences. Your concerns about the effect such changes would have on the family, as well as Dad as an individual, are probably well founded. In my own therapy, I have learned how closely I've identified with Mom in temperament as well as personality. I have a hunch that Mom will be giving up a great deal as Dad improves. I believe if there's any way to include her in your intervention, it would make it much easier for Dad to develop more fully.

Treatment began by establishing social, human connections between Bill, Frances, and the clinician. The clinician learned that Bill maintained a farm in addition to his other work, was highly skilled at carpentry, enjoyed travel, loved to cook and eat out, and had a remarkably dry sense of humor. The procedures, as discussed earlier in this chapter, were used to increase, establish, and subsequently transfer Bill's fluent speech, to develop resistance to potential fluency disrupters, to establish and maintain positive feelings about communication and himself as a communicator, and to maintain the fluency inducing effects of treatment, including behaviors, thoughts, and feelings. The initial sessions enabled Bill to explore and better understand the nature of his communication behaviors and related thoughts and feelings. Bill was given a variety of opportunities to experience speech fluency and control of his communication.

Within related assignments, Bill recorded once per day in a speech notebook a word he spoke fluently. He made this notation as soon as he could after the event as appropriate, writing down the specific word, with whom he was talking, the topic of conversation, and related thoughts and feelings about himself and the experience of control. After a social update, sessions began by having Bill summarize and describe the nature of his assignments since the previous session. In so doing, Bill discussed, and thereby internalized, the nature of fluency and the feeling of fluency control. Not long afterward, Bill said, "I want to be able to carry on a conversation. Then I wouldn't have to depend on anyone else." This statement was discussed as particularly significant because having experienced fluency success and some initial sense of control, he was beginning to imagine for himself what might become possible. Subsequent assignments enabled Bill to focus on his fluency (and later, the establishment, transfer, and maintenance of fluency facilitating control) even more often, thus providing a source of internalized and positive feedback, solidifying previous gains, and nurturing future improvements.

Experiencing success in treatment, Bill began to consider alternatives to the way he pictured himself as a person and as a communicator. Other assignments included completing hierarchies begun in treatment. He determined that the challenge of speaking fluently increased in the following order of contexts—alone, with his dog, with his wife, and with close friends. Among the most difficult were speaking to larger groups of people and on the phone.

Within 2 months, Bill's conversational rate of speech nearly doubled, from 41 to 75 fluent words per minute. Reading went from 12 to 90 fluent words per minute. Within 3 months, his use of cancellations as a fluency facilitating control increased from nonexistence to an average of 80%. The length of his longest disfluency in conversation decreased from 55 seconds to less than 5 seconds; in reading, from 90 seconds to 14 seconds. Secondary features decreased noticeably as well. Within 1 year, his rate of speech in conversation and reading reached 100 fluent words per minute. About his regular assignments in which he recorded evidence of speech fluency, fluency facilitating control, and fluency-related thoughts and feelings, Bill commented, "I've got so much fluency now. I don't have time to write it all down!" Significantly, Bill was observed in treatment to subvocalize when the clinician offered models and expansions as a form of fluency correction. This means that Bill demonstrated without vocalization the motor sequences being modeled, thus indicating that he was internalizing and processing the necessary adjustments. Frances reported that she had been receiving positive comments from family and friends about Bill's improved communication skills. Comments from those who did not know that Bill was involved in fluency intervention were particularly appreciated. Frances also noted that she had begun to have difficulty distinguishing between Bill's voice and that of their son when she made phone calls to the house. Bill and Frances both reported feeling pleased with the process and products of intervention.

Treatment continued for nearly 2 years. After 14 weekly meetings, the frequency of direct treatment was reduced steadily (biweekly, then every 3 weeks, then monthly), thus requiring increased responsibility for Bill to transfer and maintain his fluency facilitating controls. These techniques were challenged deliberately by the clinician in the treatment setting, and by Bill and others in home, work, social, and other interpersonal settings. Bill was dismissed with an explicit welcome to return anytime.

Follow-Up and Epilogue

Follow-up continued for 2 years. Bill's rate of speech in conversation and reading stabilized between 150 and 160 fluent words per minute. His frequency of disfluency remained no greater than 2% (i.e., 2 disfluent words per 100 words spoken). Bill reliably adjusted his oral postures in advance of the anticipated block (preparatory sets), although he occasionally needed to perform an adjustment while the block was occurring (pull-out). Fixations were silent, gentle, and with eyes open, lasting less than 1 second. Bill reported that he continued to ask himself the two "golden questions"—Are my articulators in the right position? If yes, go gentle. If no, what do I need to do to get there? The only remaining disfluency, therefore, was gentle prolongation of a fleeting nature. These behavioral data, combined with self-reports indicating positive feelings and thoughts about himself as a person and as a communicator and reports from Frances, other family members, and friends of maintained fluency success, all revealed significant fluency progress that was being maintained. In the later stages of treatment, Bill shared the following:

> There is no magic. You make your own magic. When I began, I had no idea I'd be where I am today. I just didn't believe it was possible. I didn't think it would be quite that hard, but it can be overcome. Take it slow and easy. And if you have to, use stretches.

A cousin who was 85 years old with whom Bill and Frances visited regularly sent me a letter after a clinical meeting in which she shared the following:

> You certainly are not the typical college professor (of course they may have changed in the last 65 years). You are easy to talk to, you have a lot of personal charm, and I might add you are handsome. I think you have found friends for life in the Rices. Frances is pleased with the improvement in Bill's personality and in life in general. There was a time he was bound up in himself by a speech impediment. He now orders his meals in the restaurant and also answers the phone. I am excited over his progress.

Guiding Principles

We return briefly to the assumptions that guide our design of intervention and its evaluation: intrafamily (personal constructs and family systems), extrafamily (interdisciplinary teaming and multicultural awareness), and psychotherapeutic (fluency shaping and stuttering modification) considerations.

Intrafamily Considerations

Bill viewed himself as a "stutterer." This was his personal construct. Stuttering was his past, his present, and the basis on which he anticipated his future. He could not imagine any other interpretation. Providing him those alternatives, not by word, but by systematic intervention planning, was the clinician's responsibility. In other words, the clinician could not convince Bill to believe differently. However, it was incumbent upon the clinician to create the necessary opportunities for him to experience success, from which Bill would draw alternative conclusions. Bill's family played an important role in the success of Bill's intervention. Bill and Frances had been married a long time. His development of fluency control was a change that potentially would alter the communication dynamics that had existed for a long time. Just because he changed through improved speech fluency and communication independence did not mean that his wife or other family members would necessarily know how to change with him. Without attending to the needs, thoughts, and feelings of the other family members, it would have been unfortunate, yet understandable, for them to feel less needed as Bill spoke more for himself. Frances and the other family members were involved regularly both inside and outside of the clinical setting to help Bill transfer and maintain his fluency; the clinician was there to help them adjust to the altered communication dynamics as Bill achieved increased fluency control.

Extrafamily Considerations

While no allied professionals participated directly in Bill's intervention program, others within Bill's communication system, including work colleagues, friends, and personal and professional associates, were involved in transfer and maintenance activities. Also, several significant multicultural considerations influenced the intervention process. Examples of these included level of education and type of professional employment, place of origin, chronological age, and religion. What could have been potential barriers to communication proved to be facilitators, creating opportunities for the clinician and client to learn from each other and, occasionally, for both to laugh at the unlikely, albeit sincere, union between people so different. Bill was a skilled factory employee who also maintained a farm; the clinician held a PhD and knew only that "hay is for horses" and milk comes from cows. The client was from the South; the clinician was from the North and never even heard of butter beans and thought "y'all" was a tool with a sharp point. The client was significantly older than the clinician, giving the clinician an opportunity to learn about passages related to Bill's health, family, and approaching retirement. The client was Christian; the clinician was Jewish and never heard of progressive dinners. In fact, the clinician thought that a progressive dinner was a liberal church function. Indeed, the client and clinician learned from each other and never ran out of things to talk about. Differences and similarities became shared topics of interest. Conversation and sincere dialogue were the mediums of intervention, presenting a context within which the participants contributed willingly to the process and learned from and with each other.

Psychotherapeutic Considerations

Bill's treatment initially emphasized fluency shaping in order to develop a measure of functional fluency and heightened motivation. Bill was given opportunities to gain control over his fluency and thereby generalize these methods to instances of disfluency. Thereafter, a combined approach favored stuttering modification for the purpose of reducing the severity of Bill's stuttering and developing increased communication independence while providing him an opportunity to identify and understand his thoughts and feelings about himself as a communicator. Treatment emphasized the fluency already contained within Bill's speech and the importance of transfer activities conducted on a daily basis between scheduled sessions to facilitate control and self-monitoring skills. All procedures encouraged Bill's active role in achievement of fluency success, heightening his understanding and thereby acceptance of himself as an effective communicator as well as transfer of fluency facilitating control and self-monitoring skills to outside settings. The people within Bill's family system participated in planning, implementing, and evaluating the treatment process, all with Bill's communication-related behaviors, thoughts, and feelings in mind. Similarly, Bill was reminded regularly of the importance of supporting the needs and feelings of his family members as he received their support. Bill came to realize that fluency and disfluency each represent active and deliberate choices available to him. He set out to achieve as much control over his communication skills as he was capable of, rather than striving toward perfect fluency. The intervention context was a positive one in which Bill actively constructed a revision of how he viewed himself and lived his life as a communicator. This context enabled Bill to achieve and maintain significant gains, providing his family with the opportunity to learn and grow together and celebrate in shared accomplishment.

Chapter Summary

This chapter presented specific strategies for assessing and treating adolescents, adults, and senior adults who stutter. In so doing, we emphasized several major points. First, clients from these three groups must understand, be in control of, and thereby increase their speech fluency before effecting reduction in their disfluency. Second, clinicians must help clients who stutter manage not only the behavioral aspects of stuttering but also their thoughts and feelings about communication and themselves as communicators. Third, effective intervention must consider and be responsive to intrafamily (personal constructs and family systems), extrafamily (interdisciplinary teaming and multicultural awareness), and psychotherapeutic (fluency shaping and stuttering modification) factors. Finally, intervention with senior adults who stutter is a positive, inviting, and enlightening opportunity. Indeed, change is realistic, desirable, and possible at any age across the life span.

We noted that adolescents, adults, and senior adults who stutter typically have been stuttering for a number of years. They often have increasingly complex behaviors, thoughts, and feelings related to the longer duration of stuttering; may have a prognosis more related to the age of their stuttering than to chronological age; and have rich stories to tell. Adolescence is an often confusing period of transition between childhood and adulthood. Adolescents demonstrate a strong desire to be like others and to be liked by others and are remarkably vulnerable even when they may appear stalwart and confident. Adulthood in mainstream United States begins between 18 and 21 years of age, typically when the individual becomes relatively independent and self-sufficient and often coinciding with leaving home or starting a career. Stuttering is thought to be fully developed in adulthood, although decreases in severity and significance, combined with reduction in speech rate, are often observed between later and senior adulthood. Senior adulthood begins roughly between 55 and 65 years of age, when one has completed one's career and when the adult children are independent. Senior adults are increasingly diverse and represent the fastest growing segment of the population. Speech–language pathologists and audiologists need to be prepared to address communication changes associated with healthy aging.

Preassessment procedures for adolescents, adults, and senior adults include completion of a case history form, review of an audio or video recording of the client engaged in family interaction, a preliminary phone call, and occasionally a preassessment conference. Assessment occurs within a supportive, nurturing, conversational context and includes a client and family interview, speech–language sampling and structured activities with and without communicative pressure, and trial management. The client and family interview begins with a social greeting and continues in an informal, conversational tone. Various topics are addressed, including the client's and family's assumptions about the assessment process and about their past, present, and future with respect to communication and the communication impairment. The speech–language sample without communicative pressure may include or be a continuation of the questions and dialogue in the client and family interview. It should be no fewer than 300 words or 5 minutes of the client's talking (10–15 minutes of real time). Structured activities without communicative pressure may include reading at different levels of complexity, recalling and describing both simple and concrete as well as complex and abstract events or things, repeating words and sentences of differing length and complexity, and responding to questions requiring answers of differing length and complexity. The speech–language sample and structured activities with communicative pressure may include activities involving time pressure, linguistic ambiguity, and violation of conversational rules. Trial management includes fluency shaping and stuttering modification techniques and enables the clinician to help the client by adjusting and exploring his behaviors, thoughts, and feelings; determine the relative effectiveness of different techniques with a particular client; and design specific treatment recommendations.

Post-assessment procedures include a thorough analysis of speech and language, leading to a determination of diagnosis, prognosis, and specific recommendations. Speech analyses address the frequency, types, molecular description, rate, secondary characteristics, severity and impact, and adaptation and consistency of the speech disfluency. The diagnosis integrates all of the information available to determine the nature of the client's speech fluency and disfluency and whether or not treatment is warranted and recommended. If intervention is indicated, the clinician estimates the client's prognosis for improvement within a proposed course of treatment. Treatment recommendations vary with each individual, particularly with respect to intrafamily, extrafamily, and psychotherapeutic considerations, and are discussed with all parties involved.

Treatment goals for adolescents, adults, and senior adults who stutter are spontaneous or controlled fluency and establishment or maintenance of a positive attitude toward communication and oneself as a communicator. Specific and comprehensive treatment recommendations were presented, discussed, and applied for the purpose of achieving the following objectives: establishing or increasing and transferring fluent speech, developing resistance to potential disrupters, establishing or maintaining positive feelings about communication and oneself as a communicator, and maintaining the fluency inducing effects of treatment on communication-related behaviors, thoughts, feelings, and attitudes. Increasing and transferring fluent speech involves establishing a "safe house," inviting treatment objectives from the client, creating opportunities for the client to experience fluency success, heightening the client's awareness of his fluent speech, developing or improving the client's use of fluency facilitating techniques during instances of stuttering, addressing the client's thoughts and feelings directly, and transferring fluency facilitating techniques to extraclinical settings. Developing resistance to potential fluency disrupters involves introducing direct fluency challenge, revisiting and advancing toward the top rung of the client's communication hierarchies, and preparing for relapse.

Establishing or maintaining positive thoughts and feelings about communication and oneself as a communicator involves addressing teasing and relapse as probabilities rather than possibilities, empowering clients with constructive strategies to withstand the potential ill effects of teasing/bullying and relapse, helping clients maintain positive thinking about communication and themselves as communicators, and talking with clients in positive ways. Finally, maintaining the fluency inducing effects of treatment involves helping the client to become his own clinician, decreasing the frequency of scheduled treatment, implementing regular maintenance checks of decreasing frequency for at least 2 years posttreatment, instituting regular client-initiated benchmarking, deliberately revisiting the past, and integrating treatment changes within the communication system.

The chapter ended with a clinical portrait of Bill Rice, a 55-year-old man, in order to apply and discuss the assessment and treatment suggestions in addition to intrafamily, extrafamily, and psychotherapeutic intervention considerations. In doing so, we discussed selected background information, an abbreviated speech–language analysis, trial management, recommendations, goals and objectives, rationale and procedural approaches to goals and objectives, a snapshot of treatment, and a follow-up and epilogue.

Chapter Ten Study Questions

1. We discussed both common and distinguishing precepts of adolescence, adulthood, and senior adulthood. What particular strengths might each of the groups bring to the treatment setting that would positively influence the treatment outcome? What special challenges might each group experience? What factors would likely motivate a person in each group to seek treatment? How might what we know about these three phases of life impact our intervention with members of the different groups? What are the dangers of stereotyping members of any group? What type of "radar" or other detection device will you utilize to prevent the inadvertent, yet frequent, experience of stereotyping?

2. Quotations by both Willa Cather (1992/1913, p. 51) ("There are only two or three human stories, and they go on repeating themselves as fiercely as if they had never happened before") and Vaclav Havel (1994) ("We live in a postmodern world, where everything is possible and almost nothing is certain") were likened in this chapter to the transitions that occur between adolescence and senior adulthood. In what ways do these quotations represent (and fail to represent) the transitions and experiences within each stage? In what ways are such transitions and experiences predictable yet unique to each individual?

3. Traditionally, senior adulthood has been conceptualized as a downward trajectory in function or competence and inevitable and irreversible loss. In what ways do

current demographic data challenge such conceptualizations? How do you define or characterize age? How did you define age when you were younger? How might your characterization of age change as you get older or gain additional experiences? In this chapter, one senior adult was quoted as saying, "I'm 84, but I still fly around the world two or three times a year. Why not? When I'm old, I can sit at home and enjoy the garden." Another stated, "I am older than most of you here, and younger than every one of you." How do these sentiments both relate to and challenge your evolving characterization of age and aging?

4. We reviewed a variety of prognostic factors and their implications for adolescents, adults, and senior adults who stutter. We stated that predicting treatment outcome is an inexact science at best. Given the concerns about the predictive validity of such factors, why do we continue to make statements of prognosis for our clients? How might a clinician's statement of prognosis affect the treatment process, its outcome, and all parties involved (e.g., client, family, clinician, interdisciplinary team)? How might one clinician's statement of prognosis affect that of another? How might a previous clinician's statement of prognosis impact your estimation of a client's potential? How might your estimation affect that of a subsequent clinician? What do you feel are the advantages and limitations of Van Riper's policy to accept at least one client who holds a "zero prognosis"? What do you feel are the advantages and limitations of Cooper's designation of Chronic Perseverative Stuttering Syndrome? Could you diagnose this syndrome within the scheduled evaluation session? What factors will you use to estimate a client's prognosis? What are the implications of such factors?

5. Numerous assessment procedures for adolescents, adults, and senior adults were discussed. Which procedures do you think are the most valuable and why? Which procedures do you feel best capture the essence of an individual's communication skills (i.e., behaviors, thoughts, and feelings)? In what ways might the assessment procedures reflect the uniqueness of the individual clinician? In what ways might the assessment procedures be tailored to the uniqueness of the individual client and the client's family?

6. The assessment process includes measuring speech fluency under conditions of communicative pressure. How can clinicians provide communicative pressure without jeopardizing the supportive, nurturing environment that is so necessary for clinical intervention, both assessment and treatment?

7. One goal of fluency intervention is establishing and maintaining positive thoughts and feelings about communication and oneself as a communicator. When discussing stuttering modification approaches, we indicated that such procedures require more advanced interpersonal and counseling skills on the part of the clinician. How are such skills acquired? When using such skills and interacting with your adult clients about a variety of topics, how will you ensure that you remain within the boundaries of your professional training? When might interacting with your client about sensitive topics (e.g., client's marriage, client's thoughts about his partner, interpersonal dynamics, family and social relationships) be within versus beyond the limits of your training? How will you remain sensitive to and detect the difference? What would you do if you found that you were approaching the limits of and extending beyond your training?

8. Four different treatment objectives were discussed for adolescents, adults, and senior adults (establish or increase and transfer fluent speech, develop resistance to potential fluency disrupters, establish or maintain positive feelings about communication and oneself as a communicator, and maintain the fluency inducing effects of treatment on the communication-related behaviors, thoughts, and feelings). Although presented separately for instructional purposes, in reality they are overlapping and interrelated. How will you integrate the treatment objectives and procedures so as to reflect your understanding and appreciation of the client as a whole and unique person? How will

your design and implementation of treatment reflect the uniqueness of each client and family on the basis of intrafamily (personal constructs and family systems), extra-family (interdisciplinary teaming and multicultural awareness), and psychotherapeutic (fluency shaping and stuttering modification) considerations?

9. A series of component operations (identification, disequilibrium, reflection, exploration, solidification of conflicting perspectives, negotiation, modification of perspective, evaluation, and construction or modification of causal theories; Shapiro & Moses, 1989, 2005) and related procedures were presented and applied to enable a client to adjust his personal construct of himself as a person and as a communicator. This same systematic, nonjudgmental, objective process can be used to resolve other novel or challenging clinical problems that frequently arise. Reflecting on a challenging clinical situation that you have observed or experienced or imagining a novel clinical situation that you might find yourself confronting, how would you use this sequence of operations and procedures for creative problem solving?

10. In this chapter, we indicated that both clinicians and clients must be and remain real and that perhaps "being real" will be empirically validated as an effective component of the clinical process and of life (see Figure 10.1). What does being real mean to you, both as a person and as a professional? What does being real mean to our clients and their families? How does being real relate to the processes of assessment and treatment and to the competencies of effective clinicians?

Unit IV

The Clinician

A Paragon of Change

Chapter Eleven

The Clinician and the Client–Clinician Relationship

*There seems to be an element of magic in stuttering therapy, an elusive,
ephemeral, and yet powerful force which most clinicians acknowledge
but few can precisely identify. The catalytic agent of this force appears to
be the interpersonal relationship between the clinician and his client, for
regardless of the particular procedures or techniques involved, changes
in the stutterer's behavior are mediated by person-to-person interaction.
(Emerick, 1974b, p. 92)*

The clinical magic (Emerick, 1974b) embodied in the interaction between a clinician
and client is the focus of the present chapter. It seems that this magic is recognizable and
powerful when it occurs, yet hard to describe and harder to re-create in identical form.
There is something intangible yet essential and absolutely unique to each master clinician. We can describe the interpersonal and intrapersonal skills that are characteristic
of the best clinicians. Nevertheless, attempts to create clinical effectiveness or those
quintessential moments of clinical magic by demonstrating the component elements
are doomed to disappointment. Clinical effectiveness is a connection between caring
clinicians and clients, involving transcendent moments of ultimate communication and
shared growth that are focused, yet timeless and placeless. Knowing that any attempt to
capture that magical experience can be an approximation at best, let us begin.

In this chapter, we will address the importance of the clinician and the client–
clinician relationship to the change process and the interpersonal and intrapersonal
competencies that are necessary for clinicians to work effectively with people who stutter and their families, emphasizing the following major points:

- The clinician is the single most critical variable in the process of change. Clients neither
  communicate nor improve communication in a vacuum. The clinician enables the client
  to imagine, work toward, and achieve communicative dreams.
- Effective clinicians who work with people who stutter have recognizable interpersonal
  characteristics—behaviors, affective attributes (i.e., manner of interaction), and language—
  that help the clinician–client relationship flourish.

▨ Effective clinicians have recognizable intrapersonal characteristics—thoughts, feelings, and beliefs; personal needs; and enduring satisfaction and internal rewards—that contribute to a productive client–clinician relationship.

▨ Once personally and professionally self-aware (i.e., aware of and in control of interpersonal and intrapersonal factors), clinicians can develop or improve their professional skills.

Importance of Clinicians to the Change Process

The clinician and the interpersonal clinical relationship are among the most significant factors influencing, if not foretelling, the outcome of treatment. Indeed, as A. T. Murphy and FitzSimons (1960) noted, "The most important single variable affecting success in the treatment of stutterers is—the clinician" (p. 27). Van Riper (1975) stated, "No matter what kind of treatment is used and no matter what its rationale may be, the clinician is always a significant part of the therapeutic dyad" (p. 455). Nevertheless, compared to the numerous investigations of children and adults who stutter, the clinician has been relatively unstudied. Van Riper (1975) observed further that "millions of words have been written about stutterers, but only a few about the clinicians who have treated them. Surely it is time to examine stuttering therapy from this other perspective" (p. 455). This blind spot in our progression as a discipline continues to the present day. Hinckley (2008) acknowledged the factors within "the great plain of clinical interaction" (p. x) as "one of the great remaining frontiers left to explore and study in the discipline of speech–language pathology" (p. x).

It is no secret that clinicians vary in professional effectiveness. This conclusion is based on the clinical literature (ASHA, 1995, 2004a, 2004b, 2004c, 2005a, 2005b, 2005c, 2009a, 2009b; Blood, Blood, McCarthy, Tellis, & Gabel, 2001; Bloodstein & Bernstein Ratner, 2008; Hayhow et al., 2002; Leahy, 2004; Plexico et al., 2005; Shapiro, 2000; Shapiro & Moses, 2005; Stewart & Richardon, 2004; Yaruss Quesal, & Murphy, 2002) and more than 30 years of working directly with and observing clients and clinicians and discussing with both what they find to be most and least effective about the clinical experience. Manning (2010) noted that there is no exclusive set of attributes that characterize an expert clinician. Indeed, clinicians' professional and personal attributes vary, as do clients' behaviors, thoughts, and feelings. Manning (2010) added,

> It is clear that some clinicians are considerably better than others at supporting and motivating their clients throughout the treatment process. The attitudes and abilities that these clinicians possess distinguish them from the clinicians who are less effective. It is the effective clinicians who are able to select appropriate therapeutic strategies and use or design related techniques. Perhaps more than any other qualities, the best clinicians are uncommonly effective in understanding, encouraging, supporting, and guiding their clients along the path of treatment. (p. 4)

Some might argue that the clinician tends to be more significant to the clinical process when treatment takes on more of a stuttering modification, or counseling, focus compared to a fluency shaping, or behavior-driven, focus (Guitar, 1998; Guitar & Peters, 2008; Manning, 2010). Others (Cooper & Cooper, 2003; Daly, 1988; Holmes, 2009; Hood, 1974; Jozefowicz, 2009; Shapiro, 1995, 2000; Shapiro et al., 2004; Van Riper, 1975) have countered that independent of the form of treatment, the clinician remains a key ingredient to its effectiveness. The following quotations indicate the importance of the clinician in the process of change:

> Workers in every phase of the helping professions recognize that the client–clinician relationship is a, if not the, crucial variable in the treatment process. (Emerick & Hood, 1974, p. vii)

The enthusiast may be influencing his patient more by his personality than by his method. The method becomes only the vehicle for this transmission. It may be that what makes a therapist an expert is an increase in his self-expressive ability through the selection and alteration of a chosen system. (Walle, 1974, p. 6)

Methods and materials used in therapy remain insignificant until touched by a spark, the individual clinician's uniqueness, which elevates them beyond the commonplace. Regardless of approach, his personal conception of the clinical interface, his attitude concerning the personal dimensions of the encounter called therapy, his blend of thinking, feeling and doing, and his way of life deeply affect both the nature of the interaction and its degree of success, be it objectively or subjectively defined. Such behavior can constitute the advocacy of a certain clinical orientation or mood, a form of attitude toward action appropriate with humans who stutter. (A. T. Murphy, 1974, p. 30)

To emphasize the importance of the clinician and the interaction within the clinical process does not negate or even challenge the importance of other aspects of the clinical process, such as understanding, planning, observing, analyzing, and integrating. Indeed, we will highlight the behavior of effective clinicians, including goals, processes, and competencies related to assessment, management, and transfer and maintenance of fluency (ASHA, 1995, 2004c, 2005c, 2009c). Many disparate kinds of treatment have resulted in communicative improvement of different kinds and degrees of durability (G. Andrews et al., 1983; Bloodstein & Bernstein Ratner, 2008; Brutten, 1993; Emerick, 1974a, 1974b; Luper, 2003; Van Riper, 1974). We know that the affective or interpersonal dimension contributes significantly to the overall clinical experience and its outcome. However, to estimate in concrete terms the relative contribution of this dimension, to date, remains conjecture. About the relative import of the interpersonal element, Emerick (1974b) noted the following:

How large a segment this interpersonal dimension occupies within the therapeutic process I do not know; some experienced clinicians suggest that at least half of what occurs in therapy is simply inspirational and elicits the release of healing processes within the individual. . . . After laboring with stutterers for over a decade, I am convinced that it is not only what I do that helps the person get better but also how I do it and who I am. (pp. 92–93)

While attempts to quantify the influence of the clinician may fail, the point remains that the clinician is at least a critical element in the client–clinician relationship. We will attempt to describe elements of that relationship and particularly interpersonal and intrapersonal factors of effective clinicians who succeed in creating clinical magic.

Interpersonal Characteristics of Effective Clinicians

Clinician Behaviors

Analyzing and describing the behaviors of effective clinicians, as will be seen, present the least degree of difficulty. The Special Interest Division on Fluency and Fluency Disorders' Guidelines for Practice in Stuttering Treatment (ASHA, 1995) addressed issues such as the following:

⚏ general guidelines for practice—timing and duration of treatment sessions; setting, duration, complexity, and cost of treatment

⚏ personal attributes of clinicians—interest and commitment, willingness to develop knowledge and skill, problem-solving skills, and flexibility

⬚ learned attributes of clinicians—an understanding of the literature, knowledge of phenomenology, a focused yet broad perspective, an understanding of the clinical process, good
communication skills

⬚ specific guidelines for practice—goals, processes, and competencies for assessment, management, and transfer and maintenance

The specific guidelines represent a comprehensive delineation of "all goals that
are considered appropriate by all philosophies of treatment currently held by speech–
language pathologists who treat people who stutter" (ASHA, 1995, p. 28), processes that
are useful for achieving specific goals and competencies (including skills and knowledge)
that clinicians can use to engage in the processes identified. The guidelines understandably are stated in behavioral terms. What remains to be addressed are the less tangible,
albeit critical, manifestations of the clinician's affective and cognitive dimensions.

Clinician Attributes and Manner of Interaction

We have long known the importance of the clinician's affective characteristics. In an
earlier publication (Shapiro, 1994a), I discussed the work of Carkhuff (1969a, 1969b);
Gazda, Asbury, Balzer, Childers, and Walters (1977); and Rogers (1957) and applied
this work to interaction analysis and self-study. The premise across these works is that
if certain facilitative conditions are present within the clinical interaction and if they
are perceived by the client, then the client will experience positive changes. Various
master clinicians have described the elements of this affective dimension, which are
recognizable yet hard to measure. Van Riper (1975) described such essential clinician
characteristics as *empathy, warmth, genuineness,* and *charisma*. Emerick (1974b) described
the critical dimensions of interpersonal sensitivity as *compatible friction, focused optimism,*
and *personal magnetism*. Because of their relevance to the importance of the interpersonal
process in the treatment of people who stutter, these elements, which overlap with one
another, will be described briefly.

Empathy

Empathy is an "authentic sensitivity for the client" (Manning, 2010, p. 11), "the ability
to imagine how it feels to be inside another person's skin" (Van Riper, 1975, p. 461), the
ability to "see with the eyes of another, hear with the ears of another, and feel with the
heart of another" (A. Adler, 1956, p. 135; also cited in Flasher & Fogle, 2004, p. 96). Van
Riper (1975) compared the empathic perceptiveness between an effective clinician and
client to that in a long and successful marriage in which each partner knows what the
other is thinking and feeling. Empathy requires objective observations that are distinct
from hypotheses or inferences. Furthermore, since all observation is selective (i.e., no
clinician can observe all behaviors of people who stutter; inherent selectivity may distort the picture), clinicians must deliberately open their field of perception and consider
alternative points of view. Empathy also requires sensitivity to clients' internal thoughts
and feelings, which may or may not be revealed by what the client does or does not
say. Empathy requires the clinician's self-awareness and the ability to observe herself
while she is observing the client. Van Riper (1975) cautioned against overidentification
or overinvolvement, noting that clinicians' and clients' circles should intersect but never
be concentric. There must always be a clear area outside the intersection to be able to
help people who stutter. In other words, in our attempt to feel the way the client feels, we
must not become so close that we take on all of these feelings or lose perspective or objectivity. Similarly, Rogers (1961) advised clinicians to retain the "as if" quality, that is,

to understand the client's angers, fears, and confusions *as if* each were our own, without letting our own angers, fears, and confusions become bound up. This is empathy.

I am doubtful that empathy can be learned; rather, I believe it is discovered and nurtured. Sometimes discovering one's own capacity for empathy is challenging, if not unsettling. Student and other novice clinicians often have expressed concern that they will become emotional in the presence of a client. "What if I cry, or totally lose it?" they say to me. I explain that our ability to relate to another person and his life is one of the reasons we decided to enter this profession. To relate to, to internalize, and even to make "as if" one's own the reality of another person: this is healthy, sound, and professional. We should not be reluctant to build our understanding of another person upon our own solid emotional foundation. This may mean that occasionally we share both a tear and a smile with someone we care for deeply. However, to lose our emotional composure (including crying uncontrollably, becoming visibly angry, or becoming internally fearful) is professionally unacceptable. Doing so inappropriately shifts the clinical focus from the client to the clinician. Typically clinicians become more comfortable with their own empathic side as they become familiar with it. Rarely have I seen a clinician who cannot develop and maintain the "as if" quality. In such few instances, I have seen clinicians sob uncontrollably in class when witnessing a person's pain (guest presentation or video recording). In only one instance that I can recall was a student counseled out of the program because of chronic overidentification with clients, despite exhaustive instructional intervention efforts (Shapiro et al., 2002).

Warmth

Warmth is a composite of behaviors including understanding, sincerity, friendliness, and respect ("unconditional positive regard"; Rogers, 1957) that, when offered, typically receives a similar response in return. I often hear warmth discussed as a tag to other affective qualities (e.g., warm and friendly, warmth and hospitality). Over the years, I have seen warmth blossom in countless clinicians. I do not believe that they had to "learn" warmth. I believe that they needed to address their own needs (e.g., anxiety, confidence, feelings of competence) before they could focus without distraction on their clients. It is that connection, that shared commitment in focused communication, that is timeless and placeless, enabling warmth to surface. Clinicians' early interviews often look like interrogations (i.e., series of staccato questions without reflection or any shared affective interaction), only to move to conversational, inviting, reflective, problem-solving dialogues. A. T. Murphy (1974) spoke of "two monologues in search of a dialogue" (p. 29). The conversational dialogue emanating from and connecting with the head and heart—this is warmth.

Van Riper (1975) noted that clients "must feel vividly that we like, respect, and care for them as persons. . . . When we could not really like a stutterer we always failed" (p. 466). Given the significant impact of clinicians' attitudes on clients' improvement (Daly, 1988), it is not surprising that the warmth conveyed by the clinician influences the client's potential communication improvement. A. T. Murphy and FitzSimons (1960) noted, "The successful clinician is the worker who is able to establish the warm relationship on which new learning is dependent" (p. 28). In most cases, clinicians have no problem relating to and liking their clients. However, what happens when clinicians are faced with a client they find unpleasant, unappealing, or otherwise unlikable as a person?

I remember one such client. He was a senior adult with a litany of medical woes. He was being treated psychiatrically for clinical depression, negativity, paranoia, and passive dependency syndrome. We were working collaboratively with family members, psychiatric services, and other allied medical and human service professionals. I remember several male and female clinicians who were well meaning, positive, perky, and young-spirited when they prepared for and began this man's treatment but who later visibly demonstrated a slow emotional crumble that ended with two broken souls leaving the treatment room. "Wait a minute," I admonished one clinician, "You are to help and support your client but not to become him." She replied, "But I don't like him. He's horrible. I think I hate him." Impressed with the student clinician's degree of self-disclosure, I needed to figuratively scrape her off the floor while impressing upon her the importance of empathic understanding and warmth.

The question remained, however. How do you express warmth, which must be sincere, to a person you don't like or respect? Fortunately, in most cases, clients and clinicians develop a sincere and positive regard for each other as the therapeutic relationship develops and progresses and as they relate to each other as people. Granted, in any relationship there are times when we may not like all of what we see in others or in ourselves. As the clinical relationship develops, its participants often become increasingly candid. Usually this candor contributes in positive ways to the development of the clinical interaction.

However, I have worked with clients who, in my presence, expressed thoughts and beliefs reflecting bigotry, racism, sexism, anti-Semitism, ego- and ethnocentrism, and other woeful constructs. I must confess that on such thankfully few occasions, my attempts to interact on the basis of our shared interests were indeed challenging and atypically deliberate. Furthermore, my manner of conveying empathy and warmth was affected by my attempts to accept a person whose views I found unacceptable. In such instances, I repeated the words I learned from a clinician whose clinical fellowship I supervised ("I know you feel that way. However, I see things differently"). By attending to communication objectives and by redirecting conversation that does not have at its heart the client as a communicator or the client's communication system, I have never referred a client to another clinician because of "personality conflicts" or "irreconcilable differences." Theoretically, however, I see this as possible and occasionally a wise professional choice. People are different. Indeed we do not need to like everything we see in or hear from our clients. But we do need to remember the value of empathy and warmth in creating a clinical climate that is conducive to meaningful change.

Genuineness

Genuineness is the ability to be one's true self as a person with a client while conveying professional competence and personal confidence. Rogers (1957, 1961) noted that the clinician's "congruence" is critical to her influence on the client. This refers to being aware, accepting, and honest about oneself and how one presents oneself to each client. In addition to personal honesty, competence is another aspect of genuineness. Clinicians must be and feel competent and be able to demonstrate this competence. Clients need to know that their clinicians are competent in order to begin to trust their clinician and believe that the clinical process really will result in meaningful change. Usually, the client's need to believe that the clinician is competent is implicit, although rarely expressed. On one occasion, however, I was intrigued by how much one adult client knew about me at the time of her diagnostic evaluation. It came out that before scheduling the appointment, she visited our university, which was 150 miles from her home, to review my professional vita, publications, and video recordings of television spots I had done for the university about my work with people who stutter. When she expressed concern that I might feel offended at the thoroughness of her investigation, I told her that I wished all prospective clients would be equally responsible and as informed as consumers. Indeed, she knew my record as she should. We were about to enter into an agreement, a clinical commitment that Van Riper (1975) referred to as "an invisible contract." Before "signing," she should know about the person with whom she is making a major decision.

All clients must be comfortable with their clinicians as people and as competent professionals. About clients' need for competent clinicians, Van Riper (1975) noted the following:

> No matter how warm and understanding and genuine we may be, they [clients] also want something more in their clinicians. They want competence. Too many amateurs have had their dirty fingers in the stutterer's pie. Stutterers demand guides who know the terrain, who know where the stutterers are in the swamp and which way they must go to get out of it. They want guides who will not abandon them, who are strong, warm, and understanding; but above all, they want their guides to be experienced and skillful and to have some kind of map. (p. 470)

Van Riper (1975) indicated that in order to gain such competence, clinicians must acquire a solid foundation of information about the nature of stuttering; personally know a large number of people who stutter; and "assume the role of a severe stutterer long enough, and in enough situations, to enable them to experience the frustrations, anxiety, shame, and other negative emotions that constitute the context of the stutterer's daily life" (p. 470). The importance of these suggestions cannot be overstated. Students in classes on fluency disorders are typically assigned to "stutter" in public in order to heighten their awareness of that reality. Students often learn as much about themselves (i.e., thoughts, feelings, attitudes) as they do about the stuttering experience. A few remain unwilling to participate in the assignment. Some explain that they feel they are mocking people who stutter; others display utter discomfort even in the anticipation of temporary deviance. How can one begin to understand the reality of another if she remains unwilling or unable to see it, to approach it, to touch it, to feel it, to experience it?

I remember how significant the experience of stuttering deliberately in public was for me. The professor of my seminar on stuttering in graduate school was Dr. Barry Guitar, for whom I hold the highest respect and regard. He and I spoke occasionally outside of class about our personal experiences as people who stutter. When the students were to report in class on an experience of stuttering in public, I didn't give the assignment much thought. I figured that I had a broad enough experiential basis from which to report on a single episode. I also figured this assignment was intended for those who didn't have any personal experience of stuttering. Shortly after I began sharing my experience in class, Barry challenged with, "David, did you do the assignment?" I began my explanation something like, "Well, Barry, actually I did stutter in public but not for this assignment," all the while masking my avoidance only to myself. Seeing right through my sorry excuse and being committed to the instructional value of stuttering deliberately in public, Barry directed, "David, leave the class and don't return until you have done the assignment." "That was direct!" I thought. Somewhat shaken and not understanding the importance of the assignment, I left reluctantly to follow his instructions. Not until completing the assignment did I realize how much I still was avoiding stuttering and how much I was permitting stuttering to impact my thoughts, feelings, and attitudes about communication and myself as a communicator. That one experience was a turning point in my life and in my development as a clinician. I share this experience with my students to help them see that I might understand their degree of reluctance and how fear may impact our behavior.

Personal Magnetism

There are certain additional personal qualities of the clinician that are attractive and arouse hope in a client. Such qualities, again easier to recognize than define, have been called personal magnetism (Emerick, 1974b; West, 1958) and charisma (Van Riper,

1975). The enchantment, sincere if not innate, that begets hope is perhaps the most critical gift of an effective clinician. It is born of the clinician's internal peace, professional knowledge, faith in the client's potential for change, and confidence in the clinical process. West (1958) described such seemingly intangible qualities in the clinician that generate the client's hope as

> that subtle, difficult-to-define thing called personal magnetism. This is a complex of impressions made upon the patient. The therapist possessed of this ability to impress the patient seems to be frank but tactful; penetrating but understanding; professional but kind; confident but humble. (p. 220)

Similarly, Emerick (1974b) described personal magnetism or charisma as a form of electromagnetic energy from the clinician to the client, a high energy output that leaves the client exhilarated and the clinician drained and exhausted. He described such magnetism as follows:

> This therapeutic approach flows from a philosophy of life that encompasses a commitment to the principles of performing everything I do at the limit of my capacity. I decided long ago that I would rather wear out than rust out. . . . Most speech clinicians I have encountered in my travels are turned-on people; they are enthusiastic about the work they do, and it shows in the way they talk about their profession. . . . Charisma or personal magnetism comes in many forms and styles but it seems essential to therapy. Without this individualized spark, the treatment process would indeed be a rather somber transaction. (pp. 99–100)

Van Riper (1973) expressed the essential nature of and critical interaction between a clinician's faith and a client's hope:

> Recognizing that hope is the very essence of motivation, the therapist must either create it or at least blow upon its faint embers until they glow. To do so, the therapist must himself have some confidence in his own abilities to help his client. If molehills or mountains are to be moved, some of the energy necessary to move them will be found in the therapist's faith in himself. This is not to say that one can always be certain of the outcome, but any therapist knows in his bones that he can do much to ease the client's suffering. Like fishermen, good therapists are optimists. Most of them have come to have a profound respect for the latent potential for self-healing that exists in all troubled souls. They resemble Michelangelo who, when asked by a bystander how he could carve such glorious angels from just a slab of stone, replied, "Oh they're already in there. I just have to chip away the stone that surrounds them." Out of the therapist's faith can come the stutterer's hope. (p. 230)

Compatible Friction

Compatible friction is another critical dimension of interpersonal sensitivity. Emerick (1974b) noted that this concept combines a philosophy of living and teaching with "an inextricable union of love and confrontation," or "a judicious wedding of positive regard and frustration" (p. 94). First, a positive tone or compatible interpersonal context is established between clinician and client, communicating that she is committed to the client's communication welfare. Then, since the clinician intends for the client to change, the clinician must disturb the equilibrium or homeostasis, introducing friction or confrontation. How is compatible friction established? Compatibility is born of empathy, warmth, and genuineness. The clinician conveys her understanding of the client's situation, from the client's own perspective, as if it were her own. The clinician expresses and demonstrates her commitment to the client and his communication needs, from which a commonality or feeling of shared identification is established. Such commitment and commonality yield the essential honesty, candor, and genuineness that transform a potentially contrived interaction into sincere human discourse of hearts and minds.

Compatibility, while essential, is not enough to achieve the objective of change. Change is stimulated by friction caused by some type of imbalance, challenge, or constructive disequilibrium (Shapiro & Moses, 1989, 2005). Emerick (1974b) noted that "man seeks imbalance as well as balance—if he is appropriately supported (compatible) during the period of disequilibrium. But it takes friction to get the gears moving in new cycles and unfamiliar patterns" (p. 96). In other words, unless a person is challenged, old patterns endure. Change requires a willingness to approach and engage in risk, knowing that a comrade is there with confidence, holding a safety net should one be necessary. Challenge or friction is calibrated to the individual client. We discussed in Chapters 8, 9, and 10 how to introduce increasing degrees of challenge within a positive context, all the while helping clients imagine and achieve communication goals otherwise considered impossible.

Realistic, Focused Optimism

Apparently, I am a positive, optimistic person. At least this is what I hear from my clients and students. One client who was a physician called me "the rah-rah man." He did not mean that I was a "sis-boom-bah" type of cheerleader. Rather, I believe he saw me as identifying his strengths and abilities, particularly when he could not, thus creating in him a positive expectation set. As a result, he came to expect that he would improve in his communication, and even more importantly, that he possessed the ability to succeed. This sharing of realistic, focused optimism inspires the client and creates faith or hope. Emerick (1974b) noted that "the concept of focused optimism involves the creation of hope or faith centered upon one or two potentials I witness in the stutterer; these serve as rallying points for the development of the achievement motive" (p. 98). And, since each client acts according to the expectations and assumptions (or personal construct) he holds about himself, clinicians must enable the client to create an alternative perspective. From structured, individually designed clinical activities, the client experiences fluency success and the feeling of communication control, on the basis of which he begins to visualize himself as a more competent, fluent communicator. Methodologies for achieving focused optimism and adjustments to one's personal construct were reviewed in the previous unit. Emerick (1974b) discussed several other valuable attitudinal considerations (pp. 98–99):

⌗ *General capacity for transcendence*: Suitably invited, supported, and challenged, a person can overcome seemingly overwhelming odds. People possess an inner urge to become something better or greater. The clinician's role is to facilitate that process of becoming.

⌗ *The clinician's attitude*: The clinician's attitude about the client's potential for change and confidence in herself as a facilitative agent for change are critical to the outcome of treatment. Emerick (1974b) noted, "The clinician's prognostic expectations have profound influence on the outcome of therapy. . . . Hope makes even an elusive goal look possible" (p. 98). Similarly, Van Riper (1975) noted,

> Whenever I see a new stutterer, I find in him so much more strength and potential than I remember having at that age that I immediately expect a favorable outcome. The feeling is this: "Lord, if that weak, miserable mess that once inhabited my skin could solve his problems and become reasonably fluent, then surely this potential client can!" Moreover, I have known other stutterers for whom the prognosis looked pretty poor but who were also able to master their tangled tongues and selves with my help. Perhaps other clinicians who create hope in their clients have similar perceptions. (p. 476)

⌗ *Treatment as work*: An effective clinician, at times, must be bold. Emerick noted that more clinicians have failed because they were timid and temporizing than because they boldly set forth a treatment plan. Similarly, Manning (2010) noted, "If clinicians, including myself, are to be faulted for any one thing, we are most likely guilty of not pushing our adult clients hard enough" (p. 24). He added that clients want and expect to be pushed hard, but that clinicians are reluctant, fearing a negative reaction. I would add, however, that as we push, clients must increasingly assume greater responsibility for the process and products of treatment.

⁙ *Dyadic, dynamic interaction*: One person's behavior in a clinical interaction influences that of the other. Emerick noted that maternal behavior on the part of the clinician will tend to elicit immaturity in the client and dependence on the clinician. Consequently, he recommended that clinicians reflect vivid expectations for improvement.

⁙ *Resilience and error*: The treatment interaction can withstand and adjust to error. Emerick spoke of a homeostatic mechanism whereby stress and resistance created in one session may be followed by relative quiescence in the next. Van Riper (1975) discussed the inevitability of error and the clinician's responsibility to identify and correct it:

> The clinician's errors in judgment show their effects very quickly in the stutterer's behavior and thus revision and correction take place. No one does any therapy without making mistakes. Competent clinicians are those who know they will make errors in judgment and are alert to their occurrence, so they can make the necessary changes in their approach to the problems encountered. Passivity, resistance, and emotional upheavals of many kinds are the signals that tell clinicians they must reassess the stutterers' needs. (pp. 476–477)

Clinician Language

Much of what we do and accomplish in speech–language pathology depends on the language we use. It is incumbent upon us to know how we talk while engaged in treatment with clients who stutter and their families. Language is a critical interpersonal variable within the client–clinician relationship. How do we become aware of our verbal and nonverbal language? That is the domain of self-study, a process by which we collect, analyze, and evaluate objective data from systematic observation of the clinical interaction. These data, or feedback, help us become aware of what we do in order to consider desired alternatives and to design and implement strategies for change (Shapiro, 1994a). Like communication behaviors among clients, our clinical behaviors can only be changed once we are aware of what is occurring. Behaviors about which we are unaware endure. There are many methods available for collecting objective data, including verbatim recording, selected verbatim recording, rating, tally, interaction analysis, nonverbal analysis, and a variety of individually designed methods (J. L. Anderson, 1988; Blood, Blood, McCarthy, et al., 2001; Casey, Smith, & Ulrich, 1988; Dowling, 2001; Ferguson, 2008; Leahy, 2004; McCrea & Brasseur, 2003; Shapiro, 1985, 1987, 1994a; Shapiro & Moses, 2005).

Having used most of the methods listed, I have found interaction analysis systems to be the most instructive (Shapiro, 1994a). In the next chapter, I will introduce such systems and discuss their use and application in professional preparation, specifically in the clinical and supervisory processes. Suffice it to say here that our best efforts to implement change are only as effective as the language we use. Heightened awareness of our verbal and nonverbal behaviors contributes significantly to the effectiveness of the change process and to our own professional growth.

Intrapersonal Characteristics of Effective Clinicians

Clinician Thoughts, Feelings, and Beliefs

Significance of Clinicians' Personal Constructs

We have emphasized the importance of clinicians understanding clients' personal constructs about communication and themselves as communicators. The thoughts and feelings that comprise the client's personal construct influence how he perceives, predicts, and interacts within his world. Of no less importance, the clinician must understand her own personal construct about communication, stuttering, people who stutter, and the processes of learning, intervention, and change. Similarly, the clinician's behavior is most influenced by her concepts about the nature of the disorder and her role within the change process (Ferguson, 2008; Hinckley, 2008; Manning, 2010; Van Riper, 1975). In other words, there is a reciprocal relationship between what clinicians think and know and what they do with people who stutter. The diversity in beliefs and attitudes, in part, accounts for the variety of intervention procedures. Addressing such variety, Van Riper (1975) noted,

> For some, the preferred cloak is that of authoritarian controller, the omniscient dispenser of punishment and reward. For others, the role of priest in the confessional may be favored. For other clinicians, the cap and gown of information giver seem to be worn most frequently. Indeed, it is possible that not only our roles as clinicians but our basic beliefs concerning the nature of stuttering as well as its treatment may be determined largely by the sort of roles we prefer or have been conditioned to accept. (p. 456)

If we take seriously that the clinicians' beliefs and attitudes influence their perceptions and how they work with people who stutter, then clinicians must become explicitly aware of such internal preconceptions before planning and implementing an intervention program. Such preconceptions deeply affect the clinical process and, in fact, whether a clinician might even choose to work with people who stutter.

Persistence of Clinicians' Negative Attitudes

That clinicians' attitudes have a significant impact on the change process is not debatable. What we need to monitor both individually and collectively, however, is the nature of that impact. We have noted that the attitudes and expectations of the clinician are highly predictive of the client's progress, and that more effective clinicians typically believe sincerely that their clients are able to succeed as a result of treatment (Daly, 1988; Emerick, 1974a, 1974b; Guitar, 2006; Manning, 2010; Van Riper, 1975). Despite such convincing arguments, the profession continues to battle negative attitudes toward stuttering and people who stutter from student clinicians and professional speech–language pathologists who feel less confident working with this population than with others (Bloodstein & Bernstein Ratner, 2008; Cooper & Cooper, 1985, 1996; Guitar, 2006; Manning, 2004, 2010; Tellis et al., 2008). Making matters worse, university training programs report that clinical practicum experiences for student clinicians and in-service training opportunities for professional speech–language pathologists are lacking in the area of fluency disorders (Quesal, 2001; Sommers & Caruso, 1995; Yaruss, 1999a; Yaruss & Quesal, 2002). Despite the justified concern over persistence of clinicians' negative attitudes about stuttering and people who stutter, change, albeit slow, seems to be happening. Cooper and Cooper (1996) found that positive change in clinicians' attitudes over an 18-year period included rejection of concepts suggesting parental causality in fluency disorders and the dangers of early intervention, as well as the perception that individuals who stutter possess characteristic personality traits. However, a significant number of clinicians continue to hold unsubstantiated beliefs regarding the personality characteristics of people who stutter, their parents, and the efficacy of early intervention with preschool children who stutter. Some clinicians also continue to feel less competent in the area of fluency disorders and believe that this feeling is shared by most clinicians working with people who stutter. Cooper and Cooper (1996) expressed their concern:

> While it is comforting to note that a shift away from viewing individuals who stutter as having psychological problems and distorted perceptions has occurred, it remains

disturbing to note that 36% of the clinicians persist in their beliefs that most people who stutter have psychological problems, that 58% believe individuals who stutter possess characteristic personality traits, and that over 63% believe those who stutter have feelings of inferiority. Where and how clinicians develop these perceptions continues to be a mystery. (p. 132)

The more recent findings of Yaruss, Quesal, and Murphy (2002) also render concern. They surveyed 200 members of the National Stuttering Association, 195 of whom reported having received treatment for stuttering. Asked about what should be done if a child presents with apparent stuttering, some respondents said "wait and see" if a child outgrows stuttering before seeking an evaluation from a speech–language pathologist— even if there is a family history of persistent stuttering. Others responded that the parents should contact a psychologist or primary care physician if a child stutters. Given that speech–language pathologists are a major source of information for people who stutter as a part of treatment, these responses give rise to concern about the information people are getting. Accurate, up-to-date information must be provided by speech–language pathologists to people who stutter (and all other constituents of the general public). Also, identifying and mitigating negative stereotypes of stuttering and people who stutter among student clinicians and professional speech–language pathologists has never been more urgent. Positive inroads to eliminate negative attitudes and stereotypes are being made (Reichel & St. Louis, 2004, 2007; St. Louis et al., 2009) and must continue to be emphasized in all aspects of professional preparation and renewal training.

Interaction of Attitudes and Professional Preparation

As just indicated, clinicians' attitudes toward stuttering and people who stutter are influenced by the professional preparation received during their undergraduate and graduate degree programs. I expressed previously my concern regarding the relative effectiveness of professional preparation to impact student clinicians' affective processes compared to their behavioral and cognitive processes. Manning (2010) noted the following:

> Our attitude about those who come to us for help and our understanding of their communication problems have a fundamental influence on how we approach them as people during both assessment and treatment. What the clinician has been told and what he or she has been able to observe about stuttering and people who stutter will determine whether he or she will even have the desire to work with such clients. (pp. 4–5)

There are clinicians who complete programs of professional preparation and "actively avoid assisting individuals who stutter" (Manning, 2010, p. 6; see also Conture, 2001; F. H. Silverman, 2004; St. Louis & Durrenberger, 1993; Van Riper, 1992). Unfortunately, as noted previously, student clinicians and professional speech–language pathologists occasionally report past instructors who have "taught" that treatment for fluency disorders is rarely successful and that students should concentrate on those clients who are more likely to make progress. What concerns me most are the clinicians who wish not to work with people who stutter and feel less than fully competent in this area and yet, for a variety reasons, continue to take on clients who stutter. This clinical arrangement is doomed to failure before it begins.

The situation just described would be less likely to exist if programs of professional preparation committed to curricula containing both depth and breadth in the area of fluency disorders. However, as of this writing, the American Speech-Language-Hearing Association (2009a, 2009b) does not mandate a minimum number of hours in the assessment or treatment of children or adults with fluency disorders, or that a student take even one course in fluency disorders. Therefore, the degree of preparedness of clinicians in the area of fluency disorders is dictated by the mission of the individual program, scheduling or other practical concerns, or preferences expressed by faculty and students. Unfortunately, I know of professional speech–language pathologists who had no clinical or academic preparation in the area of fluency disorders during their undergraduate and graduate programs. Such anecdotal reports and comprehensive analyses identifying critical areas of education that are lacking in professional preparation contribute to the movement toward upgrading current professional education of general practitioners and designing programs to educate specialists in the area of fluency disorders (ASHA, 1995, 2007d, 2009a, 2009b, 2010; St. Louis, 2001b; Tellis et al., 2008; Yaruss, 1999a; Yaruss & Quesal, 2002).

Interaction of Attitudes and Understanding of Stuttering

A clinician's attitude toward fluency, fluency disorders, and people who stutter is profoundly influenced by her understanding of the nature of stuttering. If stuttering is viewed as a mysterious disorder, clinicians understandably will be wary about treating these clients. However, if stuttering is viewed as complex, multidimensional, yet fairly rule governed, the challenge tends to be more inviting. Indeed, while we do not fully understand the nature of stuttering, we do know a lot. We understand the importance of identifying and controlling for precipitating and perpetuating factors. We know the importance of understanding and involving clients and their families in the treatment process. We know the importance of understanding clients from their own point of view and providing opportunities for success and graduated challenge. We know that many children and adults of all ages who stutter achieve great progress. Van Riper (1975) expanded as follows:

> Indeed we know a lot about the nature of stuttering even though we may not know all. We know, for example, that many of the behaviors shown by stutterers are learned responses to the expectancy or the experience of fractured fluency. We know that stutterers have fears—reasonable fears, not phobias—and a good many other negative emotions that contribute to the frequency and abnormality of the disorder. We know that there is evidence of mistiming of the sequencing of motor speech. We recognize that stutterers' self-concepts have been affected by their stuttering. We see the impact of the disorder on their language, perception, thinking, and social relationships. We have clear evidence that the frequency, duration, and kinds of their stuttering behaviors are not only variable but that they can be decreased by a variety of clinical techniques. Certainly, then, no clinician need despair of ever having a dearth of available knowledge on which to base his beliefs or therapeutic regime. What is necessary, however, is that he acquire that knowledge and then evaluate it. (pp. 457–458)

Interaction of Attitudes and Positive Observation and/or Treatment Experience

Finally, clinicians' attitudes are influenced by the treatment they have experienced or observed. This emphasizes again the importance of both the depth and breadth of professional preparation. The more students observe clinicians who are not afraid of stuttering and have had success with people who stutter, the more clinicians will be enthusiastic about intervention with people who stutter (i.e., success begets success). One of the strengths of clinical preparation—working with clients of all ages who demonstrate a wide range of communication disorders—may also be one of its limitations: not experiencing the process of change from beginning to end. In other words, student clinicians rarely follow clients throughout the entire continuum of change. This window into the clinical process available to student clinicians in graduate programs is a small one, a limitation not exclusive to student clinicians. Professional speech–language pathologists rarely follow clients beyond a few months or years after dismissal from formal treatment. Therefore, student clinicians and professional speech–language pathologists should explore opportunities to observe successful treatment and to follow the process and progress of change across the long haul.

Clinician Needs

When approaching and planning intervention, clinicians generally think about clients' needs, but rarely about their own. Surely more has been written about clients' needs. Clinicians, however, have needs too. Because clinicians' needs act like a filter through which clinical interactions are processed and interpreted, clinicians must identify, acknowledge, and address their own needs. Unless clinicians are aware of and control for their own needs, which may change over time, they run the risk of inadvertently exploiting, rather than serving, their clients. Indeed, clinicians would not exploit clients knowingly. Van Riper (1975) aptly noted,

> We have trained many clinicians in the course of a lifetime, and it is our impression that those who became the most successful were able to undergo this self-scrutiny. All of us have suffered deprivations of one sort or another in our youth and childhood, and few of us are without currently unsatisfied hungers. Perhaps we were status-deprived; if so, we should beware of our tendency toward assuming the role of authority. Perhaps we were overcontrolled in our childhood; if so, we must guard against an excessive need to control others or its opposite, the compulsion to delegate all responsibility to the client. Certainly, few of us ever got enough love, for the need to be loved seems insatiable; we must therefore be alert to the problems presented by transference. (p. 459)

I remember clearly a nontraditional (somewhat older) undergraduate student whom I interviewed before she declared her major in communication disorders. I asked her why she decided on communication disorders as an academic concentration and professional ambition. She explained that because of being physically challenged and having experienced inconvenience and ridicule as a result of using a wheelchair, she felt particularly suited to work with others who live with a handicap (communication disorder). "I can relate to them better than others who have nothing wrong with them at all," she explained. I asked her to elaborate on how she felt her personal experiences might both facilitate and inhibit her prospective functioning as a human service professional. She reiterated her sensitivity and empathic inclination for others who have a handicap, but could not conceptualize or foresee any possible limitation. I talked about how we who have or have had an exceptionality indeed experience heightened sensitivities for the human condition, and that this may serve as a professional advantage. However, a potential advantage such as this is balanced by the risk of superimposing our experiences onto another person or losing our objectivity. Doing so would assume that someone else's experiences are the same as our own, thus interpreting a client's experience from our, rather than his, assumptions and constructs. In other words, when we are unaware of and without control over our own experiences and needs, we risk treating another person as we were treated or wish we had been treated, rather than acting according to the client's strengths and needs. After discussing these issues, the student and I had an enlightening conversation about needs and competencies for effective intervention (ASHA, 1995, 2004c, 2005c, 2009a), about the nature of a clinician's personal construct (see Chapter 5), and about the importance of a clinician being aware of and in control of her personal needs. These factors and others are critical for ensuring our objective understanding of the clients we serve and for delivering individualized intervention services of the highest quality (ASHA, 2007d, 2010).

I frequently encounter any of a series of questions that result in a similar line of dialogue. These questions are as follows:

- Should a clinician who stutters treat a client who stutters?
- Can a clinician who has not stuttered be as effective as those who have in treating people who stutter?
- Aren't you more suited to treat people who stutter because you yourself have stuttered and have achieved significant fluency success?

I remain reluctant to give a blanket answer to any of these questions. Again, I view previous personal experiences as a potential advantage (sensitivity, empathy) balanced with a potential disadvantage (bias, loss of objectivity). A client who stutters would be unlikely to accuse a clinician who has stuttered or stutters that she cannot comprehend the difficulty that stuttering imposes on his life. Furthermore, clinicians who stutter typically do not approach clients who stutter with trepidation, as might clinicians who do not stutter. In fact, as Van Riper (1975) indicated,

> Stuttering clinicians, at least, are not afraid of stutterers. They know from their personal experience that they are tough animals, that they have endured and survived, and moreover that most stutterers respect a clinician who will not handle them gingerly. (p. 460)

However, a clinician's own experience with stuttering may be a disadvantage, particularly if the clinician stutters noticeably, because clients may question the clinical effectiveness of clinicians who have yet to gain control over their own fluency. I know several professional colleagues at universities who have not experienced successful fluency control and therefore voluntarily ceased to teach courses in fluency disorders or to see clients who stutter. One colleague explained to me,

> I feel like the blind leading the blind. How can I convey, "Do as I say, not as I do"? That's just not right. The field is large enough now to acknowledge that certain clinicians are more suited to work with certain clients. Knowing my limitations is a professional strength.

Among student clinicians and professional speech–language pathologists, there is debate on the question of whether clinicians who stutter without fluency control are suited to work with clients who stutter (Shapiro, Brotherton, & Ogletree, 1995). Relatively recent federal legislation has been enacted to help interpret such thorny issues (e.g., Individuals with Disabilities Education Act of 1990 [IDEA], Individuals with Disabilities Education Improvement Act of 2004; Americans with Disabilities Amendments Act of 2008). Notwithstanding their limitations, many people who stutter have made significant and lasting contributions to our profession. Van Riper (1975), discussing earlier days when training programs routinely rejected and discouraged, if not discriminated against, any person who stuttered from entering professional preparation in communication sciences and disorders, noted, "Had such a practice been universal in the early days of our profession, its development would have been markedly retarded, for stutterers have made major contributions" (p. 459).

Perhaps more important than the answer to the question of whether clinicians who stutter should treat clients who stutter is the degree to which those clinicians have truly examined their personal constructs in relation to themselves as communicators. Clinicians—all clinicians—must know themselves well before they work with clients. Clinicians prepare for, enter, and remain in the profession for different reasons. Most, however, want to make a difference in some meaningful way in the life of another person, enjoy the feeling of having the ability to relieve pain and suffering, and experience rewards when a client noticeably shows improvement. Nevertheless, clinicians have individual needs. Clinicians filter clinical interaction, in addition to all other experiences, through these needs and other components of their personal construct. Being aware of their needs, thoughts, feelings, and attitudes enables clinicians to control for them, thereby allowing them to be more open to the uniqueness of the client's experience. Novice clinicians often justify their professional commitment by expressing a motivation of altruism (selflessly serving others). Career speech–language pathologists know that helping others is both a motivation and a source of personal reward.

To be motivated and personally rewarded are needs of all people, including clinicians. Walle (1974) discussed the reciprocal relationship between clients' and clinicians' needs and behaviors:

> The therapist must achieve satisfaction from the interpersonal exchange, or his dissatisfaction may defeat the patient. . . . Who needs therapy? The therapist needs the therapy! If experiences are not therapeutic, they can be disruptive and even painful. When we choose the kinds of patients we think we can help, we are also attempting to choose those who can satisfy us. The therapeutic approach must suit the therapist; the therapist must suit the patient." (pp. 8–9)

Clinician Satisfaction and Rewards

We have already discussed the clinician's thoughts, feelings, beliefs, and needs as critical intrapersonal factors about which effective clinicians must remain aware. Other intrapersonal factors are the satisfaction and rewards experienced by clinicians. Just as some clinicians are loath to consider their own needs, erroneously fearing that so doing inhibits, rather than facilitates, addressing the client's needs, so reluctance is found among clinicians to identify sources of internal satisfaction and personal reward. I argue that clinicians must keep a finger on their own pulse of satisfaction and reward, both of which provide a sense of inherent meaning, in order to remain effective over the long run. Life must have meaning. Reminding us of our sense of inherent meaning, our satisfaction and rewards are what keep us excited, committed, and passionate about what we do professionally with people who stutter.

Van Riper (1974) eloquently described the sense of inherent meaning he found in having intimate and ultimate impact on another human being. He (1975) also expressed satisfaction in being challenged to use professional competence, learning and growing, participating in the human capacity for triumph over significant obstacles, engaging intricately in the craftsmanship of intervention, and knowing and celebrating meaningfulness. Emerick (1974a, 1974b) captured his sense of satisfaction in promoting growth in his clients, and thereby in himself, by means of continual self-confrontation. Walle (1974) discussed his satisfaction from setting in motion factors that engender hope, thereby bringing about positive changes in both the client's and clinician's life. Significantly, these and other master clinicians discuss their satisfaction and rewards as internal, or intrapersonal, factors that renew and energize. Clinicians' satisfaction and rewards differ, but clinicians must feel satisfied and rewarded in order to remain in the profession and to contribute meaningfully over their professional lifetime.

I am now in my fourth decade as a speech–language pathologist. Honestly, not a single day has passed when I have not felt thankful for the privilege of working with people who stutter and their families. I sincerely enjoy my work and believe that it is important. I appreciate the opportunity to learn and grow, on a daily basis, with and from my client, student, faculty, and administrative colleagues. At one time in my life, I hoped that I could change the world. Knowing better now, optimistically rather than in defeat, I feel fortunate to be a part of helping our clients and their families, literally across the globe, change their own communicative world. As a result, I feel a connection with the human condition that transcends any conceivable limitation, and a satisfaction in being constantly challenged to recall, apply, create, and thereby advance our knowledge of communication and its disorders. What keeps me fresh is the internal satisfaction in believing in what I do, with whom I do it, and the ultimate importance of the process and products of communication.

Discussing such aspects of communication, Gardner (1983; see also Gardner, 1993, 1995) developed the concept of personal intelligence, including both intrapersonal and interpersonal elements. Describing intrapersonal intelligence, Gardner noted,

> On the one side, there is the development of the internal aspects of a person. The core capacity at work here is access to one's own feeling life—one's range of affects or emotions: the capacity instantly to effect discriminations among these feelings and, eventually, to label them, to enmesh them in symbolic codes, to draw upon them as a means of understanding and guiding one's behavior. (1983, p. 239)

Intrapersonal knowledge is what enables clinicians and clients to understand their own feelings and those of each other. It is from this knowledge base that we think and talk introspectively about feelings, and from which we become aware of our feelings and become affectively prepared to address our clients' needs. Our intrapersonal knowledge is what enables us to come to understand our own as well as our client's personal construct.

Another aspect of personal intelligence, interpersonal knowledge, was expressed by Gardner (1983) in this way: "The other personal intelligence turns outward, to other individuals. The core capacity here is the ability to notice and make distinctions among other individuals and, in particular, among their moods, temperaments, motivations, and intentions" (p. 239). This type of knowledge is what enables clinicians to understand the intentions and desires of their clients and their families and to act upon that knowledge. We discussed in Unit III the importance of creating opportunities for clients to discuss, and thereby understand, their own objectives, thus becoming centrally involved in ("owning") the clinical process. Development of personal intelligence in clients and clinicians has at its core an emerging sense of self, an interaction between intrapersonal knowledge (inner feelings) and interpersonal (other person) knowledge.

Thus, intrapersonal and interpersonal characteristics are key to being an effective clinician. Such a development of self, in this case one's professional self, is what Gardner (1983) refers to as "the highest achievement of human beings, . . . that capacity about which individuals have the strongest and most intimate views; thus it becomes a sensitive (as well as an elusive) target to examine" (pp. 242–243). I am most grateful for the continuing opportunity to develop my intrapersonal and interpersonal knowledge, from which I accrue lasting satisfaction and internal reward.

The Clinician as Guardian Angel

The clinician's behaviors present only one aspect of the dynamic amalgam that is the clinician. Of continuing challenge for the novice and seasoned clinician alike is management of interpersonal factors such as attributes and manner of interaction and language, and intrapersonal factors such as thoughts, feelings, beliefs; needs; and satisfaction and rewards. Indeed, as Walle (1974) stated, "Qualifying for therapeutic practice is one thing; suitability is another" (p. 10). In other words, selecting and preparing for a profession is a labor-intensive endeavor in the short run. Helping clients and their families establish and realize communicative dreams while developing one's own personal and professional sense of self is a larger dynamic challenge that lasts throughout one's professional life span.

Walle (1974) discussed the importance of the clinician's capacity to appreciate the unique importance and value of each client:

> If he [the clinician] projects the attitude that this [client] is one of God's finest creations, a human being, and this person is worthy of his best efforts, his genuine interest—not only because it is his job—then the patient will pick this up and think, "I too, must give my best efforts to help him help me." This is mutual reciprocation and a kind of love . . . that opens the gates of trust. (p. 11)

Furthermore, Walle (1974) discussed the importance of both the client and clinician being willing to take a personal risk, that is, to give something of themselves, something of value in the form of a personal belief about the client's capacity for change. He advised, "If therapists can learn to care objectively and then sit still long enough to learn from the person who needs help, this—on a broad scale—could be the power to transform them both" (p. 11).

We began and now end this chapter by articulating the importance of the clinician and the client–clinician relationship to the change process. Argeropoulos (1974) presented a model depicting the relationship between one's self-concept and personal success or failure. The "tree of self-defeat" symbolizes the individual who has internalized negative qualities into his lifestyle, thus achieving little of a positive nature. In comparison, the "tree of self-realization" depicts the richness and fullness of life and positive achievement resulting from relationships of warmth and closeness. Argeropoulos likened the tree of self-defeat to a dormant tree of real life, stating, "Just as the dormant tree comes to life when the proper nurturant conditions of spring arrive, so can the defeated person come to life when the proper emotional climate is cultivated in his life" (p. 87). Such cultivation is within the domain of the effective clinician.

Many clients have a fund of positive, self-realizing forces within their communication environment (e.g., love, kindness, warmth, trust, hope, mutual support) to which the clinician contributes by helping them achieve their communication potential. These clients have internalized and retained an appropriate and positive personal construct, one focused on abilities, strengths, healing power, and self-actualization. Other clients, however, do not have such positive forces or do not perceive such forces in a positive light. These clients have internalized feelings of negativity, insecurity, fear, self-pity, and dependency. In other words, these clients have formed a personal construct based on personal limitations rather than strengths. For both clients, the clinicians' role is formidable. Particularly for the latter, the clinician might serve as an "enlightened witness" (Miller, 1990), a singular person who significantly influences another by introducing sunshine to darkness, kindness to cruelty, positive movement to negative stagnation. Miller noted that a child who has known nothing but cruelty will accept and possibly gravitate toward, rather than resist, such an environment because he has no point of comparison. He will accept such a condition as normal behavior and often repeat it. An enlightened witness, Miller noted, is someone who offers him the experience of being loved, cherished, nurtured, and accepted, thus providing a window to a positive alternative.

The clinician can be that significant other, that change agent, who introduces the sweet taste of fluency freedom that ultimately yields communicative control and independence, that moment of grace that transcends the present and impacts in the most positive ways all aspects of one's life. The clinician creates opportunities for the client to experience fluency success, thus requiring the client to reexamine his personal construct so that ultimately he can develop and nurture his own internalized prognosis for positive change. To emphasize the importance of the affective elements of the change process (e.g., love, hope, trust, nurture) minimizes neither the other interpersonal and intrapersonal factors discussed in this chapter nor the clinical procedures discussed in Chapters 8, 9, and 10. Clinical intervention both targets and utilizes affective, behavioral, and cognitive dimensions of communication.

Within this and preceding chapters, we have discussed the clinician as participating in many different professional roles. N. B. Anderson, Lee-Wilkerson, and Chabon (1995) delineated the clinician's roles as including that of environmental planner and time manager, modeler/facilitator, observer/interactor/recorder, counselor/parent advisor, collaborator/team player, and guardian angel. While all of these roles are essential, I wish to address only the final. The authors presented a touching vignette that I believe has import for working with people who stutter. When looking for a tutor for her child and after facing several dead-ends, one of the authors contacted a teacher who had written a book about helping children to achieve in school while feeling good about themselves. During the conversation, the teacher gave the parent an opportunity to share her perceptions about her son's needs and to express her own concerns. The teacher agreed to work with the boy, adding that every child needs a guardian angel and that she would like to be his. The parent reported that the teacher's statement, unexpected and unusual, gave the parent a positive lift and an immediate feeling of hope and security. N. B. Anderson et al. (1995) suggested that it may be time for clinicians to assume quietly the role of guardian angel (not unlike Miller's, 1990, concept of the enlightened witness):

> As guardian angels, we may offer acceptance, protection, guidance, and inspiration, and expect our clients to make their contributions as well. This is truly the ultimate partnership. Our guardian angels believe in us and help us to believe in ourselves. This could perhaps be our greatest role as speech–language pathologists for, in this context, . . . intervention is at its most divine. (p. 59)

Chapter Summary

This chapter addressed the clinician and the interpersonal relationship as key to effective intervention. This relationship is influenced by both intrapersonal and interpersonal factors. Once aware of and in control of such factors, clinicians can develop or improve their professional skills.

Interpersonal factors of effective clinicians include certain clinician behaviors, attributes, and features of language. Clinician behaviors refer to the goals, processes, and competencies for assessment, management, and transfer and maintenance with people who stutter that are presented in the Guidelines for Practice in Stuttering Treatment (ASHA, 1995). Attributes of effective clinicians refer to a manner of interaction characterized by empathy; warmth; genuineness; personal magnetism; compatible friction; and realistic, focused optimism. Empathy is an authentic sensitivity for another person, being able to experience, and thereby understand, the experience of another person as if it were one's own. Warmth is a composite of understanding, sincerity, friendliness, and respect that provides unconditional positive regard. Genuineness refers to the ability to be one's true self as a person with a client while conveying professional competence and personal confidence. Personal magnetism reflects those qualities of the clinician that are attractive, inviting, and arouse hope in the client. Compatible friction is the result of deliberately disturbing the client's equilibrium, which is necessary for change to occur, while the client experiences empathy, warmth, genuineness, and ongoing commitment from the clinician. Realistic, focused optimism refers to the creation of hope or faith that is centered on specific areas of the client's potential. Effective clinicians are aware of their language—their verbal and nonverbal forms of communication—when working with people who stutter and their families.

Intrapersonal factors of effective clinicians include clinician thoughts, feelings, and beliefs; needs; and satisfaction and rewards. Effective clinicians understand their own personal constructs, monitor the potential impact of their attitudes toward stuttering and people who stutter, and are aware of the potential effects of their beliefs about the nature of stuttering and their own past experience with or observation of stuttering. Effective clinicians identify, acknowledge, and address their own needs related to the clinical process. Finally, effective clinicians identify their sources of internal satisfaction and personal reward in order to retain a sense of inherent meaning in their professional practice.

The chapter closed with an acknowledgment that it is easier to become a clinician than to be one, and that qualifying for clinical practice is not necessarily synonymous with suitability for clinical practice. In her unique capacity to facilitate change and to help people who stutter and their families realize their potential, the clinician was cast as enlightened witness and as a guardian angel.

Chapter Eleven Study Questions

1. This chapter reviewed interpersonal and intrapersonal aspects of effective clinicians. What do you believe to be the ingredients of effective intervention? How might these elements be acquired? How might they be maintained? How do the factors you have identified relate to the concept of personal intelligence presented by Gardner (1983)?

2. We have discussed the multidimensionality of clinicians and clinical competence. What is clinical competence? What is the likelihood that a person who acquires the interpersonal and intrapersonal factors discussed will necessarily be clinically competent or effective as a clinician? What is meant by the distinction between qualification and suitability for clinical practice? Why is it more challenging to be a clinician than to become one? What will you do to ensure your own clinical competence and suitability after you become a clinician?

3. Clinicians wear many different hats. In what ways might a clinician be an enlightened witness for a person who stutters and his family? How might a clinician serve as a guardian angel?

4. We reviewed the attitudes of clinicians about stuttering, people who stutter, and themselves as potential change agents. We also reviewed several issues regarding current loopholes that exist in academic and clinical preparation of clinicians in the area of fluency and fluency disorders. How would you characterize both of these issues and what do you believe are their origins? Given your understanding of these issues, what recommendations do you have? What are your feelings about specialty certification in the area of fluency disorders and other areas of clinical practice?

5. In sharing my own personal construct, I distinguished between a desire to change the world and a desire to help clients and their families change their own worlds. How might each disposition influence the assessment and treatment processes? How might other personal constructs influence the processes of clinical intervention?

6. If the clinician and the client–clinician relationship are among the most significant factors that influence, if not foretell, the outcome of treatment, why have these aspects of the clinical process received relatively little empirical attention? How might an evidence-based practice perspective be applied to verify or challenge this claim? How might a clinician utilize interaction analysis or self-study to maximize her effectiveness

as a clinician? How might the processes of evidence-based practice and interaction analysis/self study be combined for the ultimate benefit of the client?

7. Positive inroads are being made to eliminate negative stereotypes of stuttering and people who stutter and to emphasize the importance of emotional intelligence as a part of professional preparation for the clinical process (Reichel, 2007; Reichel & St. Louis, 2004, 2007; St. Louis et al., 2009). Why do such stereotypes continue to exist, particularly among speech–language pathologists? What are the implications of emotional intelligence training of human service professionals? In what ways might professional preparation and renewal training maximize the positive impact on the affective, in addition to behavioral and cognitive, elements of the clinician and the clinical process?

8. This chapter addressed the importance of both intrapersonal and interpersonal factors of the clinician to the effectiveness of the clinical process. How would you evaluate yourself on the basis of each of these factors? How might your evaluation change over time? In what ways has your professional preparation contributed to the development of your intrapersonal and interpersonal skills? What other avenues are you utilizing to maximize your development as a clinician? How will you ensure peak effectiveness as a clinician over the span of your career?

Chapter Twelve

Professional Preparation and Lifelong Learning
The Making of a Clinician

No man can reveal to you aught but that which already lies half asleep in the dawning of your own knowledge. The teacher who walks in the shadow of the temple, among his followers, gives not of his wisdom but rather of his faith and his lovingness. If he is indeed wise he does not bid you enter the house of his wisdom, but rather leads you to the threshold of your own mind. (Gibran, 1923, p. 51)

How are good clinicians made? Are they born or are they cultivated? Walle (1974) distinguished between qualifications and suitability for therapeutic practice, noting that "it is easier to become a therapist than to be one" (p. 10). In the present chapter, we will address the academic, clinical, and supervisory processes by which clinical competencies are developed; highlight the increased significance of both specialization and globalization; and discuss three elements that are critical for maintaining and upgrading a clinician's competence across her professional career. In doing so, we will make the following points, among others:

- Professional preparation for clinicians who work with people who stutter must integrate experiences across the academic, clinical, and supervisory processes, and must impact the affective, behavioral, and cognitive domains.
- An explicit understanding of the academic, clinical, and supervisory processes enables its participants (namely clinicians) to contribute meaningfully to and thereby gain maximum benefit from the experience of professional preparation.
- Both specialization and globalization are important by-products of an expanding scope of practice within a diversified and instantaneously connected global community.
- Maintenance of professional competence requires internalizing the desire to learn, committing to learning as a lifelong process, and understanding and maintaining parallels in the nature and process of professional development over time.

⠵ Professional preparation and lifelong learning provide an opportunity for learners to become teachers and teachers to become learners across the interactive and dynamic journey of life.

Professional Preparation of Clinicians Who Work with People Who Stutter

The acquisition, application, creation, and advancement of knowledge relevant to stuttering and people who stutter present a formidable challenge to all participants in the academic, clinical, and supervisory processes. All participants, in my view, are learners and teachers. All participants, while serving different roles in the respective processes, are working toward similar, if not the same, objectives—to learn and grow with and from our clients and their families in order to improve the communication world in which we all live. In this section, we will consider three distinct, albeit necessarily overlapping, instructional processes—academic, clinical, and supervisory—that contribute to both becoming and being a clinician.

Traditionally, the academic process addresses the cognitive domain (thoughts and content) and the clinical and supervisory processes address the behavioral domain (procedures and application). Professional preparation may be falling short in the area of student clinicians' affective knowledge (Ferguson, 2008; Hinckley, 2008; Reichel, 2007; Reichel & St. Louis, 2004, 2007; St. Louis et al., 2009). The three domains of knowledge (affective, behavioral, and cognitive) and the instructional processes by which they are acquired (academic, clinical, and supervisory) must be integrated. Furthermore, all processes within professional preparation must deliberately impact the affective domain (feelings, beliefs, and attitudes about stuttering and people who stutter). In light of the persistent negative stereotypes held by the general public, workers in professions allied to education and medicine, and speech–language pathologists (Cooper & Cooper, 1985, 1996; Cooper & Rustin, 1985; Lass, Ruscello, Pannbacker, Schmitt, & Everly-Myers, 1989; Mallard et al., 1988; Ragsdale & Ashby, 1982; St. Louis & Durrenberger, 1993; St. Louis & Lass, 1981; Turnbaugh et al., 1979; C. L. Woods & Williams, 1971, 1976; Yairi & Williams, 1970), impacting clinicians' affective processes should be seen as a curricular imperative. To this end, each instructional process will be considered separately.

Most of you reading this chapter are student clinicians or professional speech–language pathologists. In either case, most of you are functioning both as a clinician within the clinical process (i.e., you are working with a client who stutters) and as a supervisee within the supervisory process (i.e., you are working with the support and direction of a supervisor, either in a graduate program of clinical education or within your employment setting). Some professional speech–language pathologists also may be functioning as a supervisor of other professionals or support personnel. As you read and learn more about the processes in which many of you are currently engaged, consider how you might use your heightened knowledge to effect an even greater contribution on your part to your own professional development. It is often said that we reap what we sow. Professional preparation and lifelong learning should be no exception. Therefore, consider how the frameworks, methods, and materials discussed here might be useful to your own professional development, both now and later.

Academic Process

Academic Process Defined

The academic process typically begins upon entry into a program of professional preparation and continues until completion of that program. For the purposes of this discussion, the academic process is assumed to be that which occurs within the classroom. Making such a general statement, I acknowledge that the dynamics of the classroom experience vary according to the uniqueness of and interaction among variables such as the instructor, students, methods, materials, curricula, media, and so on, and that the classroom experience necessarily relates to and must overlap with the clinical and supervisory processes.

Revision in Training Standards

Changes by the American Speech-Language-Hearing Association (ASHA) resulted in a reduction of training standards, which significantly impacted both the academic and clinical processes. Prior to 1993, ASHA required a specified number of hours of supervised clinical experience (including evaluation and treatment) for each of the basic disorder areas in speech–language pathology—articulation, language, voice, and fluency. ASHA also required that students complete requisite coursework before engaging in related clinical experiences. These two requirements necessitated that student clinicians receive both academic and clinical preparation across the spectrum of communication disorders before graduating and entering the professional arena. In 1993, however, ASHA's Council on Professional Standards (COPS) changed the requirement, mandating hours in the more generic categories of "speech disorders" and "language disorders" as opposed to requiring specified numbers of hours in individual disorder areas. This change was intended to allow programs greater flexibility in designing the academic and clinical curriculum. In practice, however, many programs cut back on coursework and clinical training in fluency disorders and voice disorders, clinical areas that are erroneously considered to be of low incidence.

While a standardized outcome measure continues to be required for all graduates of master's programs in communication disorders (i.e., the PRAXIS Examination in Speech–Language Pathology), as is demonstration of requisite knowledge and skills (ASHA, 2009a), individual programs are now more internally responsible for the nature and content of their curriculum. Various surveys, however, continue to raise serious concern about academic and clinical education in fluency disorders. Of the 159 accredited training programs surveyed in the United States, 23% indicated that they graduated students without coursework in fluency disorders and 64% without clinical practicum in fluency disorders (Yaruss & Quesal, 2002). Similarly, of 225 school-based speech–language pathologists surveyed, 47% had taken a one-semester course in fluency disorders and 54% reported feeling comfortable working with children who stutter (Tellis et al., 2008). Similar concerns exist in Canada and the United Kingdom (Kroll, Cook, De Nil, & Bernstein Ratner, 2006; Kroll & Klassen, 2007). Yaruss and Quesal (2002) identified trends toward fewer required classes in fluency disorders taught by less experienced faculty, fewer clinical hours in the assessment and treatment of fluency disorders guided by less experienced supervisors, and greater likelihood that students can graduate without any coursework or clinical practicum in fluency disorders, concluding that

> even though the scope of practice has expanded dramatically, it is still critical that we provide adequate training in specific disorders that make up the core of this field. Given the complexity of the stuttering disorder and the repeated finding that many practicing clinicians already lack sufficient comfort and competence with fluency disorders, it would seem that more training and experience, not less, is needed to prepare clinicians to help people who stutter. Present results suggest that the field does not appear to be headed in this direction, at least as far as the training that is provided in graduate programs is concerned. (Yaruss & Quesal, 2002, pp. 58–59)

These results are indeed disturbing, particularly since clinical training in the area of fluency disorders was considered insufficient even before the standards were relaxed in

1993 (Mallard et al., 1988; Sommers & Caruso, 1995; St. Louis & Durrenberger, 1993; Williams, 1971) and may be in violation of ASHA's Code of Ethics (ASHA, 2010). Recently, however, some positive advances have been made. ASHA established the Specialty Board on Fluency Disorders, which designates clinicians who are especially equipped to work with people who stutter. Also, ASHA's Special Interest Division 4 (Fluency and Fluency Disorders) has been more active and productive, providing training opportunities and heightening public and political awareness of stuttering, people who stutter, and available intervention services.

Academic Knowledge and Skills

Instructors are responsible for designing academic courses and making decisions related to objectives, content, process, and outcomes. It is important for clinicians, whether presently or previously engaged in the academic process, to understand the nature of the process and the origin of its content. Statements of curricular guidelines are found in a variety of ASHA documents, including Standards and Implementation Procedures for the Certificate of Clinical Competence in Speech–Language Pathology (ASHA 2009a) and Standards for Accreditation of Graduate Education Programs in Audiology and Speech–Language Pathology (ASHA, 2009b). A comprehensive framework for establishing objectives and content for coursework in fluency disorders is found in the Guidelines for Practice in Stuttering Treatment (ASHA, 1995). These documents and others (e.g., ASHA, 2004a, 2004b, 2004c, 2005a, 2005b, 2005c, 2009c) should be reviewed by all student clinicians and professional speech–language pathologists.

Clinical Process

Clinical Process Defined

The clinical process is defined as "that interaction that takes place between the clinician and the client" (ASHA, 1978, p. 479). When the clinical process occurs within a supervisory framework, the participants include the supervisor and the clinician, who also fills the role of the supervisee.

Clinical Knowledge and Skills

The Guidelines for Practice in Stuttering Treatment (ASHA, 1995) contain comprehensive statements of goals, processes, and competencies in the areas of assessment, management, transfer, and maintenance. These guidelines are useful to clinicians for their understanding of goals, procedures, and competencies for implementing effective intervention; for self-assessment; and for guiding continuing education and renewal training. As noted previously, the guidelines emphasize acquisition and application of knowledge within the cognitive and behavioral domains. They must be extended to include affective knowledge as well (feelings, beliefs, and attitudes about stuttering and people who stutter). All the emphasis on what is done within intervention (clinical procedures) and why it is done (clinical rationale) cannot replace the significance of how it is done (the manner in which the clinician communicates affectively her faith in the client's ability to improve and her confidence in the clinical process to achieve that change). The guidelines are also useful to people who stutter and their families for building their understanding of intervention and a framework for evaluating the services received. Cooper (1997) emphasized that clinical knowledge must include the affective element, which must be communicated to the client:

> If, from the very start, you don't like and respect your clinician, find another one. You need and deserve a clinician with whom you feel comfortable and with whom you can be open and honest about how you feel, think, and behave. If from the very first time you meet, your clinician doesn't make you feel good about being in therapy, find another.

I am not saying everything should be sweetness and light in therapy. In fact, if it is, probably nothing is happening. But I am saying your clinician should make you feel good about being there. Research reveals that effective clinicians:

⊞ express feelings openly—they let you know how they feel;

⊞ are honest—they tell it like it is;

⊞ are positive in their attitudes—they see the good where many do not;

⊞ reflect feelings rather than direct feeling—they don't presume to tell others how they should feel;

⊞ are open-minded—they are not judgmental;

⊞ are informative—they are perfectly clear about the purpose for each therapeutic activity;

⊞ are perseverative in their pursuit of goals—they hang in there; and

⊞ are detail disciplined—they don't miss a thing. (pp. 164–165)

A Model of Clinician Development

The material in this section is presented to facilitate the ongoing professional development of clinicians at all levels of experience working with people who stutter. Development of clinical competence is begun within professional preparation during the academic (student–professor interaction), clinical (client–clinician interaction), and supervisory (supervisee–supervisor interaction) processes, and is continued in renewal training, continued education, and self-study activities throughout one's career. Shapiro and Moses (1989) presented a model of clinician development (see Table 12.1)

Table 12.1   Aspects of Development in Clinical Problem Solving

Aspect	From	To
Perspective	Identifies problems in the clinical interaction that affect self (i.e., that cause personal discomfort—clinician is major focus).	Identifies problems as seen from the perspective of others and self (client is major focus).
	Tends to think of problem resolution as caused by self or other authority figure.	Views problem resolution as being the result of active and shared client–clinician interaction (i.e., goal establishment and attainment).
	Evaluates the efficacy of problem-solving procedure from self-centered perspective.	Evaluates problem-solving procedure from multiple perspectives.
Dimensions of behavior conceptualized	Conceives of behavior as unidimensional. Views problem as affecting and affected by only one dimension of behavior.	Conceives of behavior as multidimensional. Views problem as affected by many dimensions of behavior.
Possible solutions generated	Thinks of one problem-solving procedure.	Generates and reflects upon multiple problem-solving strategies.
Causal concepts	Implements problem-solving strategy, but fails to reflect upon or modify causal theories.	Implements strategy and reflects upon and modifies, if appropriate, causal theories.

Note. From "Creative Problem Solving in Public School Supervision," by D. A. Shapiro & N. Moses, 1989, *Language, Speech, and Hearing Services in Schools, 20,* p. 323. Copyright 1989 by the American Speech-Language-Hearing Association. Reprinted with permission.

containing a series of phases describing how clinicians organize and interpret information relevant to clinical planning, implementation, and problem solving. Clinical expertise implies mastery resulting from an observable and developmental sequence of skills. The model assumes that clinicians regularly engage in problem solving, which requires applying or constructing knowledge. Implicitly, construction of knowledge refers to creating ideas by reflecting on and making inferences about information and perceptions from goal-directed interaction. Explicitly, aspects of clinician development occur in four areas of problem solving: orientation of perspective, dimensions of behavior conceptualized, possible solutions generated, and causal reasoning.

Clinicians functioning at an early developmental level, challenged by novel problems encountered during clinical interaction with clients who stutter, typically center on a personal point of view about communication, stuttering, and fluency intervention; they tend to view themselves as being in control of a client's potential fluency improvement. They also tend to consider few variables when thinking about intervention strategies and causes of problems, focusing on only one aspect of a client's stuttering (e.g., behavior, thoughts, feelings). They tend to generate relatively few problem-solving procedures. For example, instead of considering multiple intervention strategies, the clinician at this developmental level might just say, "We will do airflow therapy." Finally, they fail to reflect on or modify causal assumptions after clinical intervention. If the client isn't making expected progress, for instance, the clinician might blame the client instead of reconsidering the treatment approach (e.g., "You're still too tense. That is why you stutter. We'll have to continue with airflow therapy").

At a more advanced level of clinical development, clinicians incorporate the client's perspective, viewing intervention and the change process as a shared, interactive challenge. Clinicians consider multiple variables related to intervention for and causes of stuttering, thinking about stuttering as a multidimensional problem that potentially impacts behaviors, thoughts, and feelings. Clinicians generate multiple problem-solving procedures, saying, for example,

> Why don't we consider building a foundation of fluency success so we can study and better understand all that you already do so well? That will enable you to do even more often what you do that contributes to your fluency. Then, we can study the remaining disfluencies and together decide which targets should receive focus. All the while, we can keep tabs on how you are feeling and what you are thinking as your fluency improves. What do you think about this as a preliminary plan? How does this relate to what you expressed you hoped to accomplish?

Clinicians at this more highly developed stage also reflect on and modify causal assumptions after clinical intervention:

> **Clinician:** I want to talk about your thoughts and feelings about stuttering and yourself as a communicator. This is what we call our personal construct about communication. Usually, what we think affects what we do and vice versa. Sometimes, one perpetuates the other, unless we address them directly.
>
> **Client** (later): I'm so glad you got me to think about my thoughts and feelings about stuttering and me as a communicator. I had no idea that my thinking actually was working against me, maintaining the way I communicate, particularly how, when, and where I stutter.

Further exploring their concept of clinical development, Moses and Shapiro (1996) designed a taxonomy for assessing clinician development and applied it to a microanalysis of video-recorded clinical sessions of three student clinicians. Independent raters analyzed 97 clinical problem episodes, which required a total of 3,589 classification decisions. Three developmental profiles of clinical problem solving were derived from the extensive analyses. The *novice clinician* (kitchen sink profile) oriented to herself, attended to few dimensions of behavior, and generated a limited number of possible solutions to clinical problems. The *intermediate clinician* (map reader profile) demonstrated emerging problem-solving ability reflecting inconsistency in assuming the client's perspective, referencing multiple dimensions of behavior, and generating multiple problem solutions. Finally, the *advanced clinician* (air traffic controller profile) interpreted fewer novel situations as problems, approached those that occurred from the dual perspectives of her client and herself, addressed multiple dimensions of behavior, and generated multiple problem solutions.

In a subsequent investigation, Shapiro and Moses (2005) designed a taxonomy to analyze more than 1,600 questions asked by 38 clinicians on the basis of domains of knowledge addressed (i.e., propositional, procedural, and causal) and information functions served (discovery, exploration, and understanding). *Propositional knowledge* is descriptive and defines objects and events; *procedural knowledge* is directional and serves as a guide to a solution through a sequence of steps; *causal knowledge* is explanatory and explores interrelationships among variables. *Discovery* is collection of existing knowledge to construct a foundation for more complex learning; *exploration* is further examination of the information discovered, identifying more specific characteristics, including inherent feelings, uses, similarities, and values; *understanding* contextualizes the information discovered and explored, enabling clinicians to discern relationships among variables and shift between differing perspectives. Results revealed that the domain of knowledge addressed by most of the clinicians' questions was propositional, less was procedural, and the least was causal; the information function served by most of the clinicians' questions was exploration, less was discovery, and the least was understanding. An interdependent relationship between knowledge domain and information function revealed that when the knowledge being sought was propositional, the information functions of discovery and understanding occurred more frequently than when the knowledge being sought was procedural or causal. When the knowledge being sought was either procedural or causal, the information function of exploration occurred more frequently than if the knowledge being sought was propositional. Taken together, these results indicate that clinicians pursue propositional, procedural, and causal knowledge in an effort to explore, discover, and contextualize their intellectual and professional world.

The model of clinician development (Shapiro & Moses, 1989) and the related empirical investigations (Moses & Shapiro, 1996; Shapiro & Moses, 2005) support a developmental conceptualization for improving clinical skills and becoming a master clinician from the initial experiences of professional preparation to ongoing experience and training throughout one's career. Both student clinicians and speech–language pathologists are encouraged to identify their own level of professional development and to monitor and facilitate their ongoing development over time.

Clinical Process Components

The components of the clinical process, as will be seen, are parallel to and compatible with those of the supervisory process and constitute the tools of self-supervision. The components of the clinical process (Casey et al., 1988), adapted from those described for the supervisory process (J. L. Anderson, 1988; McCrea & Brasseur, 2003), include understanding, planning, observing, analyzing, and integrating. These components are described in the following sections.

Understanding the Clinical Process.   Working effectively with people who stutter and their family requires a familiarity with the components of the clinical process and the tasks and competencies for stuttering treatment (ASHA, 1995). This familiarity is gained through coursework and continuing education related to communication and its disorders (specifically fluency and stuttering), interpersonal and technical skills, and guided observation and supervised clinical practicum. Clinicians should become aware of the observation and analysis methods that are available for documenting and describing client and clinician behavior (Moses & Shapiro, 1996; Shapiro, 1985, 1987, 1994a; Shapiro & Anderson, 1988, 1989; Shapiro & Moses, 1989, 2005). To understand the client's communication behavior, clinicians may use standardized and nonstandardized instruments to develop short- and long-term goals and related treatment plans. To understand the clinician's own communication behavior and intervention skills, she may collect and analyze baseline behaviors; use portions of the *Wisconsin Procedure for Appraisal of Clinical Competence* (W-PACC; Shriberg et al., 1975) or the *University of Texas–Dallas Competency Based Evaluation System* (UTD; Lougeay-Mottinger, Harris, Perlstein-Kaplan, & Felicetti, 1984); design individualized academic, clinical, and supervisory contracts with the supervisor (Shapiro & Anderson, 1988, 1989); or engage in other procedures discussed in the section on observing and analyzing the clinical process, below.

Planning the Clinical Process. Systematic planning is necessary for clinicians to achieve maximum growth. Casey et al. (1988) listed six steps for achieving mutual clinician and client growth, including identifying clinician and client needs and competencies related to clinical interaction, setting clinician and client short- and long-term goals, determining clinician and client baseline behaviors, identifying clinician behaviors to be used for assessing client functioning or influencing client growth, planning observation (i.e., identifying data to be collected on clinician and client skills, planning logistics of observation, identifying data collection procedures), and planning for data analysis and integration.

Observing and Analyzing the Clinical Process. Data collection, analysis, and interpretation regarding the clinical interaction are completed for different reasons (e.g., setting objectives, monitoring clinician and client change, planning for the supervisory conference, checking perceptions, engaging in self-study, and pursuing research questions). Questions about the clinical process from the clinician, client, or supervisor can be answered by collection, analysis, and interpretation of clinical data during clinician–client interaction or from video recordings. Data collection procedures include verbatim recording, selected verbatim recording, rating, tally, interaction analysis, nonverbal analysis, and individually designed methods (J. L. Anderson, 1988; ASHA, 2008a, 2008b, 2008c; Casey et al., 1988; Dowling, 2001; McCrea & Brasseur, 2003; Shapiro, 1994a). For our purposes, interaction analysis, nonverbal analysis, and individually designed methods will be reviewed briefly.

  ⌸ *Interaction analysis.* Interaction analysis systems are highly structured instruments used for collecting, analyzing, and interpreting patterns of behavior occurring during the clinical (and supervisory) process (Shapiro, 1994a). Those available for the clinical process, each with unique categories and procedures, enable the clinician or supervisor to collect clinician and client data in order to analyze the interaction. Among the many systems that are useful for heightening clinicians' understanding of the clinical process, particularly the language they use, are the *Content and Sequence Analysis of Speech and Hearing Therapy* (Boone & Prescott, 1972), the *Analysis of Behavior of Clinicians* (ABC; Schubert, Miner, & Till, 1973), and the *Hill Counselor Verbal Response Category System* (C. E. Hill, 1993). These and other systems enable clinicians to become more aware of their own verbal behavior when interacting with people who stutter and their families. Once aware, clinicians may entertain changes in order to improve the effectiveness of the clinical interaction (see also Blood, Blood, McCarthy, et al., 2001; Shapiro, 1994a).

⚙ *Nonverbal analysis.* Collecting, analyzing, and interpreting nonverbal behaviors is important because of their potential influence on the communication in the clinical session. Nonverbal behaviors might include subtleties such as smiles, head nods, touches, leans, posture changes, eye contact, or vocal stress. Van Riper (1975) noted that he observed, tallied, and discussed with the clinician the following nonverbal behaviors because they provided valuable information about the clinical session: clinician's voice quality, inflection, and rate of speaking; appropriateness of interpersonal distance between clinician and client (e.g., number of times clinician physically withdrew from client); mobility of clinician and client (e.g., how stiff their postures were); ratio between smiles and frowns; number of mirrorings shown by clinician (e.g., when the client smiles, does the clinician smile too?); and verbal (e.g., "What I mean is . . .") and nonverbal (e.g., throat clearing, head scratching, sniffing, finger shaking) tics. Other categories of nonverbal behavior, described later, are relevant to observing the clinical process as well.

⚙ *Individually designed procedures.* Observation and analysis of the clinical experience can be tailored to the uniqueness of each clinician or client, highlighting the clinician's entering level of skill, upon which individualized professional objectives are developed. The objectives may relate to any of the interpersonal or intrapersonal competencies discussed in Chapter 11. This is what I do most often. First, I identify with each clinician a handful of clinical skills that she feels are relative strengths (clinicians too often default to identifying their clinical shortcomings). Then, building on what the clinician already knows and can do, she and I identify one or two (three at most) areas that might be targeted for improvement. Assessment of the clinician's skills is done *with* (to the extent possible and individually appropriate), rather than *for*, her and may utilize resources already discussed. For each area identified for improvement, specific objectives and strategies are developed to facilitate professional growth and are documented in writing. This process enables the clinician to focus on improving specific competencies (e.g., providing clients feedback regarding fluency and disfluency, collecting data on speech behaviors as well as related thoughts and feelings, expressing warmth and genuineness, using positive verbal and nonverbal language) and enables me to provide focused, objective, and data-based feedback, rather than global feedback, on her development. I have found this method to be particularly satisfying and effective with clinicians. They feel their uniqueness as both people and professionals is not only being considered but invited, and they are participating in their own professional growth from the outset (Shapiro & Anderson, 1988, 1989).

Integrating the Components of the Clinical Process. Integrating the clinical process requires understanding, planning, observing, and analyzing its components. The supervisory conference is a catalyst for the process of integration, where the clinician reflects on the information and experiences acquired previously and how each might be applied to develop, maintain, or enhance clinical competence through self-study and ongoing professional growth.

Supervisory Process

Too often, supervisees enter supervision without knowledge of the supervisory process and, as a consequence, rely on the individual supervisor's direction without generalizing knowledge of the process to subsequent supervisory interactions. For this reason, clinicians need to be provided with an understanding of the supervisory process and prepared to function meaningfully and proactively as a supervisee.

Supervisory Process Defined

ASHA (2008b, 2008c) adopted J. L. Anderson's (1988) definition of *supervision*:

> Supervision is a process that consists of a variety of patterns of behavior, the appropriateness of which depends upon the needs, competencies, expectations and philosophies of the supervisor and the supervisee and the specifics of the situation (task, client, setting

and other variables). The goals of the supervisory process are the professional growth and development of the supervisee and the supervisor, which it is assumed will result ultimately in optimal service to clients. (J. L. Anderson, 1988, p. 12)

This definition is consistent with ASHA's position on clinical supervision (ASHA, 1985, 2008a) as effective clinical teaching or clinical education that is both a distinct area of practice in speech–language pathology and an essential component in the education of students and the continued professional growth of speech–language pathologists. To the extent that such processes involve development of self-analysis, self-evaluation, and problem solving by the individual being supervised and by the supervisor, ASHA (2008b) expanded Anderson's definition as follows:

> Professional growth and development of the supervisee and the supervisor are enhanced when supervision or clinical teaching involves self-analysis and self-evaluation. Effective clinical teaching also promotes the use of critical thinking and problem-solving skills on the part of the individual being supervised. (ASHA, 2008b, p. 3)

The primary purposes of supervision are to ensure the highest quality of clinical service (by developing skills used to assess, treat, and otherwise manage the needs of people who demonstrate communication disorders) and to ensure ongoing professional self-study, understanding, and growth (career-long acquisition, integration, and application of the information and skills necessary for quality clinical service). While there are many models and procedures for supervision, most are derivatives of clinical supervision. Originally borrowed from teacher education, clinical supervision refers to a "cycle" (Cogan, 1973) or "sequence" (Goldhammer, Anderson, & Krajewski, 1980) that emphasizes improvement of clinicians' technical and interpersonal skills. The conference is essential to the supervisory process, which includes establishing the supervisee–supervisor relationship, planning with the supervisee (i.e., clinician), planning the strategy of observation, observing therapy, analyzing the clinical and supervisory processes, planning the strategy for the conference, conducting the conference, and renewed planning. The word *clinical* conveys a face-to-face interaction between a supervisee and supervisor who are engaged in objective, data-based observation and analysis of such "intensity of focus that binds the two together in a rather intimate professional relationship" (Goldhammer, 1969, p. 55). Van Riper (1965) acknowledged clinical supervision as "the most important of all staff functions" and indicated that it is in this personal interaction with student clinicians that supervisors "turn students into clinicians" (p. 75). The central theme of clinical supervision methodology is *colleagueship*, in which the supervisee and supervisor share in all phases of planning, observation, and objective analysis of data from the clinical and supervisory processes. This partnership reportedly leads to a more analytical, problem-solving, and self-supervising supervisee (Gillam, Roussos, & Anderson, 1990; Shapiro & Anderson, 1988, 1989).

When I am invited to conduct workshops and presentations on stuttering intervention, occasionally I am asked about my ideas related to clinical supervision and colleagueship in the professional preparation of clinicians. I share that clinical supervision is a dynamic, ongoing exchange in which the participants dialogue and shift perspective to consider alternative points of view. The supervisor provides the appropriate level of guidance to facilitate the supervisee's active role in establishing and monitoring specific objectives regarding the clinical and self-supervisory skills. Colleagueship endorses clinical teaching as necessarily shared and interactive and emphasizes a philosophy of teaching and learning by which all participants engage in different but equally important roles that reflect individual skill levels along a continuum. On one such occasion, a senior faculty member stood and said, "Like hell I'll consider a student a colleague!" This outright rejection of colleagueship seemed incongruous with a key objective of supervision—to facilitate the supervisee's ability to think more independently and creatively, to problem-solve, and to self-supervise to the point where the supervisor's role becomes unnecessary. This objective is parallel to that of the clinical process, in which we nurture the client's communication independence. The assumptions that the faculty member and I held regarding the process and product of clinical instruction and professional preparation indeed were in contrast. He assumed colleagueship to be a dichotomy (one either is or is not a colleague) and that skill level alone determines colleagueship. I believe that clients, clinicians/supervisees, and supervisors are colleagues of different skill levels and engaged in different roles, all working toward heightened understanding and improved communication. The roles and responsibilities of each participant change with experience and skill improvement. The supervisee's strengths and needs are assessed and addressed individually, and evaluation is based on the supervisee's progress from a shared perspective. A collegial context also presents a vehicle for analysis and improvement of supervisors' skills. The more a supervisor becomes comfortable with and explicit about her efforts to improve her own professional skills, the more the supervisee will understand and commit to the process of ongoing and shared professional growth. Within such a dynamic, clinical, and collegial context, supervisees and supervisors learn with and from each other along the lifelong journey of professional growth.

Supervisory Knowledge and Skills

ASHA (2008c) underscored that achieving clinical competence does not imply that one has the specialized knowledge and skills to be an effective supervisor. Although ASHA does not have specific requirements for coursework or credentials to serve as a supervisor, knowledge and skills may be developed in courses or workshops on supervision, in self-study, in ASHA's Special Interest Division 11 (Administration and Supervision), and in mentored experiences. ASHA (2008c) outlined 11 core areas of knowledge and skills required for effective supervision. This document is useful for both supervisors (for guiding self-assessment as supervisors and developing professional growth plans) and supervisees (for building an understanding of the components, processes, roles, and expectations). The 11 areas of knowledge and skills are as follows: (1) preparation for the supervisory experience; (2) interpersonal communication and the supervisor–supervisor relationship; (3) development of the supervisee's critical thinking and problem-solving skills; (4) development of the supervisee's clinical competence in assessment; (5) development of the supervisee's clinical competence in intervention; (6) supervisory conferences or meetings of clinical teaching teams; (7) evaluation of the growth of the supervisee both as a clinician and as a professional; (8) knowledge of how diversity (ability, race, ethnicity, gender, age, culture, language, class, experience, and education) might influence learning, behavioral styles, and feedback mechanisms; (9) development and maintenance of clinical and supervisory documentation; (10) knowledge of ethical, regulatory, and legal requirements; and (11) knowledge of principles of mentoring. Those interested in more information are encouraged to refer to the original source (ASHA, 2008c) and to ASHA (1985) for a delineation of 13 tasks and related competencies for effective supervision, in addition to ASHA's current position statement (ASHA, 2008a) and technical report (ASHA, 2008b) on clinical supervision in speech–language pathology.

A Model of Supervisory Development

J. L. Anderson (1988; see also McCrea & Brasseur, 2003) presented a model of supervision that is consistent with the principles of clinical supervision and is sensitive to the uniqueness of what individual supervisees and supervisors bring to the supervisory interaction. The continuum of supervision, depicted in Figure 12.1, assumes that

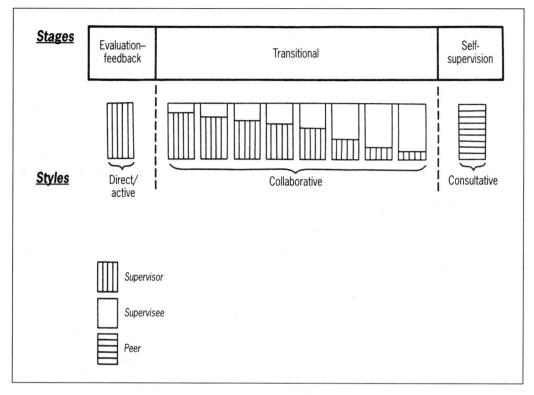

Figure 12.1.   The continuum of supervision—stages of supervision and appropriate styles for each stage. *Note.* From *The Supervisory Process in Speech–Language Pathology and Audiology* (p. 62), by J. L. Anderson, 1988, Boston: Little Brown/College-Hill. Copyright 1988 by Little Brown/ College-Hill. Reprinted with permission.

supervision exists on a continuum spanning one's professional career and that distinct styles of interaction are appropriate to each stage of the continuum. Furthermore, the continuum provides a structure for supervisors and supervisees to examine their own philosophies about supervision, identify their own behaviors, and target changes they might wish to make. Other key features of the continuum are that the component stages (i.e., evaluation–feedback, transitional, and self-supervision) are not time bound. A supervisee may find herself at any point on the continuum at any time during her career. While clinicians beginning an initial practicum generally enter the continuum at the evaluation–feedback stage, more experienced clinicians may find themselves at this beginning stage when they experience a different disorder category, type of client, work setting, technology, or procedure (J. L. Anderson, 1988; McCrea & Brasseur, 2003). The relative dominance of the supervisor decreases, while that of the supervisee increases, as they move across the continuum. Both supervisee and supervisor share responsibility for recognizing their respective placements along the continuum, for identifying and effecting necessary changes, and for progressing along the continuum. The continuum is dynamic in regard to the supervisee's and supervisor's respective stages of supervision. Different styles of supervision are appropriate to each stage. The supervisee and supervisor must adapt their individual styles as they move back and forth along the continuum as different variables require.

Evaluation–Feedback Stage.   In the evaluation–feedback stage, the supervisor assumes a relatively dominant role, providing direction, evaluation, and feedback. The supervisee assumes a relatively passive or subordinate role, primarily receiving information. As noted in Figure 12.1, the supervisor's style of interaction is direct/active; that of the supervisee is passive. A clinician/supervisee who is a novice, one who is engaged in a new type of disorder or setting, or one who is a marginal clinician (i.e., a clinician with specific academic, clinical, or combined academic and clinical deficiencies; Shapiro et al., 2002) will be at this stage of the continuum. J. L. Anderson (1988) recommended that the supervisee and supervisor should work to move out of the evaluation–feedback stage as rapidly as possible in order to facilitate the supervisee's professional development.

Transitional Stage. The relative dominance shifts in the transitional stage. The supervisee has become increasingly knowledgeable and skillful and participates in planning, implementing, and evaluating both the clinical and supervisory processes. The supervisor recognizes the supervisee's emerging competence and encourages joint problem solving. The supervisor continues to provide some direction and feedback; however, the supervisee is moving increasingly toward independence and peer interaction, which characterize self-supervision. The supervisee may move back and forth within the transitional stage depending on related experiences, skills, and needs, as noted. For example, the clinician/supervisee may be relatively comfortable designing school-based treatment plans for children who stutter but may need more direction for a child with symptoms of Tourette syndrome. A collaborative style is appropriate for the transitional stage, in which the supervisor and supervisee share responsibilities to meet common objectives. In fact, there are times when the supervisee and supervisor may reverse roles in the transitional stage, using a collaborative style. J. L. Anderson (1988) described such a situation:

> A student clinician, well-trained and with extensive experience in the clinical program and with a specific disorder area, may be working with a supervisor whose background in this area is different, limited, or not current. The supervisee might then assume a more active role in the collaboration, with the supervisor receiving the input about certain techniques or a differing philosophy. This requires openness on the part of the supervisor, and confidence, if not courage, on the part of the supervisee. (p. 59)

Self-Supervision Stage. In the self-supervision stage, the supervisee becomes even more actively involved in the clinical and supervisory processes and is relatively independent in developing and pursuing strategies for continued professional growth. A cornerstone of this stage is the supervisee's ability to observe, analyze, and alter her own clinical behavior on the basis of problem-solving skills and the objective data that she collects. The clinician/supervisee still desires a collegial (peer or consultative) type of interaction. The supervisee is now empowered to assess and make decisions about her own professional needs (e.g., identifying strengths and weaknesses, making modifications, and seeking assistance or further knowledge as appropriate). This level of independent professional functioning is the terminal objective of the supervisory process. Some clinicians achieve self-supervision by the end of their graduate degree program; others do not achieve this stage before many years of professional experience. Self-supervision is typically characterized by a consultative style, a relationship emphasizing each participant's ability to help the other and to listen, support, problem-solve, and offer suggestions where appropriate.

Supervisory Process Components

In order to achieve independent clinical skills and self-supervision across the affective, behavioral, and cognitive domains, clinicians/supervisees and supervisors must understand and be able to function within and across the components of supervision. These components, which facilitate a collaborative style used for the transitional stage of supervision, include understanding, planning, observing, analyzing, and integrating (J. L. Anderson, 1988; McCrea & Brasseur, 2003).

Understanding the Supervisory Process. The first component of the supervisory process, understanding the supervisory process, is devoted to developing a working knowledge of supervision in its entirety and its constituent elements. Building this understanding is particularly important given that supervisors and supervisees have been found to hold different perceptions of the same event (e.g., the style of supervisory interaction being used) and different expectations for the supervisory process (e.g., roles and responsibilities of each participant, related objectives) (J. L. Anderson, 1988; McCrea & Brasseur, 2003; J. E. Roberts & Smith, 1982; K. J. Smith & Anderson, 1982a, 1982b). If the supervisor expects to use a collaborative style but the supervisee expects a direct/active style, conflict is likely to occur. Preparation may take the form of dialogue between supervisees and supervisors, a component within clinical courses, or courses devoted to the supervisory process. Topics addressed might include supervisees' prior experiences in supervision and related preferences and anxieties; supervisory models, stages and styles, components, perceptions, expectations, goals, and objectives; and knowledge/skills and tasks/competencies for effective supervision (ASHA, 2008a, 2008b, 2008c).

Planning the Supervisory Process. Planning is as important for the supervisory process as it is for the clinical process. The purpose of planning is to identify objectives for the clinical and supervisory interactions. Planning is important because it establishes priorities and serves as a basis for future activity. Initial data are collected in the planning component against which progress can be measured. From these data, goals, objectives, and related strategies are established for the clinical and supervisory processes. As noted, I typically engage each clinician in self-assessment, including strengths and challenges, in order to design a professional development plan. Supervisees' strengths should serve as a foundation to and point of departure for addressing identified limitations.

Observing the Supervisory Process. Observation occurs according to the objectives and procedures specified in the planning component. An important distinction is made between observation and evaluation. Observation is the collection and recording of objective data for subsequent analysis. Evaluation implies a judgment or inference that is built upon a foundation of understanding, planning, objective observation, analysis, and integration. Observation requires application of the scientific process through systematic collection of accurate, objective, and reliable data. Observation, therefore, is not synonymous either with "watching" or "supervision." Observation is only one component of supervision. Frequently I hear supervisors say, "I've got to go supervise my clinician" when they mean, "I've got to go observe my clinician." J. L. Anderson (1988) noted that objectivity is essential in this part of the supervisory process, where data are collected and recorded by both supervisor and supervisee for further analysis and interpretation, which then lead to evaluation. The methods discussed previously for observing the clinical process apply to the supervisory process as well (verbatim recording, selected verbatim recording, rating, tally, interaction analysis, nonverbal analysis, and individually designed methods). Again, for our purposes, interaction analysis, nonverbal analysis, and individually designed procedures will be described here.

> ⟨⟩ *Interaction analysis.* Interaction analysis systems were discussed earlier in the context of methods for observing the clinical process (i.e., client–clinician interaction). Other interaction analysis systems are available for the supervisory process (i.e., supervisee–supervisor interaction). Different systems are available to suit the different purposes and questions being addressed. The systems code specific verbal behaviors that are objective and

quantifiable, yield descriptive frequency data, and require few inferences on the part of the coder, who analyzes one event at a time. Among the systems found useful for heightening supervisees' understanding of the supervisory process, and particularly the language they use within supervisory conferences, are the *System for Analyzing Supervisor–Teacher Interaction* (Blumberg, 1980), the *Underwood Category System for Analyzing Supervisor–Clinician Behavior* (Seeley, 1973; Underwood, 1979), *McCrea's Adapted Scales for the Assessment of Interpersonal Functioning in Speech Pathology Supervision Conferences* (McCrea, 1980), and *Smith's Adaptation of the Multidimensional Observational System for the Analysis of Interactions in Clinical Supervision* (MOSAICS; K. J. Smith, 1978). These (Shapiro, 1994a) and other systems (J. L. Anderson, 1988; Dowling, 2001; McCrea & Brasseur, 2003) enable supervisory participants to become more aware of their functioning within supervisory conferences and to consider changes so as to maximize supervisory effectiveness.

▦ *Nonverbal analysis.* Verbal and nonverbal behaviors, whether occurring within the clinical or supervisory interaction, are overlapping, interrelated, and interdependent. The distinction, however, is critical for training observation and interpersonal skills (Farmer & Farmer, 1989; McCready, Shapiro, & Kennedy, 1987). Farmer and Farmer noted that nonverbal behavior refers to communication events that transcend spoken or written words and may account for as much as 80% of the meaning interpreted from an intended message. Whereas verbal communication primarily conveys information, nonverbal communication primarily conveys affect. More experienced supervisees and supervisors tend to use more positive nonverbal communication than those with less experience. Farmer and Farmer (1989, pp. 165–167) suggested that supervisees and supervisors gain greater familiarity with various categories of nonverbal behaviors, including *paralinguistics* (voice quality, prosody, intonation), *kinesics* (body movement, posture, gesture, facial expression, and eye movement), *tactile communication* (touch of oneself or another person), *proxemics* (manipulating space by adjusting the room, setting, furniture, or interpersonal distance), *chronemics* (factors related to time, e.g., orientation by, reaction to, awareness of time), *color* (color of walls, floor, furniture, clothing, materials), *olfactory/gustatory sense* (smells, odors, or aromas of the environment or interpersonal context), *objects and artifacts* (clothing, jewelry, eyeglasses, hearing aids, possessions, professional or personal markers), *silence* (oral and body inactivity), *ambience* (atmosphere perceived by setting, attitudes, proxemics, colors, sounds/silence, olfactory and object messages), and *organismics* (physical attributes, e.g., height, weight, eye and skin color, body dimensions, gender, race, age, characteristics of disability). And, as noted in Chapter 6, interpretations of the appropriateness of nonverbal behaviors (such as proximity and touch) vary across cultural groups.

▦ *Individually designed procedures.* There are many individually designed procedures for observing the supervisory process. As noted previously, I design individual professional development plans with and for every clinician I supervise. Identified clinical strengths serve as a foundation for pinpointing clinical challenges and for specifying objectives, strategies, and data to be collected to facilitate these clinical skills. The same process is followed for supervisory skills. For example, a supervisee may wish to use observational data to become more independent in planning the supervisory conference agenda, monitoring her follow-through behavior, or engaging in problem solving. A supervisor may wish to collect verbal and nonverbal observational data to increase her receptivity to and use of the supervisee's ideas and to support justification provided to the supervisee (Shapiro, 1994a).

Analyzing the Supervisory Process. Analysis is a bridge between observation and evaluation. Analysis refers to objective interpretation of goal-based data reflecting events that were planned and observed. The data are examined, organized, summarized, and interpreted so as to document change and patterns of behavior relative to client, clinician/supervisee, or supervisor objectives. Data analysis increasingly moves from being a supervisor responsibility, to a joint responsibility, to a supervisee responsibility. This transition is intended to build the supervisee's independence of self-analysis and problem-solving skills within the clinical and supervisory processes, thus moving her along the continuum toward self-supervision. Assisting supervisees with ongoing objective analysis and interpretation of objective observational data is one of the tasks of effective supervision (ASHA, 1985, 2008a, 2008b, 2008c). Supervisory participants should be particularly wary of data that show consistently positive or negative outcomes. Consistently positive outcomes may reveal remarkably steady progress or insufficient challenge; consistently negative outcomes may reveal limited progress or excessive challenge. In either case, further analysis, revision, and planning are indicated.

Integrating the Supervisory Process. The supervisory conference is usually the context for integrating all that has transpired. Specifically, objectives and events that were planned, observed, and analyzed are discussed and interpreted with respect to the data collected so as to reach shared conclusions. The primary purposes of the supervisory conference are problem solving and increasing the level of the supervisee's independent functioning. Occasionally, the participants need to verify this shift in responsibility and accompanying style from direct/active (evaluation–feedback) to collaborative (transitional) to consultative (self-supervision). Given the importance of the supervisory conference, I become concerned when I see too few supervisors scheduling regular conferences with their supervisees. The most frequent justification expressed is a lack of time. Focused agendas, however, result in conferences that are meaningful and efficient. Indeed, the dynamic quality of the supervisory process, integrated and epitomized in the supervisory conference, has been described as "a process in progress" (Shapiro, 1985, p. 89).

Specialization and Globalization

There are many ways for clinicians to stay abreast of developments in the discipline of fluency disorders and to maximize the benefits of personal and professional interactions with colleagues far and wide. Based upon the academic, clinical, and supervisory processes of professional preparation described earlier, two such methods are specialization and globalization.

Specialization

Specialization was the first major topic addressed at the 1991 inaugural meeting of ASHA's Special Interest Division 4 (Fluency and Fluency Disorders). This topic was in response to proposals that resulted in elimination of the 25 hours of required practicum in fluency disorders at graduate programs of professional education, effective 1993 (St. Louis, 2001b). Having served on the Inaugural Specialty Board on Fluency Disorders, I have seen the specialty program flourish since its initiation in 1999.

One major contribution of this board, now the Specialty Board on Fluency Disorders, is to identify speech–language pathologists who voluntarily submit to extensive review of credentials and to designate these professionals as Board Recognized Fluency Specialists. However, no less significant are the implications of the questions that have arisen regarding specialization. For example, Who really is a specialist? What is specialization? What are the measurable characteristics of specialization? How are such characteristics acquired? How are they maintained? Should the characteristics of specialization reflect the nature of what the speech–language pathologist is (i.e., human *being*), what she does (human *doing*), or some combination? What characteristics of specialization transcend the individual methods being employed? Similarly, in the previous chapter, we discussed how the elements of a master clinician and an effective clinical relationship are quite other than the sum of their individual parts. St. Louis (2001b) raised related questions about how to define *specialist*. For example, is a specialist necessarily someone who is on the roster of Board Recognized Fluency Specialists? Or is a specialist anyone who expresses a focused interest, such as those on the list distributed by the Stuttering Foundation of America? St. Louis (2001b) also raised questions about the relationship between specialists and generalists: Will specialists replace generalists in the treatment of fluency disorders? What type of relationship should there be between specialists and generalists? I believe that there is a vital role both for specialists and generalists; however, the number of specialists is far too low to treat the estimated 3.5 million people who stutter in North America alone (St. Louis, 2001b). St. Louis emphasized that we must continue to work toward and lobby for better training in fluency disorders at the undergraduate and graduate levels and, with the advent of specialization, we must recognize and maximize the value of continuing education across the professional career.

The Specialty Board on Fluency Disorders currently maintains a website (see the Appendix) that is of interest for both consumers and professionals. Consumers can locate Board Recognized Fluency Specialists; professionals can learn about procedures for seeking board recognition in fluency disorders or for becoming Fluency Specialist Mentors. According to the website, the mission of the Specialty Board on Fluency Disorders is threefold:

   ▨ to promote among speech–language pathologists the highest standards for training and service delivery to impact positively the communication skills and thereby the lives of those who stutter

   ▨ to verify the knowledge of fluency disorders, commitment to treating those who stutter, and mastery of skills of professionals who seek and maintain recognition as a Board Recognized Fluency Specialist

   ▨ to publicize the benefits of working with specialists in fluency disorders and provide an up-to-date listing of individuals who maintain Board Recognized Fluency Specialist status

Also according to the website, specialists are defined as follows:

   ▨ Board Recognized Specialists in Fluency Disorders are individuals who have demonstrated a high level of clinical expertise in treating fluency disorders, advanced knowledge, and a commitment to serving people with fluency disorders. They have submitted their credentials for review and approval by a board of peers. This Specialty Recognition Program is an approved program of ASHA.

   ▨ Board Recognized Fluency Specialists who were approved since 2001 have at least two years of full-time clinical experience or its equivalent, hold the Certificate of Clinical Competence, have completed at least 100 hours of postgraduate educational training in fluency disorders, have completed at least 100 hours of guided clinical practice with people who stutter and their families under the supervision of a Board Recognized Fluency Specialist Mentor, have submitted a portfolio of clinical work for review and approval, and have passed a national fluency disorders specialty examination (note that the examination is not required after 2010, pending approval by ASHA's Council for Clinical Specialty Recognition). After approval as a Board Recognized Fluency Specialist, maintenance of this status for a 3-year period requires payment of annual fee, active engagement in direct service provision for at least 100 hours per year, completion of at least 4.5 continuing education units (45 clock hours in fluency, fluency disorders, or related areas) over a 3-year period, and verification that the applicant's CCC-SLP status is current. It is beyond present purposes to delineate all of the procedures needed to become and remain a Board Recognized Fluency Specialist or a Fluency Specialist Mentor. Eligibility requirements, procedures, and related forms are available and easily accessible on the website (Specialty Board on Fluency Disorders; see the Appendix).

Globalization

Another way to immerse oneself into the discipline of fluency disorders and to remain active and current is to build professional alliances with international colleagues. Such alliances are increasingly being made at both organizational and individual levels.

Organizationally, a significant agreement that encourages exchange of theoretical and clinical research and sharing of information on best clinical practice among speech–language pathologists went into effect January 1, 2009 (Tice & Moore, 2009). The six countries that entered into the *Agreement for the Mutual Recognition of Professional Association Credentials* (the Mutual Recognition Agreement) are the *United States* (ASHA), *Canada* (Canadian Association of Speech–Language Pathologists and Audiologists), *Ireland* (Irish Association of Speech and Language Therapists), *New Zealand* (New Zealand Speech–Language Therapists' Association), the *United Kingdom* (Royal College of Speech and Language Therapists), and *Australia* (Speech Pathology Association of Australia). This agreement establishes that speech–language pathologists who were credentialed from one of the six signatory associations will not be required to have all of their academic coursework and clinical experience evaluated when they apply for certification or full membership in the other signatory associations. While the agreement does not supersede national, state, or provincial licensing or registration requirements for practice, the agreement does benefit speech–language pathologists who wish to travel and work in other countries. Such benefits include identifying common standards of clinical competence, facilitating exchange of knowledge (e.g., research, continuing professional development, technologies), promoting international understanding of communication disorders and the role of speech–language pathologists, improving mobility of individuals with approved credentials for employment, and streamlining the reciprocal recognition of individuals who are credentialed by signatory associations. The entire Mutual Recognition Agreement with a copy of the original signatures is available from ASHA's website (see the Appendix), as is an international directory of ASHA members, a list of audiology and speech–language pathology associations outside of the United States, and an international directory of communication disorders containing a compilation of Internet resources (e.g., national and international associations, education programs, volunteer and employment opportunities, health and travel information).

Organizational globalization avenues for immersion in fluency disorders are available through affiliation with the International Fluency Association (IFA), the International Stuttering Association (IFA), and the International Cluttering Association (ICA). The *International Fluency Association* (see the Appendix for website) is an interdisciplinary organization devoted to understanding and managing fluency disorders and to improving the quality of life for people with fluency disorders. As such, the International Fluency Association brings together clinicians, researchers, people who stutter, and other interested parties from around the world through its international congresses, the *Journal of Fluency Disorders*, and ongoing electronic communications. The *International Stuttering Association* (see the Appendix) is composed of self-help organizations from around the world, all of which are working toward achieving "a world that understands stuttering." Its primary venues for communication are its international congresses, *One Voice* (its electronic newsletter), and regular electronic interactions. As noted previously, two significant forces galvanize the stuttering community and both integrate and bridge its association with the professional and research communities. The first is the *Bill of Rights and Responsibilities for People Who Stutter* (International Fluency Association & International Stuttering Association, 2001; also found on ISA's website; see the Appendix). The second is the series of Annual International Stuttering Awareness Day Online Conferences (archived and retrievable; see the Appendix for website), in which representatives from 151 different countries have participated (of the 194 recorded countries; personal communication, J. Kuster, June 25, 2009). The conferences are hosted on the Stuttering Home Page (see the Appendix). The International Stuttering Association actively affiliates with other international organizations (e.g., European League of Stuttering Associations) and member associations (e.g., Australian Speak Easy Association, British

Stammering Association, Canadian Association of People who Stutter, and the [U.S.] National Stuttering Association, among many others). The *International Cluttering Association* (see the Appendix) brings together people who clutter and their families with clinicians and researchers who are committed to understanding cluttering in order to increase public and professional awareness about this communication disorder, to encourage development and study of effective treatments, and to improve the quality of life for people who clutter.

Numerous other avenues for building professional alliances with international colleagues are available at the individual level or by person-to-person interaction. ASHA routinely publishes accounts of clinicians traveling abroad to work with people who stutter or to collaborate with colleagues for clinical service, research, and teaching. I have worked with people who stutter and their families and clinicians in all continents except Antarctica. Wonder and challenge await those who seek such international exploration of our profession, of others, and indeed, of themselves. Such experiences are not necessarily for everyone, of course. People travel and challenge the limits of their own comfort zones for different reasons. Such travel requires that one be mindful of others, respectful and accepting without judgment, inviting if not nurturing of that which is different because it genuinely reflects another's window onto the world, and seeking of points of comparison apart from one's own. One discovers that our presumed differences are far fewer than our universal similarities. Greg Mortenson (Mortenson & Relin, 2006) discussed such important lessons. After being stranded in Pakistan because of a failed attempt to climb K2 (the second highest mountain in the world), Mortenson discovered the lack of educational opportunities, particularly for girls, in that part of the world. In return for the kindness received, he returned and engaged many local people to build the first of many schools. One of the lessons he learned about local customs was the importance of building personal relationships as the most central element in all human enterprises. You have already seen how important this lesson is to me, both as a person and as a clinician. A local resident gave Mortenson the following advice:

> "If you want to thrive in Baltistan, you must respect our ways," Hali Aja said, blowing on his bowl. "The first time you share tea with a Balti, you are a stranger. The second time you take tea, you are an honored guest. The third time you share a cup of tea, you become family, and for our family, we are prepared to do anything, even die," he said, laying his hand warmly on Mortenson's own. "Doctor Greg, you must take time to share three cups of tea." (p. 150)

The message is clear. Within our personal and professional interactions, and particularly when we travel abroad, *how* we go about what we do is at least as important as *what* we do. Being is at least as important as doing. As noted previously, being is half of what we are (human beings). Why, then, do we too often focus on doing (productivity) to the exclusion of being human (focused on the nature of our presence and the manner of our interaction)? I was reminded of such lessons when I was sitting on the dirt floor of the hut of an indigenous healer in Cameroon. My hope was that I would be allowed to learn the traditional assumptions about stuttering and local intervention practices, reflecting a custom and a history that are both orally transmitted and private. In the presence of smoke, roots, and bones, I told the healer that I had come from the other side of the world to sit at his feet, if he would grant me the privilege to be his pupil. I have learned much and I am so grateful not only for the information received but also for the expression of trust, confidence, and faith; that is, for the richness of compassion and humanness provided. As a guest at Občanské sdružení LOGO in Brno, Czech Republic, I have taught and served both clinicians and people who stutter and their families. No one, however, could have learned more than I about communication, history, and humor (see Hasek, 1993). In Japan, again while teaching and serving, I learned much about Japanese values and behaviors and how they influence communication, communication disorders, and intervention, in addition to social and business relations and management styles (see Condon, 1984; Shelley, 1999). In Switzerland, after teaching a course, I received a letter from one of the participants that emphasized the importance of talking to hearts as well as to minds, shifting perspectives, being human, and teaching and learning as expressions of love.

There are so many rich opportunities to learn and grow with and from others by building professional alliances with international colleagues. A teacher in Douala, Cameroon, began the first African Stuttering Congress in 2005, sponsored by the Speak Clear Association of Cameroon, by playing his guitar and singing, "From time to time in life, birds of a feather find themselves together. Such a time is now." I urge you to find and create such times for yourselves with openness and harmony, and to write and sing such songs, in your own way, with friends and colleagues around the world. One can't know where such adventures might lead. This is good for you, for your clients, for the stuttering community, and for our discipline.

Maintenance of Professional Competence

To maintain professional competence, the clinician must internalize the desire to learn, commit to learning as a lifelong process, and understand and maintain parallels in the nature and processes of our professional development over time.

Knowing and Internalizing the Desire to Learn

Clinicians achieve tremendous strides in that period of formal professional development during which they complete their undergraduate and graduate education. The mechanism for professional development, as it currently stands, is a good process and assumed to be effective in achieving its target objectives. Efficacy data, however, are needed to document the instructional effectiveness of what we do and what we require so that we can determine how professional competence is achieved. Nevertheless, as with any good thing, there are a few inherent limitations. One such limitation is that what we do in professional preparation and how we do it may be lacking in ecological validity. In other words, some of the behaviors and attitudes being established in student clinicians may not be particularly suited for application to professional settings outside of academe.

Beukelman (1986) expressed similar concerns, stating that the experience of graduate education tends to develop in student clinicians behaviors that are "counterproductive," creating experts for the short term rather than the long term. Furthermore, he indicated that graduate education encourages learning only in structured contexts, rather than from the fire of internal motivation, thereby fostering deliberate and incomplete sharing of information, fear of losing power rather than being motivated by the sincere quest to learn and help, and feelings of territoriality and negative attitudes toward other professionals. Beukelman cautioned that the processes of professional preparation may be fostering "maladaptive" (p. 5) behaviors, thus developing "sprinters" rather than "long distance runners" (p. 8) and failing to engender sincere and professional questioning and problem-solving skills.

Adopting more of a student perspective based on her own personal experiences, Prutting (1985) described professional preparation as a "long battle for the light" (p. 5), a time during which "how you perceive yourself as an individual is a consequence of how you perform academically" (p. 5). She identified student clinicians' tendency to put themselves and their lives on hold while achieving relatively short-term objectives, often without realizing that they are missing the essence of the educational experience. She implored students to engage actively in the essential dailiness of their experiences, to immerse themselves in the science and human value of what they are about, to nurture and embrace their own exuberance, and to study how they conceptualize themselves and others within the world because that is at the core of the human spirit and how we approach all experiences within our lives (our personal construct; see Chapter 5). These two articles (Beukelman, 1986; Prutting, 1985) have proven timeless; they invite expansion of our professional experience through specialization and globalization, and should be required reading for all participants in professional preparation.

Do these observations and attendant suggestions mean that we should disparage the current process of professional preparation? I do not believe so. They do mean, however, that there are certain limitations about which we can become aware and thereby control, if not eliminate. Such limitations include artificially organizing learning into semesters or quarters rather realizing that real learning is borderless and without time limits, "mastering" whatever course we are currently taking or teaching rather than seeing the universal connections within and between all bodies of knowledge, focusing on the client to the exclusion of the communication system, and attending to the disorder rather than to the person. Such limitations tend to foster clinicians who conceive of professional preparation as an end in itself, rather than as a means to an exciting beginning. Every day with every client provides a renewed beginning, an opportunity to integrate our skills to meet the strengths and needs of people who stutter and their families. This process enables us to grow and improve, with our clients, as people and as professionals. In other words, learning must be a lifelong, internally motivated process that brings us sincere joy and excitement in our quest to understand and help others.

Learning as a Lifelong Process

When my son was 4 years old, he asked me, "What number is infinity?" Somewhat puzzled by the complexity of his question, I took him outside and, together, we looked up at the sky. I asked him to think about how far we could go into space. With little deliberation, we agreed that there was no limit. Infinity, I explained, is like that—without limit, forever, and always.

Learning as a lifelong process may be understood as similar to infinity—without limit, forever, and always. The notion of lifelong learning, which seemingly integrates a person with a process, refers to involving oneself in diverse forms of continuing education in order to remain current in a field and upgrade one's skills, thereby maintaining professional competence. It is hard, if not impossible, to credential or regulate the exuberance, or "joie de vivre" (Prutting, 1985, p. 6) that catalyzes any sincere, internal, and long-term motivation to learn. Remaining current within one's chosen profession is a significant ethical commitment we make during our own professional preparation and upon entry into our career (ASHA, 2010). Kellum and Fagan (1992) noted that human service professionals, within 10 to 12 years of receiving their professional education, were found to be approximately half as competent as they were when they graduated. They noted, "With the explosion of new knowledge and technological advances occurring in the fields of speech–language pathology and audiology, degree half-life of two to three years may well be a reality" (p. 410). That reality is now. Earning a degree and becoming a clinician mark only the beginning of one's education. Immersion into continuing education, broadly and diversely interpreted, is not a luxury, but a necessity. Kellum and Fagan noted, "The public's call for competent professionals demands it; our professional association's standards and ethical codes require it; and the individual professional's pride in his or her work should dictate it" (1992, p. 410).

Clearly, the avenues of specialized and ongoing training impacting the affective, behavioral, and cognitive domains are without limit. They involve the academic, clinical, and supervisory processes in the form of curricular offerings, externships, mentorships, applied research, distance and electronic options, and varied forms of specialization and globalization. Self-study activity and interaction analysis (J. L. Anderson, 1988; Casey et al., 1988; Dowling, 2001; McCrea & Brasseur, 2003; Shapiro, 1987, 1994a) were discussed as mechanisms for facilitating objective observations yielding heightened understanding and professional growth as clinical or supervisory participants. The motivation for lifelong learning, however, must be internally driven and continuous. Such learning is a personal and professional commitment to oneself to be and remain the best one can be. While certification (even specialty certification), licensure, and continuing education requirements are externally driven instructional mechanisms, integrating oneself with the process of lifelong professional growth requires internal motivation. Anyone can go through the motions. Only clinicians will care enough about past, present, and future clients to seek, find, seize, and create opportunities to stay current or upgrade their professional skills. The continuum of supervision (J. L. Anderson, 1988; see Figure 12.1), emphasizing professional growth leading to independent clinical functioning, self-supervision, and consultative interactions, is an ideal way to conceptualize and monitor one's development over time. The model of professional development in problem solving (Shapiro & Moses, 1989, 2005; see Table 12.1), which includes perspectives taken, dimensions of behavior conceptualized, solutions generated, and causal concepts, can also be applied to maintenance of professional competence. Models, methods, and materials are available to facilitate learning and to accommodate individual needs, circumstances, and learning styles. It is up to individual clinicians to persevere, for infinity.

Maintaining Parallels: Different Trees, Same Forest

The discussion of professional development will conclude by highlighting several pertinent and generative parallels.

The Clinical and Supervisory Processes

Historically, it has been assumed that the skills needed by supervisors are the same as those needed by clinicians. I expressed my concern about this assumption years ago (Shapiro, 1987). In fact, the Certificate of Clinical Competence continues to be the only credential issued by the American Speech-Language-Hearing Association for clinicians and supervisors (ASHA, 2008a, 2008b, 2008c). ASHA (2008c) acknowledged, "ASHA does not have specific requirements for coursework or credentials to serve as a supervisor; however, some states or settings may require coursework and/or years of experience to serve as a supervisor." I support and engage in disciplined efforts to study and understand clinical supervision as a distinct area of expertise with unique tasks and related competencies requiring specialized knowledge and skills (ASHA, 2008c; see also Shapiro et al., 2002; Shapiro & Moses, 2005) and the avenues of preparation for acquiring such specialized training (ASHA, 2008a, 2008b, 2008c). In making such statements, I am acknowledging the distinction between clinical and supervisory skills and training, though I do recognize considerable area of overlap. A number of the clinical procedures reviewed in Chapters 8, 9, and 10 are relevant to the supervisory process as well. These procedures include constructing a safe house in which learning thrives, inviting objectives, creating opportunities for success, heightening the learner's awareness of such success, developing and transferring target skills, systematically introducing and increasing levels of challenge, modeling appropriate behaviors and skills, establishing or maintaining positive feelings about oneself as a learner, facilitating empowerment, and talking with learners in positive ways.

Similarly, the interpersonal and intrapersonal factors of effective clinicians reviewed in Chapter 11 are relevant to effective supervisees and supervisors. These include clinician attributes (e.g., empathy, warmth, genuineness, personal magnetism, compatible friction, and realistic and focused optimism), in addition to clinician behavior, language, needs, and satisfaction and rewards. Like the clinician, the supervisor serves in the role of guardian angel to the supervisee. Walle's (1974) observations about being a clinician and suitability for the clinical process can be applied to supervisors and the supervisory process as well. While the clinical and supervisory processes are distinct and require unique skills, competencies, and forms of preparation, they nevertheless share a fund of knowledge that is necessary for effective practice.

Developing, Maintaining, and Upgrading Professional Competence

When considering learning and professional development as lifelong processes, we might recall the usefulness of different models and procedures reviewed in this chapter for the purpose of developing clinical and supervisory skills. These include the continuum of supervision (J. L. Anderson, 1988; McCrea & Brasseur, 2003), which is not time bound and therefore can be used to conceptualize professional development across the professional life span. Similarly, the aspects of professional development (Shapiro & Moses, 1989, 2005) applied to three clinician profiles (Moses & Shapiro, 1996) provide a mechanism for conceptualizing, observing, and monitoring continued development of problem-solving skills over time. Finally, the methods reviewed for observing and analyzing the clinical and supervisory processes within professional preparation—interaction analysis, nonverbal analysis, and individually designed methods—can be applied to maintaining or upgrading professional skills.

Back to the Beginning

The conceptual foundation built in Chapters 5, 6, and 7 for clinical intervention could also be applied to the supervisory process and to lifelong learning. First, consider the importance of the personal construct. We emphasized that the client and clinician must understand the client's personal construct (thoughts and feelings about himself as a person and as a communicator and related assumptions and values) because it is the filter through which he interprets all events within his communicative world and by which he anticipates his future. Similarly, clinicians/supervisees and supervisors must understand their own personal constructs because of the interaction between their personal viewpoints and their effectiveness as change agents, and because of the potential for conflict between constructs. These statements imply at least two critical skills. One is the ability to be honestly receptive to (by inviting, identifying, reflecting on, and genuinely considering) alternative points of view, particularly when they contrast with one's own. Another is the ability to initiate deliberate shifts from one's own perspective in order to consider alternative points of view (Moses & Shapiro, 1996; Shapiro, 1987; Shapiro & Moses, 1989, 2005). These skills will prove useful across instructional processes and over time in lifelong learning.

Second, we have emphasized that the family system is the most powerful communication network within which many of us will ever interact. Communication occurs within systems and should be addressed as such. Appreciating communication and communicators from the perspective of individual communication systems is helpful for understanding those we serve, other helpers, and ourselves.

Third, there is often strength in numbers, particularly when each person brings unique strengths and perspectives to the interdisciplinary team. Working effectively with interdisciplinary teams is consistent with the supervisory objective of achieving self-supervision and lifelong professional independence through collaboration and eventual consultative relationships with professional colleagues (J. L. Anderson, 1988; McCrea &

Brasseur, 2003). Such interdisciplinary interactions are conducive to and facilitative of the aspects of lifelong professional development—perspectives considered, dimensions of behavior conceptualized, possible solutions generated, and causal concepts. These interactions, and the aspects of professional development they generate, contribute to maintaining and improving professional (academic, clinical, and supervisory) problem-solving skills (Shapiro & Moses, 1989, 2005) within the different domains of knowledge—affective, behavioral, and cognitive.

Finally, multicultural sensitivity and understanding and openness to diversity provide but another opportunity to value people in their most dynamic forms, thus enabling us to learn about others and, therefrom, ourselves. Again, such lessons are not time bound and continue to contribute to our lifelong process of acquiring knowledge about communication and communicators within our global community.

Chapter Summary

The importance of clinicians as change agents within the clinical process was discussed in Chapter 11; the present chapter addressed the professional preparation of such persons who work with people who stutter and the process of lifelong learning. In addressing, "How are good clinicians made? Are they born or are they cultivated?" we emphasized five major points. First, professional preparation for clinicians who work with people who stutter must integrate experiences across academic, clinical, and supervisory processes, and must impact the affective, behavioral, and cognitive domains. Second, an explicit understanding of the academic, clinical, and supervisory processes enables clinicians to contribute meaningfully to and gain maximum benefit from the experience of professional preparation. Third, both specialization and globalization are important by-products of our expanding scope of practice within a diversified and instantaneously connected global community. Fourth, maintenance of clinical competence requires internalizing the desire to learn, committing to learning as a lifelong process, and understanding and maintaining parallels in the nature and process of professional development over time. Fifth, professional preparation and lifelong learning provide an opportunity for learners to become teachers and teachers to become learners across the interactive, dynamic journey of life.

Professional preparation of clinicians involves the academic, clinical, and supervisory processes, which are dynamically interrelated. The academic process is that which occurs within the classroom and has a significant impact on the clinical and supervisory processes. The clinical process is the interaction that occurs between the clinician and client and family members. Comprehensive areas of critical academic and clinical knowledge are outlined within the Guidelines for Practice in Stuttering Treatment (ASHA, 1995). Revised training standards that went into effect in 1993 continue to have significant implications for professional preparation (ASHA, 2005c, 2009a, 2009b). Models for clinician development must recognize that development of clinical competence is begun within professional preparation during the academic (student–professor interaction), clinical (client–clinician interaction), and supervisory (supervisee–supervisor interaction) processes, and is continued in renewal training, continued education, and self-study throughout one's career. One such model (Moses & Shapiro, 1996; Shapiro & Moses, 1989, 2005) was presented containing a series of developmental phases in how clinicians organize and interpret information relevant to clinical planning, implementation, and problem solving. These phases address aspects of clinician development in four areas of problem solving: orientation of perspective, dimensions of behavior conceptualized, possible solutions generated, and causal reasoning. The clinical process requires understanding, planning, observing, analyzing, and ultimately integrating all of the components inherent in the process.

The supervisory process refers to interactive forms of clinical teaching between a supervisor and supervisee, leading to improvement of the clinician's professional (technical and interpersonal) skills. Effective supervision is a distinct area of expertise, requiring at least 11 unique core areas of knowledge and skills (ASHA, 2008c; see also ASHA, 1985, for delineation of 13 tasks and related competencies). The continuum of supervision (J. L. Anderson, 1988; McCrea & Brasseur, 2003) emphasizes the importance of joint involvement and active participation of both the supervisee and supervisor in all phases of the supervisory process. The continuum is not time bound and thus presents a model of development across the career. It has three stages, each of which requires a different style of interaction—the evaluation–feedback stage (direct/active style), the transitional stage (collaborative style), and the self-supervision stage (consultative style). Parallel to the clinical process, the supervisory process requires understanding, planning, observing, analyzing, and integrating the dynamic components of supervision. Various avenues for specialized preparation and renewal training in the supervisory process are available.

There are many ways for clinicians to stay abreast of developments in the discipline of fluency disorders and to maximize the benefits of personal and professional interactions with colleagues far and wide. Based upon the academic, clinical, and supervisory processes of professional preparation, two such methods are specialization and globalization. A process is in place to designate speech–language pathologists as Board Recognized Fluency Specialists. To be considered, applicants must have 2 years of full-time clinical experience or its equivalent, the Certificate of Clinical Competence, 100 hours of postgraduate educational training in fluency disorders, 100 hours of guided clinical practice with people who stutter and their families under the supervision of a Board Recognized Fluency Specialist Mentor, and a portfolio of clinical work for review and approval. Opportunities to build professional alliances with international colleagues are available at both organizational and individual levels. Organizational opportunities include the Agreement for the Mutual Recognition of Professional Association Credentials, affiliation with international organizations (e.g., the International Fluency Association, the International Stuttering Association, and the International Cluttering Association), and participation in international meetings (on site and electronic). Individual opportunities for international affiliation were reviewed as limitless and rendering excitement, reward, wonder, and challenge.

The processes of professional preparation must set in motion a generative pattern of internally motivated, lifelong learning. In other words, maintenance of professional competence requires internalizing the desire to learn, committing to learning as a lifelong process, and understanding and maintaining parallels in the nature and process of our professional development over time.

Chapter Twelve Study Questions

1. This chapter discussed professional preparation and lifelong learning as a composite of necessary processes for the career speech–language pathologist. In what ways do you feel the academic, clinical, and supervisory processes are interrelated? How do the knowledge, skills, and competencies within each process impact one another? How do the knowledge, skills, tasks, and competencies within each process impact those of the other processes?

2. We discussed a variety of important documents—Guidelines for Practice in Stuttering Treatment (ASHA, 1995); Standards and Implementation Procedures for the Certificate of Clinical Competence in Speech–Language Pathology (ASHA, 2009a); Standards for Accreditation of Graduate Education Programs in Audiology and Speech–Language Pathology (ASHA, 2009b); and the position statement (ASHA 2008a), technical report (ASHA, 2008b), and knowledge and skills statement (ASHA, 2008c) for clinical supervision in speech–language pathology. How is the necessary knowledge within the affective, behavioral, and cognitive domains addressed within each document? Which areas of knowledge do you feel are most critical to establishing and maintaining professional competence? How might these documents prove useful to professional preparation and to lifelong learning?

3. The components of the clinical and supervisory processes include understanding, planning, observing, analyzing, and integrating the respective, dynamic components. What are the similarities and differences between the components of learning across the academic, clinical, and supervisory processes? What implications do these similarities and differences have for the processes of professional preparation and lifelong learning?

4. We reviewed a model of clinician development (Moses & Shapiro, 1996; Shapiro & Moses, 1989, 2005) that contains a series of developmental phases indicating how clinicians organize and interpret information relevant to clinical planning, implementation, and problem solving. Specifically, aspects of clinician development occur in four areas of problem solving: orientation of perspective, dimensions of behavior conceptualized, possible solutions generated, and causal reasoning. What are the similarities and differences between this model and the continuum of supervision presented by J. L. Anderson (1988)? What is the relevance of the four aspects of development to the academic, clinical, and supervisory processes? Furthermore, what is the relevance of the four aspects to professional preparation and lifelong learning?

5. In what ways are specialization and globalization related to the academic, clinical, and supervisory processes and to the affective, behavioral, and cognitive domains? How are specialization and globalization related to professional preparation and lifelong learning? What do you see as the advantages and disadvantages of specialization and globalization?

6. Eligibility requirements were outlined for the designation of Board Recognized Specialist in Fluency Disorders. Yet, the concept of specialization raises a number of significant questions. For example, how would you define *specialist*? What is specialization? What are the characteristics of specialization? How are such characteristics acquired? How are they maintained? Should such characteristics reflect the nature of who we are as people and as professionals (human *beings*), what we do (human *doings*), or some combination? What characteristics of specialization transcend the individual methods being employed in assessment and treatment? Are all those on the roster of Board Recognized Fluency Specialists really specialists? Are those not on the roster not necessarily specialists? Do your responses to these questions accord with the current procedures to become a Board Recognized Fluency Specialist? How do you think specialists in fluency disorders should be credentialed?

7. Globalization provides remarkable opportunities for those who wish to expand their knowledge of the world, the discipline of fluency disorders, and themselves both as people and as professionals through international travel and affiliation with international colleagues. Yet, I stated that "such experiences are not necessarily for everyone." Do you agree or disagree with this statement? What characteristics or qualifications do you recommend that a person have in order to explore such opportunities (i.e., characteristics that would increase the likelihood of a successful experience)? How might one systematically organize opportunities from local to global in order to diversify one's personal and professional experience, knowledge, and competence?

8. In *Three Cups of Tea: One Man's Mission to Promote Peace . . . One School at a Time* (Mortenson & Relin, 2006), Hali Aja gave Greg Mortenson essential advice. How does the advice Mr. Mortenson received in Pakistan relate to the academic, clinical, and supervisory processes; to the affective, behavioral, and cognitive domains; to becoming and being a clinician; and to you as a person?

9. Maintenance of professional competence requires internalizing the desire to learn, committing to learning as a lifelong process, and understanding and maintaining parallels in the nature and process of our professional development over time. What do these processes mean to you? For student clinicians, how are these processes being set in motion during your professional preparation? For professional speech–language pathologists, how did your professional preparation set in motion the processes that are necessary for maintenance of professional competence? What is your plan at the present time to ensure lifelong learning and maintenance of professional competence?

References

Adler, A. (1956). *The individual psychology of Alfred Adler* (H. L. Ansbacher & R. R. Ansbacher, Eds. and Trans.). New York: Harper & Row.

Adler, S. (1993). *Multicultural communication skills in the classroom.* Needham Heights, MA: Allyn & Bacon.

The age boom [Special issue]. (1997, March 9). *The New York Times Magazine,* pp. 14–78.

Ainsworth, S., & Fraser, J. (2008). *If your child stutters: A guide for parents* (Publication 11, 7th ed.). Memphis, TN: Stuttering Foundation of America.

Alm, P. A. (2004). Stuttering and the basal ganglia circuits: A critical review of possible relations. *Journal of Communication Disorders, 37,* 325–369.

Alm, P. A. (2005). *On the causal mechanisms of stuttering.* Unpublished doctoral dissertation, Lund University, Lund, Sweden.

Alm, P. A. (2007a). A new framework for understanding stuttering: The dual premotor model. In J. Au-Yeung & M. M. Leahy (Eds.), *Research, treatment, and self-help in fluency disorders: New horizons. Proceedings of the Fifth World Congress on Fluency Disorders* (pp. 77–83). Dublin: International Fluency Association.

Alm, P. A. (2007b, August). *The dual premotor model of stuttering and cluttering: A framework.* Paper presented at the 27th World Congress of the International Association of Logopedics and Phoniatrics, Copenhagen.

Ambrose, N. G. (2004, Spring). Theoretical perspectives on the cause of stuttering. *Contemporary Issues in Communication Science and Disorders, 31,* 80–91.

Ambrose, N. G., & Yairi, E. (1994). The development of awareness of stuttering in preschool children. *Journal of Fluency Disorders, 19,* 229–245.

Ambrose, N. G., & Yairi, E. (1999). Normative disfluency data for early childhood stuttering. *Journal of Speech, Language, and Hearing Research, 42,* 895–909.

Ambrose, N. G., & Yairi, E. (2002). The Tudor study: Data and ethics. *American Journal of Speech–Language Pathology, 11,* 190–203.

Ambrose, N. G., Yairi, E., & Cox, N. (1993). Genetic aspects of early childhood stuttering. *Journal of Speech and Hearing Research, 36,* 701–706.

American Psychiatric Association. (1994). *Diagnostic and statistical manual of mental disorders* (4th ed.). Washington, DC: Author.

American Speech and Hearing Association, Committee on Supervision in Speech Pathology and Audiology. (1978). Current status of supervision of speech–language pathology and audiology [Special report]. *Asha, 20,* 478–486.

American Speech-Language-Hearing Association, Committee on Supervision in Speech–Language Pathology and Audiology. (1985). Clinical supervision in speech–language pathology and audiology [Position statement]. *Asha, 27,* 57–60.

American Speech-Language-Hearing Association, Committee on the Status of Racial Minorities. (1991, May). Multicultural action agenda 2000. *Asha, 33,* 39–41.

American Speech-Language-Hearing Association. (1995). *Guidelines for practice in stuttering treatment.* Available from www.asha.org/policy.

American Speech-Language-Hearing Association. (2004a). *Evidence-based practice in communication disorders: An introduction* [Technical Report]. Available from www.asha.org/policy.

American Speech-Language-Hearing Association. (2004b). *Knowledge and skills needed by speech-language pathologists and audiologists to provide culturally and linguistically appropriate services* [Knowledge and Skills]. Available from www.asha.org/policy.

American Speech-Language-Hearing Association. (2004c). *Preferred practice patterns for the profession of speech–language pathology* [Preferred Practice Patterns]. Available from www.asha.org/policy.

American Speech-Language-Hearing Association. (2005a). *Cultural competence* [Issues in Ethics]. Available from www.asha.org/policy.

American Speech-Language-Hearing Association. (2005b). *Evidence-based practice in communication disorders* [Position statement]. Available from www.asha.org/policy.

American Speech-Language-Hearing Association. (2005c). *Quality indicators for professional service programs in audiology and speech–language pathology* [Standards/Quality Indicators]. Available from www.asha.org/policy.

American Speech-Language-Hearing Association. (2006). *Communication: The human connection* [DVD]. Rockville, MD: Author.

American Speech-Language-Hearing Association. (2007a). *Childhood apraxia of speech* [Position Statement]. Available from www.asha.org/policy.

American Speech-Language-Hearing Association. (2007b). *Childhood apraxia of speech* [Technical Report]. Available from www.asha.org/policy.

American Speech-Language-Hearing Association. (2007c, November 6). Iowa stuttering study settlement. *The ASHA Leader*, p. 8.

American Speech-Language-Hearing Association. (2007d). *Scope of practice in speech–language pathology* [Scope of Practice]. Available from www.asha.org/policy.

American Speech-Language-Hearing Association. (2008a). *Clinical supervision in speech–language pathology* [Position Statement]. Available from www.asha.org/policy.

American Speech-Language-Hearing Association. (2008b). *Clinical supervision in speech-language pathology* [Technical Report]. Available from www.asha.org/policy.

American Speech-Language-Hearing Association. (2008c). *Knowledge and skills needed by speech–language pathologists providing clinical supervision* [Knowledge and Skills]. Available from www.asha.org/policy.

American Speech-Language-Hearing Association. (2009a). *Standards and implementation procedures for the Certificate of Clinical Competence in Speech–Language Pathology* [2005 Standards for the CCC]. Available from www.asha.org/policy.

American Speech-Language-Hearing Association. (2009b). *Standards for accreditation of graduate education programs in audiology and speech–language pathology* [Chapter 3 in the 2009 Council for Academic Accreditation Manual]. Available from www.asha.org/policy.

American Speech-Language-Hearing Association. (2009c). *Strategic pathway to excellence* [ASHA's Strategic Plan]. Available from www.asha.org/policy.

American Speech-Language-Hearing Association. (2010). Code of ethics [Ethics]. Available from www.asha.org/policy.

Americans with Disabilities Amendments Act of 2008, 42 U.S.C. § 12101 *et seq.*

Amerman, J. D., & Parnell, M. M. (1992). Speech timing strategies in elderly adults. *Journal of Phonetics, 20,* 65–76.

Anderson, D. (1995). Historical perceptions of stuttering as reflected in the arts. In C. W. Starkweather & H. F. M. Peters (Eds.), *Stuttering: Proceedings of the First World Congress on Fluency Disorders, Munich* (Vol. 2, pp. 567–570). Nijmegen, The Netherlands: University of Nijmegen Press.

Anderson, J. D., & Conture, E. G. (2000). Language abilities of children who stutter: A preliminary study. *Journal of Fluency Disorders, 25,* 283–304.

Anderson, J. D., Pellowski, M. W., & Conture, E. G. (2005). Childhood stuttering and dissociations across linguistic domains. *Journal of Fluency Disorders, 30*(3), 219–253.

Anderson, J. D., Pellowski, M. W., Conture, E. G., & Kelly, E. M. (2003). Temperamental characteristics of young children who stutter. *Journal of Speech, Language and Hearing Research, 46,* 1221–1233.

Anderson, J. L. (1988). *The supervisory process in speech–language pathology and audiology.* Boston: Little, Brown/College-Hill.

Anderson, N. B., Lee-Wilkerson, D., & Chabon, S. (1995). *Preschool language disorders.* Rockville, MD: National Student Speech Language Hearing Association.

Andrews, G. (1984). Epidemiology of stuttering. In R. F. Curlee & W. H. Perkins (Eds.), *Nature and treatment of stuttering: New directions* (pp. 1–12). San Diego, CA: College-Hill.

Andrews, G., Craig, A., Feyer, A., Hoddinott, S., Howie, P., & Neilson, M. (1983). Stuttering: A review of research findings and theories circa 1982. *Journal of Speech and Hearing Disorders, 48*, 226–246.

Andrews, G., & Cutler, J. (1974). Stuttering therapy: The relation between changes in symptom level and attitudes. *Journal of Speech and Hearing Disorders, 39*, 312–319.

Andrews, G., Guitar, B., & Howie, P. (1980). Meta-analysis of the effects of stuttering treatment. *Journal of Speech and Hearing Disorders, 45*, 287–307.

Andrews, G., & Ingham, R. J. (1971). Stuttering: Considerations in the evaluation of treatment. *British Journal of Disorders of Communication, 6*, 129–138.

Andrews, G., Morris-Yates, A., Howie, P., & Martin, N. G. (1991). Genetic factors in stuttering confirmed. *Archives of General Psychiatry, 48*, 1034–1035.

Andrews, J. R., & Andrews, M. A. (1990). *Family based treatment in communicative disorders: A systemic approach.* Sandwich, IL: Janelle.

Andrews, J. R., & Andrews, M. A. (2000). *Family-based treatment in communicative disorders: A systemic approach* (2nd ed.). DeKalb, IL: Janelle.

Andrews, M. L. (2006). *Manual of voice treatment: Pediatrics through geriatrics* (3rd ed.). Clifton Park, NY: Thomson/Delmar Learning.

Andy, O. J., & Bhatnagar, S. C. (1992). Stuttering acquired from subcortical pathologies and its alleviation from thalamic perturbation. *Brain and Language, 42*, 385–401.

Annett, M. M. (2001, July 24). Article alleges 1939 study taught children to stutter. *The ASHA Leader*, pp. 1, 17.

Argeropoulos, J. (1974). Self-concept and the client–clinician relationship. In L. L. Emerick & S. B. Hood (Eds.), *The client–clinician relationship: Essays on interpersonal sensitivity in the therapeutic transaction* (pp. 84–91). Springfield, IL: Thomas.

Armson, J., & Kiefte, M. (2008). The effect of SpeechEasy on stuttering frequency, speech rate, and speech naturalness. *Journal of Fluency Disorders, 33*(2), 120–134.

Arndt, J., & Healey, E. C. (2001). Concomitant disorders in school-age children who stutter. *Language, Speech, and Hearing Services in Schools, 32*, 68–78.

Arnold, G. E. (1965). Physiology and pathology of speech and language. In R. Luchsinger & G. E. Arnold (Eds.), *Voice–speech–language, clinical communicology: Its physiology and pathology* (pp. 335–791). Belmont, CA: Wadsworth.

Aronson, A. E. (1973). *Psychogenic voice disorders: An interdisciplinary approach to detection, diagnosis, and therapy.* Philadelphia: W. B. Saunders.

Aronson, A. E., & Bless, D. M. (2009). *Clinical voice disorders* (4th ed.) New York: Thieme.

Arthur, G. (1952). *Arthur adaptation of the Leiter International Performance Scale.* Los Angeles: Western Psychological Services.

Association Parole Bégaiement. (2005). *Bégaiement: Intervention preventive précoce chez le jeune enfant.* Paris: Association Parole Bégaiement.

Attanasio, J. S. (1987a). A case of late-onset or acquired stuttering in adult life. *Journal of Fluency Disorders, 12*, 287–290.

Attanasio, J. S. (1987b). The dodo was Lewis Carroll, you see: Reflections and speculations. *Journal of Fluency Disorders, 12*, 107–118.

Attanasio, J. S. (1997). Was Moses a person who stuttered? Perhaps not. *Journal of Fluency Disorders, 22*, 65–68.

Au-Yeung, J., Howell, P., Davis, S., Charles, N., & Sackin, S. (2000). UCL survey of bilingualism and stuttering. In H.-G. Bosshardt, J. S. Yaruss, & H. F. M. Peters (Eds.), *Fluency disorders: Theory, research, treatment and self-help. Proceedings of the Third World Congress on Fluency Disorders* (pp. 129–132). Nijmegen, The Netherlands: Nijmegen University Press.

Backus, O. (1938). Incidence of stuttering among the deaf. *Annals of Otology, Rhinology, and Laryngology, 47*, 632–635.

Battle, D. E. (2002a). Communication disorders in a multicultural society. In D. E. Battle (Ed.), *Communication disorders in multicultural populations* (3rd ed., pp. 3–31). Woburn, MA: Butterworth-Heinemann.

Battle, D. E. (Ed.). (2002b). *Communication disorders in multicultural populations* (3rd ed.). Woburn, MA: Butterworth-Heinemann.

Battle, D. E. (2002c). Introduction. In D. E. Battle (Ed.), *Communication disorders in multicultural populations* (3rd ed., pp. xiii–xx). Woburn, MA: Butterworth-Heinemann.

Battle, D. E. (2005). *Interview with Delores Battle, PhD, President of the American Speech-Language-Hearing Association (ASHA)* [Diversity and Related Issues in Communication Disorders]. Available from http://www.speechpathology.com/interview/interview_detail.asp?interview_id=1052.

Baumgartner, J. M. (1999). Acquired psychogenic stuttering. In R. F. Curlee (Ed.), *Stuttering and related disorders of fluency* (2nd ed., pp. 269–288). New York: Thieme.

Benecken, J. (1995). On the nature and psychological relevance of a stigma: The "stutterer": Or what happens when "Grace Fails"? In C. W. Starkweather & H. F. M. Peters (Eds.), *Stuttering: Proceedings of the First World Congress on Fluency Disorders* (Vol. 2, pp. 548–550). Nijmegen, The Netherlands: University of Nijmegen Press.

Bengtson, V. L., & Schaie, K. W. (1989). Preface. In V. L. Bengtson & K. W. Schaie (Eds.), *The course of later life: Research and reflections* (pp. vii–xi). New York: Springer.

Benjamin, B. J. (1988). Changes in speech production and linguistic behavior with aging. In B. B. Shadden (Ed.), *Communication behavior and aging: A sourcebook for clinicians* (pp. 162–181). Baltimore: Williams & Wilkins.

Benjamin, B. J. (1997). Speech production of normally aging adults. *Seminars in Speech and Language, 18*(2), 135–141.

Bennett, E. M. (2006). *Working with people who stutter: A lifespan approach.* Upper Saddle River, NJ: Pearson Education/Merrill-Prentice Hall.

Bernstein Ratner, N. (1995). Treating the child who stutters with concomitant language or phonological impairment. *Language, Speech, and Hearing Services in Schools, 26,* 180–186.

Bernstein Ratner, N. (1997). Stuttering: A psycholinguistic perspective. In R. F. Curlee & G. M. Siegel (Eds.), *Nature and treatment of stuttering: New directions* (2nd ed., pp. 99–127). Needham Heights, MA: Allyn & Bacon.

Bernstein Ratner, N. (2001, August). Coordinator's corner. *Fluency and Fluency Disorders, 11*(3), 1–4.

Bernstein Ratner, N. (2004a, January). Caregiver–child interactions and their impact on children's fluency: Implications for treatment. *Language, Speech, and Hearing Services in Schools, 35,* 46–56.

Bernstein Ratner, N. (2004b). Fluency and stuttering in bilingual children. In B. Goldstein (Ed.), *Bilingual language development and disorders in Spanish–English speakers* (pp. 287–308). Baltimore: Brookes.

Bernstein Ratner, N. (2005a). Evidence-based practice in stuttering: Some questions to consider. *Journal of Fluency Disorders, 30,* 163–188.

Bernstein Ratner, N. (2005b). Stuttering and concomitant problems. In R. Lees & C. Stark (Eds.), *The treatment of stuttering in the young school-aged child* (pp. 163–177). Chichester, England: Whurr/Wiley.

Bernstein Ratner, N. (2006). Evidence-based practice: An examination of its ramifications for the practice of speech–language pathology. *Language, Speech, and Hearing Services in Schools, 37,* 257–267.

Bernstein Ratner, N., & Benitez, M. (1985). Linguistic analysis of a bilingual stutterer. *Journal of Fluency Disorders, 10,* 211–219.

Bernstein Ratner, N., & Guitar, B. (2006). Treatment of very early stuttering and parent-administered therapy: The state of the art. In N. Bernstein Ratner & J. Tetnowski (Eds.), *Current issues in stuttering research and practice* (pp. 99–124). Mahwah, NJ: Erlbaum.

Bernstein Ratner, N., & Healey, E. C. (Eds.). (1999). *Stuttering research and practice: Bridging the gap.* Mahwah, NJ: Erlbaum.

Bernstein Ratner, N., & Tetnowski, J. (Eds.). (2006). *Current issues in stuttering research and practice.* Mahwah, NJ: Erlbaum.

Beukelman, D. R. (1986). The transition from graduate student to speech–language pathologist in a hospital setting. *National Student Speech Language Hearing Association Journal, 14,* 5–10.

Bezemer, M., Bouwen, J., & Winkelman, C. (2006). *Stotteren: Van theorie naar therapie*. Bussum, The Netherlands: Uitgeverij Coutinho BV.

Bianco, R. (2003, February 28). Children lose a quiet, honest friend. *USA Today*, p. 5E.

Bjerkan, B. (1980). Word fragmentations and repetitions in the spontaneous speech of 2–6-yr-old children. *Journal of Fluency Disorders, 5*, 137–148.

Blanton, S. (1931). Stuttering. *Mental Hygiene, 15*, 271–282.

Blomgren, M., Roy, N., Callister, T., & Merrill, R. M. (2005). Intensive stuttering modification therapy: A multidimensional assessment of treatment outcomes. *Journal of Speech, Language, and Hearing Research, 48*, 509–523.

Blood, G. W. (1995a). A behavioral-cognitive therapy program for adults who stutter: Computers and counseling. *Journal of Communication Disorders, 28*, 165–180.

Blood, G. W. (1995b). POWER2: Relapse management with adolescents who stutter. *Language, Speech, and Hearing Services in Schools, 26*, 169–179.

Blood, G. W. (2003). *The PowerR Game: Managing stuttering*. Memphis, TN: Stuttering Foundation of America.

Blood, G. W., & Blood, I. M. (2004, Spring). Bullying in adolescents who stutter: Communicative competence and self-esteem. *Contemporary Issues in Communication Sciences and Disorders, 31*, 69–79.

Blood, G. W., Blood, I., Kreiger, J., O'Conner, S., & Qualls, C. D. (2009). Double jeopardy for children who stutter: Race and coexisting disorders. *Communication Disorders Quarterly, 30*(3), 131–141.

Blood, G. W., Blood, I. M., McCarthy, J., Tellis, G., & Gabel, R. (2001). An analysis of verbal response patterns of Charles Van Riper during stuttering modification therapy. *Journal of Fluency Disorders, 26*(2), 129–147.

Blood, G. W., Blood, I. M., Tellis, G., & Gabel, R. (2001). Communication apprehension and self-perceived communication competence in adolescents who stutter. *Journal of Fluency Disorders, 26*(3), 161–178.

Blood, G. W., Blood, I. M., Tellis, G., & Gabel, R. (2003). A preliminary study of self-esteem, stigma, and disclosure in adolescents who stutter. *Journal of Fluency Disorders, 28*(2), 143–159.

Blood, G. W., Ridenour, V. J., Qualls, C. D., & Hammer, C. S. (2003). Co-occurring disorders in children who stutter. *Journal of Communication Disorders, 36*, 427–449.

Blood, G. W., & Seider, R. (1981). The concomitant problems of young stutterers. *Journal of Speech and Hearing Disorders, 46*, 31–33.

Bloodstein, O. (1958). Stuttering as an anticipatory struggle reaction. In J. Eisenson (Ed.), *Stuttering: A symposium* (pp. 1–69). New York: Harper & Row.

Bloodstein, O. (1960a). The development of stuttering: I. Changes in nine basic features. *Journal of Speech and Hearing Disorders, 25*, 219–237.

Bloodstein, O. (1960b). The development of stuttering: II. Developmental features. *Journal of Speech and Hearing Disorders, 25*, 366–376.

Bloodstein, O. (1961). Stuttering in families of adopted stutterers. *Journal of Speech and Hearing Disorders, 26*, 395–396.

Bloodstein, O. (1975). Stuttering as tension and fragmentation. In J. Eisenson (Ed.), *Stuttering: A second symposium* (pp. 1–95). New York: Harper & Row.

Bloodstein, O. (1981). *A handbook on stuttering* (3rd ed.). Chicago: National Easter Seal Society.

Bloodstein, O. (1984). Stuttering as an anticipatory struggle disorder. In R. F. Curlee & W. H. Perkins (Eds.), *Nature and treatment of stuttering: New directions* (pp. 171–186). San Diego, CA: College-Hill.

Bloodstein, O. (1986). Semantics and beliefs. In G. H. Shames & H. Rubin (Eds.), *Stuttering then and now* (pp. 130–139). Columbus, OH: Merrill.

Bloodstein, O. (1988). Verification of stuttering in a suspected malingerer. *Journal of Fluency Disorders, 13*, 83–88.

Bloodstein, O. (1990). On pluttering, skivering, and floggering: A commentary. *Journal of Speech and Hearing Disorders, 55*, 392–393.

Bloodstein, O. (1993). *Stuttering: The search for a cause and cure*. Needham Heights, MA: Allyn & Bacon.

Bloodstein, O. (1995). *A handbook on stuttering* (5th ed.). San Diego, CA: Singular.

Bloodstein, O. (2006). Some empirical observations about early stuttering: A possible link to language development. *Journal of Communication Disorders, 39*, 185–191.

Bloodstein, O., & Bernstein Ratner, N. (2008). *A handbook on stuttering* (6th ed.). Clifton Park, NY: Thomson/Delmar Learning.

Bloom, C., & Cooperman, D. K. (1999). *Synergistic stuttering therapy: A holistic approach*. Woburn, MA: Butterworth-Heinemann.

Bluemel, C. S. (1932). Primary and secondary stammering. *Quarterly Journal of Speech, 18*, 187–200.

Bluemel, C. S. (1935). *Stammering and allied disorders*. New York: Macmillan.

Bluemel, C. S. (1957). *The riddle of stuttering*. Danville, IL: Interstate Publishing.

Blumberg, A. (1980). *Supervisors and teachers: A private cold war* (2nd ed.). Berkeley, CA: McCutchan.

Boberg, E. (1981). Maintenance of fluency: An experimental program. In E. Boberg (Ed.), *Maintenance of fluency: Proceedings of the Banff Conference* (pp. 71–112). New York: Elsevier.

Boberg, E. (2006). Behavioral transfer and maintenance programs for adolescent and adult stutterers. In J. Fraser (Ed.), *Stuttering therapy: Transfer and maintenance* (Publication 19, 2nd ed., pp. 37–56). Memphis, TN: Stuttering Foundation of America.

Boberg, E., & Kully, D. (1985). *Comprehensive stuttering treatment program*. San Diego, CA: College-Hill.

Boberg, E., & Kully, D. (1994). Long term results of an intensive treatment program for adults and adolescents who stutter. *Journal of Speech and Hearing Research, 37*, 1050–1059.

Boberg, E., Yeudall, L. T., Schopflocher, D., & Bo-Lassen, P. (1983). The effect of an intensive behavioral program on the distribution of EEG alpha power in stutterers during processing of verbal and visuospatial information. *Journal of Fluency Disorders, 8*, 245–263.

Bobrick, B. (1996). *Knotted tongues: Stuttering in history and the quest for a cure*. New York: Kodansha America/Simon & Schuster.

Boey, R. A., Wuyts, F. L., Van de Heyning, P. H., De Bodt, M. S., & Heylen, L. (2007). Characteristics of stuttering-like disfluencies in Dutch-speaking children. *Journal of Fluency Disorders, 32*, 310–329.

Boone, D. R., McFarlane, S. C., Von Berg, S. L., & Zraick, R. I. (2010). *The voice and voice therapy* (8th ed.). Boston: Pearson Education/Allyn & Bacon.

Boone, D. R., & Prescott, T. E. (1972). Content and sequence analysis of speech and hearing therapy. *Asha, 14*, 58–62.

Bothe, A. K., Davidow, J. H., Bramlett, R. E., & Ingham, R. J. (2006). Stuttering treatment research 1970–2005: I. Systematic review incorporating trial quality assessment of behavioral, cognitive, and related approaches. *American Journal of Speech–Language Pathology, 15*, 321–341.

Bothe, A. K., Ingham, R. J., & Ingham, J. C. (2010). The roles of evidence and other information in stuttering treatment. In B. Guitar & R. J. McCauley (Eds.), *Treatment of stuttering: Established and emerging interventions* (pp. 343–354). Philadelphia: Lippincott/Williams & Wilkins.

Botterill, W., & Cook, F. (1987). Personal construct theory and the treatment of adolescent dysfluency. In L. Rustin, H. Purser, & D. Rowley (Eds.), *Progress in the treatment of fluency disorders* (pp. 147–165). London: Taylor & Francis.

Botterill, W., & Kelman, E. (2010). Palin parent–child interaction. In B. Guitar & R. J. McCauley (Eds.), *Treatment of stuttering: Established and emerging interventions* (pp. 63–90). Philadelphia: Lippincott/Williams & Wilkins.

Bowen, M. (1996). Theory in the practice of psychotherapy. In P. J. Guerin, Jr. (Ed.), *Family therapy: Theory and practice* (pp. 42–90). Lake Worth, FL: Gardner.

Bradley, M. J. (2003). *Yes, your teen is crazy! Loving your kid without losing your mind*. Gig Harbor, WA: Harbor Press.

Brady, J. P. (1991). The pharmacology of stuttering: A critical review. *American Journal of Psychiatry, 148*(10), 1309–1316.

Brady, J. P. (1998). Drug-induced stuttering: A review of the literature. *Journal of Clinical Psychopharmacology, 18*(1), 50–54.

Braun, A. R., Varga, M., Stager, S., Schulz, G., Selbie, S., Maisog, J. M., et al. (1997). Altered patterns of cerebral activity during speech and language production in developmental stuttering. *Brain, 120*, 761–784.

Brawner, B. F. (2005). *Diversity.* Unpublished manuscript. Cullowhee, NC: Western Carolina University.

Breitenfeldt, D. H., & Lorenz, D. R. (1989). *Successful stuttering management program.* Cheney, WA: Eastern Washington University School of Health Sciences.

Brill, A. (1923). Speech disturbances in nervous and mental diseases. *Quarterly Journal of Speech Education, 9*, 129–135.

Brin, M. F., Stewart, C., Blitzer, A., & Diamond, B. (1994). Laryngeal botulinum toxin injections for disabling stuttering in adults. *Neurology, 44*, 2262–2266.

British Broadcasting Corporation. (1989). *John's not mad: Tourette's Syndrome* (Videocassette No. 7355: Films for the Humanities and Sciences). New York: BBC Worldwide.

British Broadcasting Corporation. (2002). *The Boy Can't Help It: Living with Tourette's Syndrome* (Videocassette No. RC375.B69: Films for the Humanities and Sciences). New York: BBC Worldwide.

Brown, S., Ingham, R. J., Ingham, J. C., Laird, A. R., & Fox, P. T. (2005). Stuttered and fluent speech production: An ALE meta-analysis of functional neuroimaging studies. *Human Brain Mapping, 25*, 105–117.

Brundage, S. B., Bothe, A. K., Lengeling, A. N., & Evans, J. J. (2006). Comparing judgments of stuttering made by students, clinicians, and highly experienced judges. *Journal of Fluency Disorders, 31*, 271–283.

Brutten, G. J. (1975). Stuttering: Topography, assessment, and behavior-change strategies. In J. Eisenson (Ed.), *Stuttering: A second symposium* (pp. 199–262). New York: Harper & Row.

Brutten, G. J. (Ed.). (1993). Proceedings of the NIDCD Workshop on Treatment Efficacy Research in Stuttering. *Journal of Fluency Disorders, 18*, 121–361.

Brutten, G. J., & Shoemaker, D. J. (1971). A two-factor learning theory of stuttering. In L. E. Travis (Ed.), *Handbook of speech pathology and audiology* (pp. 1035–1072). Englewood Cliffs, NJ: Prentice Hall.

Bruun, R. D., & Bruun, B. (1994). *A mind of its own. Tourette's Syndrome: A story and a guide.* New York: Oxford University Press.

Bunning, K. (2004). *Speech and language therapy intervention: Frameworks and processes.* London: Whurr.

Bushey, T., & Martin, R. (1988). Stuttering in children's literature. *Language, Speech, and Hearing Services in Schools, 19*, 235–250.

Butcher, J. N., Dahlstrom, W. G., Graham, J. R., Tellegen, A., & Kaemmer, B. (1989). *Minnesota multiphasic personality inventory* (2nd ed.). Bloomington, MN: NCS Pearson.

Byrd, C. T., & Gillam, R. B. (2011). Fluency disorders. In R. B. Gillam, T. P. Marquardt, & F. N. Martin (Eds.), *Communication sciences and disorders: From science to clinical practice* (2nd ed., pp. 153–180). Sudbury, MA: Jones and Bartlett.

Byrd, C. T., Wolk, L., & Davis, B. L. (2007). Role of phonology in childhood stuttering and its treatment. In E. G. Conture & R. F. Curlee (Eds.), *Stuttering and related disorders of fluency* (3rd ed., 168–182). New York: Thieme.

Byrne, A., Byrne, M. K., & Zibin, T. O. (1993). Transient neurogenic stuttering. *International Journal of Eating Disorders, 14*(4), 511–514.

Caldwell, K., Atwal, A., Copp, G., Brett-Richards, M., & Coleman, K. (2006). Preparing for practice: How well are practitioners prepared for teamwork. *British Journal of Nursing, 15*(22), 1250–1254.

Calvert, D. R., & Silverman, S. R. (1983). *Speech and deafness* (Rev. ed.). Washington, DC: Alexander Graham Bell Association for the Deaf.

Camarata, S. M. (1989). Final consonant repetition: A linguistic perspective. *Journal of Speech and Hearing Disorders, 54*, 159–162.

Canter, G. J. (1971). Observations on neurogenic stuttering: A contribution to differential diagnosis. *British Journal of Disorders of Communication, 6*(2), 139–143.

Cantwell, D., & Baker, L. (1985). Psychiatric and learning disorders with speech and language disorders: A descriptive analysis. *Advances in Learning and Behavioral Disabilities, 2*, 29–47.

Carkhuff, R. R. (1969a). *Helping and human relations: A primer for lay and professional helpers* (Vol. 1). New York: Holt, Rinehart & Winston.

Carkhuff, R. R. (1969b). *Helping and human relations: A primer for lay and professional helpers* (Vol. 2). New York: Holt, Rinehart & Winston.

Carlisle, J. A. (1985). *Tangled tongue: Living with a stutter.* Toronto: University of Toronto Press.

Carter, B., & McGoldrick, M. (Eds.). (2005). *The expanded family life cycle: Individual, family, and social perspectives* (3rd ed.). Boston: Allyn & Bacon.

Carter, E. A., & Orfanidis, M. M. (1996). Family therapy with one person and the family therapist's own family. In P. J. Guerin, Jr. (Ed.), *Family therapy: Theory and practice* (pp. 193–219). Lake Worth, FL: Gardner.

Cartwright, B. Y., Daniels, J., & Zhang, S. (2008, Summer). Assessing multicultural competence: Perceived versus demonstrated performance—Innovations in multicultural research. *Journal of Counseling and Development, 86,* 318–322.

Caruso, A. J. (2002, Spring). Editor's page. *Contemporary Issues in Communication Science and Disorder, 29,* 4.

Caruso, A. J., Max, L., & McClowry, M. T. (1999). Perspectives on stuttering as a motor speech disorder. In A. J. Caruso & E. A. Strand (Eds.), *Clinical management of motor speech disorders in children* (pp. 319–344). New York: Thieme.

Caruso, A. J., McClowry, M. T., & Max, L. (1997). Age-related effects on speech fluency. *Seminars in Speech and Language, 18*(2), 171–180.

Casey, P. L., Smith, K. J., & Ulrich, S. R. (1988). *Self-supervision: A career tool for audiologists and speech–language pathologists.* Rockville, MD: National Student Speech Language Hearing Association.

Cather, W. (1992). *O Pioneers!* New York: Vintage Books/Random House.

Centeno, J. G., Anderson, R. T., & Obler, L. K. (Eds.). (2007). *Communication disorders in Spanish speakers: Theoretical, research, and clinical aspects.* Clevedon, England: Multicultural Matters.

Chang, S.-E., Erickson, K. I., Ambrose, N. G., Hasegawa-Johnson, M. A., & Ludlow, C. L. (2008). Brain anatomy differences in childhood stuttering. *NeuroImage, 39,* 1333–1344.

Clark, R. M. (1964). Our enterprising predecessors and Charles Sydney Bluemel. *Asha, 6,* 107–114.

Clark, R. M., & Murray, F. P. (1965). Alterations in self-concept: A barometer of progress in individuals undergoing therapy for stuttering. In D. A. Barbara (Ed.), *New directions in stuttering: Theory and practice* (pp. 131–158). Springfield, IL: Thomas.

Coan, P. M. (1997). *Ellis Island interviews: Immigrants tell their own stories in their own words.* New York: Falls River Press.

Cogan, M. L. (1973). *Clinical supervision.* Boston: Houghton Mifflin.

Colburn, N., & Mysak, E. D. (1982a). Developmental disfluency and emerging grammar I. Disfluency characteristics in early syntactic utterances. *Journal of Speech and Hearing Research, 25,* 414–420.

Colburn, N., & Mysak, E. D. (1982b). Developmental disfluency and emerging grammar II. Co-occurrence of disfluency with specified semantic-syntactic structures. *Journal of Speech and Hearing Research, 25,* 421–427.

Cole, L. (1989). E pluribus pluribus: Multicultural imperatives for the 1990s and beyond. *Asha, 31*(9), 65–70.

Cole, L. (1992, May). We're serious. *Asha, 34,* 38–39.

Colligan, N. (1989, December). Recognizing Tourette Syndrome in the classroom. *School Nurse* (Brochure available from Tourette Syndrome Association, 42–40 Bell Blvd., Bayside, NY 11361).

Comings, D. E. (1995). Tourette's syndrome: A behavioral spectrum disorder. In W. J. Weiner & A. E. Lang (Eds.), *Behavioral neurology of movement disorders: Advances in Neurology Series* (Vol. 65, pp. 293–303). New York: Raven Press.

Condon, J. C. (1984). *With respect to the Japanese: A guide for Americans.* Yarmouth, ME: Intercultural Press.

Conture, E. G. (1990). Childhood stuttering: What is it and who does it? In J. A. Cooper (Ed.), *Research needs in stuttering: Roadblocks and future directions* (ASHA Report No. 18, pp. 2–14). Rockville, MD: American Speech-Language-Hearing Association.

Conture, E. G. (1997). Evaluating childhood stuttering. In R. F. Curlee & G. M. Siegel (Eds.), *Nature and treatment of stuttering: New directions* (2nd ed., pp. 239–256). Needham Heights, MA: Allyn & Bacon.

Conture, E. G. (2001). *Stuttering: Its nature, diagnosis, and treatment.* Needham Heights, MA: Allyn & Bacon.

Conture, E. G., & Curlee, R. F. (Eds.). (2007). *Stuttering and related disorders of fluency.* New York: Thieme.

Conture, E. G., & Fraser, J. (Eds.). (2007). *Stuttering and your child: Questions and answers* (Publication 22, 3rd ed.). Memphis, TN: Stuttering Foundation of America.

Conture, E. G., & Guitar, B. E. (1993). Evaluating efficacy of treatment of stuttering: School-age children. *Journal of Fluency Disorders, 18,* 253–287.

Conture, E. G., Louko, L. J., & Edwards, M. L. (1993). Simultaneously treating stuttering and disordered phonology in children: Experimental treatment, preliminary findings. *American Journal of Speech–Language Pathology, 2*(3), 72–81.

Cook, F., & Botterill, W. (2005). Family-based approach to therapy with primary school children: "Throwing the ball back." In R. Lees & C. Stark (Eds.), *The treatment of stuttering in the young school-aged child* (pp. 81–107). Chichester, England: Whurr.

Cool, L. C. (2005, May 17). Natalie's miracle. *Family Circle.* Available from www.familycircle.com.

Cooper, E. B. (1977). Controversies about stuttering therapy. *Journal of Fluency Disorders, 2,* 75–86.

Cooper, E. B. (1987a). The chronic perseverative stuttering syndrome: Incurable stuttering. *Journal of Fluency Disorders, 12,* 381–388.

Cooper, E. B. (1987b). The Cooper Personalized Fluency Control Therapy. In L. Rustin, H. Purser, & D. Rowley (Eds.), *Progress in the treatment of fluency disorders* (pp. 124–146). London: Taylor & Francis.

Cooper, E. B. (1990a). Stuttering nuggets from a perennially perplexed but persevering prospector. *The Clinical Connection, 4*(1), 1–4.

Cooper, E. B. (1990b). *Understanding stuttering: Information for parents* (Rev. ed.). Chicago: National Easter Seal Society.

Cooper, E. B. (1993a). Chronic perseverative stuttering syndrome: A harmful or helpful construct? *American Journal of Speech–Language Pathology, 2*(3), 11–15.

Cooper, E. B. (1993b). Chronic perseverative stuttering syndrome: Cooper responds to Ham. *American Journal of Speech–Language Pathology, 2*(3), 21–22.

Cooper, E. B. (1993c). Red herrings, dead horses, straw men, and blind alleys: Escaping the stuttering conundrum. *Journal of Fluency Disorders, 18,* 375–387.

Cooper, E. B. (1997). Fluency disorders. In T. A. Crowe (Ed.), *Applications of counseling in speech–language pathology and audiology* (pp. 145–166). Baltimore: Williams & Wilkins.

Cooper, E. B., & Cooper, C. S. (1985). Clinician attitudes toward stuttering: A decade of change (1973–1983). *Journal of Fluency Disorders, 10,* 19–33.

Cooper, E. B., & Cooper, C. S. (1993). Fluency disorders. In D. E. Battle (Ed.), *Communication disorders in multicultural populations* (pp. 189–211). Stoneham, MA: Andover Medical Publishers/Butterworth-Heinemann.

Cooper, E. B., & Cooper, C. S. (1995). Treating fluency disordered adolescents. *Journal of Communication Disorders, 28,* 125–142.

Cooper, E. B., & Cooper, C. S. (1996). Clinician attitudes towards stuttering: Two decades of change. *Journal of Fluency Disorders, 21,* 119–135.

Cooper, E. B., & Cooper, C. S. (2003). *Cooper personalized fluency control therapy for children* (3rd ed.). Austin, TX: PRO-ED.

Cooper, E. B., & Rustin, L. (1985). Clinician attitudes toward stuttering in the United States and Great Britain: A cross-cultural study. *Journal of Fluency Disorders, 10,* 1–17.

Corcoran, J. A., & Stewart, M. (1998). Stories of stuttering: A qualitative analysis of interview narratives. *Journal of Fluency Disorders, 23,* 247–264.

Corey, G. (2005). Theory and practice of counseling and psychotherapy (7th ed.). Belmont, CA: Brooks/Cole-Thomson Learning.

Coriat, I. H. (1928). Stammering: A psychoanalytic interpretation. *Nervous and Mental Disease Monographs, 47,* 1–68.

Corliss, R., & Lemonick, M. D. (2006). How to live to be 100. In H. Cox (Ed.), *Aging* (18th ed., 2006 Update, pp. 31–36). Dubuque, IA: McGraw-Hill/Dushkin.

Costello, J. M. (1980). Operant conditioning and the treatment of stuttering. In W. Perkins (Ed.), *Seminars in Speech, Language and Hearing* (pp. 311–325). New York: Thieme-Stratton.

Costello, J. M. (1983). Current behavioral treatments for children. In D. Prins & R. J. Ingham (Eds.), *Treatment of stuttering in early childhood: Methods and issues* (pp. 69–112). San Diego, CA: College-Hill.

Cox, M. D. (1986). The psychologically maladjusted stutterer. In K. O. St. Louis (Ed.), *The atypical stutterer: Principles and practices of rehabilitation* (pp. 93–122). Orlando, FL: Academic Press.

Cox, N. J. (1988). Molecular genetics: The key to the puzzle of stuttering? *Asha, 30*(4), 36–40.

Cox, N. J. (1993). Stuttering: A complex behavioral disorder for our times? *American Journal of Medical Genetics (Neuropsychiatric Genetics), 48*, 177–178.

Cox, N. J., & Yairi, E. (2000, November). *Genetics of stuttering: Insights and recent advances.* Paper presented at the annual meeting of the American Speech-Language-Hearing Association, Washington, DC.

Craig, A. (1998). Relapse following treatment for stuttering: A critical review and correlative data. *Journal of Fluency Disorders, 23*, 1–30.

Craig, A., & Andrews, G. (1985). The prediction and prevention of relapse in stuttering: The value of self-control techniques and locus of control measures. *Behavior Modification, 9*, 427–442.

Craig, A., Blumgart, E., & Tran, Y. (2009). The impact of stuttering on the quality of life in adults who stutter. *Journal of Fluency Disorders, 34*(2), 61–71.

Craig, A., & Hancock, K. (1995). Self-reported factors related to relapse following treatment for stuttering. *Australian Journal of Human Communication Disorders, 23*, 48–60.

Craig, A., Hancock, K., Tran, Y., & Craig, M. (2003). Anxiety levels in people who stutter: A randomized population study. *Journal of Speech, Language, and Hearing Research, 46*, 1197–1206.

Craig, A., & Tran, Y. (2005a). Epidemiology of stuttering. In R. Lees & C. Stark (Eds.), *The treatment of stuttering in the young school-aged child* (pp. 1–19). Chichester, England: Whurr/Wiley.

Craig., A., & Tran, Y. (2005b). The epidemiology of stuttering: The need for reliable estimates of prevalence and anxiety levels over the lifespan. *Advances in Speech Language Pathology, 7*, 41–46.

Crichton-Smith, I. (2002). Communicating in the real world: Accounts from people who stutter. *Journal of Fluency Disorders, 27*, 333–352.

Crowe, T. A., & Walton, J. H. (1981). Teacher attitudes toward stuttering. *Journal of Fluency Disorders, 6*, 163–174.

Culatta, R., & Goldberg, S. A. (1995). *Stuttering therapy: An integrated approach to theory and practice.* Needham Heights, MA: Allyn & Bacon.

Culatta, R., & Leeper, L. H. (1987). Disfluency in childhood: It's not always stuttering. *Journal of Childhood Communication Disorders, 10*(2), 95–106.

Culatta, R., & Leeper, L. H. (1988). Dysfluency isn't always stuttering. *Journal of Speech and Hearing Disorders, 53*, 486–488.

Culatta, R., & Leeper, L. H. (1989–1990). The differential diagnosis of disfluency. *National Student Speech Language Hearing Association Journal, 17*, 59–64.

Curlee, R. F. (1993). Preface. In R. F. Curlee (Ed.), *Stuttering and related disorders of fluency* (pp. xi–xiv). New York: Thieme.

Curlee, R. F. (2007). Identification and case selection guidelines for early childhood stuttering. In E. G. Conture & R. F. Curlee (Eds.), *Stuttering and related disorders of fluency* (pp. 3–22). New York: Thieme.

Curlee, R. F., & Perkins, W. H. (Eds.). (1984). *Nature and treatment of stuttering: New directions.* San Diego, CA: College-Hill.

Cykowski, M. D., Kochunov, P. V., Ingham, R. J., Ingham, J. C., Mangin, J.-F., Riviere, D., et al. (2007). *Cerebral cortex.* New York: Oxford University Press.

Dalton, P. (1987). Some developments in personal construct therapy with adults who stutter. In C. Levy (Ed.), *Stuttering therapies: Practical approaches* (pp. 61–70). London: Croom Helm.

Dalton, P. (1994). A personal construct approach to communication problems. In P. Dalton (Ed.), *Counseling people with communication problems* (pp. 15–27). London: Sage.

Dalton, P., & Hardcastle, W. J. (1989). *Disorders of fluency* (2nd ed.). London: Whurr.

Daly, D. A. (1986). The clutterer. In K. O. St. Louis (Ed.), *The atypical stutterer: Principles and practices of rehabilitation* (pp. 155–192). Orlando, FL: Academic Press.

Daly, D. A. (1988). A practitioner's view of stuttering. *Asha, 30*(4), 34–35.

Daly, D. A. (1992). Helping the clutterer: Therapy considerations. In F. L. Myers & K. O. St. Louis (Eds.), *Cluttering: A clinical perspective* (pp. 107–124). Kibworth, England: Far Communications.

Daly, D. A. (1993). Cluttering: Another fluency syndrome. In R. F. Curlee (Ed.), *Stuttering and related disorders of fluency* (pp. 179–204). New York: Thieme.

Daly, D. A. (1996). *The source for stuttering and cluttering*. Moline, IL: LinguiSystems.

Daly, D. A. (2006). Apraxia and stuttering/cluttering. *Perspectives on Fluency and Fluency Disorders, 16*(2), 7–10.

Daly, D. A. (2007). *Cluttering: Characteristics identified as diagnostically significant by 60 fluency experts*. Paper presented at the 10th International Stuttering Awareness Day Online Conference—Stuttering Awareness: Global Community, Local Activity. Available from http://www.mnsu.edu/comdis/isad10/papers/daly10/daly10.html.

Daly, D. A. (2008, July). *Strategies for identifying and working with difficult-to-treat cluttering clients*. Paper presented at the 8th Oxford Dysfluency Conference—Integrating the Evidence: Scientist, Clinician, and Client, Oxford, England.

Daly, D. A., & Burnett, M. L. (1999). Cluttering: Traditional views and perspectives. In R. F. Curlee (Ed.), *Stuttering and related disorders of fluency* (2nd ed., pp. 222–254). New York: Thieme.

Daly, D. A., Simon, C. A., & Burnett-Stolnack, M. (1995). Helping adolescents who stutter focus on fluency. *Language, Speech, and Hearing Services in Schools, 26*, 162–168.

Daniels, D. E., & Gabel, R. M. (2004). The impact of stuttering on identity construction. *Topics in Language Disorders, 24*(3), 200–215.

Daniels, D. E., Hagstrom, F., & Gabel, R. M. (2006). A qualitative study of how African American men who stutter attribute meaning to identity and life choices. *Journal of Fluency Disorders, 31*, 200–215.

Darley, F. L., Aronson, A. E., & Brown, J. R. (1975). *Motor speech disorders*. Philadelphia: Saunders.

Deal, J. L. (1982). Sudden onset of stuttering: A case report. *Journal of Speech and Hearing Disorders, 47*, 301–304.

Deal, J. L., & Doro, J. M. (1987). Episodic hysterical stuttering. *Journal of Speech and Hearing Disorders, 52*, 299–300.

De Buck, A. (1970). *Egyptian readingbook: Exercises and Middle Egyptian texts* (3rd ed.). Leiden, The Netherlands: Nederlands Instituut Voor Het Nabije Oosten.

Defloor, T., Van Borsel, J., & Curfs, L. (2000). Speech fluency in Prader-Willi syndrome. *Journal of Fluency Disorders, 25*, 85–98.

Dell, C. W. (1993). Treating school-age stutterers. In R. F. Curlee (Ed.), *Stuttering and related disorders of fluency* (pp. 45–67). New York: Thieme.

Dell, C. W. (2008). *Treating the school-age child who stutters: A guide for clinicians* (Publication 14, 2nd ed.). Memphis, TN: Stuttering Foundation of America.

Dempsey, G. L., & Granich, M. (1978). Hypno-behavioral therapy in the case of a traumatic stutterer: A case study. *International Journal of Clinical and Experimental Hypnosis, 26*, 125–133.

De Nil, L. F. (1999). Stuttering: A neurophysiological perspective. In N. Bernstein Ratner & E. C. Healey (Eds.), *Stuttering research and practice: Bridging the gap* (pp. 85–102). Mahwah, NJ: Erlbaum.

De Nil, L. F. (2007). *Neurogenic stuttering: So much we know, so much we still need to discover*. Paper presented at the 10th International Stuttering Awareness Day Online Conference—Stuttering

Awareness: Global Community, Local Activity. Available from http://www.mnsu.edu/comdis/isad10/papers/dunil10.html.

De Nil, L. F., Jokel, R., & Rochon, E. (2007). Etiology, symptomatology, and treatment of neurogenic stuttering. In E. G. Conture & R. F. Curlee (Eds.), *Stuttering and related disorders of fluency* (3rd ed., pp. 326–343). New York: Thieme.

De Nil, L. F., & Kroll, R. M. (2001). Searching for the neural basis of stuttering treatment outcome: Recent neuroimaging studies. *Clinical Linguistics and Phonetics, 15*(1 & 2), 163–168.

De Nil, L. F., & Sandor, P. (2008). *Stuttering and Tourette syndrome* [Brochure]. Memphis, TN: Stuttering Foundation of America.

Dewey, J. (2005). *My experience with cluttering.* Paper presented at the 8th International Stuttering Awareness Day Online Conference—Community Vision for Global Action. Available from http://www.mnsu.edu/comdis/isad8/papers/dewey8.html.

Diedrich, W. M. (1984). Cluttering: Its diagnosis. In H. Winitz (Ed.), *Treating articulation disorders* (pp. 307–323). Baltimore: University Park Press.

Diehl, C. F. (1958). *A compendium of research and theory on stuttering.* Springfield, IL: Thomas.

Dietrich, S., Jensen, K. H., & Williams, D. E. (2001). Effects of the label "stutterer" on student perceptions. *Journal of Fluency Disorders, 26,* 55–66.

DiLollo, A., & Manning, W. H. (2007). Counseling children who stutter and their parents. In E. G. Conture & R. F. Curlee (Eds.), *Stuttering and related disorders of fluency* (3rd ed., pp. 115–130). New York: Thieme.

DiLollo, A., Manning, W. H., & Neimeyer, R. A. (2003). Cognitive anxiety as a function of speaker role for fluent speakers and persons who stutter. *Journal of Fluency Disorders, 28*(3), 167–186.

DiLollo, A., Neimeyer, R. A., & Manning, W. H. (2002). A personal construct psychology view of relapse: Indications for a narrative therapy component to stuttering treatment. *Journal of Fluency Disorders, 27*(1), 19–42.

Dolby, N., & Rizvi, F. (Eds.). (2008). *Youth moves: Identities and education in global perspective.* New York: Routledge/Taylor & Francis Group.

Dollaghan, C. A. (2004). Evidence-based practice in communication disorders: What do we know, and when do we know it? *Journal of Communication Disorders, 37,* 391–400.

Donaher, J. (2006). Tourette syndrome and stuttering. *Perspectives on Fluency and Fluency Disorders, 16*(2), 5–6.

Donnan, G. A. (1979). Stuttering as a manifestation of stroke. *Medical Journal of Australia, 1*(2), 44–45.

Dorsey, M., & Guenther, R. K. (2000). Attitudes of professors and students toward college students who stutter. *Journal of Fluency Disorders, 25,* 77–83.

Douglass, E., & Quarrington, B. (1952). The differentiation of interiorized and exteriorized secondary stuttering. *Journal of Speech and Hearing Disorders, 17,* 377–385.

Dowling, S. (2001). *Supervision: Strategies for successful outcomes and productivity.* Needham Heights, MA: Allyn & Bacon/Pearson Education.

Downes, J. J., Sharp, H. M., Costall, B. M., Sagar, H. J., & Howe, J. (1993). Alternating fluency in Parkinson's disease. *Brain, 116,* 887–902.

Drayna, D. T. (1997). Genetic linkage studies of stuttering: Ready for prime time? *Journal of Fluency Disorders, 22,* 237–241.

Drayna, D. T. (2005, Fall). Newly discovered families give impetus to genetics research. *The Stuttering Foundation,* pp. 1, 12.

Drayna, D. T. (2006, Summer). New light on genetic factors. *The Stuttering Foundation,* p. 5.

Duchin, S. W., & Mysak, E. D. (1987). Disfluency and rate characteristics of young adult, middle-aged, and older males. *Journal of Communication Disorders, 20,* 245–257.

Duffy, J. R. (2005). *Motor speech disorders: Substrates, differential diagnosis, and management* (2nd ed.). St. Louis, MO: Elsevier/Mosby.

Dworkin, J. P., Culatta, R. A., Abkarian, G. G., & Meleca, R. J. (2002). Laryngeal anesthetization for the treatment of acquired disfluency: A case study. *Journal of Fluency Disorders, 27,* 215–226.

Dyer, J. (2001a, June 10). Ethics and orphans: The "Monster Study." *San Jose Mercury News.*

Dyer, J. (2001b, June 11). "Monster Experiment" taught orphans to stutter. *San Jose Mercury News*.

Education for All Handicapped Children Act of 1975, 20 U.S.C. § 1400 *et seq.* (1975).

Education for All Handicapped Children Act of 1975, 20 U.S.C. § 1400 *et seq.* (1975) (amended 1986).

Einarsdottir, J., & Ingham, R. J. (2005). Have disfluency-type measures contributed to the understanding and treatment of developmental stuttering? *American Journal of Speech–Language Pathology, 14,* 260–273.

Eisenson, J. (1958). A perseverative theory of stuttering. In J. Eisenson (Ed.), *Stuttering: A symposium* (pp. 223–271). New York: Harper & Row.

Eisenson, J. (1975). Stuttering as perseverative behavior. In J. Eisenson (Ed.), *Stuttering: A second symposium* (pp. 401–452). New York: Harper & Row.

Elders, D. (2006, April). Easter awakening: A husband who wouldn't give up and a family that never stopped praying. *Guideposts*, pp. 59–63.

Eliot, T. S. (1934). Choruses from "The Rock." In T. S. Eliot, *Collected poems: 1909–1935* (pp. 179–210). New York: Harcourt, Brace.

Emerick, L. L. (1966). Bibliotherapy for stutterers: Four case histories. *Quarterly Journal of Speech, 52*(1), 74–79.

Emerick, L. L. (1974a). Mea culpa: Failures with stutterers. In L. L. Emerick & S. B. Hood (Eds.), *The client–clinician relationship: Essays on interpersonal sensitivity in the therapeutic transaction* (pp. 109–115). Springfield, IL: Thomas.

Emerick, L. L. (1974b). Stuttering therapy: Dimensions of interpersonal sensitivity. In L. L. Emerick & S. B. Hood (Eds.), *The client–clinician relationship: Essays on interpersonal sensitivity in the therapeutic transaction* (pp. 92–102). Springfield, IL: Thomas.

Emerick, L. L., & Hood, S. B. (1974). Preface. In L. L. Emerick & S. B. Hood (Eds.), *The client–clinician relationship: Essays on interpersonal sensitivity in the therapeutic transaction* (pp. vii–viii). Springfield, IL: Thomas.

Emerson, R. W. (1876). *Nature—Addresses and lectures.* Boston: Houghton Mifflin/Riverside Press.

Epstein, N. B., & Baucom, D. H. (2002). *Enhanced cognitive-behavioral therapy for couples: A contextual approach.* Washington, DC: American Psychological Association.

Epstein, N. B., & Bishop, D. S. (1981). Problem-centered systems therapy of the family. In A. S. Gurman & D. P. Kniskern (Eds.), *Handbook of family therapy* (pp. 444–482). New York: Brunner/Mazel.

Erenberg, G. (2003). *A consumer's guide to Tourette syndrome medications.* Bayside, NY: Tourette Syndrome Association.

Ezrati-Vinacour, R., Platzky, R., & Yairi, E. (2001). The young child's awareness of stuttering-like disfluency. *Journal of Speech, Language, and Hearing Research, 44,* 368–380.

Fairbanks, G. (1954). Systematic research in experimental phonetics: 1. A theory of the speech mechanism as a servosystem. *Journal of Speech and Hearing Disorders, 19,* 133–139.

Fairbanks, G. (1960). *Voice and articulation drillbook* (2nd ed.). New York: Harper & Row.

Fantry, L. (1990, January 5). Stuttering and acquired immunodeficiency syndrome. [Letter to the Editor]. *Journal of the American Medical Association, 263*(1), 38.

Farmer, S. S., & Farmer, J. L. (1989). *Supervision in communication disorders.* Columbus, OH: Merrill.

Faulkner, R. O. (1981). *A concise dictionary of Middle Egyptian.* Oxford, England: Griffith Institute.

Felsenfeld, S. (1996). Progress and needs in the genetics of stuttering. *Journal of Fluency Disorders, 21,* 77–103.

Felsenfeld, S. (1997). Epidemiology and genetics of stuttering. In R. F. Curlee & G. M. Siegel (Eds.), *Nature and treatment of stuttering: New directions* (2nd ed., pp. 3–23). Needham Heights, MA: Allyn & Bacon.

Felsenfeld, S. (2002). Finding susceptibility genes for developmental disorders of speech: The long and winding road. *Journal of Communication Disorders, 35,* 329–345.

Felsenfeld, S., Kirk, K. M., Zhu, G., Statham, D. J., Neale, M. C., & Martin, N. G. (2000). A study of the genetic and environmental etiology of stuttering in a selected twin sample. *Behavior Genetics, 30*(5), 359–366.

Fenichel, O. (1945). *The psychoanalytic theory of neurosis*. New York: Norton.

Ferguson, A. (2008). *Expert practice: A critical discourse*. San Diego, CA: Plural.

Fey, M. E. (1986). *Language intervention with young children*. Austin, TX: PRO-ED.

Fey, M. E. (2006). Commentary on "Making Evidence-Based Decisions About Child Language Intervention in Schools" by Gilliam and Gillam. *Language, Speech, and Hearing Services in Schools, 37*, 316–319.

Fey, M. E., & Justice, L. M. (2007). Evidence-based decision making in communication intervention. In R. Paul & P. W. Cascella (Eds.), *An introduction to clinical methods in communication disorders* (2nd ed., pp. 179–202). Baltimore: Brookes.

Finkelstein, S. (1968). *Sense and nonsense of McLuhan*. New York: International Publishers.

Finn, P. (2007). Self-control and the treatment of stuttering. In E. G. Conture & R. F. Curlee (Eds.), *Stuttering and related disorders of fluency* (3rd ed., pp. 344–360). New York: Thieme.

Finn, P., & Cordes, A. K. (1997). Multicultural identification and treatment of stuttering: A continuing need for research. *Journal of Fluency Disorders, 22*, 219–236.

Fiske, S. T. (1993). Controlling other people: The impact of power on stereotyping. *American Psychologist, 48*(6), 621–628.

Flasher, L. V., & Fogle, P. T. (2004). *Counseling skills for speech–language pathologists and audiologists*. Clifton Park, NY: Thomson/Delmar Learning.

Florance, C. L. (1986, Fall). Predicting prognosis in stuttering therapy. *Hearsay: Journal of the Ohio Speech and Hearing Association*, pp. 70–73.

Flower, R. M. (1985). Asking questions. *Asha, 27*(12), 21–25.

Floyd, J., Zebrowski, P. M., & Flamme, G. A. (2007). Stages of change and stuttering: A preliminary view. *Journal of Fluency Disorders, 32*(2), 95–120.

Fogle, P. T. (2008). *Foundations of communication sciences and disorders*. Clifton Park, NY: Thomson/Delmar Learning.

Foundas, A. L., Bollich, A. M., Corey, D. M., Hurley, M., & Heilman, K. M. (2001). Anomalous anatomy of speech–language areas in adults with persistent developmental stuttering. *Neurology, 57*, 207–215.

Fox, P. T., Ingham, R. J., Ingham, J. C., Hirsch, T. B., Downs, J. H., Martin, C., Jet al. (1996). A PET study of the neural systems of stuttering. *Nature, 382*, 158–162.

Franken, M. J., Kielstra-Van der Schalk, C. J., & Boelens, H. (2005). Experimental treatment of early stuttering: A preliminary study. *Journal of Fluency Disorders, 30*, 189–199.

Franks, D., Dale, P., Hindmarsh, R., Fellows, C., Buckridge, M., & Cybinski, P. (2007). Interdisciplinary foundations: Reflecting on interdisciplinarity and three decades of teaching and research at Griffith University, Australia. *Studies in Higher Education, 32*(2), 167–185.

Fransella, F. (1972). *Personal change and reconstruction: Research on a treatment of stuttering*. London: Academic Press.

Fransella, F. (2003). From theory to research to change. In F. Fransella (Ed.), *International handbook of personal construct psychology* (pp. 211–222). Chichester, England: Wiley.

Fransella, F., & Dalton, P. (1990). *Personal construct counseling in action*. London: Sage.

Freeman, F. J., & Rosenfield, D. B. (1982). A research note on "source" in dysfluency. *Journal of Fluency Disorders, 7*, 295–296.

Freund, H. (1966). *Psychopathology and the problems of stuttering: With special consideration of clinical and historical aspects*. Springfield, IL: Thomas.

Friend, M., & Cook, L. (2010). *Interactions: Collaboration skills for school professionals* (6th ed.). Upper Saddle River, NJ: Pearson Education/Merrill.

Froeschels, E. (1955). Contribution to the relationship between stuttering and cluttering. *Logopaedie en Phoniatrie, 4*, 1–6.

Froeschels, E. (1956). [Untitled contribution]. In E. F. Hahn & E. S. Hahn (Eds.), *Stuttering: Significant theories and therapies* (2nd ed., pp. 41–47). Stanford, CA: Stanford University Press.

Froeschels, E. (1964). *Selected papers of Emil Froeschels, 1940–1964*. Amsterdam: North-Holland.

Gabel, R. M. (2006). Effects of stuttering and therapy involvement on attitudes towards people who stutter. *Journal of Fluency Disorders, 31*, 216–227.

Gabel, R. M., Blood, G. W., Tellis, G. M., & Althouse, M. T. (2004). Measuring role entrapment of people who stutter. *Journal of Fluency Disorders, 29*, 27–49.

Gardner, H. (1983). *Frames of mind: The theory of multiple intelligences.* New York: Basic Books/HarperCollins.

Gardner, H. (1993). *Multiple intelligences: The theory in practice.* New York: Basic Books/HarperCollins.

Gardner, H. (1995). *Leading minds: An anatomy of leadership.* New York: Basic Books/HarperCollins.

Garner, H. S., Uhl, M., & Cox, A. W. (1992). *Interdisciplinary teamwork training guide.* Richmond: Virginia Institute for Developmental Disabilities.

Garrard, K. R. (1990–1991). A guide for assessing young children's expressive language skills through language sampling. *National Student Speech Language Hearing Association Journal, 18,* 87–95.

Garrett, A. G. (2003). *Bullying in American schools: Causes, preventions, interventions.* Jefferson, NC: McFarland.

Gazda, G. M., Asbury, F. R., Balzer, F. J., Childers, W. C., & Walters, R. P. (1977). *Human relations development—A manual for educators* (2nd ed.). Boston: Allyn & Bacon.

Geffner, R. A., Loring, M., & Young, C. (Eds.). (2001). *Bullying behavior: Current issues, research, and interventions.* Binghamton, NY: Hayworth Press.

Gibran, K. (1923). *The prophet.* New York: Knopf.

Gillam, R. B., Roussos, C. S., & Anderson, J. L. (1990). Facilitating changes in supervisees' clinical behaviors: An experimental investigation of supervisory effectiveness. *Journal of Speech and Hearing Disorders, 55,* 729–739.

Gilles de la Tourette, G. (1885). Étude sur une affection nerveuse caracterisée par de l'incoordination motrice accompagnée d'écholalie et de copralalie. *Archives Neurologiques* (Paris), *9,* 19–42, 158–200.

Giraud, A.-L., Keumann, K., Bachoud-Levi, A.-C., von Gudenberg, A. W., Euler, H. A., Lanfermann, H., & Preibisch, C. (2008). Severity of dysfluency correlates with basal ganglia activity in persistent developmental stuttering. *Brain and Language, 104,* 190–199.

Gladding, S. T. (2007). *Family therapy: History, theory, and practice* (4th ed.). Upper Saddle River, NJ: Pearson Education/Merrill, Prentice Hall.

Glauber, P. (1958). The psychoanalysis of stuttering. In J. Eisenson (Ed.), *Stuttering: A symposium* (pp. 71–119). New York: Harper & Row.

Glennen, S. (2002). Language development and delay in internationally adopted infants and toddlers: A review. *American Journal of Speech–Language Pathology, 11,* 333–339.

Glennen, S. (2007). International adoption speech and language mythbusters. *Perspectives on Communication Disorders and Sciences in Clinically and Linguistically Diverse Populations, 14*(3), 3–8.

Glennen, S. (2008, December 16). Speech and language "mythbusters" for internationally adopted children. *The ASHA Leader,* pp. 10–13.

Glennen, S., & Masters, M. G. (2002). Typical and atypical language development in infants and toddlers adopted from Eastern Europe. *American Journal of Speech–Language Pathology, 11,* 417–433.

Goberman, A. M., & Blomgren, M. (2003). Parkinsonian speech disfluencies: Effects of L-dopa-related fluctuations. *Journal of Fluency Disorders, 28,* 55–70.

Goldberg, B. (1989, June/July). Historic treatments for stuttering: From pebbles to psychoanalysis. *Asha, 31,* 71.

Goldhammer, R. (1969). *Clinical supervision: Special methods for the supervision of teachers.* New York: Holt, Rinehart & Winston.

Goldhammer, R., Anderson, R. H., & Krajewski, R. J. (1980). *Clinical supervision: Special methods for the supervision of teachers* (2nd ed.). New York: Holt, Rinehart & Winston.

Goldiamond, I. (1965). Stuttering and fluency as manipulable operant responses classes. In L. Krasner & L. P. Ullmann (Eds.), *Research in behavior modification: New developments and implications* (pp. 106–156). New York: Holt, Rinehart & Winston.

Gordon, P. A., & Luper, H. L. (1992a). The early identification of beginning stuttering I: Protocols. *American Journal of Speech–Language Pathology, 1*(3), 43–53.

Gordon, P. A., & Luper, H. L. (1992b). The early identification of beginning stuttering II: Problems. *American Journal of Speech–Language Pathology, 1*(4), 49–55.

Gottwald, S. R. (1999). Family communication patterns and stuttering development: An analysis of the research literature. In N. Bernstein Ratner & E. C. Healey (Eds.), *Stuttering research and practice: Bridging the gap* (pp. 175–192). Mahwah, NJ: Erlbaum.

Gottwald, S. R. (2010). Stuttering prevention and early intervention: A multidimensional approach. In B. Guitar & R. J. McCauley (Eds.), *Treatment of stuttering: Established and emerging interventions* (pp. 91–117). Philadelphia: Lippincott/Williams & Wilkins.

Gottwald, S. R., & Hall, N. (2003). Stuttering treatment in schools: Developing family and teacher partnerships. *Seminars in Speech and Language, 23,* 41–46.

Gottwald, S. R., & Starkweather, C. W. (1984, November). *Stuttering prevention: Rationale and method.* Short course presented at the annual meeting of the American Speech-Language-Hearing Association, San Francisco.

Gottwald, S. R., & Starkweather, C. W. (1995). Fluency intervention for preschoolers and their families in the public schools. *Language, Speech, and Hearing Services in Schools, 26,* 117–126.

Gouge, C. G., & Shapiro, D. A. (1989–1990). A concurrent approach to fluency treatment. *National Student Speech Language Hearing Association Journal, 17,* 72–76.

Grant, A. C., Biousse, V., Cook, A. A., & Newman, N. J. (1999). Stroke-associated stuttering. *Archives of Neurology, 56*(5), 624–627.

Gregory, H. H. (1979). Controversial issues: Statement and review of the literature. In H. H. Gregory (Ed.), *Controversies about stuttering therapy* (pp. 1–62). Baltimore: University Park Press.

Gregory, H. H. (1986). *Stuttering: Differential evaluation and therapy.* Austin, TX: PRO-ED.

Gregory, H. H. (1995). Analysis and commentary. *Language, Speech, and Hearing Services in Schools, 26,* 196–200.

Gregory, H. H. (2003). *Stuttering therapy: Rationale and procedures.* Boston: Allyn & Bacon-Pearson Education.

Gregory, H. H. (2007). What is involved in therapy? In E. G. Conture & J. Fraser (Eds.), *Stuttering and your child: Questions and answers* (Publication 22, 3rd ed., pp. 38–47). Memphis, TN: Stuttering Foundation of America.

Gruber, L. (1986). Moses: His impediment and behavior therapy. *Journal of Psychology and Judaism, 10*(1), 5–13.

Guenther, F. H. (2008). Neuroimaging of normal speech production. In R. J. Ingham (Ed.), *Neuroimaging in communication sciences and disorders* (pp. 1–51). San Diego, CA: Plural.

Guitar, B. (1976). Pretreatment factors associated with the outcome of stuttering therapy. *Journal of Speech and Hearing Research, 19,* 590–600.

Guitar, B. (1997). Therapy for children's stuttering and emotions. In R. F. Curlee & G. M. Siegel (Eds.), *Nature and treatment of stuttering: New directions* (2nd ed., pp. 280–291). Needham Heights, MA: Allyn & Bacon.

Guitar, B. (1998). *Stuttering: An integrated approach to its nature and treatment* (2nd ed.). Baltimore: Williams & Wilkins.

Guitar, B. (2006). *Stuttering: An integrated approach to its nature and treatment* (3rd ed.). Baltimore: Lippincott/Williams & Wilkins.

Guitar, B., & Bass, C. (1978). Stuttering therapy: The relation between attitude change and long-term outcome. *Journal of Speech and Hearing Disorders, 43,* 392–400.

Guitar, B., & Guitar, C. (2008). *Stuttering and your child: Help for parents* [DVD]. Memphis, TN: Stuttering Foundation of America.

Guitar, B., & Peters, T. J. (2008). *Stuttering: An integration of contemporary therapies* (Publication 16, 4th ed.). Memphis, TN: Stuttering Foundation of America.

Guyette, T. W., & Baumgartner, J. M. (1988). Stuttering in the adult. In N. J. Lass, L. V. McReynolds, J. L. Northern, & D. E. Yoder (Eds.), *Handbook of speech–language pathology and audiology* (pp. 640–654). Toronto: B. C. Decker.

Hage, A. (2001). Is there a link between the development of cognitive–linguistic abilities in children and the course of stuttering? In H.-G. Bosshardt, J. S. Yaruss, & H. F. M. Peters (Eds.), *Fluency disorders: Theory, research, treatment and self-help. Proceedings of the Third World Congress on Fluency Disorders* (pp. 192–194). Nijmegen, The Nethlerlands: Nijmegen University Press.

Hahn, E. F., & Hahn, E. S. (1956). *Stuttering: Significant theories and therapies* (2nd ed.). Stanford, CA: Stanford University Press.

Hall, D. E., Wray, D. F., & Conti, D. M. (1986, Fall). The language–disfluency relationship: A case study. *Hearsay: Journal of the Ohio Speech and Hearing Association*, pp. 110–113.

Hall, N. E. (2007). Fluency in childhood apraxia of speech. *Perspectives on fluency and fluency disorders, 17*(2), 9–14.

Hall, N. E., Wagovich, S. A., & Bernstein Ratner, N. (2007). Language consideration in early childhood. In E. G. Conture & R. F. Curlee (Eds.), *Stuttering and related disorders of fluency* (3rd ed., pp. 153–167). New York: Thieme.

Hall, P. K. (1977). The occurrence of disfluencies in language-disordered school-age children. *Journal of Speech and Hearing Disorders, 42*, 364–369.

Halvorson, J. (1999). *Abandoned: Now stutter my orphan*. Hager City, WI: Jerry Halvorson/Halvorson Farms.

Halvorson, J. (2008). *Regression therapy for stuttering*. Hager City, WI: Jerry Halvorson/Halvorson Farms.

Ham, R. E. (1990). *Therapy of stuttering: Preschool through adolescence*. Englewood Cliffs, NJ: Prentice Hall.

Ham, R. E. (1999). *Clinical management of stuttering in older children and adolescents*. Gaithersburg, MD: Aspen.

Hammer, C. S., Detwiler, J. S., Detwiler, J., Blood, G. W., & Qualls, C. D. (2004). Speech–language pathologists' training and confidence in serving Spanish–English bilingual children. *Journal of Communication Disorders, 37*, 91–108.

Harms, M. A., & Malone, J. Y. (1939). The relationship of hearing acuity to stammering. *Journal of Speech Disorders, 4*, 363–370.

Harrington, J. (1988). Stuttering, delayed auditory feedback, and linguistic rhythm. *Journal of Speech and Hearing Research, 31*, 36–47.

Harris, V., Onslow, M., Packman, A., Harrison, E., & Menzies, R. (2002). An experimental investigation of the impact of the Lidcombe Program on early stuttering. *Journal of Fluency Disorders, 27*, 203–214.

Harrison, E., & Onslow, M. (2010). The Lidcombe Program for preschool children who sutter. In B. Guitar & R. J. McCauley (Eds.), *Treatment of stuttering: Established and emerging interventions* (pp. 118–140). Philadelphia: Lippincott/Williams & Wilkins.

Harrison, E., Onslow, M., & Rousseau, I. (2007). Lidcombe Program 2007: Clinical tales and clinical trials. In E. G. Conture & R. F. Curlee (Eds.), *Stuttering and related disorders of fluency* (3rd ed., pp. 55–75). New York: Thieme.

Hartman, A., & Laird, J. (1983). *Family-centered social work practice*. New York: Free Press/Macmillan.

Hašek, J. (1993). *The good soldier Švejk and his fortunes in the world war*. New York: Knopf.

Havel, V. (1994, July 4). *The need for transcendence in the postmodern world*. Speech presented in Independence Hall, Philadelphia. Available from http://www.worldtrans.org/whole/havelspeech.html.

Hayhow, R., Cray, A. M., & Enderby, P. (2002). Stammering and therapy views of people who stammer. *Journal of Fluency Disorders, 27*, 1–17.

Haynes, W. O., & Pindzola, R. H. (2008). *Diagnosis and evaluation in speech pathology* (7th ed.). Boston: Pearson/Allyn & Bacon.

Haynes, W. O., Pindzola, R. H., & Emerick, L. L. (1992). *Diagnosis and evaluation in speech pathology* (4th ed.). Englewood Cliffs, NJ: Prentice Hall.

Healey, E. C. (2007). A multidimensional approach to the assessment of children who stutter. *Perspectives on Fluency and Fluency Disorders, 17*(3), 6–9.

Healey, E. C., Reid, R., & Donaher, J. (2005). Treating children who stutter with coexisting learning, behavioral or cognitive challenges. In R. Lees & C. Stark (Eds.), *The treatment of stuttering in the young school-aged child* (pp. 178–196). Chichester, England: Whurr/Wiley.

Healey, E. C., & Scott, L. A. (1995). Strategies for treating elementary school-age children who stutter: An integrative approach. *Language, Speech, and Hearing Services in Schools, 26*, 151–161.

Healey, E. C., Trautman, L. S., & Susca, M. (2004, Spring). Clinical applications of a multidimensional approach for the assessment and treatment of stuttering. *Contemporary Issues in Communication Science and Disorders, 31,* 40–48.

Helm, N. A., Butler, R. B., & Benson, D. F. (1978). Acquired stuttering. *Neurology, 28,* 1159–1165.

Helm, N. A., Butler, R. B., & Canter, G. J. (1980). Neurogenic acquired stuttering. *Journal of Fluency Disorders, 5,* 269–279.

Helm-Estabrooks, N. (1986). Diagnosis and management of neurogenic stuttering in adults. In K. O. St. Louis (Ed.), *The atypical stutterer: Principles and practices of rehabilitation* (pp. 193–217). Orlando, FL: Academic Press.

Helm-Estabrooks, N. (1993). Stuttering associated with acquired neurological disease. In R. F. Curlee (Ed.), *Stuttering and related disorders of fluency* (pp. 205–219). New York: Thieme.

Helm-Estabrooks, N. (1999). Stuttering associated with acquired neurological disorders. In R. F. Curlee (Ed.), *Stuttering and related disorders of fluency* (2nd ed., pp. 255–268). New York: Thieme.

Helm-Estabrooks, N., & Hotz, G. (1998). Sudden onset of "stuttering" in an adult: Neurogenic or psychogenic? *Seminars in Speech and Language, 19*(1), 23–29.

Helm-Estabrooks, N., Yeo, R., Geschwind, N., Freedman, M., & Weinstein, C. (1986, August). Stuttering: Disappearance and reappearance with acquired brain lesions. *Neurology, 36,* 1109–1112.

Higdon, C. W. (2002, May 14). Non-traditional clinical experience in Costa Rica. *The ASHA Leader,* pp. 4–6, 16.

Hill, C. E. (1993). *Manual for Hill Counselor Verbal Response Category System.* College Park: University of Maryland.

Hill, D. G. (2003). Differential treatment of stuttering in the early stages of development. In H. H. Gregory (Ed.), *Stuttering therapy: Rationale and procedures* (pp. 142–185). Boston: Allyn & Bacon/Pearson Education.

Hillary, E. (2004, February). Just back from Boston. *Travel and Leisure, 34*(2), 192.

Himes, C. L. (2006). Elderly Americans. In H. Cox (Ed.). *Aging* (18th ed., 2006 Update, pp. 2–6). Dubuque, IA: McGraw-Hill/Dushkin.

Hinckley, J. J. (2008). *Narrative-based practice in speech–language pathology: Stories of a clinical life.* San Diego, CA: Plural.

Hirschberg, S., & Hirschberg, T. (Eds.). (2007). *One world, many cultures* (6th ed.). New York: Pearson Education/Longman.

Hodson, B., & Paden, E. (1991). *Teaching intelligible speech: A phonological approach to remediation* (2nd ed.). Austin, TX: PRO-ED.

Holland, A. L. (2007). *Counseling in communication disorders: A wellness perspective.* San Diego, CA: Plural.

Holmes, L. (2009, July 14). Lessons from Stephanie: A clinical perspective. *The ASHA Leader,* p. 16.

Hood, S. B. (1974). Clients, clinicians and therapy. In L. L. Emerick & S. B. Hood (Eds.), *The client–clinician relationship: Essays on interpersonal sensitivity in the therapeutic transaction* (pp. 45–59). Springfield, IL: Thomas.

Hooper, C. R. (1996, Winter). Forming a therapeutic alliance with older adults. *Asha, 38*(1), 43–45.

Howell, P. (2004, Spring). Assessment of some contemporary theories of stuttering that apply to spontaneous speech. *Contemporary Issues in Communication Science and Disorders, 31,* 123–140.

Howell, P., Sackin, S., & Williams, R. (1999). Differential effects of frequency-shifted feedback between child and adult stutterers. *Journal of Fluency Disorders, 24,* 127–136.

Howie, P. M. (1981). Concordance for stuttering in monozygotic and dizygotic twin pairs. *Journal of Speech and Hearing Disorders, 24,* 317–321.

Huer, M. B., & Saenz, T. I. (2003). Challenges and strategies for conducting survey and focus group research with culturally diverse groups. *American Journal of Speech–Language Pathology, 12,* 209–220.

Huinck, W. J., Langevin, M. J., Kully, D., Graamans, K., Peters, H. F., & Hulstijn, W. (2006). The relationship between pre-treatment clinical profile and treatment outcome in an integrated stuttering program. *Journal of Fluency Disorders, 31*, 43–63.

Humphrey, B., & Van Borsel, J. (2001). *Word-final dysfluencies: Ten infrequently asked questions.* Paper presented at the 4th International Stuttering Awareness Day Online Conference—You Are Not Alone: Transforming Perceptions. Available from http://www.mnsu.edu/comdis/isad4/papers/humphrey.html.

Individuals with Disabilities Education Act of 1990, 20 U.S.C. § 1400 *et seq.*

Individuals with Disabilities Education Act of 1990, 20 U.S.C. § 1400 *et seq.* (1990) (amended 1997).

Individuals with Disabilities Education Improvement Act of 2004, 20 U.S.C. § 1400 *et seq.* (2004).

Ingham, R. J. (1999). Performance-contingent management of stuttering in adolescents and adults. In R. F. Curlee (Ed.), *Stuttering and related disorders of fluency* (2nd ed., pp. 200–221). New York: Thieme.

Ingham, R. J. (2001). Brain imaging studies of developmental stuttering. *Journal of Communication Disorders, 34*, 493–516.

Ingham, R. J. (2010, October). Comments on article by Maguire et al.: Pagoclone trial: Questionable findings for stuttering treatment. *Journal of Clinical Psychopharmocology, 30*(5).

Ingham, R. J., Cykowski, M., Ingham, J. C., & Fox, P. T. (2008). In R. J. Ingham (Ed.), *Neuroimaging in communication sciences and disorders* (pp. 53–85). San Diego, CA: Plural.

Ingham, R. J., Ingham, J. C., Finn, P., & Fox, P. T. (2003). Towards a functional neural systems model of developmental stuttering. *Journal of Fluency Disorders, 28*, 297–319.

International Fluency Association and International Stuttering Association. (2001). *The bill of rights and responsibilities for people who stutter.* Available from www.stutterisa.org/Mission_R&R .html#billofrights.

Irwin, M. (2007). Terminology—How should stuttering be defined? and Why? In J. Au-Yeung & M. M. Leahy (Eds.), *Research, treatment, and self-help in fluency disorders: New horizons. Proceedings of the Fifth World Congress on Fluency Disorders* (pp. 41–45). Dublin: International Fluency Association.

Isaac, K. (2002). *Speech pathology in cultural and linguistic diversity.* London: Whurr.

Iverach, L., Jones, M., O'Brian, S., Block, S., Lincoln, M., Harrison, E., et al. (2009). The relationship between mental health disorders and treatment outcomes among adults who stutter. *Journal of Fluency Disorders, 34*, 29–43.

Ivoškuvienė, R., & Makauskienė, V. (2009). Experiences of teachers working with children who stammer. *Special Education, 1*(20), 93–100.

Jancke, L., Hanggi, J., & Steinmetz, H. (2004). Morphological brain differences between adult stutterers and non-stutterers. *BMC Neurology, 4*(23). Available from www.biomed.com.

Janssen, P., Kloth, S., Kraaimaat, F., & Brutten, G. J. (1996). Genetic factors in stuttering: A replication of Ambrose, Yairi, and Cox's (1993) study with adult probands. *Journal of Fluency Disorders, 21*, 105–108.

Jeffreys, M. R. (2006). *Teaching cultural competence in nursing and health care: Inquiry, action, and innovation.* New York: Springer.

Jewett, J. (2003, May 23). A labor of love in Bosnia. *The ASHA Leader*, pp. 20–21, 27.

Jewett, J., Gallagher, J., & Taggart, A. (2002, March 19). A winning battle in Bosnia. *The ASHA Leader*, pp. 1, 20–22.

Jewish Publication Society of America. (1965). *The holy scriptures* (rev. ed.). Philadelphia: Jewish Publication Society of America/World Publishing.

Jezer, M. (1997). *Stuttering: A life bound up in words.* New York: Basic Books/Harper & Row.

Jobs, S. (2005, June 14). *In praise of dropping out* (Commencement Address, Stanford University). Available from http://slashdot.org/comments.pl?sid=152625&cid=12810404.

Johnson, B. A., & Mata-Pistokache, T. (1996). Introduction to multicultural issues: Identifying, assessing, and treating children of various cultural backgrounds. In B. A. Johnson, *Language disorders in children: An introductory clinical perspective* (pp. 265–339). Albany, NY: Delmar.

Johnson, C. J. (2006). Getting started in evidence-based practice for childhood speech–language disorders. *American Journal of Speech–Language Pathology, 15,* 20–35.

Johnson, E., Sickels, E. R., & Sayers, F. C. (1970). *Anthology of children's literature* (4th ed.). Boston: Houghton Mifflin.

Johnson, W. (1930). *Because I stutter.* New York: Appleton.

Johnson, W. (1939). The treatment of stuttering. *The Journal of Speech Disorders, 4,* 170–172.

Johnson, W. (1942). A study of the onset and development of stuttering. *Journal of Speech Disorders, 7,* 251–257.

Johnson, W. (1944). The Indians have no word for it. I. Stuttering in children. *Quarterly Journal of Speech, 30,* 330–337.

Johnson, W. (1958). *Toward understanding stuttering.* Chicago: National Society for Crippled Children and Adults.

Johnson, W. (1961). *Stuttering and what you can do about it.* Danville, IL: Interstate.

Johnson, W., & Associates. (1959). *The onset of stuttering: Research findings and implications.* Minneapolis: University of Minnesota Press.

Johnston, J. R. (1983). What is language intervention? The role of theory. In J. Miller, D. E. Yoder, & R. Schiefelbusch (Eds.), *Contemporary issues in language intervention* (pp. 52–57). Rockville, MD: American Speech-Language-Hearing Association.

Jokel, R., De Nil, L., & Sharpe, K. (2007). Speech disfluencies in adults with neurogenic stuttering associated with stroke and traumatic brain injury. *Journal of Medical Speech–Language Pathology, 15*(3), 243–261.

Jones, J. E. (2005, June). Finding my voice. *Time Magazine,* p. F14.

Jones, J. E., & Niven, P. (1993). *Voices and silences.* New York: Charles Scribner's Sons.

Jones, M., Onslow, M., Harrison, E., & Packman, A. (2000). Treating stuttering in young children: Predicting treatment time in the Lidcombe Program. *Journal of Speech, Language, and Hearing Research, 43,* 1440–1450.

Jones, M., Onslow, M., Packman, A., Williams, S., Ormond, T., Schwartz, I., & Gebski, V. (2005). A randomized controlled trial of the Lidcombe Program for Early Stuttering Intervention. *British Medical Journal, 331,* 659–661.

Jozefowicz, S. (2009, July 14). TBI: An insider's journey. *The ASHA Leader,* pp. 14–16.

Kalinowski, J. S., & Saltuklaroglu, T. (2006). *Stuttering.* San Diego, CA: Plural.

Kamhi, A. G. (2006). Prologue: Combining research and reason to make treatment decisions. *Language, Speech, and Hearing Services in Schools, 37,* 255–256.

Karniol, R. (1992). Stuttering out of bilingualism. *First Language, 12,* 255–283.

Karinol, R. (1995). Stuttering, language, and cognition: A review and a model of stuttering as suprasegmental sentence plan alignment (SPA). *Psychological Bulletin, 117,* 104–124.

Kart, C. S., & Kinney, J. M. (2001). *The realities of aging: An introduction to gerontology* (6th ed.). Needham Heights, MA: Pearson Education/Allyn & Bacon.

Kathard, H. (1998). *Issues of culture and stuttering: A South African perspective.* International Stuttering Awareness Day Online Conference (Power Your Voice). Available from http://www.mnsu.edu/comdis/isad/papers/kathard.html.

Kauffman, J. M., & Hallahan, D. P. (Eds.). (2005). *The illusion of full inclusion: A comprehensive critique of a current special education bandwagon* (2nd ed.). Austin, TX: PRO-ED.

Kellum, G. D., & Fagan, E. C. (1992). Continuing education. In J. A. Rassi & M. D. McElroy (Eds.), *The education of audiologists and speech–language pathologists* (pp. 409–420). Timonium, MD: York Press.

Kelly, E. M., & Conture, E. G. (1992). Speaking rates, response time latencies, and interrupting behaviors of young stutterers, nonstutterers, and their mothers. *Journal of Speech and Hearing Research, 35,* 1256–1267.

Kelly, G. A. (1955a). *The psychology of personal constructs. Vol. 1: A theory of personality.* New York: Norton.

Kelly, G. A. (1955b). *The psychology of personal constructs. Vol. 2: Clinical diagnosis and psychotherapy.* New York: Norton.

Kent, R. D. (1989–1990). Fragmentation of clinical service and clinical science in communication disorders. *National Student Speech Language Hearing Association Journal, 17,* 4–16.

Kent, R. D. (2006). Evidence-based practice in communication disorders: Progress not perfection. *Language, Speech, and Hearing Services in Schools, 37,* 268–270.

Kidd, K. K. (1984). Stuttering as a genetic disorder. In R. F. Curlee & W. H. Perkins (Eds.), *Nature and treatment of stuttering: New directions* (pp. 149–169). San Diego, CA: College-Hill.

Kindlon, D., & Thompson, M. (2000). *Raising Cain: Protecting the emotional life of boys.* New York: Ballantine Books/Random House.

Klein, J. F., & Hood, S. B. (2004). The impact of stuttering on employment opportunities and job performance. *Journal of Fluency Disorders, 29*(4), 255–273.

Klein, S. D., & Schive, K. (2001). *You will dream new dreams: Inspiring personal stories by parents of children with disabilities.* New York: Kensington Books.

Klingbeil, G. M. (1939). The historical background of the modern speech clinic. *Journal of Speech Disorders, 4,* 115–132.

Klompas, M., & Ross, E. (2004). Life experiences of people who stutter, and the perceived impact of stuttering on quality of life: Personal accounts of South African individuals. *Journal of Fluency Disorders, 29*(4), 275–305.

Kloth, S. A. M., Kraaimaat, F. W., Janssen, P., & Brutten, G. J. (1999). Persistence and remission of incipient stuttering among high-risk children. *Journal of Fluency Disorders, 24,* 253–265.

Kolk, H., & Postma, A. (1997). Stuttering as a covert repair phenomenon. In R. F. Curlee & G. Siegel (Eds.), *Nature and treatment of stuttering: New directions* (2nd ed., pp. 182–203). Boston: Allyn & Bacon.

Krah, B. (2002, August 6). The anatomy of a tic: From the point of view of a person with TS. *The ASHA Leader,* pp. 5, 7.

Kroll, R. M., Cook, F., De Nil, L., & Bernstein Ratner, N. (2006). *Preparing clinicians to treat stuttering.* Paper presented in the 9th International Stuttering Awareness Day Online Conference. Available from http://www.mnsu.edu/comdis/isad9/papers/kroll9.html.

Kroll, R. M., & Klassen, T. R. (2007). Ensuring the effectiveness of academic and clinical preparation for stuttering treatment. In J. Au-Yeung & M. M. Leahy (Eds.), *Research, treatment, and self-help in fluency disorders: New horizons. Proceedings of the Fifth World Congress on Fluency Disorders* (pp. 292–297). Dublin: International Fluency Association.

Kully, D. A., & Langevin, M. J. (1999). Intensive treatment for stuttering adolescents. In R. F. Curlee (Ed.), *Stuttering and related disorders of fluency* (2nd ed., pp. 139–159). New York: Thieme.

Kully, D. A., Langevin, M. J., & Lomheim, H. (2007). Intensive treatment of adolescents and adults who stutter. In E. G. Conture & R. F. Curlee (Eds.), *Stuttering and related disorders of fluency* (3rd ed., pp. 213–232). New York: Thieme.

Kussmaul, A. (1877). Disturbances of speech. In H. von Ziemssen (Ed.), *Cyclopedia of the practice of medicine* (Vol. 14). New York: William Wood.

Kuster, J. (2005). *Folk myths about stuttering.* (The Stuttering Home Page.) Available from http://www.mnsu.edu/comdis/kuster/Infostuttering/folkmyths.html.

Kwak, C., & Jankovic, J. (2002, August 6). The neurology of a tic: From the point of view of the scientist. *The ASHA Leader,* pp. 4, 6–7, 36.

Langdon, H. W. (2008). *Assessment and intervention for communication disorders in culturally and linguistically diverse populations.* Clifton Park, NY: Thomson/Delmar Learning.

Langevin, M. J. (2009). The Peer Attitudes Toward Children Who Stutter scale: Reliability, known groups validity, and negativity of elementary school-age children's attitudes. *Journal of Fluency Disorders, 34*(2), 72–86.

Langevin, M. J., Bortnick, K., Hammer, T., & Wiebe, E. (1998). Teasing/bullying experienced by children who stutter: Toward development of a questionnaire. *Contemporary Issues in Communication Science and Disorders, 25,* 12–24.

Langevin, M. J., Huinck, W. J., Kully, D., Peters, H. F. M., Lomheim, H., & Tellers, M. (2006). A cross-cultural, long-term outcome evaluation of the ISTAR Comprehensive Stuttering Program across Dutch and Canadian adults who stutter. *Journal of Fluency Disorders, 31,* 229–256.

Langevin, M. J., & Kully, D. (2003). Evidence-based treatment of stuttering: III. Evidence-based practice in a clinical setting. *Journal of Fluency Disorders, 28*(3), 219–236.

Langevin, M. J., Kully, D. A., & Ross-Harold, B. (2007). The Comprehensive Stuttering Program for School-Age Children with strategies for managing teasing and bullying. In E. G. Conture & R. F. Curlee (Eds.), *Stuttering and related disorders of fluency* (3rd ed., pp. 131–149). New York: Thieme.

Langevin, M. J., Packman, A., & Onslow, M. (2009). Peer responses to stuttering in the preschool setting. *American Journal of Speech–Language Pathology, 18*(3), 264–276.

Lass, N. J., Ruscello, D. M., Pannbacker, M. D., Schmitt, J. F., & Everly-Myers, D. S. (1989). Speech–language pathologists' perceptions of child and adult female and male stutterers. *Journal of Fluency Disorders, 14*, 127–134.

Lass, N. J., Ruscello, D. M., Pannbacker, M., Schmitt, J. F., Kiser, A. M., Mussa, A. M., & Lockhart, P. (1994). School administrators' perceptions of people who stutter. *Language, Speech, and Hearing Services in Schools, 25*(2), 90–93.

Lass, N. J., Ruscello, D. M., Schmitt, J. F., Pannbacker, M. D., Orlando, M. B., Dean, K. A., et al. (1992). Teachers' perceptions of stutterers. *Language, Speech, and Hearing Services in Schools, 23*(1), 78–81.

Leahy, M. M. (2004, January). Therapy talk: Analyzing therapeutic discourse. *Language, Speech, and Hearing Services in Schools, 35*, 70–81.

Lebrun, Y., & Van Borsel, J. (1990). Final sound repetitions. *Journal of Fluency Disorders, 15*, 107–113.

Leith, W. R. (1986). Treating the stutterer with atypical cultural influences. In K. O. St. Louis (Ed.), *The atypical stutterer: Principles and practices of rehabilitation* (pp. 9–34). Orlando, FL: Academic Press.

Levis, B., Ricci, D., Lukong, J., & Drayna, D. (2004). Genetic linkage studies in a large West African kindred. *American Journal of Human Genetics, 75*, S2026.

Lew, E. (1995, July/August). *My stuttering saved my life: Letting go.* Anaheim Hills, CA: National Stuttering Project.

Lewis, G. A. (1899). *The origin and treatment of stammering.* Detroit: Phono-Meter Press.

Lichtheim, M. (1973). *Ancient Egyptian literature: A book of readings* (Vol. 1). Berkeley: University of California Press.

Lickley, R. J., Hartsuiker, R. J., Corley, M., Russell, M., & Nelson, R. (2005). Judgment of disfluency in people who stutter and people who do not stutter: Results from magnitude estimation. *Language and Speech, 48*(3), 299–312.

Liles, B. Z., Lerman, J., Christensen, L., & St. Ledger, J. (1992). A case description of verbal and signed disfluencies of a 10-year-old boy who is retarded. *Language, Speech, and Hearing Services in Schools, 23*, 107–112.

Lincoln, M., Packman, A., & Onslow, M. (2006). Altered auditory feedback and the treatment of stuttering: A review. *Journal of Fluency Disorders, 31*(2), 71–89.

Logan, K. J. (2003). The effect of syntactic structure upon speech initiation times of stuttering and nonstuttering speakers. *Journal of Fluency Disorders, 28*, 17–35.

Logan, K. J., & Conture, E. G. (1995). Length, grammatical complexity, and rate differences in stuttered and fluent conversational utterances of children who stutter. *Journal of Fluency Disorders, 20*, 35–61.

Logan, K. J., & LaSalle, L. R. (2003). Developing intervention programs for children with stuttering and concomitant impairments. *Seminars in Speech and Language, 24*(1), 13–20.

Logan, K. J., & Yaruss, J. S. (1999, Spring). Helping parents address attitudinal and emotional factors with young children who stutter. *Contemporary Issues in Communication Science and Disorders, 26*, 69–81.

Lohr, J. B., & Wisniewski, A. A. (1987). *Movement disorders: A neuropsychiatric approach.* New York: Guilford Press.

Lopez, O. L., Becker, J. T., Dew, M. A., Banks, G., Dorst, S. K., & McNeil, M. (1994, November). Speech motor control disorder after HIV infection. *Neurology, 44*, 2187–2189.

Lougeay-Mottinger, J., Harris, M. R., Perlstein-Kaplan, K. E., & Felicetti, T. (1984). UTD competency based evaluation system. *Asha, 26*(11), 39–43.

Lubinski, R., & Welland, R. J. (1997). Normal aging and environmental effects on communication. *Seminars in Speech and Language, 18*(2), 107–126.

Ludlow, C. L. (1990). Treatment of speech and voice disorders with botulinum toxin. *Journal of the American Medical Association, 264,* 2671–2675.

Ludlow, C. L., & Braun, A. (1993). Research evaluating the use of neuropharmacological agents for treating stuttering: Possibilities and problems. *Journal of Fluency Disorders, 18,* 169–182.

Luper, H. L. (Ed.). (2003). *Stuttering: Successes and failures in therapy* (Publication 6). Memphis, TN: Stuttering Foundation of America.

Luper, H. L., & Mulder, R. L. (1964). *Stuttering: Therapy for children.* Englewood Cliffs, NJ: Prentice Hall.

Luterman, D. M. (2008). *Counseling persons with communication disorders and their families* (5th ed.). Austin, TX: PRO-ED.

Lynch, E. W., & Hanson, M. J. (Eds.). (1997). *Developing cross-cultural competence: A guide for working with children and their families* (2nd ed.). Baltimore: Brookes.

Macauley, B. L., & Steckol, K. D. (2004, October 5). Musical stuttering: A true scenario and a genuine phenomenon. *The ASHA Leader,* pp. 8, 18.

MacKinnon, S. P., Hall, S., & MacIntyre, P. D. (2007). Origins of the stuttering stereotype: Stereotype formation through anchoring-adjustment. *Journal of Fluency Disorders, 32,* 297–309.

Maguire, G. A. (2007, Summer). New drugs for stuttering may be on the horizon. *Stuttering Foundation of America Newsletter,* p. 3.

Maguire, G. A., Franklin, D., Vatakis, N. G., Morgenshtern, E., Denko, T., Yaruss, J. S., et al. (2010, February). Exploratory randomized clinical study of pagoclone in persistent developmental stuttering: The Examining Pagoclone for Persistent Developmental Stuttering Study. *Journal of Clinical Psychopharmocology, 30*(1), 48–56.

Maguire, G. A., Riley, G., Franklin, D. L., & Gumusaneli, E. (2010). The physiologic basis and pharmacologic treatment of stuttering. In B. Guitar & R. J. McCauley (Eds.), *Treatment of stuttering: Established and emerging interventions* (pp. 329–342). Philadelphia: Lippincott/Williams & Wilkins.

Maguire, G., Riley, G., Franklin, D., Maguire, M., Nguyen, C., & Brojeni, P. (2004). Olanzapine in the treatment of developmental stuttering: A double-blind, placebo-controlled trial. *Annals of Clinical Psychiatry, 16*(2), 63–67.

Mahr, G., & Leith, W. (1992). Psychogenic stuttering of adult onset. *Journal of Speech and Hearing Research, 35,* 283–286.

Makauskienė, V. (2008). *Designing intervention for stuttering pupils within the child centered education paradigm.* Unpublished doctoral dissertation, Šiauliai University, Šiauliai, Lithuania.

Mallard, A. R., Gardner, L. S., & Downey, C. S. (1988). Clinical training in stuttering for school clinicians. *Journal of Fluency Disorders, 13,* 253–259.

Mandela, N. (1995). *The long walk to freedom: The autobiography of Nelson Mandela.* New York: Bay Back Books/Little, Brown.

Manning, W. H. (Ed.). (2000). The demands and capacities model. *Journal of Fluency Disorders, 25,* 317–383.

Manning, W. H. (2001). *Clinical decision making in fluency disorders* (2nd ed.). San Diego, CA: Singular/Thomson.

Manning, W. H. (2004, Spring). How can you understand stuttering? You don't stutter! *Contemporary Issues in Communication Sciences and Disorders, 31,* 58–68.

Manning, W. H. (2006). Therapeutic change and the nature of our evidence. In N. Bernstein Ratner & J. Tetnowski (Eds.), *Current issues in stuttering research and practice* (pp. 125–158). Mahwah, NJ: Erlbaum.

Manning, W. H. (2010). *Clinical decision making in fluency disorders* (3rd ed.). Clifton Park, NY: Delmar/Cengage Learning.

Manning, W. H., & Monte, K. L. (1981). Fluency breaks in older speakers: Implications for a model of stuttering throughout the life cycle. *Journal of Fluency Disorders, 6,* 35–48.

Manning, W. H., & Shirkey, E. A. (1981). Fluency and the aging process. In D. S. Beasley & G. A. Davis (Eds.), *Aging: Communication processes and disorders* (pp. 175–189). New York: Grune & Stratton.

Mansson, H. (2000). Childhood stuttering: Incidence and development. *Journal of Fluency Disorders, 25,* 47–57.

Market, K. E., Montague, J. C., Buffalo, M. D., & Drummond, S. S. (1990). Acquired stuttering: Descriptive data and treatment outcome. *Journal of Fluency Disorders, 15,* 21–33.

Marshall, C. (2003). A reconsideration of Moses' speech disorder [Letter to the Editor]. *Journal of Fluency Disorders, 28,* 71–73.

May, H. G., & Metzger, B. M. (1962). *The holy Bible: Revised standard version containing the Old and New Testaments.* New York: Oxford University Press.

McAllister, J., & Kingston, M. (2005). Final part-word repetitions in school-age children: Two case studies. *Journal of Fluency Disorders, 30,* 255–267.

McCarthy, M. M. (1981). Speech effect of theophylline [Letter to the Editor]. *Pediatrics, 68*(5), 749–750.

McCrea, E. S. (1980). Supervisee ability to self-explore and four facilitative dimensions of supervisor behavior in individual conferences in speech–language pathology (Doctoral dissertation, Indiana University, 1980). *Dissertation Abstracts International, 41,* 2134B.

McCrea, E. S., & Brasseur, J. A. (2003). *The supervisory process in speech–language pathology and audiology.* Boston: Allyn & Bacon/Pearson Education.

McCready, V., Shapiro, D., & Kennedy, K. (1987). Identifying hidden dynamics in supervision: Four scenarios. In M. B. Crago & M. Pickering (Eds.), *Supervision in human communication disorders: Perspectives on a process* (pp. 169–201). Boston: Little, Brown/College-Hill.

McGoldrick, M., & Carter, B. (2003). The family life cycle. In F. Walsh (Ed.), *Normal family processes: Growing diversity and complexity* (3rd ed., pp. 375–398). New York: Guilford Press.

McGoldrick, M., & Carter, E. A. (1982). The family life cycle. In F. Walsh (Ed.), *Normal family processes* (pp. 167–195). New York: Guilford Press.

McLeod, S. (Ed.). (2007). *The international guide to speech acquisition.* Clifton Park, NY: Thomson/Delmar Learning.

McLuhan, M. (1964). *Understanding media: The extensions of man.* New York: McGraw-Hill.

McLuhan, M., & Fiore, Q. (1967). *The medium is the massage.* New York: Random House.

Meline, T. (2006, Spring). Selecting studies for systematic review: Inclusion and exclusion criteria. *Contemporary Issues in Communication Science and Disorders, 33,* 21–27.

Meltzer, A. (1992). Horn stuttering. *Journal of Fluency Disorders, 17,* 257–264.

Merrill, J. C., & Lowenstein, R. L. (1971). *Media, messages, and men: New perspectives in communication.* New York: David McKay.

Messick, S. (1980). Test validity and the ethics of assessment. *American Psychologist, 35*(11), 1012–1027.

Meyers, S. C., & Freeman, F. J. (1985a). Interruptions as a variable in stuttering and disfluency. *Journal of Speech and Hearing Research, 28,* 428–435.

Meyers, S. C., & Freeman, F. J. (1985b). Mother and child speech rates as a variable in stuttering and disfluency. *Journal of Speech and Hearing Research, 28,* 436–444.

Miles, S., & Bernstein Ratner, N. (2001). Parental language input to children at stuttering onset. *Journal of Speech, Language and Hearing Research, 44,* 1116–1130.

Millard, S. K., Nicholas, A., & Cook, F. M. (2008). Is parent–child interaction therapy effective in reducing stuttering? *Journal of Speech, Language, and Hearing Research, 51,* 636–650.

Miller, A. (1990). *Banished knowledge: Facing childhood injuries.* New York: Doubleday.

Milner, M. (2004). *Freaks, geeks, and cool kids: America's teenagers, schools, and the culture of consumption.* New York: Routledge/Taylor & Francis Group.

Miyamoto, S., Hayasaka, K., & Shapiro, D. (2007, July). An examination of the checklist for possible cluttering in Japan. In J. Au-Yeung & M. M. Leahy (Eds.), *Research, treatment, and self-help in fluency disorders: New horizons. Proceedings of the Fifth World Congress on Fluency Disorders* (pp. 279–282). Dublin: International Fluency Association.

Molt, L. (Ed.). (2005, October 18). International focus on stuttering [Special issue]. *The ASHA Leader,* pp. 2, 19.

Montgomery, B. M., & Fitch, J. L. (1988). The prevalence of stuttering in the hearing-impaired school age population. *Journal of Speech and Hearing Disorders, 53,* 131–135.

Montgomery, C. S. (2006). The treatment of stuttering: From the hub to the spoke: Description and evaluation of an integrated therapy program. In N. Bernstein Ratner & J. Tetnowski

(Eds.), *Current issues in stuttering research and practice* (pp. 159–204). Mahwah, NJ: Erlbaum.

Moore, B. J., & Montgomery, J. K. (2008). *Making a difference for America's children: Speech–language pathologists in public schools* (2nd ed.). Austin, TX: PRO-ED.

Moore, W. H. (1984). Hemispheric alpha asymmetries during an electromyographic biofeedback procedure for stuttering. *Journal of Fluency Disorders, 17,* 143–162.

Morris, R., & Brown, W. S. (1987). Age-related voice measures among adult women. *Journal of Voice, 1,* 38–43.

Mortenson, G., & Relin, D. O. (2006). *Three cups of tea: One man's mission to promote peace . . . One school at a time.* New York: Penguin Books.

Moscicki, E. K. (1984, August). The prevalence of "incidence" is too high. *Asha, 26*(8), 39–40.

Moses, N., & Shapiro, D. A. (1996). A developmental conceptualization of clinical problem solving. *Journal of Communication Disorders, 29,* 199–221.

Motluck, A. (1997). Cutting out stuttering. *New Scientist, 153*(2067), 32–35.

Movsessian, P. (2005). Neuropharmacology of theophylline induced stuttering: The role of dopamine, adenosine and GABA. *Medical Hypotheses, 64*(2), 290–297.

Mowrer, D. E. (1987). Repetition of final consonants in the speech of a young child. *Journal of Speech and Hearing Disorders, 52,* 174–178.

Mowrer, D. E., & Younts, J. (2001). Sudden onset of excessive repetitions in the speech of a patient with multiple sclerosis: A case report. *Journal of Fluency Disorders, 26,* 269–309.

Mueller, P. B. (1982). Voice characteristics of octogenarian and nonagenarian persons. *Ear, Nose and Throat Journal, 61,* 33–37.

Mueller, P. B. (1997). The aging voice. *Seminars in Speech and Language, 18*(2), 159–169.

Muma, J. (1978). Connell, Spradlin, and McReynolds: Right but wrong! [Letter to the Editor]. *Journal of Speech and Hearing Disorders, 43,* 549–552.

Murphy, A. T. (1974). The quiet hyena: Two monologues in search of a dialogue. In L. L. Emerick & S. B. Hood (Eds.), *The client–clinician relationship: Essays on interpersonal sensitivity in the therapeutic transaction* (pp. 29–44). Springfield, IL: Thomas.

Murphy, A. T., & FitzSimons, R. M. (1960). *Stuttering and personality dynamics: Play therapy, projective therapy, and counseling.* New York: Ronald Press.

Murphy, B. (2005). Dealing with guilt and shame. [DVD #9505; *The Child Who Stutters*]. Memphis, TN: Stuttering Foundation of America.

Murphy, W. P., & Quesal, R. W. (2004, Spring). Best practices for preparing students to work with people who stutter: *Contemporary Issues in Communication Science and Disorders, 31,* 25–39.

Murphy, W. P., Yaruss, J. S., & Quesal, R. W. (2007a). Enhancing treatment for school-age children who stutter: I. Reducing negative reactions through desensitization and cognitive restructuring. *Journal of Fluency Disorders, 32*(2), 121–138.

Murphy, W. P., Yaruss, J. S., & Quesal, R. W. (2007b). Enhancing treatment for school-age children who stutter: II. Reducing bullying through role-playing and self-disclosure. *Journal of Fluency Disorders, 32*(2), 139–162.

Murray, F. P. (2008). *A stutterer's story* (2nd ed.). Memphis, TN: Stuttering Foundation of America.

Myers, F. L., & Kissagizlis, P. (2007). *Putting cluttering on the world map: Formation of the International Cluttering Association (ICA).* Paper presented at the 10th International Stuttering Awareness Day Online Conference—Stuttering Awareness: Global Community, Local Activity. Available from http://www.mnsu.edu/comdis/isad10/papers/myers10.html.

Myers, F. L., & St. Louis, K. O. (2006). Disfluency and speaking rate in cluttering: Perceptual judgments versus counts. *Bulgarian Journal of Communication Disorders, 1*(1), 28–35.

Myers, F. L., & St. Louis, K. O. (2007). *Cluttering* [DVD, #9700]. Memphis, TN: Stuttering Foundation of America.

National Center for Health Statistics. (2009). *Health, United States, 2008.* Hyattsville, MD: Author.

Natke, U., Grosser, J., & Kalveram, K. T. (2001). Fluency, fundamental frequency, and speech rate under frequency-shifted auditory feedback in stuttering and nonstuttering persons. *Journal of Fluency Disorders, 26*(3), 227–241.

Nellum-Davis, P., Gentry, B., & Hubbard-Wiley, P. (2002). Clinical practice issues. In D. E. Battle (Ed.), *Communication disorders in multicultural populations* (3rd ed., pp. 461–486). Woburn, MA: Butterworth-Heinemann.

Nelson, L. A. (2002). Language formulation related to disfluency and stuttering. In J. Fraser (Ed.), *Stuttering therapy: Prevention and intervention with children* (pp. 19–38). Memphis, TN: Stuttering Foundation of America.

Nelson, N. W. (2007, June 19). "Be-attitudes" for managing change in school-based practice. *The ASHA Leader*, pp. 20–21.

Neumann, K., Euler, H. A., von Gudenberg, A. W., Giraud, A.-L., Lanfermann, H., Gall, V., & Preibisch, C. (2003). The nature and treatment of stuttering as revealed by fMRI: A within- and between-group comparison. *Journal of Fluency Disorders, 28*, 381–410.

Nichols, K. (1987). *Feelings of Western Carolina University students toward stutterers and stuttering.* Unpublished manuscript. Cullowhee, NC: Western Carolina University.

Nichols, M. P. (2004). *Family therapy: Concepts and methods* (6th ed.). Boston: Pearson Education/Allyn & Bacon.

Nichols, S. L., & Good, T. L. (2004). *America's teenagers—Myths and realities: Media images, schooling, and the social costs of careless indifference.* Mahwah, NJ: Erlbaum.

Nicolosi, L., Harryman, E., & Kresheck, J. (2004). *Terminology of communication disorders: Speech–language–hearing* (5th ed.). Baltimore: Lippincott/Williams & Wilkins.

Nippold, M. A. (1990). Concomitant speech and language disorders in stuttering children: A critique of the literature. *Journal of Speech and Hearing Disorders, 55*, 51–60.

Nippold, M. A. (2002). Stuttering and phonology: Is there an interaction? *American Journal of Speech–Language Pathology, 11*, 99–110.

No Child Left Behind Act of 2001, 20 U.S.C. 70 § 6301 *et seq.* (2002).

Novak, J. M. (Ed.). (2002a, Spring). Counseling and intervention with diverse populations [Special issue]. *Contemporary Issues in Communication Science and Disorders, 29*, 5–110.

Novak, J. M. (2002b, Spring). Improving communication in adolescents with language/learning disorders: Clinician considerations and adolescent skills. *Contemporary Issues in Communication Science and Disorders, 29*, 79–90.

Nurnberg, H. G., & Greenwald, B. (1981). Stuttering: An unusual side effect of phenothiazines. *American Journal of Psychiatry, 138*(3), 386–387.

O'Donnell, J. J., Armson, J., & Kiefte, M. (2008). The effectiveness of SpeechEasy during situations of daily living. *Journal of Fluency Disorders, 33*(2), 99–119.

Ogletree, B. T. (1999). Introduction to teaming. In B. T. Ogletree, M. A. Fischer, & J. B. Schulz (Eds.), *Bridging the family–professional gap: Facilitating interdisciplinary services for children with disabilities* (pp. 3–11). Springfield, IL: Thomas.

Ogletree, B. T., & Daniels, D. B. (1995). Communication-based assessment and intervention for prelinguistic infants and toddlers: Strategies and issues. In J. A. Blackman (Ed.), *Identification and assessment in early intervention* (pp. 222–234). Gaithersburg, MD: Aspen.

Ogletree, B. T, Fischer, M. A., & Schulz, J. B. (Eds.). (1999). *Bridging the family–professional gap: Facilitating interdisciplinary services for children with disabilities.* Springfield, IL: Thomas.

Ogletree, B. T., Saddler, Y. N., & Bowers, L. S. (1995). Speech–language pathology. In B. A. Thyer & N. P. Kropf (Eds.), *Developmental disabilities: A handbook for interdisciplinary practice* (pp. 217–233). Cambridge, MA: Brookline Books.

O'Neill, G. (2009). The baby boom age wave: Population success or tsunami? In R. B. Hudson (Ed.), *Boomer bust? Economic and political issues of the graying society* (pp. 3–21). Westport, CT: Praeger.

Onslow, M. (2003). Evidence based treatment of stuttering: IV. Empowerment through evidence-based treatment practices. *Journal of Fluency Disorders, 28*, 237–245.

Onslow, M. (2004). Advice to students of stuttering treatment. *Contemporary Issues in Communication Sciences and Disorders, 31*, 5–24.

Onslow, M., & Packman, A. (1999). The Lidcombe Program of early stuttering intervention. In N. Bernstein Ratner & E. C. Healey (Eds.), *Stuttering research and practice: Bridging the gap* (pp. 193–210). Mahwah, NJ: Erlbaum.

Onslow, M., Packman, A., & Harrison, E. (2003). *The Lidcombe Program of early stuttering intervention: A clinician's guide.* Austin, TX: PRO-ED.

Onslow, M., & Yaruss, J. S. (2007). Differing perspectives on what to do with a stuttering preschooler and why. *American Journal of Speech–Language Pathology, 16,* 65–68.

Ooki, S. (2005). Genetic and environmental influences on stuttering and tics in Japanese twin children. *Twin Research and Human Genetics, 8*(1), 69–75.

Oyler, M. E. (1996). Vulnerability in stuttering children. *Dissertation Abstracts International Section A: Humanities and Social Sciences, 56*(9-A), 3374.

Packman, A., & Onslow, M. (1999). Fluency disruption in speech and in wind instrument playing. *Journal of Fluency Disorders, 24,* 293–298.

Packman, A., Onslow, M., & Attanasio, J. (2004). The demands and capacities model: Implications for evidence-based practice in the treatment of stuttering. In A. K. Bothe (Ed.), *Evidence-based treatment of stuttering: Empirical bases and clinical applications* (pp. 65–79). Mahwah, NJ: Erlbaum.

Packman, A., Onslow, M., Richard, F., & van Doorn, J. (1996). Syllabic stress and variability: A model of stuttering. *Clinical Linguistics and Phonetics, 10,* 235–263.

Paden, E. P. (2005). Development of phonological ability. In E. Yairi & N. G. Ambrose, *Early childhood stuttering* (pp. 197–234). Austin, TX: PRO-ED.

Palmer, P. J. (1997). The grace of great things: Reclaiming the sacred in knowing, teaching, and learning. *Holistic Education Review, 10*(3), 8–16.

Palmer, S. (2007). Inspiration or affliction? *BBC Knowledge,* pp. 58–61.

Palmer, T. R., & Hunter, M. B. (2007). Issues in geriatric medicine. In A. F. Johnson & B. H. Jacobson (Eds.), *Medical speech–language pathology: A practitioners guide* (2nd ed., pp. 301–314). New York: Thieme.

Panagiotopoulos, C. (2001, September 25). The Jeddah Institute for Speech and Hearing: Where Middle East meets West. *The ASHA Leader,* pp. 11–12.

Paul, R. (2007). *Language disorders from infancy through adolescence: Assessment and intervention* (3rd ed.). St. Louis, MO: Mosby/Elsevier.

Pauls, D. L., Leckman, J. F., & Cohen, D. J. (1993). Familial relationship between Gilles de la Tourette's Syndrome, attention deficit disorder, learning disabilities, speech disorders, and stuttering. *Journal of the American Academy of Child and Adolescent Psychiatry, 32*(5), 1044–1050.

Peacher, W. G., & Harris, W. E. (1946). Speech disorders in World War II: VIII. Stuttering. *Journal of Speech Disorders, 11,* 303–308.

Perkins, W. H. (1973a). Replacement of stuttering with normal speech: I. Rationale. *Journal of Speech and Hearing Disorders, 38,* 283–294.

Perkins, W. H. (1973b). Replacement of stuttering with normal speech: II. Clinical procedures. *Journal of Speech and Hearing Disorders, 38,* 295–303.

Perkins, W. H. (1978). *Human perspectives in speech and language disorders.* St. Louis, MO: Mosby.

Perkins, W. H. (1979). From psychoanalysis to discoordination. In H. H. Gregory (Ed.), *Controversies about stuttering therapy* (pp. 97–127). Baltimore: University Park Press.

Perkins, W. H. (1990a). What is stuttering? *Journal of Speech and Hearing Disorders, 55,* 370–382.

Perkins, W. H. (1990b). Gratitude, good intentions, and red herrings: A response to commentaries. *Journal of Speech and Hearing Disorders, 55,* 402–404.

Perkins, W. H. (2000). Stuttering vs. fluency. In J. Fraser (Ed.), *Counseling those who stutter* (Publication 18, pp. 59–68). Memphis, TN: Stuttering Foundation of America.

Perkins, W. H. (2006). An alternative to automatic fluency. In J. Fraser (Ed.), *Stuttering therapy: Transfer and maintenance* (Publication 19, 2nd ed., pp. 57–67). Memphis, TN: Stuttering Foundation of America.

Perkins, W. H., Kent, R. D., & Curlee, R. F. (1991). A theory of neuropsycholinguistic function in stuttering. *Journal of Speech and Hearing Research, 34,* 734–752.

Perkins, W. H., Rudas, J., Johnson, L., Michael, W. B., & Curlee, R. F. (1974). Replacement of stuttering with normal speech: III. Clinical effectiveness. *Journal of Speech and Hearing Disorders, 39,* 416–428.

Pietranton, A. A. (2006). An evidence-based practice primer: Implications and challenges for the treatment of fluency disorders. In N. Bernstein Ratner & J. Tetnowski (Eds.), *Current issues in stuttering research and practice* (pp. 47–60). Mahwah, NJ: Erlbaum.

Pindzola, R. H., Jenkins, M. M., & Lokken, K. J. (1989). Speaking rates of young children. *Language, Speech, and Hearing Services in Schools, 20*(2), 133–138.

Pindzola, R. H., & White, D. T. (1986). A protocol for differentiating the incipient stutterer. *Language, Speech, and Hearing Services in Schools, 17*(1), 2–15.

Plante, E. (2004). Evidence-based practice in communication sciences and disorders. *Journal of Communication Disorders, 37,* 389–465.

Platzky, R., & Girson, J. (1993). Indigenous healers and stuttering. *South African Journal of Communication Disorders, 30,* 43–47.

Plexico, L. W., Manning, W. H., & DiLollo, A. (2005). A phenomenological understanding of successful stuttering management. *Journal of Fluency Disorders, 30,* 1–22.

Plexico, L. W., Manning, W. H., & Levitt, H. (2009a). Coping responses by adults who stutter: Part I. Protecting the self and others. *Journal of Fluency Disorders, 34*(2), 87–107.

Plexico, L. W., Manning, W. H., & Levitt, H. (2009b). Coping responses by adults who sutter: Part II. Approaching the problem and achieving agency. *Journal of Fluency Disorders, 34*(2), 108–126.

Pollack, W. (1999). *Real boys: Rescuing our sons from the myths of boyhood.* New York: Holt/First Owl Books.

Pollard, R., Ellis, J. B., Finan, D., & Ramig, P. R. (2009). Effects of the SpeechEasy on objective and perceived aspects of stuttering: A 6-month, phase I clinical trial in naturalistic environments. *Journal of Speech, Language, and Hearing Research, 52,* 516–533.

Pool, K. D., Devous, M. D., Freeman, F. J., Watson, B. C., & Finitzo, T. (1991). Regional cerebral blood flow in developmental stutterers. *Archives of Neurology, 48,* 509–512.

Portnuff, C. (2006, November 7). A partnership for communication: A personal journey through Amyotropic Lateral Sclerosis. *The ASHA Leader,* pp. 8, 32.

Post, J. G., & Leith, W. R. (1983). I'd rather tell a story than be one. *Asha, 25*(4), 23–26.

Postma, A., & Kolk, H. (1993). The covert repair hypothesis: Prearticulatory repair processes in normal and stuttered disfluencies. *Journal of Speech and Hearing Research, 36,* 472–487.

Prins, D. (1993). Management of stuttering: Treatment of adolescents and adults. In R. F. Curlee (Ed.), *Stuttering and related disorders of fluency* (pp. 115–138). New York: Thieme.

Prins, D., & Ingham, R. J. (2009). Evidence-based treatment and stuttering—Historical perspective. *Journal of Speech, Language, and Hearing Research, 52,* 254–263.

Prutting, C. A. (1985). The long battle for the light. *National Student Speech Language Hearing Association Journal, 13,* 5–9.

Quader, S. E. (1977). Dysarthria: An unusual side effect of tricyclic antidepressants. *British Medical Journal, 2,* 97.

Quesal, R. W. (2001, December). How do students learn if clients aren't there? *Fluency and Fluency Disorders, 11*(4), 8–11.

Quesal, R. W. (2007). Data-based assessment of adolescents and adults who stutter. In E. G. Conture & R. F. Curlee (Eds.), *Stuttering and related disorders of fluency* (3rd ed., pp. 39–51). New York: Thieme.

Quinn, P. T., & Andrews, G. (1977). Neurological stuttering—A clinical entity? *Journal of Neurology, Neurosurgery, and Psychiatry, 40,* 699–701.

Quinn, P. T., & Peachey, E. C. (1973). Haloperidol in the treatment of stutterers. [Letter to the Editor]. *British Journal of Psychiatry, 123,* 247–248.

Rabinowitz, A. (2001). *Beyond the last village.* Washington, DC: Island Press/Shearwater Books.

Rabinowitz, A. (2005). *Keynote address* [DVD]. Memphis, TN: Stuttering Foundation of America.

Ragsdale, J. D., & Ashby, J. K. (1982). Speech–language pathologists' connotations of stuttering. *Journal of Speech and Hearing Research, 25,* 75–80.

Rakowski, W., & Pearlman, D. N. (1995). Demographic aspects of aging: Current and future trends. In W. Reichel (Ed.), *Care of the elderly: Clinical aspects of aging* (4th ed., pp. 488–495). Baltimore: Williams & Wilkins.

Ramig, P. R., & Bennett, E. M. (1995). Working with 7- to 12-year-old children who stutter: Ideas for intervention in the public schools. *Language, Speech, and Hearing Services in Schools, 26,* 138–150.

Ramig, P. R., & Dodge, D. M. (2010). *The child and adolescent stuttering treatment and activity resource guide* (2nd ed.). Clifton Park, NY: Delmar/Cengage Learning.

Ramig, P. R., Ellis, J. B., & Polland, R. (2010). Application of the SpeechEasy to stuttering treatment: Introduction, background, and preliminary observations. In B. Guitar & R. J. McCauley (Eds.), *Treatment of stuttering: Established and emerging interventions* (pp. 312–328). Philadelphia: Lippincott/Williams & Wilkins.

Reeves, L. (2006). The role of self-help/mutual aid in addressing the needs of individuals who stutter. In N. Bernstein Ratner & J. Tetnowski (Eds.), *Current issues in stuttering research and practice* (pp. 255–278). Mahwah, NJ: Erlbaum.

Rehabilitation Act of 1973, 29 U.S.C. § 701 *et seq.*

Reichel, I. (2005). *Development of emotional intelligence module in graduate fluency disorders courses.* Unpublished doctoral dissertation, Nova Southeastern University, Ft. Lauderdale, FL.

Reichel, I. (2007). *Emotional intelligence and stuttering intervention.* Paper presented for International Stuttering Awareness Day Online Conference-Stuttering Awareness: Global Community, Local Activity. Available from http://www.mnsu.edu/comdis/isad10/papers/reichel10.html.

Reichel, I. K., & Bakker, K. (2009, July). Global landscape of cluttering. *Perspectives on Fluency and Fluency Disorders, 19,* 62–66.

Reichel, I. K., & St. Louis, K. O. (2004). The effects of emotional intelligence training in fluency disorders classes. In A. Packman, A. Meltzer, & H. F. M. Peters (Eds.), *Theory, research, and therapy in fluency disorders. Proceedings of the Fourth World Congress on Fluency Disorders* (pp. 474–481). Nijmegen, The Netherlands: Nijmegen University Press.

Reichel, I. K., & St. Louis, K. O. (2007). Mitigating negative stereotyping of stuttering in a fluency disorders class. In J. Au-Yeung & M. M. Leahy (Eds.), *Research, treatment, and self-help in fluency disorders: New horizons. Proceedings of the Fifth World Congress on Fluency Disorders* (pp. 236–243). Dublin: International Fluency Association.

Reinhardt, S. (2005, May 8). After coma, Mother's Day is sweeter for woman and her family. *Asheville Citizens-Times,* pp. B1, B5.

Reitzes, P. (2006). *Fifty great activities for children who stutter: Lessons, insights, and ideas for therapy success.* Austin, TX: PRO-ED.

Remington, T., & Fagan, S. C. (2007). Drug-induced communication and swallowing disorders. In A. F. Johnson & B. H. Johnson (Eds.), *Medical speech–language pathology: A practitioner's guide* (2nd ed., pp. 363–378). New York: Thieme.

Rentschler, G. J., Driver, L. E., & Callaway, E. A. (1984). The onset of stuttering following drug overdose. *Journal of Fluency Disorders, 9,* 265–284.

Retzinger, M. J. (2001, December). Johnson/Tudor study of orphans. *Fluency and Fluency Disorders, 11*(4), 19–20.

Riaz, N., Steinberg, S., Ahmad, J., Pluzhnikov, A., Riazuddin, S., Cox, N. J., & Drayna, D. (2005). Genomewide significant linkage to stuttering on chromosome 12. *American Journal of Human Genetics, 76,* 647–651.

Riley, G. D. (1981). *Stuttering prediction instrument for young children.* Austin, TX: PRO-ED.

Riley, G. D. (1994). *Stuttering severity instrument for children and adults* (3rd ed.). Austin, TX: PRO-ED.

Riley, G. D. (2009). *Stuttering severity instrument* (4th ed.). Austin, TX: PRO-ED.

Riley, G. D., & Riley, J. (1979). A component model for diagnosing and treating children who stutter. *Journal of Fluency Disorders, 4,* 279–293.

Riley, G. D., & Riley, J. (2000, Fall). A revised component model for diagnosing and treating children who stutter. *Contemporary Issues in Communication Science and Disorders, 27,* 188–199.

Rivara, J. B., Jaffe, K. M., Fay, G. C., Polissar, N. L., Martin, K. M., Shurtleff, H. A., & Liao, S. (1993). Family functioning and injury severity as predictors of child functioning 1 year following traumatic brain injury. *Archives of Physical Medicine and Rehabilitation, 74,* 1047–1055.

Roberts, J. E., & Smith, K. J. (1982). Supervisor–supervisee role differences and consistency of behavior in supervisory conferences. *Journal of Speech and Hearing Research, 25,* 428–434.

Roberts, P. M., & Shenker, R. C. (2007). Assessment and treatment of stuttering in bilingual speakers. In E. G. Conture & R. F. Curlee (Eds.), *Stuttering and related disorders of fluency* (3rd ed., 183–209). New York: Thieme.

Robey, R. R. (2004). A five-phase model for clinical-outcome research. *Journal of Communication Disorders, 37*, 401–411.

Robinson, T. L., & Crowe, T. A. (1998). Culture-based considerations in programming for stuttering intervention with African American clients and their families. *Language, Speech, and Hearing Services in Schools, 29*, 172–179.

Robinson, T. L., & Crowe, T. (2000). Multicultural issues and speech fluency. In T. J. Coleman (Ed.), *Clinical management of communication disorders in culturally diverse children* (pp. 251–269). Needham Heights, MA: Allyn & Bacon/Pearson Education.

Robinson, T. L., Davis, J. G., & Crowe, T. A. (2000, Fall). Disfluency in nonstuttering African American preschoolers during conversation and narrative discourse. *Contemporary Issues in Communication Science and Disorders, 27*, 164–171.

Rogers, C. R. (1957). The necessary and sufficient conditions of therapeutic personality change. *Journal of Consulting Psychology, 21*, 95–103.

Rogers, C. R. (1961). *On becoming a person.* Boston: Houghton Mifflin.

Rokusek, C. (1995). An introduction to the concept of interdisciplinary practice. In B. A. Thyer & N. P. Kropf (Eds.), *Developmental disabilities: A handbook for interdisciplinary practice* (pp. 1–12). Cambridge, MA: Brookline.

Rollin, W. J. (1987). *The psychology of communication disorders in individuals and their families.* Englewood Cliffs, NJ: Prentice Hall.

Rollin, W. J. (2000). *Counseling individuals with communication disorders: Psychodynamic and family aspects* (2nd ed.). Woburn, MA: Butterworth-Heinemann.

Rommel, D., Hage, A., Kalehne, P., & Johannsen, H. (2000). Development, maintenance and recovery in childhood stuttering: Prospective longitudinal data 3 years after first contact? In K. Baker, L. Rustin, & F. Cook (Eds.), *Proceedings of the Fifth Oxford Dysfluency Conference* (pp. 168–182). Windsor: Chappell Gardner.

Roseberry-McKibbin, C. (2007). *Language disorders in children: A multicultural and case perspective.* Boston: Pearson/Allyn & Bacon.

Rosenbek, J. C. (1984). Stuttering secondary to nervous system damage. In R. F. Curlee & W. H. Perkins (Eds.), *Nature and treatment of stuttering: New directions* (pp. 31–48). San Diego, CA: College-Hill.

Rosenbek, J. C., McNeil, M. R., Lemme, M. L., Prescott, T. E., & Alfrey, A. C. (1975). Speech and language findings in a chronic hemodialysis patient: A case report. *Journal of Speech and Hearing Disorders, 40*, 245–252.

Rosenbek, J. C., Messert, B., Collins, M., & Wertz, R. T. (1978). Stuttering following brain damage. *Brain and Language, 6*, 82–96.

Rosenfield, D. B., & Freeman, F. J. (1983). Stuttering onset after laryngectomy. *Journal of Fluency Disorders, 8*, 265–268.

Rosenfield, D. B., McCarthy, M., McKinney, K., & Viswanath, N. S. (1994). Stuttering induced by theophylline. *Ear Nose Throat Journal, 73*, 914–920.

Rosenfield, D. B., & Nudelman, H. B. (1991). Fluency, dysfluency, and aging. In D. N. Ripich (Ed.), *Handbook of geriatric communication disorders* (pp. 227–238). Austin, TX: PRO-ED.

Roth, C. R., Aronson, A. E., & Davis, L. J. (1989). Clinical studies in psychogenic stuttering of adult onset. *Journal of Speech and Hearing Disorders, 54*, 634–646.

Rousseau, I., Packman, A., Onslow, M., Harrison, E., & Jones, M. (2007). Language, phonology, and treatment time in the Lidcombe Program: A prospective study in a Phase II trial. *Journal of Communication Disorders, 40*(5), 382–397.

Runyan, C. M., & Runyan, S. E. (2007). The fluency rules program for school-age children who stutter. In E. G. Conture & R. F. Curlee (Eds.), *Stuttering and related disorders of fluency* (3rd ed., pp. 100–114). New York: Thieme.

Runyan, C. M., & Runyan, S. E. (2010). The fluency rules program. In B. Guitar & R. J. McCauley (Eds.), *Treatment of stuttering: Established and emerging interventions* (pp. 167–187). Philadelphia: Lippincott/Williams & Wilkins.

Ruscello, D. M., Lass, N. J., & Brown, J. (1988). College students' perceptions of stutterers. *National Student Speech Language Hearing Association Journal, 16*, 115–120.

Rush, W. L., & The League of Human Dignity. (n.d.). *Write with dignity: Reporting on people with disabilities.* Lincoln, NE: Hitchcock Center.

Russo, F. (2005, June 20). Who cares more for mom? *Time*, pp. F7–F8, F10.

Rustin, L. (1987). The treatment of childhood dysfluency through active parental involvement. In L. Rustin, H. Purser, & D. Rowley (Eds.), *Progress in the treatment of fluency disorders* (pp. 166–180). London: Taylor & Francis.

Rustin, L., Botterill, W., & Kelman, E. (1996). *Assessment and therapy for young dysfluent children: Family interaction.* San Diego, CA: Singular.

Rustin, L., & Purser, H. (1991). Child development, families, and the problem of stuttering. In L. Rustin (Ed.), *Parents, families, and the stuttering child* (pp. 1–24). San Diego, CA: Singular.

Ryan, B. P. (1974). *Programmed therapy for stuttering in children and adults.* Springfield, IL: Thomas.

Ryan, B. P. (1992). Articulation, language, rate, and fluency characteristics of stuttering and non-stuttering preschool children. *Journal of Speech and Hearing Research, 35,* 333–342.

Ryan, B. P. (2001). *Programmed therapy for stuttering in children and adults* (2nd ed.). Spingfield, IL: Thomas.

Ryan, B. P. (2003, Summer). Response to Coordinator's Corner (August, 2002). *Perspectives on Fluency and Fluency Disorders, 13,* 36–37.

Ryan, B. P. (2006). Response to Blomgren, Roy, Callister, and Merrill (2005). *Journal of Speech, Language, and Hearing Research, 49,* 1412–1414.

Ryan, B. P., & Van Kirk, B. (1971). *Programmed conditioning for fluency: Program book.* Monterey, CA: Behavioral Sciences Institute.

Ryan, B. P., & Van Kirk, B. (1978). *Monterey fluency program.* Monterey, CA: Monterey Learning Systems.

Sackett, D. L., Rosenberg, W. M., Gray, J. A., Haynes, R. B., & Richardson, W. S. (1996). Evidence based medicine: What it is and what it isn't. *British Medical Journal, 312,* 71–72.

Sacks, O. (1985). *The man who mistook his wife for a hat and other clinical tales.* New York: Summit Books/Simon & Schuster.

Sacks, O. (1995). *An anthropologist on Mars: Seven paradoxical tales.* New York: Knopf.

Samelson, W. (2006). *Beyond anger: Chronicle of a life reclaimed.* Baltimore: Publish America.

Sandburg, C. (1955). Prologue. In E. Steichen (Ed.), *The family of man* (pp. 2–3). New York: Museum of Modern Art.

Satir, V. (1983). *Conjoint family therapy* (3rd ed.). Palo Alto, CA: Science and Behavior Books.

Sawyer, J., & Yairi, E. (2006). The effect of sample size on the assessment of stuttering severity. *American Journal of Speech–Language Pathology, 15,* 36–44.

Saxon, K. G., & Ludlow, C. L. (2007). A critical review of the effect of drugs on stuttering. In E. G. Conture & R. F. Curlee (Eds.), *Stuttering and related disorders of fluency* (3rd ed., pp. 277–293). New York: Thieme.

Scahill, L., Lynch, K. A., & Ort, S. I. (1995). Tourette Syndrome: Update and review. *Journal of School Nursing, 11*(2), 26–32.

Schneider, P. (2004). *Transcending stuttering: The inside story* [DVD]. New York: Philip Schneider. (Available from the National Stuttering Association, 119 W. 40th Street, 14th Floor, New York, NY 10018)

Schubert, G. W., Miner, A. L., & Till, J. A. (1973). *The analysis of behavior of clinicians (ABC) system.* Unpublished manuscript, University of North Dakota, Grand Forks.

Schulz, G. M., Varga, M., Jeffires, K., Ludlow, C. L., & Braun, A. R. (2005). Functional neuroanatomy of human vocalization: An H 2 15 O PET study. *Cerebral Cortex, 15,* 1835–1847.

Schulz, J. B. (1993). Heroes in disguise. In A. P. Turnbull, J. M. Patterson, S. K. Behr, D. L. Murphy, J. G. Marquis, & M. J. Blue-Banning (Eds.), *Cognitive coping, families, and disability* (pp. 31–41). Baltimore: Brookes.

Schulz, J. B. (2008). *Grown man now.* Kingsport, TN: in2Wit Publishing.

Schwartz, H. D. (1993). Adolescents who stutter. *Journal of Fluency Disorders, 18,* 289–302.

Schwartz, H. D., & Conture, E. G. (1988). Subgrouping young stutterers: Preliminary behavioral observations. *Journal of Speech and Hearing Research, 31,* 62–71.

Schwartz, H. D., Zebrowski, P. M., & Conture, E. G. (1990). Behaviors at the onset of stuttering. *Journal of Fluency Disorders, 15,* 77–86.

Schweinfurth, J. M., Billante, M., & Courey, M. S. (2002). Risk factors and demographics in patients with spasmodic dysphonia. *Larnygoscope, 112*(2), 220–223.

Schwenk, K. A., Conture, E. G., & Walden, T. A. (2007). Reaction to background stimulation of preschool children who do and do not stutter. *Journal of Communication Disorders, 40,* 129–141.

Screen, R. M., & Anderson, N. B. (1994). *Multicultural perspectives in communication disorders.* San Diego, CA: Singular.

Searl, J. P., Gabel, R. M., & Fulks, J. S. (2002). Speech disfluency in centenarians. *Journal of Communication Disorders, 35,* 383–392.

Seeley, J. U. (1973). Interaction analysis between the supervisor and the speech and hearing clinician (Doctoral dissertation, University of Denver, 1973). *Dissertation Abstracts International, 34,* 2995B.

Seery, C. H. (2005). Differential diagnosis of stuttering for forensic purposes. *American Journal of Speech–Language Pathology, 14,* 284–297.

Seery, C. H., Watkins, R. V., Mangelsdorf, S. C., Shigeto, A. (2007). Subtyping stuttering II: Contributions from language and temperament. *Journal of Fluency Disorders, 32,* 197–217.

Shadden, B. B. (1997). Discourse behaviors in older adults. *Seminars in Speech and Language, 18*(2), 143–157.

Shakespeare, W. (2007). *The complete works of William Shakespeare* (Wordsworth Library Collection). Hertfordshire, England: Wordsworth Editions Ltd.

Shames, G. H. (1975). Operant conditioning and stuttering. In J. Eisenson (Ed.), *Stuttering: A second symposium* (pp. 263–332). New York: Harper & Row.

Shames, G. H. (2006). *Counseling the communicatively disabled and their families: A manual for clinicians* (2nd ed.). Mahwah, NJ: Erlbaum.

Shames, G. H., & Florance, C. L. (1980). *Stutter-free speech: A goal for therapy.* Columbus, OH: Merrill.

Shames, G. H., & Rubin, H. (Eds.). (1986). *Stuttering then and now.* Columbus, OH: Merrill.

Shapiro, D. A. (1985). Clinical supervision: A process in progress. *National Student Speech Language Hearing Association Journal, 13,* 89–108.

Shapiro, D. A. (1987, Fall). Myths in the method to the madness of supervision. *Hearsay: Journal of the Ohio Speech and Hearing Association,* pp. 78–83.

Shapiro, D. A. (1994a). Interaction analysis and self-study: A single-case comparison of four methods of analyzing supervisory conferences. *Language, Speech, and Hearing Services in Schools, 25,* 67–75.

Shapiro, D. A. (1994b). Tender gender issues. *Asha, 36*(11), 46–49.

Shapiro, D. A. (1995, March). A way through the forest: One boy's story with a happy ending. *The Staff,* pp. 2, 7. (Available from Aaron's Associates, 6114 Waterway, Garland, TX 75043)

Shapiro, D. A. (2000, June). *Redefined CCCs for clinical training in stuttering.* Keynote presentation at the 7th Annual Leadership Conference of ASHA's Special Interest Division 4, Fluency and Fluency Disorders (Clinical Training in Stuttering), Charleston, SC.

Shapiro, D. A. (2002a, September). Au coeur de la communication: Traitement des enfants d'âge scolaire qui bégaient. *Rééducation Orthophonique, 211,* 75–94.

Shapiro, D. A. (2002b). Stuttering: Part I. *Our Purple & Gold, 6*(1), 3, 6. (Alumni publication available from Western Carolina University, Cullowhee, NC)

Shapiro, D. A. (2002c). Stuttering: Part II. *Our Purple & Gold, 6*(2), 3. (Alumni publication available from Western Carolina University, Cullowhee, NC)

Shapiro, D. A. (2004a). Achieving fluency freedom with school-age children who stutter. *ACQuiring Knowledge in Speech, Language, and Hearing* [Australia], *6*(3), 158–161.

Shapiro, D. A. (2004b). Beyond speech fluency: Lessons learned in pursuit of communication freedom. *Stuttering Now* [Japan Stuttering Project], *121,* 1–8. (Available from Shinji Ito, B-1526, 919–1, Uchiage, Neyagawa, Osaka 572–0802 Japan; English translation available from shapiro@email.wcu.edu)

Shapiro, D. A. (2004c). Dosažení plynulé řeči u dospívajících a dospělých balbutiků. *Papoušek: Čtvrtletník Občanského sdružení LOGO, 3* (Prosinec), 4–7. (Available from Eva Neubauerová, Občanské sdružení LOGO, Vsetínská 20, 639 00 Brno, Czech Republic; English translation available from shapiro@email.wcu.edu)

Shapiro, D. A. (2004d). Dosažení volně plynulé řeči u dětí školního věku, které koktají. *Papoušek: Čtvrtletník Občanské sdružení LOGO, 4* (květen), 5–7. (Available from Eva Neubauerová,

Občanské sdružení LOGO, Vsetinska 20, 639 00 Brno, Czech Republic; English translation available from shapiro@email.wcu.edu)

Shapiro, D. A. (2004e). *Just the way you are.* Seventh International Stuttering Awareness Day Online Conference: International Year of the Child Who Stutters (J. Kuster, Conference Chair, Minnesota State University, Mankato). Available from http://www.mnsu.edu/comdis/isad7/papers/bridgebuilders7/shapiro7.html.

Shapiro, D. A. (2004f). Talefrihet for barn som stammer: Et opplegg med samarbeid, suksess og moro—del 1. *Stamposten—Norsk interesseforening for stamme, 3/04*, 15–17. (Available from Liv Marit Dalen, Vestre Vadmyra 4, N-5172 Loddfjord, Norway; English translation available from shapiro@email.wcu.edu)

Shapiro, D. A. (2004g). Verdenskongressen 2004: Et internasjonalt slektsstevne. *Stamposten—Norsk interesseforening for stamme, 2/04*, 9–11. (Available from Liv Marit Dalen, Vestre Vadmyra 4, N-5172 Loddfjord, Norway; English translation available from shapiro@email.wcu.edu)

Shapiro, D. A. (2005). Talefrihet for barn som stammer: Et opplegg med samarbeid, suksess og moro—del 2. *Stamposten—Norsk interesseforening for stamme, 1/05*, 12–15. (Available from Liv Marit Dalen, Vestre Vadmyra 4, N-5172 Loddfjord, Norway; English translation available from shapiro@email.wcu.edu)

Shapiro, D. A. (2006). Un chemin á travers la forêt: L'histoire d'un garçon qui se termine bien. *Lettre Parole Bégaiement, 41*, 5–6. (Available from Anne-Marie Simon, 4 bis, rue Cécile Vallet, 92340 Bourg-La-Reine, France; English translation available from shapiro@email.wcu.edu)

Shapiro, D. A. (2007a). *Being real.* Tenth International Stuttering Awareness Day Online Conference: Stuttering Awareness—Global Community, Local Activity (J. Kuster, Conference Chair, Minnesota State University, Mankato). Available from http://www.mnsu.edu/comdis/isad10/papers/messages10/shapiro10.html.

Shapiro, D. A. (2007b). Terapia zajakavosti v školskom veku. *Efeta, 17*(3), 23–28. (Available from Viktor Lechta, Cerovská 149, SK-900 81 Šenkvice, Slovak Republic; English translation available from shapiro@email.wcu.edu)

Shapiro, D. A. (2008). Cesta lesem Příběh jednoho chlapce se šťastným koncem. *Papoušek, 3.* (Available from Eva Neubauerová, ředitelka sdružení, Občanské sdružení LOGO, Vsetínská 20, 639 00 Brno, Czech Republic; English translation available from shapiro@email.wcu.edu)

Shapiro, D. A., Abbink, M., Bortz, M., Bruna, A. V., Cook, F., Dhu, P., et al., (2004). A multinational investigation of stuttering intervention: Assumptions, practices, and lessons. In A. Packman, A. Meltzer, & H. F. M. Peters (Eds.), *Theory, research and therapy in fluency disorders: Proceedings of the Fourth World Congress on Fluency Disorders* (pp. 123–138). Nijmegen, The Netherlands: Nijmegen University Press.

Shapiro, D. A., & Anderson, J. L. (1988). An analysis of commitments made by student clinicians in speech–language pathology and audiology. *Journal of Speech and Hearing Disorders, 53*, 202–210.

Shapiro, D. A., & Anderson, J. L. (1989). One measure of supervisory effectiveness in speech–language pathology and audiology. *Journal of Speech and Hearing Disorders, 54*, 549–557.

Shapiro, D. A., Brotherton, W. D., & Ogletree, B. T. (1995). The graduate student with marginal abilities in communication disorders: Concept and intervention strategies. *The Supervisors' Forum, 2*, 64–70.

Shapiro, D. A., Molt, L. F., Lundberg, A., Reichel, I., Ohashi, Y., Simon, A. M., & Wahlhaus, M. M. (2000). Multinational understanding through stuttering intervention: Diverse influences and global lessons. In H.-G. Bosshardt, J. S. Yaruss, & H. F. M. Peters (Eds.), *Fluency disorders: Theory, research, treatment and self-help: Proceedings of the Third World Congress on Fluency Disorders* (pp. 505–512). Nijmegen, The Netherlands: Nijmegen University Press.

Shapiro, D. A., Molt, L. F., Lundberg, A., Reichel, I., Ohashi, Y., Simon, A., & Wahlhaus, M. (2001, June). Le traitement du bégaiement: Son approche selon différents pays, influences diverses et leçons générales. *Rééducation Orthophonique, 206*, 113–126.

Shapiro, D. A., & Moses, N. (1989). Creative problem solving in public school supervision. *Language, Speech, and Hearing Services in Schools, 20*, 320–332.

Shapiro, D. A., & Moses, N. (2005). Clinicians' questioning behavior: Achieving intellectual intimacy in a postmodern professional era. *Contemporary Issues in Communication Science and Disorders, 32,* 64–76.

Shapiro, D. A., Ogletree, B. T., & Brotherton, W. D. (2002). Graduate students with marginal abilities in communication sciences and disorders: Prevalence, profiles, and solutions. *Journal of Communication Disorders, 35,* 421–451.

Shapiro, E. J., & Dempsey, C. J. (2008). Conflict resolution in team teaching: A case study in interdisciplinary teaching. *College Teaching, 56*(3), 157–162.

Sheehan, J. G. (1958). Conflict theory of stuttering. In J. Eisenson (Ed.), *Stuttering: A symposium* (pp. 121–166). New York: Harper & Row.

Sheehan, J. G. (1970). *Stuttering: Research and therapy.* New York: Harper & Row.

Sheehan, J. G. (1975). Conflict theory and avoidance-reduction therapy. In J. Eisenson (Ed.), *Stuttering: A second symposium* (pp. 97–198). New York: Harper & Row.

Sheehy, G. (2006). *Passages: Predictable crises of adult life.* New York: Random House.

Shelley, R. (1999). *Culture shock! A guide to customs and etiquette.* Portland, OR: Graphic Arts Center Publishing.

Shenker, R. C. (2004). Bilingualism in early stuttering: Empirical issues and clinical implications. In A. K. Bothe (Ed.), *Evidence-based treatment of stuttering: Empirical bases and clinical applications* (pp. 81–115). Mahwah, NJ: Erlbaum.

Shine, R. E. (1980). Direct management of the beginning stutterer. In W. Perkins (Ed.), *Seminars in speech, language and hearing* (pp. 339–350). New York: Thieme-Stratton.

Shine, R. E. (1984). Assessment and fluency training with the young stutterer. In M. Peins (Ed.), *Contemporary approaches in stuttering therapy* (pp. 173–216). Boston: Little, Brown.

Shipley, K. G., & McAfee, J. G. (2009). *Assessment in speech–language pathology: A resource manual* (4th ed.). Clifton Park, NY: Delmar/Cengage Learning.

Shipley, K. G., & Roseberry-McKibbin, C. (2006). *Interviewing and counseling in communicative disorders: Principles and procedures* (3rd ed.). Austin, TX: PRO-ED.

Shirkey, E. A. (1987). Forensic verification of stuttering. *Journal of Fluency Disorders, 12,* 197–203.

Shriberg, L. D., Filley, F. S., Hayes, D. M., Kwiatkowski, J., Schatz, J. A., Simmons, K. M., & Smith, M. E. (1975). The Wisconsin procedure for appraisal of clinical competence (W–PACC): Model and data. *Asha, 17,* 158–165.

Shugart, Y. Y., Mundorff, J., Kilshaw, J., Doheny, K., Doan, B., Wanyee, J., et al. (2004). Results of a genome-wide linkage scan for stuttering. *American Journal of Medical Genetics, 124A,* 133–135.

Siegel, G. M. (1990). Moses the stutterer: An interpretation of Deuteronomy 3:23. In J. Albach (Ed.), *To say what is ours: The best of 10 years of Letting Go* (pp. VII-7–VII-12). San Francisco: National Stuttering Project.

Siegel, G. M. (2000). Demands and capacities or demands and performance? *Journal of Fluency Disorders, 25,* 321–327.

Silverman, E.-M. (1982). Speech–language clinicians' and university students' impressions of women and girls who stutter. *Journal of Fluency Disorders, 7,* 469–478.

Silverman, F. H. (1988). The "monster" study. *Journal of Fluency Disorders, 13,* 225–231.

Silverman, F. H. (2004). *Stuttering and other fluency disorders* (3rd ed.). Long Grove, IL: Waveland.

Silverman, F. H., & Bohlman, P. (1988). Flute stuttering. *Journal of Fluency Disorders, 13,* 427–428.

Silverman, F. H., & Bongey, T. A. (1997). Nurses' attitudes toward physicians who stutter. *Journal of Fluency Disorders, 22,* 61–62.

Silverman, F. H., & Silverman, E.-M. (1971). Stutter-like behavior in the manual communication of the deaf. *Perceptual and Motor Skills, 33,* 45–46.

Silverman, S. W., & Bernstein Ratner, N. (2002). Measuring lexical diversity in children who stutter: Applications of vocd. *Journal of Fluency Disorders, 27,* 289–305.

Simon, A.-M. (1999). *Paroles de parents: Prévention du bégaiement et des risques de chronicisation.* Isbergues, France: L'Ortho-Edition.

Skott-Myhre, H. A. (2008). *Youth and subculture as creative force: Creating new spaces for radical youth work.* Toronto: University of Toronto Press.

Smith, A. (1999). Stuttering: A unified approach to a multifactorial, dynamic disorder. In N. Bernstein Ratner & E. C. Healey (Eds.), *Stuttering research and practice: Bridging the gap* (pp. 27–44). Mahwah, NJ: Erlbaum.

Smith, K. J. (1978). Identification of perceived effectiveness components in the individual supervisory conference in speech pathology and an evaluation of the relationship between ratings and content in the conferences (Doctoral dissertation, Indiana University, 1977). *Dissertation Abstracts International, 39,* 680B.

Smith, K. J., & Anderson, J. L. (1982a). Development and validation of an individual supervisory conference rating scale for use in speech–language pathology. *Journal of Speech and Hearing Research, 25,* 243–251.

Smith, K. J., & Anderson, J. L. (1982b). Relationship of perceived effectiveness to verbal interaction/content variables in supervisory conferences in speech–language pathology. *Journal of Speech and Hearing Research, 25,* 252–261.

Smits-Bandstra, S., & De Nil, L. F. (2007). Sequence skill learning in persons who stutter: Implications for cortico-striato-thalamo-cortical dysfunction. *Journal of Fluency Disorders, 32*(4), 251–278.

Snyder, G. (2006). *The existence of stuttering in sign language and other forms of expressive communication: Sufficient cause for the emergence of a new stuttering paradigm?* Research paper presented in the 9th International Stuttering Awareness Day Online Conference. Available from http://www.mnsu.edu/comdis/isad9/papers/snyder9.html.

Sokoly, M. M., & Dokecki, P. R. (1992). Ethical perspectives on family-centered early intervention. *Infants and Young Children, 4*(4), 23–32.

Sommer, M., Koch, M. A., Paulus, W., Weiller, C., & Buchel, C. (2002). Disconnection of speech-relevant brain areas in persistent developmental stuttering. *The Lancet, 360,* 380–383.

Sommers, R. K., & Caruso, A. J. (1995). Inservice training in speech–language pathology: Are we meeting the needs for fluency training? *American Journal of Speech–Language Pathology, 4*(3), 22–28.

Stager, S. V., Calis, K., Grothe, D., Bloch, M., Berensen, N. M., Smith, P. J., & Braun, A. (2005). Treatment with medications affecting dopaminergic and serotonergic mechanisms: Effects on fluency and anxiety in persons who stutter. *Journal of Fluency Disorders, 30,* 319–335.

Stager, S. V., & Ludlow, C. (1994). Responses of stutterers and vocal tremor patients to treatment with botulinum toxin. In J. Jankovic & M. Hallatt (Eds.), *Therapy with botulinum toxin* (pp. 481–490). New York: Marcel Dekker.

Stansfield, J. (1995). Word-final disfluencies in adults with learning difficulties. *Journal of Fluency Disorders, 20,* 1–10.

Starkweather, C. W. (1984). On fluency. *National Student Speech Language Hearing Association Journal, 12,* 30–37.

Starkweather, C. W. (1987). *Fluency and stuttering.* Englewood Cliffs, NJ: Prentice Hall.

Starkweather, C. W. (1993). Issues in the efficacy of treatment for fluency disorders. *Journal of Fluency Disorders, 18,* 151–168.

Starkweather, C. W. (1997). Therapy for younger children. In R. F. Curlee & G. M. Siegel (Eds.), *Nature and treatment of stuttering: New directions* (2nd ed., pp. 257–279). Needham Heights, MA: Allyn & Bacon.

Starkweather, C. W. (2002a). The development of fluency in normal children. In H. H. Gregory (Ed.), *Stuttering therapy: Prevention and intervention with children* (pp. 67–100). Memphis, TN: Stuttering Foundation of America.

Starkweather, C. W. (2002b). The epigenesis of stuttering. *Journal of Fluency Disorders, 27,* 269–288.

Starkweather, C. W., & Givens-Ackerman, J. (1997). *Stuttering.* Austin, TX: PRO-ED.

Starkweather, C. W., Gottwald, S. R., & Halfond, M. M. (1990). *Stuttering prevention: A clinical method.* Englewood Cliffs, NJ: Prentice Hall.

Stewart, T., & Richardson, G. (2004). A qualitative study of therapeutic effect from a user's perspective. *Journal of Fluency Disorders, 29,* 95–108.

Stewart, T., & Rowley, D. (1996). Acquired stammering in Great Britain. *European Journal of Disorders of Communication, 31,* 1–9.

St. Louis, K. O. (Ed.). (1996). Research and opinion on cluttering: State of the art and science. *Journal of Fluency Disorders, 21,* 171–371.

St. Louis, K. O. (1999). Person-first labeling and stuttering. *Journal of Fluency Disorders, 24,* 1–24.

St. Louis, K. O. (2001a). *Living with stuttering: Stories, basics, resources, and hope.* Morgantown, WV: Populore.

St. Louis, K. O. (2001b, December). Specialization: Implications for training specialists and generalists—A brief history of specialization. *Fluency and Fluency Disorders, 11*(4), 12–16.

St. Louis, K. O. (2005, October 18). A global project to measure public attitudes about stuttering. *The ASHA Leader,* pp. 12–13, 22.

St. Louis K. O. (2006). Measurement issues in fluency disorders. In N. Bernstein Ratner & J. Tetnowski (Eds.), *Current issues in stuttering research and practice* (pp. 61–86). Mahwah, NJ: Erlbaum.

St. Louis, K. O., & Durrenberger, C. H. (1993, December). What communication disorders do experienced clinicians prefer to manage? *Asha, 35,* 23–31.

St. Louis, K. O., & Lass, N. J. (1981). A survey of communicative disorders students' attitudes toward stuttering. *Journal of Fluency Disorders, 6,* 49–79.

St. Louis, K. O., & Myers, F. L. (1997). Management of cluttering and related fluency disorders. In R. F. Curlee & G. M. Siegel (Eds.), *Nature and treatment of stuttering: New directions* (2nd ed., pp. 313–332). Needham Heights, MA: Allyn & Bacon.

St. Louis, K. O., Myers, F. L., Bakker, K., & Raphael, L. J. (2007). Understanding and treating cluttering. In E. G. Conture & R. F. Curlee (Eds.), *Stuttering and related disorders of fluency* (3rd ed., pp. 297–325). New York: Thieme.

St. Louis, K. O., Myers, F. L., Faragasso, K., Townsend, P. S., & Gallaher, A. J. (2004). Perceptual aspects of cluttered speech. *Journal of Fluency Disorders, 29,* 213–235.

St. Louis, K. O., Raphael, L. J., Myers, F. L., & Bakker, K. (2003, November 18). Cluttering updated. *The ASHA Leader,* pp. 4–5, 20–22.

St. Louis, K. O., Reichel, I. K., Yaruss, J. S., & Lubker, B. B. (2009). Construct and concurrent validity of a prototype questionnaire to survey public attitudes toward stuttering. *Journal of Fluency Disorders, 34*(1), 11–28.

Stockman, I. J., Boult, J., & Robinson, G. C. (2008). Multicultural/multilingual instruction in educational programs: A survey of perceived faculty practices and outcomes. *American Journal of Speech–Language Pathology, 17,* 241–264.

Stoneman, Z., & Malone, D. M. (1995). The changing nature of interdisciplinary practice. In B. A. Thyer & N. P. Kropf (Eds.), *Developmental disabilities: A handbook for interdisciplinary practice* (pp. 234–247). Cambridge, MA: Brookline Books.

Strauss, R. (2008, Nov. 25). Making the bilingual connection. *The ASHA Leader,* pp. 30–32.

Stuart, A., Kalinowski, J., Rastatter, M., Saltuklaroglu, T., & Dayalu, V. (2004). Investigations of the impact of altered auditory feedback in-the-ear devices on the speech of people who stutter: Initial fitting and 4-month follow-up. *International Journal of Language and Communication Disorders, 39*(1), 93–113.

Sturm, J. A., & Seery, C. H. (2007). Speech and articulatory rates of school-age children in conversation and narrative contexts. *Language, Speech, and Hearing Services in Schools, 38,* 47–59.

Suresh, R., Ambrose, N., Roe, C., Pluzhnikov, A., Wittke-Thompson, J. K., Ng, M. C.-Y, et al. (2006). New complexities in the genetics of stuttering: Significant sex-specific linkage signals. *American Journal of Human Genetics, 78,* 554–563.

Tanner, D. C. (2001, April 3). Hooray for Hollywood: Communication disorders and the motion picture industry. *The ASHA Leader,* pp. 10–11, 29.

Tanner, D. C. (2003). *Exploring communication disorders: A 21st century introduction through literature and media.* Boston: Allyn & Bacon.

Tapia, F. (1969). Haldol in the treatment of children with tics and stutterers—and an incidental finding. *Psychiatric Quarterly, 43,* 647–649.

Taylor, O. L. (1986). Historical perspectives and conceptual framework. In O. L. Taylor (Ed.), *Treatment of communication disorders in culturally and linguistically diverse populations* (pp. 3–19). San Diego, CA: College-Hill.

Taylor, O. L. (1993). Forward. In D. E. Battle (Ed.), *Communication disorders in multicultural populations* (pp. xii–xiii). Stoneham, MA: Andover Medical Publishers/Butterworth-Heinemann.

Tellis, G. M., Bressler, L., & Emerick, K. (2008). An exploration of clinicians' views about assessment and treatment of stuttering. *Perspectives on Fluency and Fluency Disorders, 18*, 16–23.

Terry, W. (1994, December 25). When his sound was silenced. *Parade Magazine*, pp. 12–13.

Tetnowski, J., & Schagen, A. J. (2001). A comparison of listener and speaker perception of stuttering events. *Journal of Speech–Language Pathology and Audiology, 25*, 8–18.

Theys, C., van Wieringen, A., & De Nil, L. (2008). A clinician survey of speech and non-speech characteristics of neurogenic stuttering. *Journal of Fluency Disorders, 33*, 1–23.

Thompson, D. A., Arora, T., & Sharp, S. (2002). *Bullying: Effective strategies for long-term improvement*. New York: Routledge/Falmer.

Throneburg, R. N., & Yairi, E. (2001). Durational, proportionate, and absolute frequency characteristics of disfluencies: A longitudinal study regarding persistence and recovery. *Journal of Speech, Language, and Hearing Research, 44*, 38–51.

Thyer, B. A., & Kropf, N. P. (1995). Preface. In B. A. Thyer & N. P. Kropf (Eds.), *Developmental disabilities: A handbook for interdisciplinary practice* (pp. i–iii). Cambridge, MA: Brookline.

Tice, P, & Moore, M. (2009, January 20). Six nations now participate in certification recognition. *The ASHA Leader*, pp. 34–35.

Tiger, R. J., Irvine, T. L., & Reis, R. P. (1980). Cluttering as a complex of learning disabilities. *Language, Speech, and Hearing Services in Schools, 11*(1), 3–14.

Tillis, M., & Wagner, W. (1984). *Stutterin' boy*. New York: Rawson Associates.

Tolchard, B. (1995). Treatment of Gilles de la Tourette Syndrome using behavioural psychotherapy: A single case example. *Journal of Psychiatric and Mental Health Nursing, 2*(4), 233–236.

Toner, M. A., & Shadden, B. B. (2002, Spring). Counseling challenges: Working with older clients and caregivers. *Contemporary Issues in Communication Science and Disorders, 29*, 68–78.

Tourette Syndrome Association. (2005). *The genetics of Tourette Syndrome: Who it affects and how it occurs in families*. Bayside, NY: Tourette Syndrome Association.

Tourette Syndrome Association. (2006). *Questions and answers about Tourette Syndrome*. Bayside, NY: Tourette Syndrome Association.

Travis, L. E. (1971). The unspeakable feelings of people with special reference to stuttering. In L. E. Travis (Ed.), *Handbook of speech pathology and audiology* (pp. 1009–1033). Englewood Cliffs, NJ: Prentice Hall.

Travis, L. E. (1978). The cerebral dominance theory of stuttering: 1931–1978. *Journal of Speech and Hearing Disorders, 43*, 278–281.

Tudor, M. (1939). *An experimental study of the effect of evaluative labeling on speech fluency*. Unpublished master's thesis, University of Iowa.

Turnbaugh, K. R., Guitar, B. E., & Hoffman, P. R. (1979). Speech clinicians' attribution of personality traits as a function of stuttering severity. *Journal of Speech and Hearing Research, 22*, 37–45.

Turnbull, A. P., Patterson, J. M., Behr, S. K., Murphy, D. L., Marquis, J. G., & Blue-Banning, M. J. (Eds.). (1993). *Cognitive coping, families, and disability*. Baltimore: Brookes.

Turnbull, A. P., & Turnbull, H. R., III. (1990). *Families, professionals, and exceptionality: A special partnership* (2nd ed.). Columbus, OH: Merrill.

Turnbull, A. P., Turnbull, R., Erwin, E. J., & Soodak, L. C. (2006). *Families, professionals, and exceptionality: Positive outcomes through partnerships and trust* (5th ed.). Upper Saddle River, NJ: Prentice Hall.

Turnbull, A. P., Turnbull, R., & Wehmeyer, M. L. (2007). *Exceptional lives: Special education in today's schools* (5th ed.). Upper Saddle River, NJ: Prentice Hall.

Underwood, J. K. (1979). *Underwood category system for analyzing supervisor–clinician behavior*. Unpublished manuscript, University of Northern Colorado, Greeley.

U.S. Census Bureau. (2000). *Statistical abstract of the United States* (120th ed.). Washington, DC: Author.

Van Bloss, N. (2006). *Busy body: My life with Tourette's Syndrome*. London: Fusion Press/Satin Publications.

Van Borsel, J. (1997). Neurogenic stuttering: A review. *Journal of Clinical Speech and Language Studies*, 7, 17–33.

Van Borsel, J. (2006). Fluency disorders in genetic syndromes. *Bulgarian Journal of Communication Disorders*, 1(1), 38–50.

Van Borsel, J., & de Britto Pereira, M. M. (2005). Assessment of stuttering in a familiar versus an unfamiliar language. *Journal of Fluency Disorders*, 30, 109–124.

Van Borsel, J., Jozefien, M., Charlotte, M., Rijke, R., Evy Van, L., & Van Tineke, R. (2006). Prevalence of stuttering in regular and special school populations in Belgium based on teacher perceptions. *Folio Phoniatrica*, 58, 289–302.

Van Borsel, J., Maes, E., & Foulon, S. (2001). Stuttering and bilingualism: A review. *Journal of Fluency Disorders*, 26, 179–205.

Van Borsel, J., & Tetnowski, J. (2007). Fluency disorders in genetic syndromes. *Journal of Fluency Disorders*, 32(4), 279–296.

Van Borsel, J., Van Coster, R., & Van Lierde, K. (1996). Repetitions in final position in a 9-year-old boy with focal brain damage. *Journal of Fluency Disorders*, 21(2), 137–146.

Van Borsel, J., Van Lierde, K., Van Cauwenberge, P., Guldemont, I., & Van Orshoven, M. (1998). Severe acquired stuttering following injury to the left supplementary motor region: A case report. *Journal of Fluency Disorders*, 23, 49–58.

Van Riper, C. (1965). Supervision of clinical practice. *Asha*, 7, 75–77.

Van Riper, C. (1972). *Speech correction: Principles and methods* (5th ed.). Englewood Cliffs, NJ: Prentice Hall.

Van Riper, C. (1973). *The treatment of stuttering*. Englewood Cliffs, NJ: Prentice Hall.

Van Riper, C. (1974). Success and failure in speech therapy. In L. L. Emerick & S. B. Hood (Eds.), *The client–clinician relationship: Essays on interpersonal sensitivity in the therapeutic transaction* (pp. 103–106). Springfield, IL: Thomas..

Van Riper, C. (1975). The stutterer's clinician. In J. Eisenson (Ed.), *Stuttering: A second symposium* (pp. 453–492). New York: Harper & Row.

Van Riper, C. (1982). *The nature of stuttering* (2nd ed.). Englewood Cliffs, NJ: Prentice Hall.

Van Riper, C. (1991, April). A message from Charles Van Riper. *Letting Go*, 11(4), 1.

Van Riper, C. (1992). Some ancient history. *Journal of Fluency Disorders*, 17, 25–28.

Vanryckeghem, M., Brutten, G. J., & Hernandez, L. M. (2005). A comparative investigation of the speech-associated attitude of preschool and kindergarten children who do and do not stutter. *Journal of Fluency Disorders*, 30, 307–318.

Venable, G. P. (2006, November 7). How a sister (and SLP) learned the right questions to ask. *The ASHA Leader*, p. 9.

Vierck, E., & Hodges, K. (2005). *Aging: Lifestyles, work, and money*. Westport, CT: Greenwood Press.

Villa, R. A., & Thousand, J. S. (Eds.). (2005). *Creating an inclusive school* (2nd ed.). Alexandria, VA: Association for Supervision and Curriculum Development.

Vinnard, R. T. (1990a, January). AIDS-related acquired stuttering. *Quo Vadis*, 2(2), 6.

Vinnard, R. T. (1990b, September). Dr. Comings writes on Tourette's. *Quo Vadis*, 2(5), 1, 3.

Viswanath, N., Lee, H. S., & Chakraborty, R. (2004). Evidence for a major gene influence on persistent developmental stuttering. *Human Biology*, 76(3), 401–412.

Voelker, E. S., & Voelker, C. H. (1937). Spasmophemia in dyslallia cophotica. *Annals of Otology, Rhinology, and Laryngology*, 46, 740–743.

Von Drehle, D. (2007, August 6). The myth about boys. *Time*, 170(6), 38–47.

Wall, M. J., & Myers, F. L. (1995). *Clinical management of childhood stuttering* (2nd ed.). Austin, TX: PRO-ED.

Walle, E. L. (1974). A journey in experiences in interpersonal relations with sociopathic criminals. In L. L. Emerick & S. B. Hood (Eds.), *The client–clinician relationship: Essays on interpersonal sensitivity in the therapeutic transaction* (pp. 3–28). Springfield, IL: Thomas.

Walle, E. L. (1976). *Prevention of stuttering [Part 1]: Identifying the danger signs*. [Videotape]. Memphis, TN: Stuttering Foundation of America.

Wallen, V. (1961). Primary stuttering in a 28-year-old adult. *Journal of Speech and Hearing Disorders,* *26,* 394–395.

Walsh, F. (Ed.). (2003). *Normal family processes: Growing diversity and complexity* (3rd ed.). New York: Guilford Press.

Walsh, F. (2006). *Strengthening family resilience* (2nd ed.). New York: Guilford Press.

Wand, R. R., Matazow, G. S., Shady, G. A., Furer, P., & Staley, D. (1993). Tourette Syndrome: Associated symptoms and most disabling features. *Neuroscience and Biobehavioral Reviews,* *17*(3), 271–275.

Watkins, K. E., Smith, S. M., Davis, S., & Howell, P. (2008). *Brain, 131,* 50–59.

Watkins, R. V. (2005). Language abilities of young children who stutter. In E. Yairi & N. G. Ambrose, *Early childhood stuttering: For clinicians by clinicians* (pp. 235–251). Austin, TX: PRO-ED.

Watkins, R. V., Yairi, E., & Ambrose, N. G. (1999). Early childhood stuttering III: Initial status of expressive language abilities. *Journal of Speech, Language, and Hearing Research, 42,* 1125–1135.

Watson, J. B. (1995). Exploring the attitudes of adults who stutter. *Journal of Communication Disorders, 28,* 143–164.

Way, N., & Chu, J. Y. (Eds.). (2004). *Adolescent boys: Exploring diverse cultures of boyhood.* New York: New York University Press.

Webber, M., & Onslow, M. (2003). Maintenance of treatment effects. In M. Onslow, A. Packman, & E. Harrison (Eds.), *The Lidcombe Program of early stuttering intervention: A clinician's guide* (pp. 81–90). Austin, TX: PRO-ED.

Weber, L. (2007). *The Holocaust chronicle: A history in words and pictures.* Lincolnwood, IL: Publications International/Legacy.

Webster, E. J. (1977). *Counseling with parents of handicapped children: Guidelines for improving communication.* New York: Grune & Stratton.

Webster, R. L. (1979). Empirical considerations regarding stuttering therapy. In H. H. Gregory (Ed.), *Controversies about stuttering therapy* (pp. 209–239). Baltimore: University Park Press.

Weiner, A. E. (1981). A case of adult onset of stuttering. *Journal of Fluency Disorders, 6,* 181–186.

Weiss, D. A. (1964). *Cluttering.* Englewood Cliffs, NJ: Prentice Hall.

Wells, P. G., & Malcolm, M. T. (1971). Controlled trial of the treatment of 36 stutterers. *British Journal of Psychiatry, 119,* 603–604.

West, R. (1958). An agnostic's speculations about stuttering. In J. Eisenson (Ed.), *Stuttering: A symposium* (pp. 167–222). New York: Harper & Row.

Westby, C. E. (2000). Multicultural issues in speech and language assessment. In J. B. Tomblin, H. L. Morris, & D. C. Spriestersbach (Eds.), *Diagnosis in speech–language pathology* (2nd ed., pp. 35–62). San Diego, CA: Singular.

Westling, D. L., & Fox, L. (2009). *Teaching students with severe disabilities* (4th ed.). Upper Saddle River, NJ: Pearson Education/Merrill.

Wexler, K. B. (1982). Developmental disfluency in 2-, 4-, and 6-year-old boys in neutral and stress situations. *Journal of Speech and Hearing Research, 25,* 229–234.

Whitaker, C. (1996). A family is a four-dimensional relationship. In P. J. Guerin, Jr. (Ed.), *Family therapy: Theory and practice* (pp. 182–192). Fort Worth, FL: Gardner Press.

Whitbourne, S. K. (2008). *Adult development and aging: Biophychosocial perspectives* (3rd ed.). Hoboken, NJ: Wiley.

Whitebread, G. (2004). *Stuck on the tip of my thumb: Stuttering in American Sign Language.* Unpublished Honors Thesis, Gallaudet University, 2004.

Williams, D. E. (1957). A point of view about "stuttering." *Journal of Speech and Hearing Disorders, 22*(3), 390–397.

Williams, D. E. (1971). Stuttering therapy for children. In L. E. Travis (Ed.), *Handbook of speech pathology and audiology* (pp. 1073–1093). Englewood Cliffs, NJ: Prentice Hall.

Williams, D. E. (1978). Differential diagnosis of disorders of fluency. In F. L. Darley & D. C. Spriestersbach (Eds.), *Diagnostic methods in speech pathology* (2nd ed., pp. 409–438). New York: Harper & Row.

Williams, D. E. (1979). A perspective on approaches to stuttering therapy. In H. H. Gregory (Ed.), *Controversies about stuttering therapy* (pp. 241–268). Baltimore: University Park Press.

Williams, D. E. (2003). Talking with children who stutter. In J. Fraser (Ed.), *Effective counseling in stuttering therapy* (Publication 18, pp. 53–64). Memphis, TN: Stuttering Foundation of America.

Williams, D. E. (2004). *The genius of Dean Williams* (Publication 425). Memphis, TN: Stuttering Foundation of America.

Williams, D. E. (2006). Working with children in the school environment. In J. Fraser (Ed.), *Stuttering therapy: Transfer and maintenance* (Publication 19, 2nd ed., pp. 25–35). Memphis, TN: Stuttering Foundation of America.

Williams, D. E., Darley, F. L., & Spriestersbach, D. C. (1978). Appraisal of rate and fluency. In F. L. Darley & D. C. Spriestersbach (Eds.), *Diagnostic methods in speech pathology* (2nd ed., pp. 256–283). New York: Harper & Row.

Wilmoth, J. M., & Longino, C. F. (2007). Demographic perspectives on aging. In J. M. Wilmoth & K. F. Ferraro (Eds.), *Gerontology: Perspectives and Issues* (3rd ed., pp. 35–55). New York: Springer.

Wingate, M. E. (1964). A standard definition of stuttering. *Journal of Speech and Hearing Disorders, 29*, 484–489.

Wingate, M. E. (1969). Sound and pattern in "artificial" fluency. *Journal of Speech and Hearing Research, 12*, 677–686.

Wingate, M. E. (1976). *Stuttering: Theory and treatment.* New York: Irvington Publishers/Halsted Press.

Wingate, M. E. (1983). Speaking unassisted: Comments on a paper by Andrews et al. *Journal of Speech and Hearing Disorders, 48*, 255–263.

Wingate, M. E. (1988). *The structure of stuttering: A psycholinguistic analysis.* New York: Springer-Verlag.

Wingate, M. E. (1997). *Stuttering: A short history of a curious disorder.* Westport, CT: Bergin & Garvey.

Wingate, M. E. (2001). SLD is not stuttering. *Journal of Speech, Language, and Hearing Research, 44*, 381–384.

Winslow, M., & Guitar, B. (1994). The effects of structured turn-taking on disfluencies: A case study. *Language, Speech, and Hearing Services in Schools, 25*, 251–257.

Wischner, G. J. (1950). Stuttering behavior and learning: A preliminary theoretical formulation. *Journal of Speech and Hearing Disorders, 15*, 324–335.

Wischner, G. J. (1952). An experimental approach to expectancy and anxiety in stuttering behavior. *Journal of Speech and Hearing Disorders, 17*, 139–154.

Wolf, A. E. (1991). *Get out of my life, but first could you drive me and Cheryl to the mall? A parent's guide to the new teenager.* New York: Noonday Press.

Wolk, L. (1998). Intervention strategies for children who exhibit coexisting phonological and fluency disorders: A clinical note. *Child Language Teaching and Therapy, 14*, 69–82.

Wolk, L., Edwards, M. L., & Conture, E. G. (1993). Coexistence of stuttering and disordered phonology in young children. *Journal of Speech and Hearing Research, 36*, 906–917.

Wood, F., Stump, D., McKeehan, A., Sheldon, S., & Proctor, J. (1980). Patterns of regional cerebral blood flow during attempted reading aloud by stutterers both on and off haloperidol medication: Evidence for inadequate left frontal activation during stuttering. *Brain and Language, 9*, 141–144.

Woods, C. L., & Williams, D. E. (1971). Speech clinicians' conceptions of boys and men who stutter. *Journal of Speech and Hearing Disorders, 36*, 225–234.

Woods, C. L., & Williams, D. E. (1976). Traits attributed to stuttering and normally fluent males. *Journal of Speech and Hearing Research, 19*, 267–278.

Woods, S., Shearsby, J., Onslow, M., & Burnham, D. (2002). Psychological impact of the Lidcombe Program of early stuttering intervention. *International Journal of Language and Communication Disorders, 37*(1), 31–40.

World Health Organization. (1977). *Manual of the international statistical classification of diseases, injuries, and causes of death.* Vol. 1. Geneva: Author.

World Health Organization. (1980). *International classification of impairments, disabilities, and handicaps: A manual of classification relating to the consequences of disease*. Geneva: Author.

World Health Organization. (2001). *International classification of functioning, disability, and health*. Geneva: Author.

World Health Organization. (2010). *The ICD-10, Classification of mental and behavioral disorders: Clinical descriptions and diagnostic guidelines*. Geneva: Author. Available from www.who.int/classifications/icd/en/bluebook.pdf.

Worrall, L. E., & Hickson, L. M. (2003). *Communication disability in aging: From prevention to intervention*. Clifton Park, NY: Thomson/Delmar Learning.

Yairi, E. (1981). Disfluencies of normally speaking two-year-old children. *Journal of Speech and Hearing Research, 24*, 490–495.

Yairi, E. (1993). Epidemiologic and other considerations in treatment efficacy research with preschool age children who stutter. *Journal of Fluency Disorders, 18*, 197–219.

Yairi, E. (1997). Disfluency characteristics of childhood stuttering. In R. F. Curlee & G. M. Siegel (Eds.), *Nature and treatment of stuttering: New directions* (2nd ed., pp. 49–78). Needham Heights, MA: Allyn & Bacon.

Yairi, E. (2004). The formative years of stuttering: A changing portrait. *Contemporary Issues in Communication Sciences and Disorders, 31*, 92–104.

Yairi, E. (2005, Fall). On the gender factor in stuttering. *The Stuttering Foundation of America*, p. 5.

Yairi, E. (2006, Summer). Genetics of stuttering: New developments. *The Stuttering Foundation of America*, pp. 2, 6.

Yairi, E. (2007). Subtyping stuttering I: A review. *Journal of Fluency Disorders, 32*, 165–196.

Yairi, E., & Ambrose, N. (1992a). A longitudinal study of stuttering in children: A preliminary report. *Journal of Speech and Hearing Research, 35*, 755–760.

Yairi, E., & Ambrose, N. (1992b). Onset of stuttering in preschool children: Selected factors. *Journal of Speech and Hearing Research, 35*, 782–788.

Yairi, E., & Ambrose, N. G. (1999). Early childhood stuttering I: Persistency and recovery rates. *Journal of Speech, Language, and Hearing Research, 42*, 1097–1112.

Yairi, I., & Ambrose, N. G. (2001, July 24). The Tudor Experiment and Wendell Johnson: Science and Ethics Reexamined. *The ASHA Leader*, p. 17.

Yairi, E., & Ambrose, N. G. (2005). *Early childhood stuttering*. Austin, TX: PRO-ED.

Yairi, E., Ambrose, N. G., & Cox, N. (1996). Genetics of stuttering: A critical review. *Journal of Speech and Hearing Research, 39*, 771–784.

Yairi, E., Ambrose, N. G., & Niermann, R. (1993). The early months of stuttering: A developmental study. *Journal of Speech and Hearing Research, 36*, 521–528.

Yairi, E., & Carrico, D. M. (1992). Early childhood stuttering: Pediatricians' attitudes and practices. *American Journal of Speech–Language Pathology, 1*(3), 54–62.

Yairi, E., & Clifton, N. F., Jr. (1972). Disfluent speech behavior of preschool children, high school seniors, and geriatric persons. *Journal of Speech and Hearing Research, 15*, 714–719.

Yairi, E., & Seery, C. H. (2011). *Stuttering: Foundations and clinical implications*. Upper Saddle River, NJ: Pearson Education.

Yairi, E., Watkins, R., Ambrose, N., & Paden, E. (2001). What is stuttering? *Journal of Speech, Language, and Hearing Research, 44*, 585–592.

Yairi, E., & Williams, D. E. (1970). Speech clinicians' stereotypes of elementary-school boys who stutter. *Journal of Communication Disorders, 3*, 161–170.

Yairi, E., & Williams, D. E. (1971). Reports of parental attitudes by stuttering and by nonstuttering children. *Journal of Speech and Hearing Research, 14*, 596–604.

Yaruss, J. S. (1998). Treatment outcomes in stuttering: Finding value in clinical data. In A. Cordes & R. Ingham (Eds.), *Toward treatment efficacy in stuttering: A search for empirical bases* (pp. 213–242). Austin, TX: PRO-ED.

Yaruss, J. S. (1999a). Current status of academic and clinical education in fluency disorders at ASHA-accredited training programs. *Journal of Fluency Disorders, 24*, 169–183.

Yaruss, J. S. (1999b). Utterance length, syntactic complexity, and childhood stuttering. *Journal of Speech and Hearing Research, 42*, 329–344.

Yaruss, J. S. (2000). Converting between word and syllable counts in children's conversational speech samples. *Journal of Fluency Disorders, 25*, 305–316.

Yaruss, J. S. (2001). Evaluating treatment outcomes for adults who stutter. *Journal of Communication Disorders, 34*, 163–182.

Yaruss, J. S., Coleman, C., & Hammer, D. (2006). Treating preschool children who stutter: Description and preliminary evaluation of a family-focused treatment approach. *Language, Speech, and Hearing Services in Schools, 37*, 118–136.

Yaruss, J. S., & Conture, E. G. (1996). Stuttering and phonological disorders in children: Examination of the Covert Repair Hypothesis. *Journal of Speech and Hearing Research, 39*, 349–364.

Yaruss, J. S., LaSalle, L. R., & Conture, E. G. (1998). Evaluating stuttering in children: Diagnostic data. *American Journal of Speech–Language Pathology, 7*(4), 62–76.

Yaruss, J. S., Murphy, B., Quesal, R. W., & Reardon, N. A. (2004). *Bullying and teasing: Helping children who stutter.* New York: National Stuttering Association.

Yaruss, J. S., & Pelczarski, K. (2007). Evidence-based practice for school-age stuttering: Balancing existing research with clinical practice. *EBP Briefs, 2*(4), 1–8.

Yaruss, J. S., Pelczarski, K., & Quesal, R. W. (2010). Comprehensive treatment for school-age children who stutter: Treating the entire disorder. In B. Guitar & R. J. McCauley (Eds.), *Treatment of stuttering: Established and emerging interventions* (pp. 215–244). Philadelphia: Lippincott/Williams & Wilkins.

Yaruss, J. S., & Quesal, R. W. (2001). Developing instruments for documenting stuttering treatment outcomes. In H.–G. Bosshardt, J. S. Yaruss, & H. F. M. Peters (Eds.), *Fluency disorders: Theory, research, treatment, and self-help. Procedings of the Third World Congress on Fluency Disorders* (pp. 227–231). Nijmegen, The Netherlands: Nijemegen University Press.

Yaruss, J. S., & Quesal, R. W. (2002). Academic and clinical education in fluency disorders: An update. *Journal of Fluency Disorders, 27*, 43–63.

Yaruss, J. S., & Quesal, R. W. (2004a). Partnerships between clinicians, researchers, and people who stutter in the evaluation of stuttering treatment outcomes. *Stammering Research, 1*(1), 1–15.

Yaruss, J. S., & Quesal, R. W. (2004b). Stuttering and the International Classification of Functioning, Disability, and Health (ICF): An update. *Journal of Communication Disorders, 37*, 35–52.

Yaruss, J. S., & Quesal, R. W. (2006). Overall Assessment of the Speaker's Experience of Stuttering (OASES): Documenting multiple outcomes in stuttering treatment. *Journal of Fluency Disorders, 31*, 90–115.

Yaruss, J. S., & Quesal, R. W. (2008). *OASES: Overall assessment of the speaker's experience of stuttering.* Bloomington, MN: Pearson/AGS.

Yaruss, J. S., Quesal, R. W., & Murphy, B. (2002). National Stuttering Association members' opinions about stuttering treatment. *Journal of Fluency Disorders, 27*, 227–242.

Yaruss, J. S., Quesal, R. W., Reeves, L. (2007). Self-help and mutual aid groups as an adjunct to stuttering therapy. In E. G. Conture & R. F. Curlee (Eds.), *Stuttering and related disorders of fluency* (3rd ed., pp. 256–276). New York: Thieme.

Yaruss, J. S., Quesal, R. W., Reeves, L., Molt, L. F., Kluetz, B., Caruso, A. J., et al. (2002). Speech treatment and support group experiences of people who participate in the National Stuttering Association. *Journal of Fluency Disorders, 27*, 115–134.

Yaruss, J. S., & Reardon-Reeves, N. A. (2006). *Young children who stutter (Ages 2–6): Information and support for parents (Five steps to help you help your child)* (4th ed.). New York: National Stuttering Association.

Yeakle, M. K., & Cooper, E. B. (1986). Teacher perceptions of stuttering. *Journal of Fluency Disorders, 11*, 345–359.

Young, M. A. (1985). Increasing the frequency of stuttering. *Journal of Speech and Hearing Research, 28*, 282–293.

Zarski, J. J., DePompei, R., & Zook, A., II (1988). Traumatic head injury: Dimensions of family responsivity. *Journal of Head Trauma Rehabilitation, 3*(4), 31–41.

Zebrowski, P. M. (1994). Stuttering. In J. B. Tomblin, H. L. Morris, & D. C. Spriestersbach (Eds.), *Diagnosis in speech–language pathology* (pp. 215–245). San Diego, CA: Singular.

Zebrowski, P. M. (1995). The topography of beginning stuttering. *Journal of Communication Disorders, 28*, 75–91.

Zebrowski, P. M. (1997). Assisting young children who stutter and their families: Defining the role of the speech–language pathologist. *American Journal of Speech–Language Pathology, 6*(2), 19–28.

Zebrowski, P. M. (2002, Spring). Building clinical relationships with teenagers who stutter. *Contemporary Issues in Communication Science and Disorders, 29*, 91–100.

Zebrowski, P. M. (2003). Understanding and coping with emotions: Counseling teenagers who stutter. In J. Fraser (Ed.), *Effective counseling in stuttering therapy* (Publication 18, pp. 85–94). Memphis, TN: Stuttering Foundation of America.

Zebrowski, P. M. (2007). Treatment factors that influence therapy outcomes of children who stutter. In E. G. Conture & R. F. Curlee (Eds.), *Stuttering and related disorders of fluency* (3rd ed., pp. 23–38). New York: Thieme.

Zimmermann, G. (1980a). Articulatory dynamics of fluent utterances of stutterers and nonstutterers. *Journal of Speech and Hearing Research, 23*, 95–107.

Zimmermann, G. (1980b). Stuttering: A disorder of movement. *Journal of Speech and Hearing Research, 23*, 122–136.

Zimmermann, G. (1984). Articulatory dynamics of stutterers. In R. F. Curlee & W. H. Perkins (Eds.), *Nature and treatment of stuttering: New directions* (pp. 131–147). San Diego, CA: College-Hill.

Zimmermann, G., Liljeblad, S., Frank, A., & Cleeland, C. (1983). The Indians have many terms for it: Stuttering among the Bannock-Shoshoni. *Journal of Speech and Hearing Research, 26*, 315–318.

Zimmermann, G. N., Smith, A., & Hanley, J. M. (1981). Stuttering: In need of a unifying conceptual framework. *Journal of Speech and Hearing Research, 24*, 25–31.

Zimmerman, I., Steiner, V., & Pond, R. (1979). *Preschool language scale.* San Antonio, TX: Psychological Corp.

Zraick, R. I., Gregg, B. A., & Whitehouse, E. L. (2006). Speech and voice characteristics of geriatric speakers: A review of the literature and a call for research and training. Journal of Medical Speech–Language Pathology, *14*(3), 133–142.

Appendix

Helpful Websites

American Speech-Language-Hearing Association

http://www.asha.org/

ASHA is the professional, scientific, and credentialing association at the national level in the United States for audiologists, speech–language pathologists, and speech, language, and hearing scientists. ASHA also is an information resource for the public and helps locate service providers in any geographic location.

Bill of Rights and Responsibilities for People Who Stutter

http://www.stutterisa.org/Mission_R&R.html#billofrights/

The Bill of Rights and Responsibilities for People Who Stutter is a joint project by people who stutter, professional clinicians, and researchers. It provides a framework for building a more humane, just, and compassionate world for the millions of people who stutter.

Friends: The National Association of Young People Who Stutter

http://www.friendswhostutter.org/

Friends is a national organization created to provide a network of support and empowerment for children and teenagers who stutter. Members include young people who stutter (in addition to adults who stutter), their families, and the speech–language pathologists who work with them.

International Cluttering Association

http://associations.missouristate.edu/ICA/

The International Cluttering Association brings together people who clutter and their families with clinicians and researchers who are committed to understanding cluttering. Its mission is to increase public and professional awareness about this communication disorder, to encourage development and study of effective treatments, and to improve the quality of life for people who clutter.

International Fluency Association

http://www.theifa.org/

The International Fluency Association is an interdisciplinary organization devoted to understanding and managing fluency disorders and to improving the quality of life for people with fluency disorders. As such, IFA brings together clinicians, researchers, people who stutter, and other interested parties from around the world through its international congresses, the *Journal of Fluency Disorders*, and ongoing electronic communications.

International Stuttering Association

http://www.stutterisa.org/

The International Stuttering Association is composed of self-help organizations from around the world. Members include people who stutter, speech–language pathologists, and others who together are working toward achieving "a world that understands stuttering." Its primary venues for communication are its international congresses, *One Voice* (its electronic newsletter), and regular electronic interactions. ISA actively affiliates with other international organizations (e.g., European League of Stuttering Associations) and member associations (e.g., Australian Speak Easy Association, British Stammering Association, Canadian Association of People who Stutter, and the National Stuttering Association, among many others).

International Stuttering Awareness Day Online Conferences

http://www.mnsu.edu/comdis/kuster/isadarchive/onlineconference.html

These annual international conferences about stuttering have been held since 1998. Hosted on the Stuttering Home Page, they are open for active participation by any interested individual at no cost from October 1 to 22 of each year. Thereafter, they are archived for permanent retrieval.

National Stuttering Association

http://www.WeStutter.org/

The National Stuttering Association is the largest self-help organization in the United States for people who stutter. Their mission is to bring "hope, dignity, support, education, and empowerment to children and adults who stutter, and their families."

The Specialty Board on Fluency Disorders

http://www.stutteringspecialists.org/

The Specialty Board on Fluency Disorders is of use for both consumers and professionals. Consumers can locate Board Recognized Fluency Specialists. Professionals can learn and pursue procedures for seeking board recognition in fluency disorders or for becoming Fluency Specialist Mentors. This Specialty Recognition Program is an approved program of ASHA.

Stuttering Foundation of America

http://www.stutteringhelp.org/ (English), http://www.tartamudez.org/ (Spanish)

The Stuttering Foundation of America provides free online resources, services, and support, in both English and Spanish, to people who stutter and their families, and supports research into the causes of stuttering. It provides books and other instructional materials for consumers (people of all ages who stutter and their families) and for speech–language pathologists.

The Stuttering Home Page

http://www.stutteringhomepage.com/

This website, created by Judith Maginnis Kuster and maintained at Minnesota State University, Mankato, is dedicated to providing information about stuttering for both consumers and professionals who work with people who stutter. It includes information about research, therapy, self-help organizations, and conferences and other events. It contains the most comprehensive series of links to other homepages about stuttering.

Tourette Syndrome Association

http://tsa-usa.org/

The Tourette Syndrome Association is committed to raising public awareness about Tourette syndrome and offers resources and referrals to help people and their families cope with this disorder. Members include individuals, families, relatives, and medical and allied professionals working in the field.

Author Index

Subject Index

ABC (*Analysis of Behavior of Clinicians*), 472
Academic preparation of clinicians, 466–468, 488–489
Acceptable stuttering, 208
Acquired disfluency following laryngectomy, 141
Acquired immunodeficiency syndrome. *See* AIDS
Active listening, 422
Adaptability of families, 170
Adaptation, 60, 220, 266–267, 313, 394
Adderall, 138
Adductor spasmodic dysphonia, 140–141
ADHD, 138
Adolescents
  assessment of, 382–392, 439
  attitudes and feelings of, 394, 414, 417–423
  awareness of speech fluency in treatment of, 412
  benchmarking for, 424–425
  client and family interview with, 383–387
  decreasing frequency of scheduled treatment for, 423–424
  diagnosis of, 395
  experiences of fluency success in treatment of, 411–412
  extraclinical assignments for, 412–413
  extrafamily considerations for, 408–409
  fluency facilitating techniques for, 413–414
  fluency shaping for, 391
  general precepts about, 372–374
  goals and objectives for treatment of, 406, 411
  helping client become his own clinician, 423
  increase and transfer of fluent speech, 410–415
  informational resources for, 406
  integration of treatment changes within communication system of, 428–429
  intrafamily considerations for, 407–408
  maintenance of speech fluency by, 423–431
  personal construct theory and, 407, 425–428
  positive feelings about communication and oneself as communicator in treatment of, 417–419, 421–422
  post-assessment procedures for, 392–406, 439
  preassessment procedures for, 379–382, 439
  primary role of conversational partners of, 429–431
  procedures for treatment of, 409–431
  prognosis and recommendations for, 395–404
  psychotherapeutic considerations on, 409
  rate of speech, 393–394
  rationale underlying treatment of, 406–409
  relapse prevention for, 416–417, 419–421
  resistance to fluency disrupters in treatment of, 415–417
  "safe house" for treatment of, 410
  speech analysis of, 393–395
  speech-language samples and structured activities for, 387–390
  study questions, 440–442
  stuttering modification for, 391–392
  summary on, 438–440
  talking with, in positive ways, 423
  teasing and, 419–421
  treatment of, 406–431, 439–440
  trial management for, 390–392
Adults. *See also* Senior adults
  assessment of, 382–392, 439
  attitudes and feelings of, 394, 414, 417–423
  awareness of speech fluency in treatment of, 412
  benchmarking for, 424–425
  client and family interview with, 383–387
  clinical portrait, 431–438
  decreasing frequency of scheduled treatment for, 423–424
  diagnosis of, 395
  experiences of fluency success in treatment of, 411–412
  extraclinical assignments for, 412–413
  extrafamily considerations for, 408–409, 437–438

About the Author

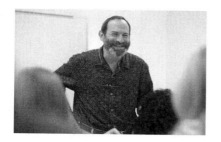

David A. Shapiro, PhD, CCC-SLP, ASHA Fellow, is Western Carolina University's first Robert Lee Madison Distinguished Professor. Affiliated with WCU since 1984, Dr. Shapiro teaches undergraduate and graduate courses, provides clinical service and instruction to people who stutter and their families, engages in research related to stuttering and professional preparation, and serves the university community.

Now in his fourth decade of providing clinical service, Dr. Shapiro is a regular presenter at national and international conferences and has taught, provided clinical service, and conducted research in six continents. In addition to being the author of the present text, Dr. Shapiro researches multinational approaches to stuttering intervention and has numerous publications in international journals. Dr. Shapiro serves as an editorial reviewer of manuscripts submitted for publication and was appointed as an external reviewer for the Australian Stuttering Research Center (University of Sydney, Australia) and as a member of the editorial board for *Specialusis Ugdymas* (*Special Education*, a journal published by the Research Centre of Special Education of Šiauliai University, Šiauliai, Lithuania).

Dr. Shapiro is actively involved in numerous organizations, including the International Fluency Association (IFA) and the International Stuttering Association (ISA). He is a Board Recognized Specialist in Fluency Disorders and received IFA's Award of Distinction for Outstanding Clinician (Dublin, Ireland, 2006). Other recognitions include Fellow of the American Speech-Language-Hearing Association, the University of North Carolina Board of Governors' Award for Excellence in Teaching, and the University (WCU) Scholar Award.

Dr. Shapiro remains actively engaged in continuing education and served as an elected member of the Inaugural Specialty Board on Fluency Disorders. He has participated in all of the World Congresses of the International Fluency Association and the African Stuttering Conference in Cameroon (2005) and Burkina Faso (2008); he was the only representative from North America and, with a colleague from France, provided clinical service and instruction to people who stutter from 20 African nations. At IFA's 4th World Congress, Dr. Shapiro presented "A Multinational Investigation of Stuttering Intervention," representing a commitment of 17 coauthor/clinician–researchers from 15 countries across six continents. His current research into stuttering intervention is expanding to former Soviet-bloc countries and to the assumptions and practices of indigenous healers.

Dr. Shapiro and his wife, Kay, live in Cullowhee, North Carolina, near the Great Smoky Mountains National Park. They have two children, Sarah and Aaron, who are now young adults. Dr. Shapiro enjoys spending time with his family and hiking, camping, fly fishing, bicycling, and traveling.